TEACH Instructor Resource Manual
Christensen & Kockrow

Adult Health Nursing

Sixth Edition

Kim D. Cooper, MSN
Nursing Department Program Chair
Ivy Tech Community College
Terre Haute, Indiana

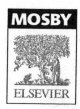

MOSBY

ELSEVIER

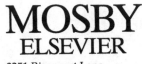

3251 Riverport Lane
St. Louis, Missouri 63043

TEACH INSTRUCTOR RESOURCE MANUAL FOR
ADULT HEALTH NURSING, SIXTH EDITION   978-0-323-06769-0

Notices

Knowledge and best practice in this field are constantly changing. As new research and experience broaden our understanding, changes in research methods, professional practices, or medical treatment may become necessary.

Practitioners and researchers must always rely on their own experience and knowledge in evaluating and using any information, methods, compounds, or experiments described herein. In using such information or methods they should be mindful of their own safety and the safety of others, including parties for whom they have a professional responsibility.

With respect to any drug or pharmaceutical products identified, readers are advised to check the most current information provided (i) on procedures featured or (ii) by the manufacturer of each product to be administered, to verify the recommended dose or formula, the method and duration of administration, and contraindications. It is the responsibility of practitioners, relying on their own experience and knowledge of their patients, to make diagnoses, to determine dosages and the best treatment for each individual patient, and to take all appropriate safety precautions.

To the fullest extent of the law, neither the Publisher nor the authors, contributors, or editors, assume any liability for any injury and/or damage to persons or property as a matter of products liability, negligence or otherwise, or from any use or operation of any methods, products, instructions, or ideas contained in the material herein.

Vice President and Publisher: Tom Wilhelm
Managing Editor: Jill Ferguson
Developmental Editor: Tiffany Trautwein
Associate Developmental Editor: Jennifer Hermes
Publishing Services Manager: Jeffrey Patterson
Senior Project Manager: Mary G. Stueck
Book Designer: Margaret Reid

Printed in the United States of America

Last digit is the print number: 9 8 7 6 5 4 3 2 1

How to Use the TEACH Instructor Resource Manual

WELCOME TO TEACH, YOUR TOTAL CURRICULUM SOLUTION!

The TEACH Instructor Resource Manual is designed to help you prepare for class lectures for *Adult Health Nursing*. We hope it will reduce your lesson preparation time, give you new and creative ideas to promote student learning, and help you to make full use of the rich array of resources in the Christensen & Kockrow teaching package.

ORGANIZATION

The TEACH Instructor Resource Manual includes lessons that correspond with each chapter from your *Adult Health Nursing* textbook and includes the following two sections:

1. **Lesson Plan:** Includes several class preparation checklists and a 50-minute lesson that provide you with the building blocks for your curriculum.
2. **Lecture Outline:** Consists of a 50-minute lecture outline that incorporates the PowerPoint® Presentations.

Lesson Plans and Lecture Outlines are also available on Evolve at http://evolve.elsevier.com/Christensen/ adult.

Lesson Plans

The Lesson Plans are designed to promote active student learning and get students involved in class discussions and activities. They include preparation checklists for you, individual lesson(s), and performance evaluation tools to help you gauge your students' understanding of the course material and adapt lessons to their needs.

Checklists

The introduction of each Lesson Plan includes the following checklists to ensure that you are well-prepared for class:

- **Teaching Focus:** Identifies key student learning goals for the chapter
- **Materials and Resources:** Lists materials needed for each lesson within the chapter
- **Lesson Checklist:** Includes instructor preparation suggestions
- **Key Terms:** Provides page references for each key term in the chapter
- **Additional Resources:** Lists instructor resources available for the chapter

Lessons

Each Lesson Plan includes one or more 50-minute lessons—building blocks that can be sequenced to fit your class schedule. The Lesson Plans are available in electronic format on Evolve so you can customize them to fit the requirements of your course. Every lesson includes a wide variety of teaching resources. In many cases, our subject matter experts have provided more resources and activities than can be covered in a 50-minute lesson. We encourage you to choose activities that match the needs of your students and your curriculum, and the materials and resources available at your school.

Lesson Plans can be a valuable tool for documenting how your curriculum covers learning objectives in compliance with accrediting organizations. Some accrediting organizations require that learning resources be integrated into a program's curriculum, to enhance students' learning experiences. The activities in this Lesson Plan Manual will help your students use available resources, such as the library or the Internet, to complement their textbook.

Each lesson includes the following sections:

- **Pretest and Background Assessment:** The first lesson in each chapter includes a Pretest and Background Assessment questions designed to help you gauge your students' readiness for the lesson. Depending on students' responses, you may wish to modify your lesson. Students who are comfortable with the topic may need more challenging activities. Students who have difficulty with the topic may need to start by addressing more fundamental concepts.
- **Critical Thinking Question:** Every lesson includes a Critical Thinking Question to motivate students by demonstrating real-world applications of the lesson content.
- **Lesson Guide:** The heart of the TEACH lesson plan is the three-column Lesson Guide that links Objectives and content from *Adult Health Nursing* with appropriate Teaching Resources. Teaching Resources reference all the elements of the ancillary package and include additional teaching tips such as class activities, discussion topics, and much more. This section correlates your textbook and its ancillary materials with the objectives upon which your course is based.
- **Homework/Assignments and Instructor's Notes/Student Feedback:** These sections are provided for you to add your own notes for assignments, for recording student feedback, and for other notes relating to the lesson.

Lecture Outlines

The Lecture Outlines include PowerPoint slides to provide a compelling visual presentation and summary of the main chapter points. Lecture notes for each slide highlight key topics and provide questions for discussion—to help create an interactive classroom environment.

We encourage you to select material from the TEACH Instructor Resource Manual that meets your students' needs, integrate TEACH into your existing lesson plans, and put your own teaching approach into the plans. We hope TEACH will be an invaluable tool in your classroom!

Lesson Plan

1 Introduction to Anatomy and Physiology

TEACHING FOCUS

In this chapter, the student will be introduced to the basics of anatomy and physiology, including the basic structure and function of the cell; the various types of tissues, organs, and systems; and the two types of epithelial membranes. The student will have the opportunity to learn in detail about the 11 major organ systems of the body, along with the principles of active and passive transport processes. Finally, the student will explore the principal directional terms used in describing the body, along with the abdominopelvic regions and quadrants.

MATERIALS AND RESOURCES

- ☐ Computer/overhead projector (Lessons 1.1 and 1.2)
- ☐ White/black board and marker/chalk (Lessons 1.1 and 1.2)
- ☐ Blank note cards, one per student (Lesson 1.1)
- ☐ Drawing of the body in anatomical position (Lesson 1.1)
- ☐ Unlabeled diagrams of the abdomen, one per student (Lesson 1.1)
- ☐ Small, soft ball or pillow that can be tossed from student to student (Lesson 1.1)
- ☐ Several clear plastic or glass beakers containing water; several colored sugar cubes (Lesson 1.2)
- ☐ Chart with three columns labeled Tissue, Location, and Function (Lesson 1.2)

LESSON CHECKLIST

Preparations for this lesson include:

- • Lecture

KEY TERMS

active transport (FAAHN p. 1244, AHN p. 8)
anatomy (FAAHN p. 1237, AHN p. 1)
cell (FAAHN p. 1240, AHN p. 4)
cytoplasm (FAAHN p. 1242, AHN p. 6)
diffusion (FAAHN p. 1245, AHN p. 9)
dorsal (FAAHN p. 1237, AHN p. 1)
filtration (FAAHN p. 1245, AHN p. 9)
homeostasis (FAAHN p. 1241, AHN p. 5)
membrane (FAAHN p. 1248 , AHN p. 12)
mitosis (FAAHN p. 1243, AHN p. 7)
nucleus (FAAHN p. 1242, AHN p. 6)

organ (FAAHN p. 1248, AHN p. 12)
osmosis (FAAHN p. 1245 AHN p. 9)
passive transport (FAAHN p. 1244, AHN p. 8)
phagocytosis (FAAHN p. 1244, AHN p. 8)
physiology (FAAHN p. 1237, AHN p. 1)
pinocytosis (FAAHN p. 1244, AHN p. 8)
system (FAAHN p. 1241, AHN p. 5)
tissue (FAAHN p. 1241, AHN p. 5)
ventral (FAAHN p. 1237, AHN p. 1)

ADDITIONAL RESOURCES (AHN)

PPT Ch. 41, 1 through 40 FAAHN (Ch. 1, 1 through 40 AHN)
EILR IC images Ch. 41, 1 through 13 FAAHN (Ch. 1, 1through 13 AHN)
EILR TB questions Ch. 41, 1 through 34 FAAHN (Ch. 1, 1 through 34 AHN)
EILR Open Book Quiz Ch. 41, 1 through 10 FAAHN (Ch. 1, 1 through 10 AHN)
ESLR Review Questions for the NCLEX® Examination Ch. 41, 41-01 through 41-10 FAAHN (Ch. 1, 01-01 through 01-10 AHN)

Legend

PPT PowerPoint Slides	**EILR** EVOLVE Instructor Learning Resources: Image Collection, Test Bank, Open Book Quizzes	**ESLR** EVOLVE Student Learning Resources: Review Questions for the NCLEX Examination	**SG** Study Guide	**NCP CTQ** Nursing Care Plan Critical Thinking Question

Class Activities are indicated in *bold italic*.

ELSEVIER

Adult Health Nursing, 6th ed.
Christensen & Kockrow

LESSON 1.1

PRETEST

1. The plane of the body running lengthwise from front to back is known as:
   a. distal.
   b. proximal.
   c. sagittal.
   d. coronal.

2. The abdominal cavity contains which of the following body organs?
   a. Stomach, liver, gallbladder, spleen, and appendix
   b. Stomach, gallbladder, spleen, small intestine, and bladder
   c. Liver, gallbladder, spleen, colon, and rectum
   d. Stomach, liver, gallbladder, and pancreas

3. _____ is the term used to refer to the body when it is in an erect position with the arms at the sides and the palms forward.
   a. Lateral position
   b. Anatomical position
   c. Superficial position
   d. Coronal position

4. The division of cells acting in unity to carry out a common function is known as:
   a. tissues.
   b. systems.
   c. cytoplasm.
   d. organs.

5. The smallest complete units of matter are called:
   a. tissues.
   b. organs.
   c. molecules.
   d. atoms.

6. When body cells trap large protein molecules, a process known as _____ occurs.
   a. phagocytosis
   b. calcium pumping
   c. pinocytosis
   d. mitosis

7. Which of the following statements best describes the processes associated with diffusion?
   a. The movement of water through a membrane by a force of pressure or gravity
   b. The passage of water across a permeable membrane
   c. The movement of fluid from an area of higher concentration to an area of lower concentration
   d. The movement of solid particles in a fluid from an area of higher concentration to an area of lower concentration

8. _____ is the movement of water and particles through a membrane by a force from either pressure or gravity.
   a. Filtration
   b. Diffusion
   c. Osmosis
   d. Active transport

9. The types of primary tissues that make up the body's organs are:
   a. epithelial, connective, muscle, and nervous tissues.
   b. connective, muscle, striated, and nervous tissues.
   c. muscle, adipose, epithelial, and nervous tissues.
   d. nervous, adipose, areolar, and muscular tissues.

10. The three types of muscle tissue in the body are:
    a. skeletal, cardiac, and visceral tissue.
    b. skeletal, connective, and visceral tissue.
    c. cardiac, fibrous, and hematopoietic tissue.
    d. visceral, fibrous, and hematopoietic tissue.

Answers:

1. c	2. d	3. b	4. a	5. d
6. c	7. d	8. a	9. a	10. a

BACKGROUND ASSESSMENT

Question: You have been assigned a patient who is being admitted to the medical surgical unit. She is complaining of abdominal pain. During the assessment, when asked the location of her pain, she points to her lower abdomen. When asked if it is concentrated more to the left or the right side, she states it is more centered. She reports the pain is sharper on the left side than the right when touched. No tenderness is present on the top of the stomach. Palpation of the abdomen reveals it is soft. After completing the assessment, you must chart the findings. How will you refer to the body locations using the appropriate terminology?

Answer: The abdomen is soft with areas of tenderness. Pain is noted in the hypogastric region. The left lower quadrant demonstrates sharp pain with palpation. The right lower quadrant is least tender. The hypochondriac and epigastric regions are absent of discomfort.

Question: Many of the body's surfaces that open to the outside are lined by mucous membranes. These membranes secrete a thin mucous film. Body surface areas having these characteristics include the nose, mouth, and urinary tract. What is the purpose of the mucous secretion? What other areas of the body share similar characteristics?

Answer: Mucous membranes produce a lubricating, moisturizing substance. In addition to lubrication, protection against bacteria is also provided. Body surfaces open to the environment have mucous membranes. Other examples include the respiratory, gastrointestinal, and reproductive tracts.

CRITICAL THINKING QUESTION

When the body is exposed to bacteria or a virus, illness can result. In response, the body's natural defenses attempt to recover and rid the body of the invading organism. How does the body use its inborn defenses to handle infections?

Guidelines: When the body is exposed to toxins and becomes infected, it often has the ability to purge itself of the invader. In response to these toxins, the body produces white blood cells whose function is to protect the body from infection. The response to an illness is an increase of white blood cells. These white blood cells travel through the blood system and attack the foreign matter, trapping it. Once the bacteria is trapped, the process of phagocytosis occurs to rid the body of toxins and infections.

OBJECTIVES	CONTENT	TEACHING RESOURCES
Define the difference between anatomy and physiology.	■ Introduction (FAAHN p. 1237 AHN p. 1)	☒■ PPT 1 through 2, Ch. 41 FAAHN (Ch. 1 PPT 1 through 2 AHN) ⬛ EILR TB Ch. 41 questions 11, 12 FAAHN (Ch. 1 questions 11, 12 AHN) SG Anatomy and Physiology Ch. 41 pp. 313-314 FAAHN (Ch. 1 pp. 1-2 AHN)

OBJECTIVES	CONTENT	TEACHING RESOURCES
		‣ Discuss the differences between anatomy and physiology.
		‣ Discuss the relationship between anatomy and physiology.
		Class Activity Provide a small note card to each student. Ask each person to record what he/she believes anatomy and physiology are and how the study of these two subjects is important to nursing. When the cards are completed, collect them and review them. Use the cards to determine if students have an appropriate level of comprehension of the subjects.
Define the term anatomical position.	■ Anatomical terminology (FAAHN p. 1237, AHN p. 1)	PPT 3 Ch. 41 FAAHN (Ch. 1 PPT 3 AHN)
		EILR IC Ch. 41 image 1FAAHN (Ch. 1 image 1 AHN)
		EILR TB Ch. 41 questions 1, 16, 18, 28 FAAHN (Ch. 1 questions 1, 16, 18, 28 AHN)
		ESLR Review Questions for the NCLEX Examination Ch. 41 question 6 FAAHN (Ch. 1 question 6 AHN)
		SG Positions of the Body Ch. 41 pp. 313-314 FAAHN (Ch. 1 pp. 1-2 AHN)
		BOOK RESOURCES
		Fig. 41-1 Anatomical position (FAAHN p. 1238) (Fig. 1-1 AHN p. 2)
		‣ Discuss the need to refer to the body with anatomical terms in the health care profession.
		‣ Discuss the physical positioning when referring to anatomical position.
		Class Activity Ask the class to stand. Using the rules and principles from the children's game "Simon Says," ask the students to touch or point toward the areas indicated using the anatomical position terms.

OBJECTIVES	CONTENT	TEACHING RESOURCES
List and define the principal directional terms and sections (planes) used in describing the body and the relationship of body parts to one another.	■ Anatomical terminology (FAAHN p. 1237, AHN p. 1) □ Body planes (FAAHN p. 1238, AHN p. 2)	⊠ PPT 3 through 5, Ch. 41 FAAHN (Ch. 1 PPT 3 through 5 AHN) *e* EILR IC Ch. 41 images 2 through 5 FAAHN (Ch. 1 images 2 through 5 AHN) *e* EILR TB Ch. 41 question 1, 17, 28 FAAHN (Ch. 1 questions 1, 17, 28 AHN) *e* ESLR Review Questions for the NCLEX Examination Ch. 41 question 7 FAAHN (Ch. 1 question 7 AHN) SG Anatomical Terms Ch. 41 pp. 314-315 FAAHN (Ch. 1 pp. 2-3 AHN) **BOOK RESOURCES** Fig. 41-2 Directions and planes of the body (FAAHN p. 1238) (Fig. 1-2 AHN p. 2) ▸ Discuss the three planes used to divide the body. ▸ Discuss the relationships of body parts in relation to each other. *Class Activity Provide a drawing of the body in anatomical position. Ask the students to identify the planes of the body. Once labeling is done, ask the students to refer to the diagram to determine physical relationships of body parts to one another.*

Use each word of a given list of anatomical terms in a sentence.	■ Anatomical terminology (FAAHN p. 1237, AHN p. 1)
	
	□ Body planes (FAAHN p. 1238, AHN p. 2)
	
	□ Body cavities (FAAHN p. 1238, AHN p. 2)
	
	  – Ventral cavity (FAAHN p. 1238, AHN p. 2)
	
	  – Dorsal cavity (FAAHN p. 1238, AHN p. 2)
		⊠ PPT 3 through 5, Ch. 41 FAAHN (Ch. 1 PPT 3 through 5 AHN)
		
		e EILR IC Ch. 41 image 3 FAAHN (Ch. 1 image 3 AHN)
		
		e EILR TB Ch. 41 question 32 FAAHN (Ch. 1 question 32AHN)
		
		e EILR Open Book Quiz Ch. 41 question 1 FAAHN (Ch. 1 question 1 AHN)
		
		SG Anatomical Terms Ch. 41 pp. 313-314 FAAHN (Ch. 1 pp. 1-2 AHN)
		
		BOOK RESOURCES
		
		Fig. 41-3 Location and subdivisions of the dorsal and ventral body cavities as viewed from the front and the side (FAAHN p. 1239) (Fig. 1-3 AHN p. 3)

OBJECTIVES	CONTENT	TEACHING RESOURCES
		Table 41-1 Body Cavities (FAAHN p. 1239) (Table 1-1 AHN p. 3) ▶ Discuss the appropriate use of medical terminology when referring to the body. *Class Activity Divide the class into small groups (three to five students). Assign each group two or three anatomical terms. Ask each group to develop two fill-in-the-blank questions and one multiple choice question using its assigned terms. Collect the questions when done. Use them in a review session for the chapter.*
List the nine abdominopelvic regions and the abdominopelvic quadrants.	■ Abdominal regions (FAAHN p. 1239, AHN p. 3) ■ Abdominopelvic quadrants (FAAHN p. 1239, AHN p. 3)	PPT 6 through 12, Ch. 41 FAAHN (Ch. 1 PPT 6 through 12 AHN) EILR IC Ch. 41 images 4, 5 FAAHN (Ch. 1 images 4, 5 AHN) EILR TB Ch. 41 questions 4, 10, 13 FAAHN (Ch. 1 questions 4, 10, 13 AHN) EILR Open Book Quiz Ch. 41 questions 2, 3 FAAHN (Ch. 1 questions 2, 3 AHN) ESLR Review Questions for the NCLEX Examination Ch. 41 question 2 FAAHN (Ch. 1 question 2 AHN) SG Facing the Patient Ch. 41 pp. 319-320 FAAHN (Ch. 1 pp. 7-8 AHN) **BOOK RESOURCES** Fig. 41-4 The nine regions of the abdominopelvic cavity (FAAHN p. 1239) (Fig. 1-4 AHN p. 3) Fig. 41-5 Horizontal and vertical line passing through the umbilicus divides the abdomen into right and left upper quadrants and right and left lower quadrants (FAAHN p. 1240) (Fig. 1-5 AHN p. 4) ▶ Discuss the use of the abdominopelvic quadrants when performing a physical assessment. ▶ Discuss documentation relating to the use of the abdominopelvic quadrants. *Class Activity Provide each student with unlabeled diagrams of the human abdomen. Ask the students to label the quadrants and abdominopelvic regions.*

OBJECTIVES	CONTENT	TEACHING RESOURCES
List and discuss in order of increasing complexity the levels of organization of the body.	■ Structural levels of organization (FAAHN p. 1239, AHN p. 3)	PPT 13, Ch. 41 FAAHN (Ch. 1 PPT 13 AHN)
		EILR IC Ch. 41 image 6 FAAHN (Ch. 1 image 6 AHN)
		EILR TB Ch. 41 questions 14, 29, 30 FAAHN (Ch. 1 questions 14, 29, 30 AHN)
		EILR Open Book Quiz Ch. 41 question 4 FAAHN (Ch. 1 question 4 AHN)
		ESLR Review Questions for the NCLEX Examination Ch. 41 question 1 FAAHN (Ch. 1 question 1 AHN)
		SG Body Systems Ch. 41 p. 315 FAAHN (Ch. 1 p. 3 AHN)
		BOOK RESOURCES
		Fig. 41-6 Structural levels of organization in the body (FAAHN p. 1240) (Fig. 1-6 AHN p. 4)
		▶ Discuss the hierarchy of atoms, molecules, cells, tissues, and organs.
		▶ Discuss the systems of the body. How does the increasing level of complexity relate to the functionality of the body systems?
		Class Activity Tell each student to select a partner. Ask the members of the class to stand. Toss a small object, such as a ball, around the room. As each pair catches the ball, they will be asked to name a body system. The next pair will be asked to name an organ of that system. Once that system's organs have been identified, the next pair will name a different body system. This will continue until the body is completed.

1.1 Homework/Assignments:

1.1 Instructor's Notes/Student Feedback:

LESSON 1.2

CRITICAL THINKING QUESTION

Human beings begin as the union of two cells. The repeated division is responsible for the growth that eventually becomes a living being. Does cellular reproduction result in identical body cells? Does the continued cellular reproduction result in an overabundance of body cells? Why or why not?

Guidelines: While mitosis does result in the replication of body cells, the cells produced are not identical. During fetal development, the body cells become specialized. For example, some of the cells are designed to function in the digestive system, some in the integumentary system, and still others in the skeletal system. It is necessary for cellular reproduction to take place for growth and development. Some of the cells being reproduced will be used to replace cells that are old or no longer functional. The life span of the body's cells can vary by type and system. Age and overall health status play a role in the rate of cellular reproduction and life span.

OBJECTIVES	CONTENT	TEACHING RESOURCES
Identify and define three major components of the cell.	■ Structural levels of organization (FAAHN p. 1239, AHN p. 3) ☐ Cells (FAAHN p. 1241, AHN p. 5) – Structural parts of cells (FAAHN p. 1241, AHN p. 5) – Protein synthesis (FAAHN p. 1243, AHN p. 7)	PPT 14 through 18, Ch. 41 FAAHN (Ch. 1 PPT 14 through 18 AHN) EILR IC Ch. 41 image 7 FAAHN (Ch. 1 image 7 AHN) EILR TB Ch. 41 question 2, 3, 15, 33 FAAHN (Ch. 1 question 2, 3, 15, 33 AHN) ESLR Review Questions for the NCLEX Examination Ch. 41 question 3 FAAHN (Ch. 1 question 3 AHN) SG Cell Art Ch. 41 p. 315 FAAHN (Ch. 1 p. 3 AHN) **BOOK RESOURCES** Fig. 41-7 A typical cell (FAAHN p. 1241) (Fig. 1-7 AHN p. 5) Table 41-2 Some Major Cell Structures and Their Functions (FAAHN p. 1242) (Table 1-2 AHN p. 6) Fig. 41-8 DNA molecule (FAAHN p. 1244) (Fig. 1-8 AHN p. 8) ▸ Discuss the function of the components of a cell. ▸ Discuss the impact of impaired cell functioning on the body as a whole. *Class Activity To review the content in preparation for a quiz, ask each student to develop three quiz-style questions relating to the cell and its components and bring them to the next class session. During the next class, separate the students into groups of three or four. Ask the students to review the questions submitted by their peers.*

Adult Health Nursing, 6th ed.

Christensen & Kockrow

OBJECTIVES	CONTENT	TEACHING RESOURCES
Discuss the stages of mitosis and explain the importance of cellular reproduction.	– Cell division (FAAHN p. 1243, AHN p. 7) – Movement of materials across cell membranes (FAAHN p. 1244, AHN p. 8)	PPT 19, Ch. 41 FAAHN (Ch. 1 PPT 19 AHN) EILR IC Ch. 41 images 8, 9 FAAHN (Ch. 1 images 8, 9 AHN) EILR TB Ch. 41 questions 5, 6 FAAHN (Ch. 1 questions 5, 6 AHN) EILR Open Book Quiz Ch. 41 questions 5, 6 FAAHN (Ch. 1 questions 5, 6 AHN) ESLR Review Questions for the NCLEX Examination Ch. 41 question 8 FAAHN (Ch. 1 question 8 AHN) SG Phases of Mitosis Ch. 41 p. 316 FAAHN (Ch. 1 p. 4 AHN) **BOOK RESOURCES** Fig. 41-9 Mitosis (FAAHN p. 1245) (Fig. 1-9 AHN p. 9) ▶ Discuss the three phases of cellular reproduction. ▶ Discuss the importance of mitosis. ▶ Discuss the process of cellular reproduction *Class Activity **Lead the class in a discussion of how our characteristics (e.g., hair color, eye color, size of nose) are passed down through generations.***
Differentiate between active and passive transport processes that act to move substances through cell membranes, and give two examples of each.	– Movement of materials across cell membranes (FAAHN p. 1244, AHN p. 8)	PPT 20 through 23, Ch. 41 FAAHN (Ch. 1 PPT 20 through 23 AHN) EILR IC Ch. 41 images 10, 11 FAAHN (Ch. 1 images 10, 11 AHN) EILR TB Ch. 41 questions 19, 23, 24, 25 FAAHN (Ch. 1 questions 19, 23, 24, 25 AHN) EILR Open Book Quiz Ch. 41 question 7 FAAHN (Ch. 1 question 7 AHN) ESLR Review Questions for the NCLEX Examination Ch. 41 questions 4, 9 FAAHN (Ch. 1 questions 4, 9 AHN) SG Movement Ch. 41 p. 318-319 FAAHN (Ch. 1 p. 6-7 AHN)

OBJECTIVES	CONTENT	TEACHING RESOURCES
		BOOK RESOURCES
		Table 41-3 Active Transport Processes (FAAHN p. 1244) (Table 1-3 AHN p. 8)
		Table 41-4 Passive Transport Processes (FAAHN p. 1245) (Table 1-4 AHN p. 9)
		Fig. 41-10 Diffusion (FAAHN p. 1245) (Fig. 1-10 AHN p. 9)
		Fig. 41-11 Osmosis (FAAHN p. 1246) (Fig. 1-11 AHN p. 10)
		▸ Discuss the role of the cell's membrane during the transport process.
		▸ Discuss and define the passive transport processes.
		▸ Discuss and define the active transport processes.
		Class Activity Place several clear plastic or glass beakers containing water throughout the room. Invite the students to go to the beaker of their choice. Instruct the students to drop a single sugar cube of colored sugar in the water. As the cube dissolves, ask the students to observe and record what takes place next. After the sugar is dissolved, explain they have viewed diffusion. The sugar entered the water in a large concentration. After being introduced to the water, the sugar dissolved and became more evenly distributed to areas of lower concentration. NOTE: If you can't find colored sugar cubes, add some food coloring to white sugar cubes.
Differentiate among tissues, organs, and systems.	☐ Tissues (FAAHN p. 1245, AHN p. 9) – Epithelial tissue (FAAHN p. 1247, AHN p. 11) – Connective tissue (FAAHN p. 1247, AHN p. 11) – Muscle tissue (FAAHN p. 1247, AHN p. 11) – Nervous tissue (FAAHN p. 1247, AHN p. 11) ☐ Membranes (FAAHN p. 1248, AHN p. 12)	PPT 24 through 40, Ch. 41 FAAHN (Ch. 1 PPT 24 through 40 AHN) EILR IC Ch. 41 image 12 FAAHN (Ch. 1 image 12 AHN) EILR TB Ch. 41 questions 8, 9, 20, 21, 31 FAAHN (Ch. 1 questions 8, 9, 20, 21, 31 AHN) ESLR Review Questions for the NCLEX Examination Ch. 41 question 10 FAAHN (Ch. 1 question 10 AHN) SG Body Systems Ch. 41 p. 315 FAAHN (Ch. 1 p. 3 AHN)

ELSEVIER

OBJECTIVES	CONTENT	TEACHING RESOURCES
	– Epithelial membranes (FAAHN p. 1248, AHN p. 12) – Mucous membranes (FAAHN p. 1248, AHN p. 12) – Serous membranes (FAAHN p. 1248, AHN p. 12) – Connective tissue membranes (synovial membranes) (FAAHN p. 1248, AHN p. 12) ☐ Organs/systems (FAAHN p. 1248, AHN p. 12)	**BOOK RESOURCES** Table 41-5 Tissues (FAAHN p. 1246) (Table 1-5 AHN p. 10) Fig. 41-12 Types of muscles (FAAHN p. 1247) (Fig. 1-12 AHN p. 11) ▶ Discuss the organization of the body's systems. What generalized role do tissues and organs play in each system? *Class Activity **Divide the students into four groups. Assign each group one of the types of tissue. Each group is instructed to locate a scientific or nursing journal article, discussing the assigned tissue type. The group is then to write a brief (two or three paragraphs) review on the tissue and its role in the body. The groups will then present their findings to the class.***
Describe the four types of body tissues.	☐ Tissues (FAAHN p. 1245, AHN p. 9) – Epithelial tissue (FAAHN p. 1247, AHN p. 11) – Connective tissue (FAAHN p. 1247, AHN p. 11) – Muscle tissue (FAAHN p. 1247, AHN p. 11) – Nervous tissue (FAAHN p. 1247, AHN p. 11)	▦ PPT 24 through 28, Ch. 41 FAAHN (Ch. 1 PPT 24 through 28 AHN) 𝒆 EILR IC Ch. 41 images 20 through 22 FAAHN (Ch. 1 images 20 through 22 AHN) 𝒆 EILR TB Ch. 41 questions 7 through 9, 20 through 22, 26, 27 FAAHN (Ch. 1 questions 7 through 9, 20 through 22, 26, 27 AHN) 𝒆 EILR Open Book Quiz Ch. 41 questions 8, 9 FAAHN (Ch. 1 questions 8, 9 AHN) 𝒆 ESLR Review Questions for the NCLEX Examination Ch. 41 question 5 FAAHN (Ch. 1 question 5 AHN) SG Types of Muscles Ch. 41 p. 318 FAAHN (Ch. 1 p. 6 AHN) ▶ Discuss the different types of tissues in the body. Where are each of these types located? ▶ Discuss how the functions of the types of tissues are similar and how they are different. *Class Activity **Develop a chart. The chart will need three columns. The columns are to be labeled "TISSUE," "LOCATION," and "FUNCTION." Lead a class discussion to complete the chart. Make copies of the completed chart to distribute to the students to be used as a study guide for the content.***

Adult Health Nursing, 6ᵗʰ ed.

Mosby items and derived items © 2011 by Mosby, Inc., an affiliate of Elsevier Inc. Some material was previously published.

Christensen & Kockrow

OBJECTIVES	CONTENT	TEACHING RESOURCES
Discuss the two types of epithelial membranes.	☐ Membranes (FAAHN p. 1248, AHN p. 12) – Epithelial membranes (FAAHN p. 1248, AHN p. 12) – Connective tissue membranes (synovial membranes) (FAAHN p. 1248, AHN p. 12)	PPT 29 through 31, Ch. 41 FAAHN (Ch. 1 PPT 29 through 31 AHN) EILR Open Book Quiz Ch. 41 question 10 FAAHN (Ch. 1 question 10 AHN) SG Identify Types of Membranes Ch. 41 pp. 316-317 FAAHN (Ch. 1 pp. 4-5 AHN) ▶ Discuss the function of the body's membranes. ▶ Discuss the two types of epithelial membranes. How do they differ?
List the 11 major organ systems of the body and briefly describe the major functions of each.	☐ Organs/systems (FAAHN p. 1248, AHN p. 12	PPT 32 through 40, Ch. 41 FAAHN (Ch. 1 PPT 32 through 40 AHN) EILR IC Ch. 41 image 13 FAAHN (Ch. 1 image 13 AHN) EILR TB Ch. 41 question 29 FAAHN (Ch. 1 question 29 AHN) EILR Open Book Quiz Ch. 41 question 1 FAAHN (Ch. 1 question 1 AHN) SG Major Systems—Patient Observation Ch. 41 p. 317 FAAHN (Ch. 1 p. 5 AHN) **BOOK RESOURCES** Table 41-6 Organ Systems and Their Functions (FAAHN p. 1248) (Table 1-7 AHN p. 12) ▶ Discuss the major body systems. What functions is each system responsible for? ▶ Discuss the organs that compose each of the body systems. *Class Activity Lead a class discussion concerning each of the body systems. Review the functions of each of the systems. Investigate the interrelationship between the body systems.*
Performance Evaluation		EILR TB Ch. 41 questions 1 through 34 FAAHN (Ch. 1 questions 1 through 34 AHN) EILR Open Book Quiz Ch. 41 questions 1 through 10 FAAHN (Ch. 1 questions 1 through 10 AHN) ESLR Review Questions for the NCLEX Examination Ch. 41 questions 1 through 10 FAAHN (Ch. 1 questions 1 through 10 AHN)

OBJECTIVES	CONTENT	TEACHING RESOURCES
		SG Ch. 41 pp. 313-320 FAAHN (Ch. 1 pp. 1-8 AHN) **BOOK RESOURCES** Review Questions for the NCLEX Examination Ch. 41, questions 1 through 30 FAAHN (Ch. 1 questions 1 through 30 AHN)

1.2 Homework/Assignments:

1.2 Instructor's Notes/Student Feedback:

Christensen & Kockrow

Slide 1

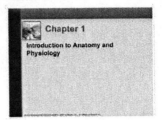

Slide 2

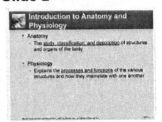

- Anatomy and physiology share an intertwined relationship. Review the connection between the two sciences.

Slide 3

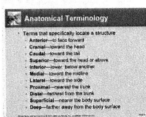

- When studying anatomy, a series of terms are used to refer to locations within the body. How should the body be positioned to appropriately utilize the terms?

Slide 4

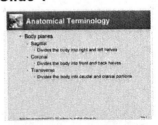

- The body is divided into planes to aid in the study of anatomy and physiology.

Slide 5

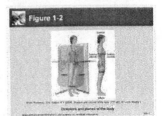

Slide 6

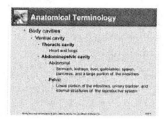

- Unlike the outer solid appearance, internally the body contains cavities. What physiological function do the body cavities have?

Slide 7

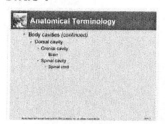

- What are some organs in each body cavity?

Slide 8

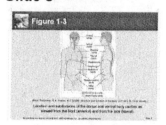

- There are seven cavities in the body. How are the cavities divided?

Slide 9

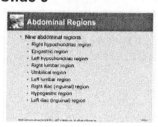

- The abdomen is subdivided into nine regions.
- How do these regions aid the practitioner when performing a physical assessment?
- How are findings documented when referring to the abdominal regions?

Slide 10

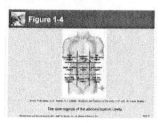

- Review the abdominal regions in relation to the diagram.
- What organs are found in each of the regions?

Slide 11

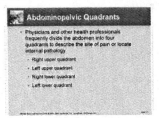

- Physical assessments of the abdomen can be further clarified by referring to the quadrants when conducting an examination.

- Identify the abbreviations that are used to denote each of the quadrants.

Slide 12

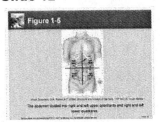

- Review the quadrants of the abdomen.

- What organs are found in each of the quadrants?

Slide 13

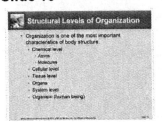

- The body consists of interrelated organization levels. Each of the levels is responsible for a specific set of functions. Although the levels have differing functions, their components are quite similar.

- What type of interdependence exists between the body's organization levels? Does impairment in one level impact the others?

Slide 14

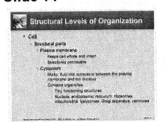

- The smallest known unit of structure and function in the body is the cell.

- Cells are located throughout the body. Despite their location, they all have the same characteristics. What are the five shared cellular characteristics?

Slide 15

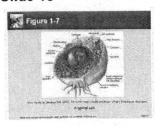

- Each part of the cell has special functions.

ELSEVIER

Mosby items and derived items © 2011, 2007 by Mosby, Inc., an affiliate of Elsevier Inc.
Some material was previously published.

Adult Health Nursing, 6th ed.
Christensen & Kockrow

Slide 16

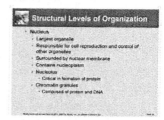

- The activities of the cell are regulated by the nucleus.

- The nucleus also contains the chromatin granules. They are made of DNA. What major role does DNA play in the body?

Slide 17

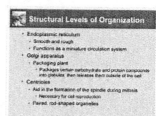

- Supportive organelles within the cell include the endoplasmic reticulum, Golgi apparatus, and the centrioles. Given their roles, what would the impact on the cell be if its function was impaired? How would this affect the body as a whole?

Slide 18

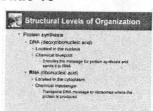

- DNA is found in the cell's nucleus. RNA is located in the cytoplasm.

- Discuss the relationship between the cell's DNA and RNA.

Slide 19

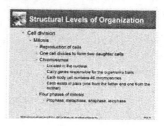

- To maintain bodily functions, cells must continually reproduce. This process is known as mitosis. During mitosis, a single cell divides into two cells.

- Mitosis consists of four phases. What occurs in each of the phases?

- What is the result on the cell's future if any one of the phases does not occur normally?

Slide 20

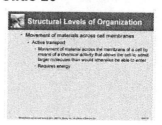

- Survival requires a cell to receive food and oxygen. There must also be a means to relieve cellular waste products. Functions that enable these life-sustaining actions to take place are known as transport.

- There are both active transport and passive transport functions. How do they differ?

ELSEVIER

Adult Health Nursing, 6th ed.
Christensen & Kockrow

Slide 21

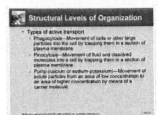

- Active transport functions include phagocytosis, pinocytosis, and pump (calcium or sodium-potassium).

- In addition to the requirement of energy to complete their functions, what do they have in common?

Slide 22

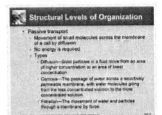

- Cellular energy is not needed for the body to carry out passive transport.

- Examples of passive transport include diffusion, osmosis, and filtration.

- What is the catalyst that allows passive transport to take place?

Slide 23

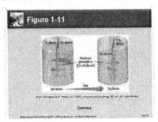

- Figure 1-11 is an example of osmosis.

- Note the concentration of water and albumin in each of the cylinders. Why is the membrane permeable to water but not albumin?

- What is the general direction of osmosis with regard to the concentration of the solution?

Slide 24

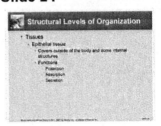

- Tissues are groups of cells working together to serve a specific function.

- Epithelial tissue has three basic functions. Describe ways epithelial tissue conducts the functions of protection, absorption, and secretion.

Slide 25

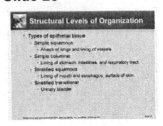

- Epithelial tissues typically do not have blood vessels. Their nourishment comes from underlying tissues.

- There are four types of epithelial tissue. Study their names. What method has been used to classify them?

ELSEVIER

Slide 26

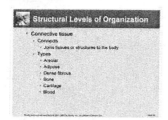

- Connective tissue is the most common tissue in the body. Functions of this tissue include support and protection.
- Study the types and locations of the varying types of connective tissue. How do the differing types of connective tissues perform their functions?

Slide 27

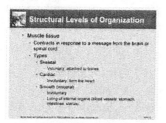

- Muscle tissue contracts in reaction to messages sent from the brain or spinal cord.
- What actions are needed by the muscle fibers to produce movement?
- Some muscle tissue is striated. What are striations?

Slide 28

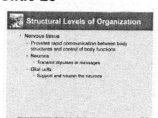

- The chief responsibility of nervous tissue is communication.
- Where is nervous tissue located?

Slide 29

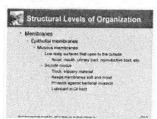

- Epithelial membranes are made of a lower layer of connective tissue that supports a thin layer of epithelial cells.
- There are two types of epithelial membranes.

Slide 30

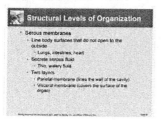

Christensen & Kockrow

Slide 31

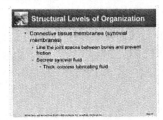

- Connective tissue membranes are smooth and slick.

- What function does the synovial fluid they secrete play?

- How do they differ from serous and mucous membranes?

Slide 32

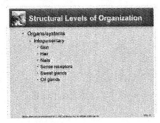

- Organs are formed when different tissues join to perform a higher function. When organs group with other organs to execute even greater levels of functioning, a system results.

- The body has 10 systems. What are the general functions of each of the body systems?

- What will occur if one or more of the organs in a system becomes unable to perform its normal role? What could the impact be on other systems?

- Which body systems work closest together?

Slide 33

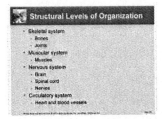

Slide 34

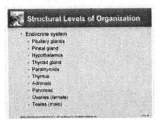

Slide 35

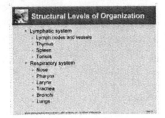

Slide 36

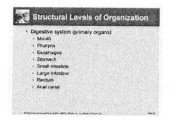

Slide 37

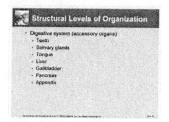

Slide 38

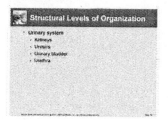

Slide 39

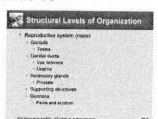

Slide 40

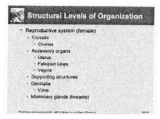

TEACHING FOCUS

In this chapter, the student will be introduced to the role of the nurse in the care of the surgical patient, beginning with the purposes and types of surgery, and continuing with preoperative tasks, various types of sedation and anesthesia, the roles of the circulating nurse and scrub nurse during surgery, and considerations for older surgical patients. The student also will have the opportunity to learn about postoperative care, including turning, breathing, coughing, and exercises; the prevention of postoperative complications; and preparations for discharge.

MATERIALS AND RESOURCES

- ☐ Computer/overhead projector (all lessons)
- ☐ White/black board and marker/chalk (all lessons)
- ☐ Blank note cards for each student (Lesson 2.1)
- ☐ Several copies of blank nursing care plan forms (Lessons 2.1 and 2.2)
- ☐ Blank sheet of paper (Lesson 2.2)
- ☐ Four patient scenarios (Lesson 2.3)

LESSON CHECKLIST

Preparations for this lesson include:
- Lecture
- Invite a respiratory therapist to class to discuss his/her role in the care of the postoperative patient.

TERMS & DEFINITIONS

ablation (FAAHN p. 1254, AHN p. 18)

anesthesia (FAAHN p. 1273, AHN p. 37)

atelectasis (FAAHN p. 1285, AHN p. 49)

cachexia (FAAHN p. 1284, AHN p. 48)

catabolism (FAAHN p. 1288, AHN p. 52)

conscious sedation (FAAHN p. 1276, AHN p. 40)

dehiscence (FAAHN p. 1284, AHN p. 48)

drainage (FAAHN p. 1281, AHN p. 45)

embolus (FAAHN p. 1269, AHN p. 33)

evisceration (FAAHN p. 1284, AHN p. 48)

extubate (FAAHN p. 1281, AHN p. 45)

exudate (FAAHN p. 1281, AHN p. 45)

incentive spirometry (FAAHN p. 1264, AHN p. 28)

incisions (FAAHN p. 1271, AHN p. 35)

infarct (FAAHN p. 1269, AHN p. 33)

informed consent (FAAHN p. 1260, AHN p. 24)

intraoperative (FAAHN p. 1254, AHN p. 18)

palliative (FAAHN p. 1254, AHN p. 18)

paralytic ileus (FAAHN p. 1288, AHN p. 52)

perioperative (FAAHN p. 1254, AHN p. 18)

postoperative (FAAHN p. 1254, AHN p. 18)

preoperative (FAAHN p. 1254, AHN p. 18)

prosthesis (FAAHN p. 1277, AHN p. 41)

singultus (FAAHN p. 1288, AHN p. 52)

surgery (FAAHN p. 1253, AHN p. 17)

surgical asepsis (FAAHN p. 1280, AHN p. 44)

thrombus (FAAHN p. 1268, AHN p. 32)

ADDITIONAL RESOURCES (AHN)

PPT Ch. 42, 1 through 62 FAAHN (Ch. 2, 1 through 62 AHN)

EILR IC images Ch. 42, 1 through 18 FAAHN (Ch. 2, 1 through 18 AHN)

EILR TB questions Ch. 42, 1 through 41 FAAHN (Ch. 2, 1 through 41 AHN)

EILR Open Book Quiz Ch. 42, 1 through 10 FAAHN (Ch. 2, 1 through 10 AHN)

ESLR Review Questions for the NCLEX® Examination Ch. 42, 42-01 through 42-10 FAAHN (Ch. 2, 02-01 through 02-10 AHN)

Legend

PPT
PowerPoint
Slides

EILR
EVOLVE Instructor
Learning Resources:
Image Collection, Test
Bank, Open Book Quizzes

ESLR
EVOLVE Student
Learning Resources:
Review Questions
for the NCLEX
Examination

SG
Study Guide

NCP CTQ
Nursing Care Plan
Critical Thinking
Question

Class Activities are indicated in ***bold italic***.

LESSON 2.1

PRETEST

1. During the admission process for a surgery scheduled the following morning, the patient discloses he has been taking St. John's wort to manage his depression for the past 2 years. When questioned further, he reveals that his physician has not been made aware of this regimen. Based upon your knowledge, you:
   a. are not concerned as St. John's wort is a safe, natural method to manage depression and there is no potential impact for a patient undergoing surgery.
   b. immediately notify the physician because of the increase in bleeding times associated with the use of St. John's wort.
   c. notify the physician because of concerns relating to potential interrelationships with other medications that may be prescribed for a surgical patient.
   d. are not concerned but encourage the patient to discontinue the medication to be "on the safe side."

2. Which of the following patients is at greater risk for developing complications postoperatively due to an interrelationship between his herbal remedies and the analgesics administered to manage his pain?
   a. The patient taking ginger for motion sickness
   b. The patient taking valerian root to manage insomnia
   c. The patient taking large amounts of feverfew
   d. The patient taking moderate amounts of St. John's wort to manage chronic back pain

3. Which of the following ethnic groups is known for avoiding eye contact due to the belief that eye contact signals disrespect?
   a. African-Americans
   b. Native Americans
   c. Vietnamese-Americans
   d. Southeast Asians

4. When preparing to complete a surgical consent for a patient scheduled to undergo an exploratory surgery, which of the following individuals would require a guardian to sign the surgical consent?
   a. A hearing-impaired patient, age 100
   b. A married 17-year-old female
   c. An intermittently confused 22-year-old male
   d. A 91-year-old patient who recently suffered a stroke

5. While you are working in the emergency room, a 15-year-old female arrives to the unit. She is badly hurt and might require surgery. Attempts to locate her parents have been futile. After her condition worsens, the physician asks you to prepare her for surgery. How will the issues related to the consent for surgery be handled?
   a. The surgery can take place as this is a justifiable emergency.
   b. The law requires that the surgeon wait until her parents can be notified.
   c. There are provisions in the law allowing the hospital's attorney to provide consent for the surgery in the case of an emergency.
   d. The patient is able to understand the consent and may sign the papers due to the emergent situation.

Mosby items and derived items © 2011 by Mosby, Inc., an affiliate of Elsevier Inc.
Some material was previously published.

6. When considering patients at risk for latex allergies, which of the following presents the highest risk?
   a. There is a history of allergy to melons and tomatoes.
   b. There is a history of allergy to poinsettia plants.
   c. The patient works at a paper mill.
   d. The patient has a history of gastrointestinal disorders.

7. When planning the operative care for a patient who is at high risk for an allergic response to latex exposure, which of the following elements must be included in the plan of care?
   a. Administer intravenous prophylactic steroid treatment.
   b. Administer intramuscular injection of a prophylactic anti-inflammatory medication.
   c. Use latex-safe supplies.
   d. Administer intravenous steroids and antihistamines preoperatively.

8. A complication known as a(n) _____ may occur due to the blood slowing, resulting in an accumulation of platelets, fibrin, clotting factors, and cellular elements of the blood attached to the wall of the vessel.
   a. infarct
   b. thrombus
   c. embolus
   d. transient ischemic attack

9. During the preoperative period, the anesthesiologist prescribes Versed 3.5 mg to be administered IM. This medication, when prescribed prior to surgery, serves which important function?
   a. The medication aids in the reduction of postoperative pain.
   b. The anticoagulation effects of the medication reduce operative bleeding.
   c. The bactericidal actions aid in preventing infection.
   d. The administration of this medication promotes sedation.

10. A 78-year-old patient is concerned about the impact her insulin-dependent diabetes will have on her postoperative recovery experience. She asks about her insulin needs during the first day after surgery. Which of the following facts will the nurse include in the teaching session?
    a. There should be no change in her body's postoperative insulin needs.
    b. Insulin needs are usually reduced due to the body's stress response.
    c. Insulin needs will be slightly elevated due to the administration of intravenous fluids.
    d. Insulin needs will be greatly increased due to the physiological stress of the anesthesia and surgery.

Answers:

1. c	2. b	3. d	4. c	5. a
6. b	7. c	8. b	9. d	10. b

BACKGROUND ASSESSMENT

Question: An 82-year-old patient is scheduled to undergo a total hip replacement. During the preoperative interview process, he voices concerns about the impact his advanced age may have on his recovery time. What bearing will his age have on his recuperation?

Answer: Older surgical patients face a set of unique circumstances. In addition to the normally anticipated milestones and tasks associated with the postoperative period, older adults undergoing surgery have a higher morbidity and mortality rate. The aging process is associated with physiological changes that weaken body systems. This normal weakening often results in the onset of chronic diseases. Comorbid conditions can also occur with advancing age. Weaknesses and disease processes affecting the immune, cardiovascular, and respiratory systems increase the risk of aspiration, atelectasis, pneumonia, thrombus, and infection. Medications administered during the preoperative, operative, and postoperative periods may not be metabolized as effectively in older patients. This might cause disorientation or toxicity.

Question: This country is known for being both a social and cultural melting pot. In the course of their daily work lives, nurses face challenges caring for individuals having differing beliefs and cultural values. At times, these beliefs and values could be contradictory to those held by the nurse. What responsibilities does

ELSEVIER

Mosby items and derived items © 2011 by Mosby, Inc., an affiliate of Elsevier Inc.
Some material was previously published.

Adult Health Nursing, 6th ed.
Christensen & Kockrow

the nurse have when providing care to patients of different cultural and ethnic backgrounds? How does culture influence patient care and outcomes?

Answer: Cultural influences may have a vast effect on a patient's progress during illness. These beliefs help shape the patient's responses to health, illness, and the health care system. Reactions to pain, figures of authority, nonverbal behaviors, and medication therapies are affected by cultural background. Differing ethnic groups face health care challenges in conflicting ways. Given the importance of these factors to the recovery of a patient, nurses must attempt to investigate a patient's personal wishes. If possible, these desires should be incorporated into the plan of care. Nurses are also challenged to be aware of potential patient behaviors that can be a result of the patient's cultural or ethnic belief system and act accordingly.

CRITICAL THINKING QUESTION

After the decision is made to have surgery, there are a number of tasks the patient must complete. During the preoperative phase, the patient will require education concerning the admission process, surgery, and recovery periods. How should preoperative education be conducted and what impact might it have on the total surgical experience?

Guidelines: Preoperative education should occur at least 1 to 2 days before the surgical procedure. The education should be conducted in a comfortable and private environment. The nurse should use clear, easy- to-understand terms, clarifying terms and procedures the patient could encounter during the process. The nurse should evaluate the readiness to learn and special learning needs of the patient. Preoperative education is vital to answer questions the patient and family might have. Answering the questions provides not only information but also emotional support. Education and knowledge aid in reducing fears held concerning the surgery. A reduction in fear and anxiety can aid the patient in understanding the process and promote healthier behaviors. Further anxiety could increase pain. Thus, reduced anxiety might aid in achieving increased comfort.

OBJECTIVES	CONTENT	TEACHING RESOURCES
Identify the purposes of surgery.	■ Introduction (FAAHN p. 1253, AHN p. 17)	PPT 2 through 5, Ch. 42 FAAHN (Ch. 2 PPT 2 through 5 AHN)
		EILR TB Ch. 42 question 2 FAAHN (Ch. 2 question 2 AHN)
		EILR Open Book Quiz Ch. 42 question 1 FAAHN (Ch. 2 question 1 AHN)
		SG Purposes of Surgery, Ch. 42 p. 321 FAAHN (Ch. 2 p. 9, AHN)
		BOOK RESOURCES
		Table 42-1 Classification for Surgical Procedures (FAAHN p. 1254) (Table 2-1 AHN p. 18)
		Table 42-2 Surgical Terminology (FAAHN p. 1255) (Table 2-2 AHN p. 19)
		Box 42-1 Common Surgical Settings (FAAHN p. 1255) (Box 2-1 AHN p. 19)
		▶ Discuss current trends in surgery. This discussion should include the impact of insurance.

ELSEVIER

Adult Health Nursing, 6th ed.
Christensen & Kockrow

OBJECTIVES	CONTENT	TEACHING RESOURCES
		▸ Discuss the differences between diagnostic, palliative, elective, and therapeutic surgical procedures.
		Class Activity Provide note cards to the class. Ask each student to list four types of surgical procedures on the card. After allowing the students 5 minutes to complete the task, ask the students to trade cards with someone sitting near them. The students are then asked to decide if each of the surgical procedures is diagnostic, palliative, elective, or therapeutic.
Distinguish among elective, urgent, and emergency surgery.	☐ Introduction (FAAHN p. 1253, AHN p. 17)	PPT 3 Ch. 42 FAAHN (Ch. 2 PPT 3 AHN) 🖲 EILR TB Ch. 42 questions 24, 36 FAAHN (Ch. 2 questions 24, 36 AHN) 🖲 EILR Open Book Quiz Ch. 42 question 1 FAAHN (Ch. 2 question 1 AHN) 📕 SG Surgery Urgency, Ch. 42 pp. 9-10 FAAHN (Ch. 2 pp. 321-322 AHN) *Class Activity Generate a discussion about the impact of the large number of reality television programs involved in surgical care issues. How have these programs influenced the public's perceptions regarding surgery?*
Explain the concept of perioperative nursing	☐ Perioperative nursing (FAAHN p. 1254, AHN p. 18)	PPT 6, Ch. 42 FAAHN (Ch. 2 PPT 6 AHN) 🖲 EILR TB Ch. 42 question 36 FAAHN (Ch. 2 question 36 AHN) 🖲 EILR Open Book Quiz Ch. 42 question 3 FAAHN (Ch. 2 question 3 AHN) 📕 SG Perioperative Nursing, Ch. 42 p. 322 FAAHN (Ch. 2 p. 10 AHN) *Class Activity Divide the students into small groups of three to four. Instruct each student group to develop a list of tasks that can be delegated to assistive personnel. Compare the lists. Review the factors that must be taken into consideration when delegating patient care responsibilities.*

Christensen & Kockrow

Discuss the factors that influence an individual's ability to tolerate surgery.	☐ Influencing factors (FAAHN p. 1255, AHN p. 19)
	
	   – Age (FAAHN p. 1255, AHN p. 19)
	
	   – Physical condition (FAAHN p. 1255, AHN p. 19)
	
	   – Nutritional factors (FAAHN p. 1256, AHN p. 20)
	
	☐ Psychosocial needs (FAAHN p. 1256, AHN p. 20)
	
	☐ Socioeconomic and cultural needs (FAAHN p. 1256, AHN p. 20)
	
	☐ Medications (FAAHN p. 1257, AHN p. 21)
	
	☐ Education and experience (FAAHN p. 1259, AHN p. 23)
		PPT 7 through 12, Ch. 42 FAAHN (Ch. 2 PPT 7 through 12 AHN)
		
		EILR IC Ch. 42 image 1 FAAHN (Ch. 2 image 1 AHN)
		
		EILR TB Ch. 42 questions 15, 25, 31, 34, 38, FAAHN (Ch. 2 questions 15, 25, 31, 34, 38, AHN)
		
		EILR Open Book Quiz Ch. 42 question 3, 4 FAAHN (Ch. 2 question 3, 4 AHN)
		
		ESLR Review Questions for the NCLEX Examination Ch. 42 question 2 FAAHN (Ch. 2 question 2AHN)
		
		SG Tolerance Factors Ch. 42 pp. 322-323 FAAHN (Ch. 2 pp. 10-11 AHN)
		
		BOOK RESOURCES
		
		Box 42-3 ABCDE Mnemonic Device to Ascertain Serious Illness or Trauma in the Preoperative Patient (FAAHN p. 1256) (Box 2-3 AHN p. 20)
		
		Box 42-4 Common Fears Associated with Surgery (FAAHN p. 1257) (Box 2-4 AHN p. 21)
		
		Cultural Considerations The Surgical Patient (FAAHN p. 1258) (AHN p. 22)
		
		Table 42-3 Preoperative Considerations for Commonly Ingested Herbs (FAAHN p. 1258) (Table 2-3 AHN p. 22)
		
		Table 42-4 Surgical Effects on Body Systems (FAAHN p. 1259) (Table 2-4 AHN p. 23)
		
		Fig. 42-1 Often knowledge deficits occur when the patient is undergoing her first surgical experience (FAAHN p. 1257) (Fig. 2-1 AHN p. 21)
		
		Patient Teaching Preoperative Care (FAAHN p. 1257) (AHN p. 21)
		
		▶ Discuss the impact of culture on the surgical experience. How do different ethnic groups view the health care experience? What are the responsibilities of the nurse when faced with cultural differences that impact the plan of care?
		
		▶ Discuss the impact of existing health problems on the surgical experience.

Christensen & Kockrow

		Class Activity **Provide copies of nursing care plan forms to the members of the class. Allow students to gather in small groups (two to four students) and develop a plan of care for the patient undergoing surgery for hysterectomy, bowel resection, total hip replacement, or carpal tunnel repair.**
Discuss considerations for the older adult surgical patient.	☐ Influencing factors (FAAHN p. 1255, AHN p. 19) – Age (FAAHN p. 1255, AHN p. 19)	⊠▬ PPT 7, Ch. 42 FAAHN (Ch. 2 PPT 7 AHN) *e* EILR TB Ch. 42 questions 7, 37 FAAHN (Ch. 2 questions 7, 37 AHN) *e* ESLR Review Questions for the NCLEX Examination Ch. 42 question 1 FAAHN (Ch. 2 question 1 AHN) SG Tolerance Factors, Ch. 42 pp. 322-323 FAAHN (Ch. 2 pp. 10-11 AHN) ▸ Discuss potential needs of the older adult patient when planning the preoperative teaching session. ▸ Discuss preadmission evaluations that might be needed by the older adult patient contemplating surgery. *Class Activity* **Recruit three or four people. The recruits will assist in a role-play exercise and pretend to be older patients of varying ages planning to undergo surgery. The groups of students will obtain preadmission surgery assessment information. This information and its implications will be discussed with the entire group after the interviews are completed.**

2.1 Homework/Assignments:

2.1 Instructor's Notes/Student Feedback:

Adult Health Nursing, 6th ed.
Christensen & Kockrow

LESSON 2.2

CRITICAL THINKING QUESTION

A 73-year-old patient is scheduled to have elective surgery. The patient is a widow and lives alone. She has signed the consent for surgery, and the preoperative teaching has been completed. She appears to have an understanding of the concepts presented. Just prior to the surgery, the patient's daughter comes to the nurse's station and requests to have the surgery cancelled. She states that her mother is old and is not in her right mind to make such big decisions. Furthermore, she is questioning the ability of her mother to sign the surgical consent. In her agitation, she states, "Whoever witnessed that signature is really going to be in trouble!" What should be done at this time?

Guidelines: Despite her advanced age, the patient is still within her rights to consent to medical care, including surgery. Age does not reduce her legal rights to make health care decisions. By signing the surgical consent, the patient is stating an understanding of the surgical procedure including the care, risks, benefits, and possible alternative therapies. The witness identified on the consent is only supporting the claims that the patient who signed the consent did so without coercion.

At this time, there is no reason to cancel the surgery. The nurse should notify her supervisor and attempt to calm the situation. The physician might need to be contacted if concerns remain.

OBJECTIVES	CONTENT	TEACHING RESOURCES
Describe the preoperative checklist.	■ Preoperative phase (FAAHN p. 1259, AHN p. 23) □ Preoperative teaching (FAAHN p. 1260, AHN p. 24) □ Preoperative preparation (FAAHN p. 1260, AHN p. 24) – Laboratory tests and diagnostic imaging (FAAHN p. 1260, AHN p. 24) – Informed consent (FAAHN p. 1260, AHN p. 24) – Gastrointestinal preparation (FAAHN p. 1261, AHN p. 25) – Skin preparation (FAAHN p. 1261, AHN p. 25) – Latex allergy considerations (FAAHN p. 1262, AHN p. 26) – Respiratory preparation (FAAHN p. 1264, AHN p. 28) – Cardiovascular considerations (FAAHN p. 1268, AHN p. 32) – Vital signs (FAAHN p. 1269, AHN p. 33) – Genitourinary considerations (FAAHN p. 1271, AHN p. 35) – Surgical wounds (FAAHN p. 1271, AHN p. 35)	PPT 8 through 31, Ch. 42 FAAHN (Ch. 2 PPT 8 through 31 AHN) EILR IC Ch. 42 images 2 through 9 FAAHN (Ch. 2 images 2 through 9 AHN) EILR TB Ch. 42 questions 16, 20, 32, 40 FAAHN (Ch. 2 questions 16, 20, 32, 40 AHN) EILR Open Book Quiz Ch. 42 questions 5, 7 FAAHN (Ch. 2 questions 5, 7 AHN) ESLR Review Questions for the NCLEX Examination Ch. 42 questions 3, 4, 7FAAHN (Ch. 2 questions 3, 4, 7 AHN) SG Preoperative Information, Ch. 42 pp. 323-324 FAAHN (Ch. 2 pp. 11-12 AHN) **BOOK RESOURCES** Box 42-2 Delegation Considerations in Perioperative Nursing (FAAHN p. 1255) (Box 2-2 AHN p. 19) Table 42-4 Surgical Effects on Body Systems (FAAHN p 1259) (Table 2-4 AHN p. 23) Fig. 42-2 Skin preparation for surgery on various body areas (FAAHN p. 1263) (Fig. 2-2 AHN p. 27) Skill 42-1 Performing a Surgical Skin Preparation (FAAHN p. 1262) (Skill 2-1 AHN p. 26)

ELSEVIER

OBJECTIVES	CONTENT	TEACHING RESOURCES
	− Pain (FAAHN p. 1271, AHN p. 35) − Tubes (FAAHN p. 1271, AHN p. 35) − Preoperative medication (FAAHN p. 1271, AHN p. 35) − Anesthesia (FAAHN p. 1273, AHN p. 37) − Preoperative checklist (FAAHN p. 1277, AHN p. 41) − Transport to the operating room (FAAHN p. 1279, AHN p. 43) − Preparing for the postoperative patient (FAAHN p. 1279, AHN p. 43)	Box 42-5 Responding to a Patient's Risk for Latex Allergy (FAAHN p. 1264) (Box 2-5 AHN p. 28) Skill 42-2 Incentive Spirometry or Positive Expiratory Pressure Therapy and "Huff" Coughing (FAAHN p. 1264) (Skill 2-2 AHN p. 28) Patient Teaching box Incentive Spirometry (FAAHN p. 1264) (AHN p. 28) Patient Teaching box Controlled Coughing Technique (FAAHN p. 1266) (AHN p. 30) Fig. 42-3 Volume-oriented spirometer (FAAHN p. 1266) (Fig. 2-3 AHN p. 30) Skill 42-5 Applying Thromboembolic Deterrent Stockings and Sequential Compression Devices (FAAHN p. 1269) (Skill 2-5 AHN p. 33) Fig. 42-4 Applying antiembolism stockings (FAAHN p. 1270) (Fig. 2-4 AHN p. 34) Fig. 42-5 Application of sequential compression devices (FAAHN p. 1270) (Fig. 2-5 AHN p. 34) Fig. 42-6 Assess the bladder by palpating the lower abdomen for distention (FAAHN p. 1271) (Fig. 2-6 AHN p. 35) Drug Table 42-1 Perioperative Medications and Their Purposes (FAAHN pp. 1272-1273) (Drug Table 2-1 AHN pp. 36-37) Table 42-5 Medications with Special Implications for the Surgical Patient (FAAHN p. 1274) (Table 2-5 AHN p. 38) Fig. 42-7 Possible airways used during surgery (FAAHN p. 1273) (Fig. 2-7 AHN p. 37) Fig. 42-9 Common perioperative positions and the padding provided to relieve pressure in each position (FAAHN p. 1277) (Fig. 2-9 AHN p. 41) Fig. 42-10 Preoperative assessment form (FAAHN p. 1278) (Fig. 2-10 AHN p. 42) ▶ Discuss the importance of the surgical preoperative check list. How is it used by the surgical department after completion?

OBJECTIVES	CONTENT	TEACHING RESOURCES
		▸ Discuss common laboratory tests that could be completed prior to surgery. What is the significance of these particular tests? *Class Activity Divide the students into pairs and assign roles. One will be the patient and the other, the nurse. Ask the students to role-play a preoperative education session. Be sure to include all of the skills listed above.*
Explain the importance of informed consent for surgery.	– Informed consent (FAAHN p. 1260, AHN p. 24)	PPT 14, Ch. 42 FAAHN (Ch. 2 PPT 14 AHN) EILR TB Ch. 42 questions 3, 4, 29 FAAHN (Ch. 2 question 3, 4, 29 AHN) ESLR Review Questions for the NCLEX Examination Ch. 42 question 5 FAAHN (Ch. 2 question 5 AHN) SG Informed Consent, Ch. 42 pp. 324-325 FAAHN (Ch. 2 pp. 12-13 AHN) ▸ Discuss the purpose of informed consent. Who does it protect? ▸ Discuss patient attributes the nurse should look for to determine if the criteria of informed consent have been met. *Class Activity Pass a sheet of paper around the class. Ask each student to write any questions about the elements of informed consent and the role of the nurse in obtaining the consent. After all students have had the opportunity to identify questions, read them aloud to the entire class. Encourage group input.*
Explain the procedure for turning, deep breathing, coughing, and leg exercises for postoperative patients.	– Respiratory preparation (FAAHN p. 1264, AHN p. 28)	PPT 15 through 16, Ch. 42 FAAHN (Ch. 2 PPT 15 through 16 AHN) EILR IC Ch. 42 images 3 FAAHN (Ch. 2 images 3 AHN) EILR TB Ch. 42 question 8, 15, 26, 28 FAAHN (Ch. 2 question 8, 15, 26, 28 AHN) EILR Open Book Quiz Ch. 42 questions 4, 5, 6 FAAHN (Ch. 2 questions 4, 5, 6 AHN) ESLR Review Questions for the NCLEX Examination Ch. 42 question 6 FAAHN (Ch. 2 question 6 AHN)

OBJECTIVES	CONTENT	TEACHING RESOURCES
		▣ SG Turning, Coughing, Deep-Breathing, and Leg Exercises, Ch. 42 p. 324 FAAHN (Ch. 2 p. 12 AHN)
		BOOK RESOURCES
		Skill 42-3 Teaching Controlled Coughing (FAAHN pp. 1266-1267) (Skill 2-3 AHN pp. 30-31)
		Patient Teaching Controlled Coughing Technique (FAAHN p. 1266) (AHN p. 30)
		Skill 42-4 Teaching Postoperative Breathing Techniques, Leg Exercises, and Turning (FAAHN pp. 1267-1268) (Skill 2-4 AHN p. 31-31)
		Patient Teaching Use of Thromboembolic Deterrent Stockings and Sequential Compression Devices (FAAHN p. 1269) (AHN p. 33)
		Box 42-6 Surgeries for Which Coughing is Contraindicated or Modified (FAAHN p. 1269) (Box 2-6 AHN p. 33)
		▸ Discuss why postoperative breathing exercises are necessary.
		▸ Discuss preoperative interventions and education that can be provided to reduce postoperative respiratory complications.
		*Class Activity **Invite a respiratory therapist to be a guest speaker at the class. Ask the therapist to discuss his/her role in the care of the postoperative patient.***
Differentiate among general, regional, and local anesthesia.	− Anesthesia (FAAHN p. 1273, AHN p. 37)	▨ PPT 27 through 29, Ch. 42 FAAHN (Ch. 2 PPT 27 through 29 AHN)
		✎ EILR IC Ch. 42 image 8 FAAHN (Ch. 2 image 8 AHN)
		✎ EILR TB Ch. 42 questions 5, 6 FAAHN (Ch. 2 questions 5, 6 AHN)
		✎ EILR Open Book Quiz Ch. 42 questions 8, 9 FAAHN (Ch. 2 questions 8, 9 AHN)
		✎ ESLR Review Questions for the NCLEX Examination Ch. 42 question 8 FAAHN (Ch. 2 question 8 AHN)

OBJECTIVES	CONTENT	TEACHING RESOURCES
		📖 SG Anesthesia During the Surgical Experience, Ch. 42 pp. 325-326 FAAHN (Ch. 2 pp. 13-14 AHN)
		BOOK RESOURCES
		Fig. 42-8 Spinal column(FAAHN p. 1275) (Fig. 2-8 AHN p. 39).
		▶ Discuss the psychological implications and needs for the patient undergoing spinal or epidural anesthesia.
		▶ Discuss the four stages of general anesthesia administration.
		▶ Discuss the differing tactile sensations experienced by patients undergoing spinal, local, and epidural anesthesia.
		Class Activity Ask the class to list several types of surgery. Write the surgeries on the board. Next, ask the class to determine if the procedure would most likely be done using general, regional, or local anesthesia.
Explain conscious sedation.	– Anesthesia (FAAHN p. 1273, AHN p. 37)	📺 PPT 29, Ch. 42 FAAHN (Ch. 2 PPT 29 AHN)
		💿 EILR TB Ch. 42 question 6 FAAHN (Ch. 2 question 6 AHN)
		💿 ESLR Review Questions for the NCLEX Examination Ch. 42 question 9 FAAHN (Ch. 2 question 9 AHN)
		📖 SG Anesthesia During the Surgical Experience, Ch. 42 pp. 325-326 FAAHN (Ch. 2 pp. 13-14 AHN)
		▶ Discuss the types of procedures that might require conscious sedation.
		▶ Discuss the advantages of conscious sedation over general anesthesia.
		Class Activity Distribute nursing care plan forms. Ask each student to develop a brief care plan for the patient undergoing a procedure with conscious sedation. Have students identify the role of the LPN/LVN in conscious sedation of a patient.

2.2 Homework/Assignments:

2.2 Instructor's Notes/Student Feedback:

LESSON 2.3

CRITICAL THINKING QUESTION

A 43-year-old female patient has just returned from the Postanesthesia Care Unit. She underwent a total hysterectomy earlier in the day. As you begin to outline the plans for her care, she states that she is too tired to move and does not wish to be disturbed until the following day. Based upon your knowledge, this inactivity will increase her risk factors for postoperative complications. When you attempt to explain that she will have increased risk of complications, she responds by stating, "I don't understand what a little extended bed rest can possibly do to hurt me." What actions should be taken?
Guidelines: The patient is at increased risk for postoperative complications if her inactivity is allowed to continue. The first step is to determine specifically why she is not willing to participate in her plan of care. After that is done, it is possible to focus on her reasoning and possibly change her mind. She might also be unaware of the detriment that could result from her inactivity. She should be advised that her risk of respiratory complications, including pneumonia and hypoventilation, is increased with her decision. There are also problems involving venous stasis. The lack of movement will promote reduced blood flow to the extremities, thus increasing the risk of thrombus formation. If she remains unwilling to participate in the preventative care plan, perhaps you can develop a compromise with her. She might consider taking some pain medicine, followed by a rest period, and then agree to begin turning, coughing, and deep breathing. Despite what the outcome of this interaction is, the conversations, the patient's refusal, and the nursing actions taken must be documented in the patient's record. Repeated attempts to engage the patient should be made.

OBJECTIVES	CONTENT	TEACHING RESOURCES
Describe the role of the circulating nurse and the scrub nurse during surgery.	■ Intraoperative phase (FAAHN p. 1279, AHN p. 43) ■ Holding area (FAAHN p. 1279, AHN p. 43) ■ The nurse's role (FAAHN p. 1280, AHN p. 44)	PPT 35 through 39, Ch. 42 FAAHN (Ch. 2 PPT 35 through 39 AHN) EILR IC Ch. 42 images 11, 12, 13 FAAHN (Ch. 2 images 11, 12, 13 AHN) EILR TB Ch. 42 question 21 FAAHN (Ch. 2 question 21 AHN) SG Nurse's Responsibilities, Ch. 42 p. 327 FAAHN (Ch. 2 p. 15 AHN) **BOOK RESOURCES** Fig. 42-11 Traditional operating room (FAAHN p. 1279) (Fig. 2-11 AHN p. 43) Box 42-7 Responsibilities of the Circulating Nurse and the Scrub Nurse (FAAHN p. 1280) (Box 2-7 AHN p. 44) Fig. 42-12 Safe, effective intraoperative care requires a team effort (FAAHN p. 1280) (Fig. 2-12 AHN p. 44) Fig. 42-13 Nurse in a postanesthesia care unit (FAAHN p. 1281) (Fig. 2-13 AHN p. 45) ▶ Discuss the special training needed by the circulating nurse and scrub nurse in surgery. ▶ Discuss how the roles of the circulating and scrub nurse differ.

Adult Health Nursing, 6th ed.
Christensen & Kockrow

OBJECTIVES	CONTENT	TEACHING RESOURCES
		Class Activity Assign the students in groups of three or four. Each group will be required to locate an article in a professional nursing journal regarding surgical nursing. Each group will then be asked to provide a 5- to 10-minute overview of their findings.
Discuss the initial nursing assessment and management immediately after transfer from the postanesthesia care unit.	■ Postoperative phase (FAAHN p. 1280, AHN p. 44) ☐ Immediate postoperative phase (FAAHN p. 1280, AHN p. 44)	⊠ PPT 40 through 41, Ch. 42 FAAHN (Ch. 2 PPT 40 through 41 AHN) 🔁 EILR TB Ch. 42 questions 9, 12, 13, 14, 22, 23, 30, 41 FAAHN (Ch. 2 questions 9, 12, 13, 14, 22, 23, 30, 41 AHN) 🔁 ESLR Review Questions for the NCLEX Examination Ch. 42 question 10 FAAHN (Ch. 2 question 10 AHN) SG Postoperative Care, Ch. 42 p. 328 FAAHN (Ch. 2 p. 16 AHN) **BOOK RESOURCES** Table 42-6 Interventions Associated with the ABCs of Immediate Recovery (FAAHN p. 1281) (Table 2-6 AHN p. 45) Table 42-7 Temperature Assessment and Intervention (FAAHN p. 1282) (Table 2-7 AHN p. 46) ▸ Discuss the prioritization of care required in the postanesthesia unit. What assessments are of the highest priority? ▸ Discuss interventions that can be expected of the nurse working in the postanesthesia unit. ▸ Discuss the frequency of assessments in the postanesthesia care unit. *Class Activity Have students as a group develop specific questions for an interviewee who has had surgery, about recollections of the postanesthesia period. See Homework box at end of lesson.*

Mosby items and derived items © 2011 by Mosby, Inc., an affiliate of Elsevier Inc.
Some material was previously published.

OBJECTIVES	CONTENT	TEACHING RESOURCES

List assessment data for the surgical patient	☐ Later postoperative phase (FAAHN p. 1282, AHN p. 46)
	
	  – Immediate assessments (FAAHN p. 1282, AHN p. 46)
	
	  – Incision (FAAHN p. 1284, AHN p. 48)
	
	  – Ventilation (FAAHN p. 1284, AHN p. 48)
	
	  – Pain (FAAHN p. 1285, AHN p. 49)
	
	  – Urinary function (FAAHN p. 1286, AHN p. 50)
	
	  – Venous stasis (FAAHN p. 1286, AHN p. 50)
	
	  – Activity (FAAHN p. 1287, AHN p. 51)
	
	☐ Gastrointestinal status (FAAHN p. 1288, AHN p. 52)
	
	☐ Fluids and electrolytes (FAAHN p. 1288, AHN p. 52)
		🔲 SG Nursing Process, Ch. 42 p. 330 FAAHN (Ch. 2 p. 18 AHN)
		
		BOOK RESOURCES
		
		Box 42-2 Delegation Considerations in Perioperative Nursing (FAAHN p. 1255) (Box 2-2 AHN p. 19)
		
		Box 42-3 ABCDE Mnemonic Device to Ascertain Serious Illness or Trauma in the Preoperative Patient (FAAHN p. 1256) (Box 2-3 AHN p. 20)
		
		▸ Discuss elements of the nursing assessment of the surgical patient.
		
		▸ Discuss the prioritization of the nursing assessment for the surgical patient.

Identify the rationale for nursing interventions designed to prevent postoperative complications.	☐ Later postoperative phase (FAAHN p. 1282, AHN p. 46)
	
	  – Immediate assessments (FAAHN p. 1282, AHN p. 46)
	
	  – Incision (FAAHN p. 1284, AHN p. 48)
	
	  – Ventilation (FAAHN p. 1284, AHN p. 48)
	
	  – Pain (FAAHN p. 1285, AHN p. 49)
	
	  – Urinary function (FAAHN p. 1286, AHN p. 50)
	
	  – Venous stasis (FAAHN p. 1286, AHN p. 50)
	
	  – Activity (FAAHN p. 1287, AHN p. 51)
	
	☐ Gastrointestinal status (FAAHN p. 1288, AHN p. 52)
	
	☐ Fluids and electrolytes (FAAHN p. 1288, AHN p. 52)
		🔲 PPT 40 through 57, Ch. 42 FAAHN (Ch. 2 PPT 40 through 57 AHN)
		
		💾 EILR IC Ch. 42 images 15, 16, 17 FAAHN (Ch. 2 images 15, 16, 17 AHN)
		
		💾 EILR TB Ch. 42 questions 1, 10, 11, 15, 17, 18, 19, 23, 28 FAAHN (Ch. 2 questions 1, 10, 11, 15, 17, 18, 19, 23, 28 AHN)
		
		🔲 SG Rationale for Nursing Intervenntions, Ch. 42 p. 329 FAAHN (Ch. 2 p. 17 AHN)
		
		BOOK RESOURCES
		
		Table 42-7 Temperature assessment and Intervention (FAAHN p. 1282) (Table 2-7 AHN p. 46)
		
		Fig. 42-14 Postoperative assessment form (FAAHN p. 1283) (Table 2-8 AHN p. 47)
		
		Box 42-8 Possible Causes of Postoperative Shock (FAAHN p. 1284) (Box 2-8 AHN p. 48)
		
		Fig. 42-15 Wound dehiscence and Evisceration (FAAHN p. 1284) (Fig. 2-15 AHN p. 48)

OBJECTIVES	CONTENT	TEACHING RESOURCES
		Box 42-9 Postoperative Comfort Measures for Pain (FAAHN p. 1285) (Box 2-9 AHN p. 49)
		Fig. 42-16 Transcutaneous electric nerve stimulation (TENS) unit (FAAHN p. 1286) (Fig. 2-16 AHN p. 50)
		Box 42-10 Effects of Early Postoperative Ambulation (FAAHN p. 1287) (Box 2-10 AHN p. 51)
		Fig. 42-17 Progression in levels of postoperative activity promotes tissue perfusion (FAAHN p. 1287) (Fig. 2-17 AHN p. 51)
		▸ Discuss the use of the pain scale for postoperative patients and documentation of the patient's perception of pain.
		▸ Discuss nonpharmacological methods that can be used to manage pain in the postoperative patient.
		▸ Discuss the possible causes of postoperative shock.
		Class Activity Ask each student to record his/her definition of pain. After students have recorded the definition, ask them to record the nurse's responsibility in managing this pain. Encourage the students to give consideration beyond medication management. After a brief period, allow the students to discuss their recordings to the class at large.
Discuss the nursing process as it pertains to the surgical patient.	☐ Nursing process for the surgical patient (FAAHN p. 1289, AHN p. 53) – Assessment (FAAHN p. 1289, AHN p. 53) – Nursing diagnoses (FAAHN p. 1289, AHN p. 53) – Expected outcomes and planning (FAAHN p. 1289, AHN p. 53) – Implementation (FAAHN p. 1289, AHN p. 53) – Evaluation (FAAHN p. 1289, AHN p. 53)	▣ PPT 55 through 58, Ch. 42 FAAHN (Ch. 2 PPT 55 through 58 AHN) 🖥 EILR TB Ch. 42 questions 14, 27 FAAHN (Ch. 2 questions 14, 27 AHN) 📕 SG Nursing Process, Ch. 42 p. 330 FAAHN (Ch. 2 p. 18 AHN) **BOOK RESOURCES** Box 42-11 Preoperative Nursing Diagnoses (FAAHN p. 1289) (Box 2-11 AHN p. 53) Box 42-12 Postoperative Nursing Diagnoses (FAAHN p. 1290) (Box 2-12 AHN p. 54) Nursing Care Plan The Postoperative Patient (FAAHN pp. 1290-1291) (AHN pp. 54-55) ▸ Discuss potential nursing diagnoses for the patient who has recently undergone surgery.

Christensen & Kockrow

OBJECTIVES	CONTENT	TEACHING RESOURCES
		▸ Discuss and review goal setting for the postoperative patient. What goals are realistic? How can these goals be evaluated?
		Class Activity Develop four patient scenarios. Put students into groups of three or four. Require that the students select groups not sitting near them in the classroom. Assign each group a patient scenario. Ask each group to determine the priorities of care for each of the patients. The rationale for the priorities selected should be provided by the group as well.

Identify the information needed for the postoperative patient in preparation for discharge.	☐ Discharge: providing general information (FAAHN p. 1291, AHN p. 55)
	
	  – Ambulatory surgery discharge (FAAHN p. 1291, AHN p. 55)
		PPT 61 through 62, Ch. 42 FAAHN (Ch. 2 PPT 61 through 62 AHN)
		
		  EILR IC Ch. 42 image 18 FAAHN (Ch. 2 image 18 AHN)
		
		  EILR TB Ch. 42 questions 35, 39 FAAHN (Ch. 2 questions 35, 39 AHN)
		
		  SG Preparation for Discharge Ch. 42 p. 330 FAAHN (Ch. 2 p. 18 AHN)
		
		BOOK RESOURCES
		
		Box 42-13 Vital Information for the Discharged Patient (FAAHN p. 1292) (Box 2-13 AHN p. 56)
		
		Fig. 42-18 Reviewing discharge planning instructions (FAAHN p. 1292) (Box 2-18 AHN p. 56)
		
		▸ Discuss promoting an environment that is conducive to learning.
		
		▸ Discuss assessment of the patient's readiness to learn.
		
		Class Activity Ask each student to develop a list of common postoperative discharge questions and concerns. These questions will be gathered and reviewed as a class.

ELSEVIER

Adult Health Nursing, 6th ed.
Christensen & Kockrow

| Performance Evaluation | | EILR TB Ch. 42 questions 1 through 41 FAAHN (Ch. 2 questions 1 through 41 AHN)
| | | EILR Open Book Quiz Ch. 42 question 1 through 10 FAAHN (Ch. 2 question 1 through 10 AHN)
| | | ESLR Review Questions for the NCLEX Examination Ch. 42 question 1 through 10 FAAHN (Ch. 2 question 1 through 10 AHN)
| | | SG Ch. 42 pp. 321 through 332 FAAHN (Ch. 2 pp. 9 through 20 AHN)
| | | **BOOK RESOURCES**
| | | Review Questions for the NCLEX Examination Ch. 42 questions 1 through 25 FAAHN (Ch. 2 questions 1 through 25 AHN)

2.3 Homework/Assignments:

1. Have each student interview an acquaintance who has had surgery. Then discuss in class.

2.3 Instructor's Notes/Student Feedback:

Christensen & Kockrow

Slide 1

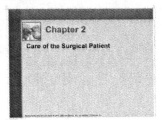

Slide 2

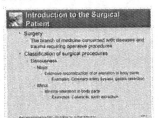

- Surgery has changed greatly since it became a medical specialty in the mid-19th century. What changes and health care advances have influenced the growth of surgery? Include asepsis, technology, and anesthesiology in the discussion.

- Describe the role of the nurse in the early days of surgery.

Slide 3

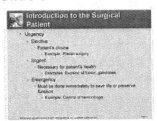

- How do the types of surgery differ?

- What special emotional support might be indicated for patients in the differing types of surgery? Are the psychosocial needs of the patient undergoing emergency surgery different from those planning an elective procedure?

Slide 4

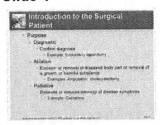

- As surgery has changed, the settings for surgery have changed. What alternatives to the traditional hospital environment for surgical procedures are available?

- *Examples include physician offices and surgery centers.*

Slide 5

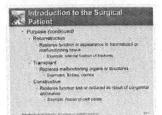

Slide 6

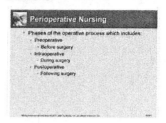

- The term perioperative encompasses all phases of surgery.
- What are the responsibilities of the nurse in the preoperative period?
- Which actions can be delegated to assistive personnel?

Slide 7

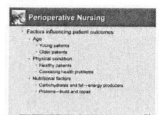

- Older adults and children do not adapt to the physiologic stressors associated with surgery as well as young and middle-aged adults do.
- What metabolic needs influence the outcomes of older and younger aged patients?
- Examine disease conditions associated with older adulthood that might hinder a rapid postoperative recovery.
- Why are young children at a higher surgical risk?
- What measures can the nurse implement to increase the patient's response to surgery?

Slide 8

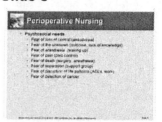

- What is the impact fear can have on the patient's response to surgery?
- Review the interrelationship between fear and pain.
- What role does nursing play in coping with the patient's perioperative fears?

Slide 9

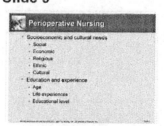

- The patient's reaction and adaptation to a health care crisis are influenced by the patient's environment.
- Review the nursing role in meeting the socioeconomic and cultural needs of the patient.
- How do life experiences impact the patient's response to surgery?

Slide 10

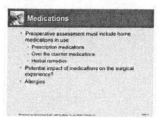

- What common medications may be taken more frequently in the older adult? How can these medication influence surgical outcomes?
- Discontinuation of medications may be ordered after consultation with the physician and the anesthesiologist.

ELSEVIER

Adult Health Nursing, 6th ed.
Christensen & Kockrow

Slide 11

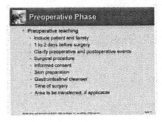

- Why is 1 to 2 days prior to surgery the ideal time to complete patient education?
- Converse about the characteristics of the ideal preoperative teaching environment.

Slide 12

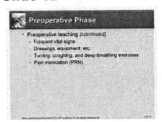

- Continue discussion from slide 11.

Slide 13

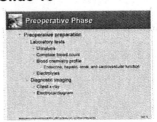

- Preoperative testing aids in determining the condition of the patient before the surgical procedure. It also provides baseline health data.
- What abnormalities would need to be reported to the physician before surgery?

Slide 14

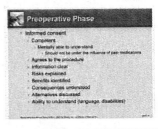

- Informed consent is necessary to determine if the patient is aware of the planned procedure. What are the responsibilities of the nurse when determining informed consent?
- What attributes are necessary to give informed consent for a surgical procedure?
- Review the steps that must be taken in an emergency situation in which the patient or guardians are not able or available to provide informed consent.

Slide 15

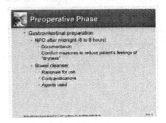

- In preparation for the surgical procedure, an empty gastrointestinal tract is frequently desired. This will reduce the chance of emesis or aspiration.
- What education should be given to the patient regarding NPO status?
- In some surgeries the patient may be able to have fluid intake the day after the procedure.
- Bowel cleansing regimens might be implemented. There are, however, surgical procedures or patient conditions in which bowel cleansing is contraindicated. Identify some of these procedures.

Adult Health Nursing, 6th ed.

Christensen & Kockrow

Slide 16

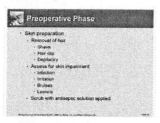

- Skin preparations are completed to clean and prepare the surgical site. This aids in reducing the risk of infection.

- What are differing options for preparing the skin before surgery?

- During the skin preparation, it is the role of the nurse to assess the area for lesions, bruises, irritation, or signs of infection.

- Certain populations bring special challenges to skin preparation. Discuss the unique issues of older adults and children.

Slide 17

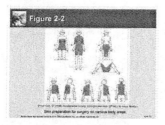

Slide 18

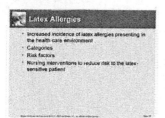

- The assessment of the risk factors must include the patient's experience with the allergy response.

- Review the different categories of reaction associated with latex sensitivity

Slide 19

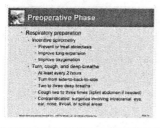

- Respiratory complications can occur after surgery. This is due to the reduced ability of the lungs to expand during the procedure.

- What should the patient be told preoperatively concerning respiratory care?

Slide 20

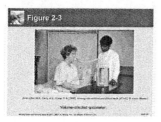

- Outline the purpose and use of the incentive spirometer.

- Demonstrate use of the incentive spirometer.

ELSEVIER

Mosby items and derived items © 2011, 2007 by Mosby, Inc., an affiliate of Elsevier Inc.
Some material was previously published.

Adult Health Nursing, 6th ed.
Christensen & Kockrow

Slide 21

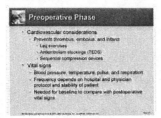

- Blood stasis during surgery promotes the risk of cardiovascular complications.
- What interventions can be employed to reduce cardiovascular complications?
- What patient attributes might increase the risk of cardiovascular complications?

Slide 22

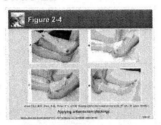

- Review the use of antiembolism stockings. How do they reduce cardiovascular complications?
- What assessments should be performed after the stockings are applied?
- Review the locations to measure the patient's legs to ensure a safe fit.

Slide 23

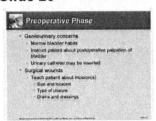

- Review the types of surgeries necessitating the placement of a urinary catheter.
- When in the preoperative experience will the catheter be inserted?
- What information can be given to the patient about what the insertion will feel like?
- How do sutures, staples, and Steri-Strips differ?

Slide 24

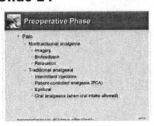

- Discuss the use of a pain scale.
- How can a pain scale be used for children who do not understand numerical concepts?
- What responsibilities does the nurse have concerning the documentation of pain?

Slide 25

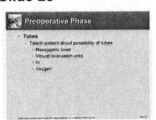

- Discuss the types of drainage tubes that might be placed during the surgical procedure.
- What purpose do these tubes serve?

Adult Health Nursing, 6th ed.

Christensen & Kockrow

Slide 26

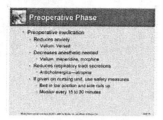

- What types of preoperative medications are administered?
- What are their desired effects?
- What responsibilities does the nurse have regarding the administration of preoperative medications?

Slide 27

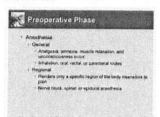

- Anesthesia means the absence of feeling.
- Review the three categories of anesthesia.
- What types of surgeries might be candidates for general anesthesia?
- What types of surgeries might be candidates for regional anesthesia?

Slide 28

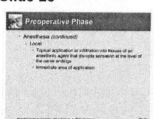

- What are the types of surgeries that would be eligible for local anesthesia?

Slide 29

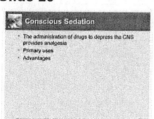

- When caring for the patient undergoing conscious sedation, what is the role of the nurse?
- The nurse caring for the patient undergoing conscious sedation must be knowledgeable about physiology, cardiac dysrhythmias, procedural complications, and pharmacologic principles of medication administration.

Slide 30

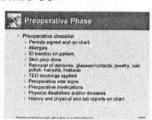

- What is the purpose of the preoperative checklist?
- Who is responsible for completion of the preoperative checklist?
- Review the time frame in which the preoperative checklist should be completed prior to the onset of surgery.

ELSEVIER

Adult Health Nursing, 6th ed.
Christensen & Kockrow

Slide 31

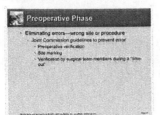

Slide 32

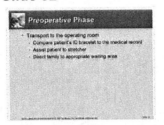

Slide 33

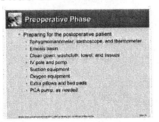

- After the patient has been transported to the surgical department, the floor nurse begins preparations for his return. Advance planning reduces or eliminates time lost waiting by the patient for the supplies needed early in the postoperative period.

- Consult the physician's order sheet to identify items needed.

- A review of postoperative orders is still needed after the patient returns from the recovery room. This will enable the nurse to assess for unexpected changes in the plan of treatment.

- What items can be anticipated? Review a list of supplies to gather.

Slide 34

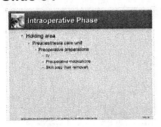

- Some facilities might have a holding area known as a Preanesthesia Care Unit.

- Outline the role of the nurse during this period.

- What emotional needs does the patient have during this time? How can nurses work to meet the needs of the patient awaiting surgery?

Slide 35

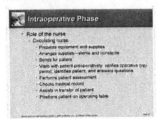

- What is the role of the circulating nurse?

Adult Health Nursing, 6th ed.
Christensen & Kockrow

Slide 36

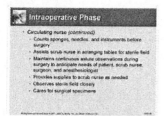

- What is the role of the circulating nurse?

Slide 37

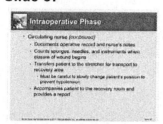

- Discuss student interest in observation of or future employment as a circulating nurse

Slide 38

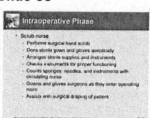

- What is the role of the scrub nurse?

- Discuss student interest in observation of or future employment as a scrub nurse.

Slide 39

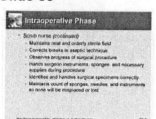

- What is the role of the scrub nurse?

- Discuss student interest in observation of or future employment as a scrub nurse.

Slide 40

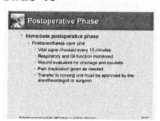

- Immediately after surgery, the patient is transported to the Postanesthesia Care Unit.

- Review the nursing interventions associated with the ABCs of immediate recovery. How long will the patient remain in the Postanesthesia Care Unit?

- What criterion indicates the patient is ready to be transferred to the nursing floor?

Slide 41

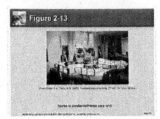

- Discuss student interest in an observation experience or employment in a Postanesthesia Care Unit.

Slide 42

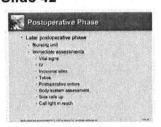

- After release from the Postanesthesia Care Unit, the patient is returned to the nursing unit. Review the responsibility of the nurse accepting transfer of the patient from the Postanesthesia Care Unit.

- The frequency of the assessment once the patient has been received to the unit utilizes the "times-four" factor. Review the timing of this plan.

- What findings in the postoperative assessment are considered abnormal? Interpret the significance of these abnormal findings.

- What safety interventions should be instituted?

Slide 43

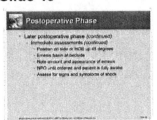

- How is the patient to be positioned after surgery? What determines optimal positioning during the postoperative period? Discuss surgical procedures that require alternative positioning in the postoperative period.

- Why is shock a risk factor for the later postoperative period? Review the manifestations associated with shock (increased HR, thready pulse, reduced B/P, cool and clammy skin, reduced urinary output, changes in LOC)

- What are nursing documentation requirements after the patient assessment is completed?

Slide 44

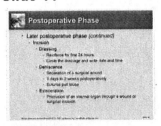

- During the initial 24 hours after surgery, the incision is typically covered with a dressing. The length of time the incision remains covered beyond that point varies by physician.

- What can bleeding from the incision signal? (Hemorrhage. The dressing requires monitoring for drainage.)

- What actions will the nurse take if the dressing becomes soiled?

- What wound complications are associated with impaired healing?

Slide 45

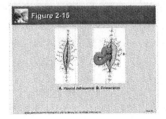

Christensen & Kockrow

Slide 46

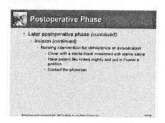

- In the event of a complication associated with impaired wound healing, what patient education is needed?
- Review the required nursing documentation in the event of a wound complication.

Slide 47

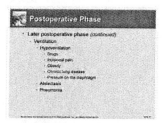

- Respiratory compromise is a surgical complication. Timely nursing assessments and interventions are vital to preventing postoperative complications.
- Why does surgical intervention reduce respiratory function?
- What should the nurse assess regarding respiratory function?
- Identify potential respiratory-related postoperative complications.

Slide 48

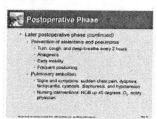

- Preventative interventions often cause discomfort in the patient. What can the nurse do to reduce the discomfort experienced by the patient?
- If the patient does not comply with the respiratory preventative care interventions, the nurse has additional responsibilities relating to continued assessment, education, and documentation. What are these responsibilities?

Slide 49

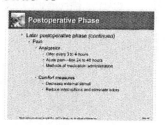

- Pain is one of the largest concerns and complaints of the postoperative period.
- Nurses have the responsibility to assess and medicate the patient as indicated.
- What are the pros and cons of intermittent injections, PCA pump, epidural, and oral analgesics?
- At what point in the postoperative period are each of the preceding methods of analgesic administration most commonly utilized?

Slide 50

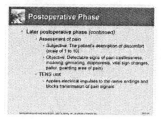

- Some patients might not vocalize feelings of pain. What nonverbal behaviors are indicative of pain?
- What should the nurse do if the patient's reports of pain levels are not consistent with the behaviors being observed?
- Review nonpharmacological methods to reduce/manage pain.

Slide 51

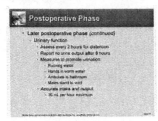

- Why is urinary function a postoperative concern?

- Discuss measures to promote urination.

- Fluid intake and output measurements continue for the first few days after surgery. When should the nurse become concerned about urinary function?

Slide 52

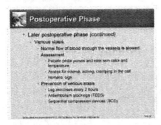

- The inactivity associated with surgical intervention promotes venous stasis. Venous stasis is the underlying cause of thrombus formation.

- What pharmacological therapies can be used to prevent thrombus formation?

- What signs and symptoms indicate the potential development of deep vein thrombosis?

- What are some nursing interventions that can reduce venous complications?

Slide 53

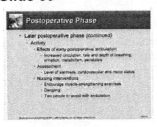

- What are safety interventions that are necessary in the early postoperative period as the patient begins to ambulate?

Slide 54

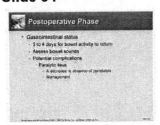

- Surgical manipulation and medications slow the normal peristaltic action of the bowel.

- What elements should be evaluated during the nursing assessment of the gastrointestinal system?

- What interventions might be required to manage gastrointestinal complications?

Slide 55

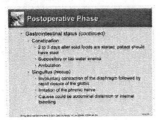

- What effect does narcotic administration have on bowel function?

Slide 56

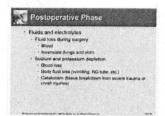

- The patient's reduced dietary intake, combined with the fluid and blood losses of surgery, can result in electrolyte imbalances.
- Surgery stressors and body responses to trauma compound the situation.

Slide 57

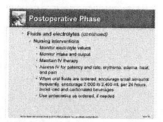

- What physiological and psychological cues might indicate the patient is ready to begin dietary intake?
- What process should be used to reintroduce fluids and solids into the patient's diet?
- Review laboratory studies that can be used to evaluate electrolyte balance in the postoperative period.

Slide 58

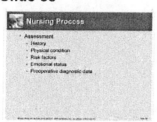

- What is the role of the LPN/LVN in relation to the nursing process and the surgical process?

Slide 59

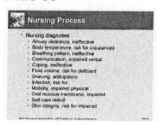

- Develop a nursing diagnosis focusing on common postoperative diagnoses.

Slide 60

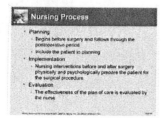

Christensen & Kockrow

Slide 61

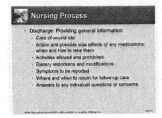

- Review the information needed by the patient prior to discharge.

- What setting is optimal for giving discharge teaching? What behaviors indicate a readiness to learn? Who should be included in the teaching session?

Slide 62

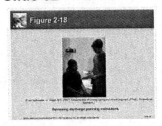

Adult Health Nursing, 6th ed.
Christensen & Kockrow

Mosby items and derived items © 2011, 2007 by Mosby, Inc., an affiliate of Elsevier Inc.
Some material was previously published.

Lesson Plan

3 Care of the Patient with an Integumentary Disorder

TEACHING FOCUS

In this chapter, the student will be introduced to the structure and function of the integumentary system. Next, the student will explore the nurse's role in the care of the patient's integumentary system, beginning with the general assessment and continuing to skin disorders, including viral, bacterial, fungal, inflammatory, and parasitic disorders. The student then will have the opportunity to learn the disorders associated with various appendages of the skin. Finally, the student will explore the care of the burn patient, beginning with the pathophysiology of a burn injury and continuing to the stages of burn care and the classification of a burn injury.

MATERIALS AND RESOURCES

- ☐ Computer/overhead projector (all lessons)
- ☐ White/black board and marker/chalk (all lessons)
- ☐ Photograph of the structures of the skin (Lesson 3.1)
- ☐ Small, soft ball or pillow that can be tossed around the room (Lesson 3.2)
- ☐ About a dozen sheets of easel-size paper (Lesson 3.2)
- ☐ Note cards labeled with clinical manifestations, treatment, or nursing interventions for scabies and pediculosis (Lesson 3.3)
- ☐ Blank nursing care form (Lesson 3.3)
- ☐ Blank note cards for each student (Lesson 3.3)
- ☐ Easel-size sheets, each with a figure outline and a brief description of the location of the body burned (Lesson 3.3)

LESSON CHECKLIST

Preparations for this lesson include:
- Lecture

KEY TERMS

alopecia (FAAHN p. 1330, AHN p. 94)
autograft (FAAHN p. 1336, AHN p. 100)
contracture (FAAHN p. 1334, AHN p. 98)
Curling's ulcer (FAAHN p. 1334, AHN p. 98)
debridement (FAAHN p. 1335, AHN p. 99)
eschar (FAAHN p. 1335, AHN p. 99)
excoriation (FAAHN p. 1308, AHN p. 72)
exudate (FAAHN p. 1305, AHN p. 69)
heterograft (xenograft) (FAAHN p. 1336, AHN p. 100)
homograft (allograft) (FAAHN p. 1336, AHN p. 100)
keloids (FAAHN p. 1326, AHN p. 90)
macules (FAAHN p. 1312, AHN p. 76)

nevi (FAAHN p. 1327, AHN p. 91)
papules (FAAHN p. 1315, AHN p. 79)
pediculosis (FAAHN p. 1323, AHN p. 87)
pruritus (FAAHN p. 1297, AHN p. 61)
pustulant vesicles (FAAHN p. 1312, AHN p. 76)
rule of nines (FAAHN p. 1332, AHN p. 96)
suppuration (FAAHN p. 1313, AHN p. 77)
urticaria (FAAHN p. 1317, AHN p. 81)
verruca (FAAHN p. 1327, AHN p. 91)
vesicle (FAAHN p. 1304, AHN p. 68)
wheals (FAAHN p. 1317, AHN p. 81)

ADDITIONAL RESOURCES

PPT Ch. 43, 1 through 80 FAAHN (Ch. 3, 1 through 80 AHN)
EILR IC images Ch. 43, 1 through 25 FAAHN (Ch. 3, 1 through 25 AHN)
EILR TB questions Ch. 43, 1 through 41 FAAHN (Ch. 3, 1 through 41 AHN)
EILR Open Book Quiz Ch. 43, 1 through 10 FAAHN (Ch. 3, 1 through 10 AHN)
ESLR Review Questions for the NCLEX® Examination Ch. 43, 43-01 through 43-10 FAAHN (Ch. 3, 03-01 through 03-10 AHN)

Legend

PPT
PowerPoint
Slides

EILR
EVOLVE Instructor
Learning Resources:
Image Collection, Test
Bank, Open Book Quizzes

ESLR
EVOLVE Student
Learning Resources:
Review Questions
for the NCLEX
Examination

SG
Study Guide

NCP CTQ
Nursing Care Plan
Critical Thinking
Question

Class Activities are indicated in ***bold italic***.

LESSON 3.1

PRETEST

1. A patient presents to the ambulatory care clinic with complaints of an "itchy rash." When preparing to examine the rash, the nurse should use what type of lighting?
   a. Fluorescent lighting
   b. Natural lighting
   c. A wood light
   d. A penlight

2. A patient of African-American ancestry having brown skin tones is hospitalized. The physician makes a diagnosis of anemia. What skin tones can be found during assessment to support this diagnosis?
   a. Ashen or gray
   b. Pale pink
   c. Yellow toned
   d. Ruddy

3. After suffering from a condition in which chronic pruritus and scratching occurred, which of the following might be an anticipated finding?
   a. Fissure development
   b. Scars
   c. Keloid scarring
   d. Lichenification

4. Education for the patient who has been prescribed Benadryl should include the following instructions:
   a. Do not operate heavy machinery while taking the medication.
   b. Avoid exposure to sunlight during the medication therapy.
   c. This medication can alter liver functioning.
   d. Discontinue use if excessive drying and peeling of skin occurs.

5. Drug therapy for the patient experiencing an outbreak of herpes simplex could include:
   a. Acyclovir.
   b. Vistaril.
   c. Atarax.
   d. Lidex.

6. The primary mode of transmission for herpes simplex is:
   a. airborne.
   b. skin-to-skin contact.
   c. contact with infected personal articles.
   d. reactivation of a dormant virus.

7. Upon removal of the thick crust associated with impetigo contagiosa, the skin will appear:
   a. dry and discolored.
   b. bruised and torn.
   c. red and smooth.
   d. moist and draining.

8. During the data collection interview, the patient states she has noticed a grouping of red and swollen areas with yellowed centers on her back. She reports they are painful. Based upon your knowledge you anticipate a diagnosis of:
    a. herpes zoster.
    b. carbuncles.
    c. felons.
    d. furuncles.

9. A patient diagnosed with tinea pedis is prescribed Burow's solution soaks. The patient asks how this medication will work. The following should be included in the teaching plan:
    a. Burow's solution has antimicrobial properties.
    b. This medication will reduce inflammation.
    c. Soaking in this medication will act as a skin emollient.
    d. Burow's solution has astringent characteristics.

10. After experiencing concerns with a growth on her neck, a patient seeks care. During the assessment, you document the growth as a firm, nodular lesion with a crusted top. Based upon your knowledge, you anticipate a diagnosis of:
    a. malignant melanoma.
    b. squamous cell carcinoma.
    c. basal cell carcinoma.
    d. keloids.

Answers:

1. b	2. c	3. d	4. a	5. a
6. b	7. c	8. b	9. d	10. b

BACKGROUND ASSESSMENT

Question: What factors influence the incidence of acne?

Answer: There are many misconceptions concerning acne. Acne is associated with an increase in oil production. Oil production is most increased during puberty. These oil glands become clogged, resulting in the characteristic lesions. Stress and heredity can also play a role. There is no scientific support for the impact of hygiene, sex, or chocolate on acne incidence.

Question: A patient is diagnosed with ringworm. The patient's mother is concerned and reports she that always ensures her daughter washes with soap and water after playing in the dirt or sandbox. She asks how the worms still infected the child. What response should be given by the nurse?

Answer: The misconceptions held by the patient's mother should be addressed and corrected. Ringworm is a fungal infection in which the lesions characteristically form a ring-like shape. Ringworm is not a parasitic infection. Playing in the dirt does not increase the risk factors for development of the disorder.

CRITICAL THINKING QUESTION

A female patient, age 15, is diagnosed with herpes simplex. She voices concerns about how she got this condition and how it will be "cured." What are the nursing interventions and education that should be provided this patient?

Guidelines: Herpes simplex is transmitted by skin-to-skin contact with infected individuals. The patient should also be advised how this condition will be managed and treated. There is no cure for herpes simplex. Treatment could include antiviral therapy with acyclovir (Zovirax). Analgesics may be indicated during the initial outbreak. The patient should be advised to keep the lesions clean and to practice good self-hygiene. Her education should also include avoidance of sexual contact during outbreak periods. She should be instructed to practice safe sex at all times.

Adult Health Nursing, 6th ed.
Christensen & Kockrow

OBJECTIVES	CONTENT	TEACHING RESOURCES
Discuss the primary functions of the integumentary system.	■ Overview of anatomy and physiology (FAAHN p. 1295, AHN p. 59) □ Functions of the skin (FAAHN p. 1295, AHN p. 59) – Protection (FAAHN p. 1296, AHN p. 60) – Temperature regulation (FAAHN p. 1296, AHN p. 60) – Vitamin D synthesis (FAAHN p. 1296, AHN p. 60)	PPT 1, 2, Ch. 43 FAAHN (Ch. 3 PPT 1, 2 AHN) EILR IC Ch. 43 image 1 FAAHN (Ch. 3 image 1 AHN) EILR TB Ch. 43 question 35 FAAHN (Ch. 3 question 35 AHN) EILR Open Book Quiz Ch. 43 question 1 FAAHN (Ch. 3 question 1 AHN) SG Protection, Ch. 43 p. 333 FAAHN (Ch. 3 p. 21 AHN) **BOOK RESOURCES** Box 43-1 Functions of the Skin (FAAHN p. 1295) (Box 3-1 AHN p. 59) ▶ Discuss how each of the functions of the skin takes place in the body. ▶ Discuss the effects on the body if any of the skin's functions do not occur or are impaired. *Class Activity **Divide the class into groups. Assign each group one of the skin's vital functions. Instruct each group to identify conditions in which the selected skin function is impaired.***
Describe the differences between the epidermis and the dermis.	□ Structure of the skin (FAAHN p. 1296, AHN p. 60) – Epidermis (FAAHN p. 1296, AHN p. 60) –Dermis (FAAHN p. 1297, AHN p. 61) – Subcutaneous layer (FAAHN p. 1297, AHN p. 61)	PPT 2, 3, Ch. 43 FAAHN (Ch. 3 PPT 2, 3 AHN) EILR TB Ch. 43 question 33 FAAHN (Ch. 3 question 33 AHN) EILR Open Book Quiz Ch. 43 question 2 FAAHN (Ch. 3 question 2 AHN) SG Structures of the Skin, Ch. 43 p. 333 FAAHN (Ch. 3 p. 21 AHN) **BOOK RESOURCES** Fig. 43-1 Structures of the skin (FAAHN p. 1296) (Fig. 3-1 AHN p. 60) ▶ Discuss differences between the layers of the epidermis. How are they structurally different? Do their functions differ as well? ▶ Discuss the physiological factors that influence the skin's color. Review the disease conditions that can impact skin color.

OBJECTIVES	CONTENT	TEACHING RESOURCES
		Class Activity Provide a photograph of the structures of the skin. Ask students to label the structures and layers.
Discuss the functions of the three major glands located in the skin.	☐ Appendages of the skin (FAAHN p. 1297, AHN p. 61) − Sudoriferous glands (FAAHN p. 1297, AHN p. 61) − Ceruminous glands (FAAHN p. 1297, AHN p. 61) − Sebaceous glands (FAAHN p. 1297, AHN p. 61) − Hair and nails (FAAHN p. 1297, AHN p. 61)	▨ PPT 5, Ch. 43 FAAHN (Ch. 3 PPT 5 AHN) 🖙 EILR TB Ch. 43 question 34 FAAHN (Ch. 3 question 34 AHN) 🖙 EILR Open Book Quiz Ch. 43 question 3 FAAHN (Ch. 3 question 3 AHN) 📖 SG Protection, Ch. 43 p. 333 FAAHN (Ch. 3 p. 21 AHN) ▸ Discuss the composition of hair and nails. In addition to the social importance of these appendages, what function do they serve for the human body? What is the psychosocial impact on a patient in which the hair or nails are impaired in function or appearance? ▸ Discuss what is secreted by the glands of the skin. How does age impact the level of secretion by the glands?
Discuss the general assessment of the skin.	■ Assessment of the skin (FAAHN p. 1297, AHN p. 61) ☐ Inspection and palpation (FAAHN p. 1297, AHN p. 61) − Assessment of dark skin (FAAHN p. 1303, AHN p. 67) ☐ Chief complaint (FAAHN p. 1303, AHN p. 67) ■ Psychosocial assessment (FAAHN p. 1304, AHN p. 68)	▨ PPT 6 through 12, Ch. 43 FAAHN (Ch. 3 PPT 6 through 12 AHN) 🖙 EILR TB Ch. 43 questions 6, 7, 26 FAAHN (Ch. 3 questions 6, 7, 26 AHN) 🖙 EILR Open Book Quiz Ch. 43 question 5 FAAHN (Ch. 3 question 5 AHN) 🖙 ESLR Review Questions for the NCLEX Examination Ch. 43 questions 1, 2 FAAHN (Ch. 3 questions 1, 2 AHN) 📖 SG Assessing Skin Disorders Ch. 43 p. 335 FAAHN (Ch. 3 p. 23 AHN) **BOOK RESOURCES** Table 43-1 Primary Skin Lesions (FAAHN pp. 1298-1303 (Table 3-1 AHN pp. 62-67) Cultural Considerations: Skin Care (FAAHN p. 1304) (AHN p. 68) ▸ Discuss the characteristics of each of the skin lesions. What characteristics are associated with abnormal skin lesions? ▸ Discuss the types of conditions associated with the skin lesions reviewed.

Adult Health Nursing, 6th ed.
Christensen & Kockrow

OBJECTIVES	CONTENT	TEACHING RESOURCES
		▶ Discuss the observation of skin color. Where should a baseline skin color assessment be located?
		▶ Discuss the data collection process for a chief integumentary complaint.
		***Class Activity** Ask students to select a partner. Identify one as the patient and the other as the nurse. Instruct each pair to role-play the data collection phase of the patient interview for someone experiencing an integumentary disorder.*

3.1 Homework/Assignments:

3.1 Instructor's Notes/Student Feedback:

LESSON 3.2

CRITICAL THINKING QUESTION

A patient presents to the clinic with complaints of a skin rash and itching. The patient reports it just "suddenly appeared." An assessment of the rash reveals numerous reddened papules along her arms and torso. After an initial diagnosis of contact dermatitis, the physician prescribes a corticosteroid cream and oral antihistamines. Upon receipt of the prescriptions, the patient voices concerns. She states, "I don't see why these medications have been prescribed for my condition. What good will these antihistamines do? It's not as if I have a cold." What information should be provided to her? What are potential causes of the dermatitis? What can she do to pinpoint the cause of the skin eruptions?

Guidelines: Contact dermatitis can be caused by a variety of factors. In an attempt to identify the culprit, the patient should be asked to recall the previous 48 hours. Information should include soaps and detergents used, any change in personal hygiene items, travel, or exposure to plants and flowers. The pharmacological treatment plan is appropriate. Corticosteroids are used to reduce inflammation, and antihistamines reduce the histamine release and aid in reducing symptoms. The use of antihistamines is not limited to cold symptoms.

OBJECTIVES	CONTENT	TEACHING RESOURCES
Discuss the viral disorders of the skin.	■ Viral disorders of the skin (FAAHN p. 1304, AHN p. 68) ☐ Herpes simplex (FAAHN p. 1304, AHN p. 68) – Etiology and pathophysiology (FAAHN p. 1304, AHN p. 68) – Clinical manifestations (FAAHN p. 1304, AHN p. 68) – Assessment (FAAHN p. 1305, AHN p. 69) – Diagnostic tests (FAAHN p. 1305, AHN p. 69) – Medical management (FAAHN p. 1305, AHN p. 69) – Nursing interventions and patient teaching (FAAHN p. 1305, AHN p. 69) – Prognosis (FAAHN p. 1305, AHN p. 69) ☐ Herpes zoster (shingles) (FAAHN p. 1308, AHN p. 72) – Etiology and pathophysiology (FAAHN p. 1308, AHN p. 72) – Clinical manifestations (FAAHN p. 1308, AHN p. 72) – Assessment (FAAHN p. 1308, AHN p. 72)	🖼 PPT 13 through 23, Ch. 43 FAAHN (Ch. 3 PPT 13 through 23 AHN) 📧 EILR IC Ch. 43 images 2 through 5 FAAHN (Ch. 3 images 2 through 5 AHN) 📧 EILR TB Ch. 43 questions 2, 3, 20, 31 FAAHN (Ch. 3 questions 2, 3, 20, 31 AHN) 📧 EILR Open Book Quiz Ch. 43 question 6 FAAHN (Ch. 3 question 6 AHN) 📧 ESLR Review Questions for the NCLEX Examination Ch. 43 questions 3, 4 FAAHN (Ch. 3 questions 3, 4 AHN) 📙 SG Viral Disorders of the Skin, Ch. 43 p. 336 FAAHN (Ch. 3 p. 24 AHN) **BOOK RESOURCES** Fig. 43-2 Herpex simplex (FAAHN p. 1305) (Fig. 3-2 AHN p. 69) Table 43-2 Medications for the integumentary system (FAAHN pp. 1306-1307) (Table 3-2 AHN pp. 70-71) Fig. 43-3 Herpes zoster (FAAHN p. 1308) (Fig. 3-3 AHN p. 72) Nursing Care Plan 43-1 The Patient with Herpes Zoster (FAAHN p. 1309) (NCP 3-1 AHN p. 73)

OBJECTIVES	CONTENT	TEACHING RESOURCES
	– Diagnostic tests (FAAHN p. 1308, AHN p. 72) – Medical management (FAAHN p. 1308, AHN p. 72) ☐ Pityriasis rosea (FAAHN p. 1310, AHN p. 74) – Etiology and pathophysiology (FAAHN p. 1310, AHN p. 74) – Clinical manifestations (FAAHN p. 1310, AHN p. 74) – Assessment (FAAHN p. 1310, AHN p. 74) – Diagnostic tests (FAAHN p. 1310, AHN p. 74) – Medical management (FAAHN p. 1310, AHN p. 74) – Nursing interventions (FAAHN p. 1310, AHN p. 74) – Prognosis (FAAHN p. 1310, AHN p. 74)	Fig. 43-4 Pityriasis rosea herald patch (FAAHN p. 1310) (Fig. 3-4 AHN p. 74) ▶ Discuss how viral disorders differ from bacterial skin disorders; include treatment concerns and etiology. ▶ Discuss the characteristic appearance of each of the viral infections. ▶ Discuss the medical and nursing management of each of the viral infection conditions. *Class Activity Pass a small, soft ball or pillow around the room. As it goes to each student, ask questions about the viral skin infections. Once a student answers the question, he/she passes the object on to another and the process continues.*
Discuss the bacterial, fungal, and inflammatory disorders of the skin.	■ Bacterial disorders of the skin (FAAHN p. 1310, AHN p. 74) ☐ Cellulitis (FAAHN p. 1310, AHN p. 74) – Etiology and pathophysiology (FAAHN p. 1310, AHN p. 74) – Clinical manifestations (FAAHN p. 1311, AHN p. 75) – Assessment (FAAHN p. 1311, AHN p. 75) – Diagnostic tests (FAAHN p. 1311, AHN p. 75) – Medical management (FAAHN p. 1311, AHN p. 75) – Nursing interventions and patient teaching (FAAHN p. 1311, AHN p. 75) – Prognosis (FAAHN p. 1311, AHN p. 75) ☐ Impetigo contagiosa (FAAHN p. 1311, AHN p. 75)	PPT 24 through 56, Ch. 43 FAAHN (Ch. 3 PPT 24 through 56 AHN) EILR IC Ch. 43 images 6 through 11 FAAHN (Ch. 3 images 6 through 11 AHN) EILR TB Ch. 43 questions 1, 4 through 9, 17, 21, 22, 27, 29, 30, 37 FAAHN (Ch. 3 questions 1, 4 through 9, 17, 21, 22, 27, 29, 30, 37 AHN) EILR Open Book Quiz Ch. 43 questions 7 through 9 FAAHN (Ch. 3 questions 7 through 9, AHN) ESLR Review Questions for the NCLEX Examination Ch. 43 questions 5 through 10 FAAHN (Ch. 3 questions 5 through 10 AHN) SG Bacterial, Fungal, and Inflammatory Disorders of the Skin Ch. 43 p. 336 FAAHN (Ch. 3 p. 24 AHN) **BOOK RESOURCES** Fig. 43-5 Impetigo and herpes simplex (FAAHN p. 1312) (Fig. 3-5 AHN p. 76)

OBJECTIVES	CONTENT	TEACHING RESOURCES
	– Etiology and pathophysiology (FAAHN p. 1311, AHN p. 75)	Fig. 43-6 Furuncle of the forearm (FAAHN p. 1313) (Fig. 3-6 AHN p. 77)
	– Clinical manifestations (FAAHN p. 1312, AHN p. 76)	Fig. 43-7 Tinea capitis (FAAHN p. 1314) (Fig. 3-7 AHN p. 78)
	– Assessment (FAAHN p. 1312, AHN p. 76)	Fig. 43-8 Tinea corporis (FAAHN p. 1314) (Fig. 3-8 AHN p. 79)
	– Diagnostic tests (FAAHN p. 1312, AHN p. 76)	Fig. 43-9 Acne vulgaris (FAAHN p. 1319) (Fig. 3-9 AHN p. 83)
	– Medical management (FAAHN p. 1312, AHN p. 76)	Health Promotion Healthy Skin (FAAHN p. 1320) (AHN p. 84)
	– Nursing interventions and patient teaching (FAAHN p. 1312, AHN p. 76)	Fig. 43-10 Psoriasis (FAAHN p. 1320) (Fig. 3-10 AHN p. 84)
	– Prognosis (FAAHN p. 1312, AHN p. 76)	Fig. 43-11 Systemic lupus erythematosus flare (FAAHN p. 1321) (Fig. 3-11 AHN p. 85)
	☐ Folliculitis, furuncles, carbuncles, and felons (FAAHN p. 1313, AHN p. 77)	Box 43-2 Pathogenic Conditions and Clinical Manifestations in Body Systems of Persons with Systemic Lupus Erythematosus (FAAHN p. 1322) (Box 3-2 AHN p. 86)
	– Etiology and pathophysiology (FAAHN p. 1313, AHN p. 77)	Box 43-3 Diagnostic Tests for Systemic Lupus Erythematosus (FAAHN p. 1322) (Box 3-3 AHN p. 86)
	– Clinical manifestations (FAAHN p. 1313, AHN p. 77)	
	– Assessment (FAAHN p. 1313, AHN p. 77)	Nursing Care Plan 43-2 The Patient with Systemic Lupus Erythematosus (FAAHN p. 1324) (NCP 3-2 AHN p. 88)
	– Diagnostic tests (FAAHN p. 1313, AHN p. 77)	▶ Discuss the differences in the management of bacterial, fungal, and inflammatory integumentary conditions.
	– Medical management (FAAHN p. 1313, AHN p. 77)	▶ Discuss the characteristic appearance of each of the bacterial infections of the skin.
	– Nursing interventions and patient teaching (FAAHN p. 1313, AHN p. 77)	▶ Discuss the characteristic appearance of each of the inflammatory and fungal conditions of the skin.
	– Prognosis (FAAHN p. 1313, AHN p. 77)	▶ Discuss the transmission of each of the bacterial, inflammatory, and fungal conditions of the skin.
	■ Fungal infections of the skin (FAAHN p. 1314, AHN p. 78)	▶ Discuss the nursing and medical management of each of the bacterial, inflammatory, and fungal conditions of the skin.
	– Etiology and pathophysiology (FAAHN p. 1314, AHN p. 78)	
	– Clinical manifestations (FAAHN p. 1314, AHN p. 78)	▶ Discuss patient teaching that should be provided by the nurse for the patients experiencing each of the bacterial, inflammatory, and fungal conditions of the skin.
	– Assessment (FAAHN p. 1314, AHN p. 78)	

Christensen & Kockrow

OBJECTIVES	CONTENT	TEACHING RESOURCES
	– Diagnostic tests (FAAHN p. 1314, AHN p. 78) – Medical management (FAAHN p. 1314, AHN p. 78) – Nursing interventions and patient teaching (FAAHN p. 1314, AHN p. 78) – Prognosis (FAAHN p. 1315, AHN p. 79) ☐ Inflammatory disorders of the skin (FAAHN p. 1315, AHN p. 79) ☐ Contact dermatitis (FAAHN p. 1315, AHN p. 79) – Etiology and pathophysiology (FAAHN p. 1315, AHN p. 79) – Clinical manifestations (FAAHN p. 1315, AHN p. 79) – Assessment (FAAHN p. 1315, AHN p. 79) – Diagnostic tests (FAAHN p. 1315, AHN p. 79) – Medical management (FAAHN p. 1315, AHN p. 79) – Nursing interventions and patient teaching (FAAHN p. 1315, AHN p. 79) – Prognosis (FAAHN p. 1316, AHN p. 80) ☐ Dermatitis venenata, exfoliative dermatitis, and dermatitis medicamentosa (FAAHN p. 1316, AHN p. 80) – Etiology and pathophysiology (FAAHN p. 1316, AHN p. 80) – Clinical manifestations (FAAHN p. 1316, AHN p. 80) – Assessment (FAAHN p. 1316, AHN p. 80) – Diagnostic tests (FAAHN p. 1316, AHN p. 80)	▸ Discuss the pathogenic occurrences and clinical manifestations in each of the body systems in a patient diagnosed with lupus. *Class Activity Place easel chart paper around the room. Provide one or two sheets per integumentary condition. Divide students into small groups; instruct each group to discuss each condition and list populations who are at risk for each of the disorders.* *Class Activity Divide students into small groups. Ask each group to develop an elimination diet that might be used for a patient with a pending diagnosis of eczema. How would this diet differ for a child?*

OBJECTIVES	CONTENT	TEACHING RESOURCES

	– Medical management (FAAHN p. 1316, AHN p. 80)
	
	    – Nursing interventions and patient teaching (FAAHN p. 1316, AHN p. 80)
	
	    – Prognosis (FAAHN p. 1317, AHN p. 81)
	
	☐ Urticaria (FAAHN p. 1317, AHN p. 81)
	
	    – Etiology and pathophysiology (FAAHN p. 1317, AHN p. 81)
	
	    – Clinical manifestations (FAAHN p. 1317, AHN p. 81)
	
	    – Assessment (FAAHN p. 1317, AHN p. 81)
	
	    – Diagnostic tests (FAAHN p. 1317, AHN p. 81)
	
	    – Medical management (FAAHN p. 1317, AHN p. 81)
	
	    – Nursing interventions and patient teaching (FAAHN p. 1317, AHN p. 81)
	
	    – Prognosis (FAAHN p. 1317, AHN p. 81)
	
	☐ Angioedema (FAAHN p. 1317, AHN p. 81)
	
	    – Etiology and pathophysiology (FAAHN p. 1317, AHN p. 81)
	
	    – Assessment (FAAHN p. 1317, AHN p. 81)
	
	    – Diagnostic tests (FAAHN p. 1317, AHN p. 81)
	
	    – Medical management (FAAHN p. 1317, AHN p. 81)
	
	    – Nursing interventions and patient teaching (FAAHN p. 1318, AHN p. 82)
	
	    – Prognosis (FAAHN p. 1318, AHN p. 82)
	
	☐ Eczema (atopic dermatitis) (FAAHN p. 1318, AHN p. 82)	

Adult Health Nursing, 6th ed.

Christensen & Kockrow

OBJECTIVES	CONTENT	TEACHING RESOURCES
	– Etiology and pathophysiology (FAAHN p. 1318, AHN p. 82)	
	– Clinical manifestations (FAAHN p. 1318, AHN p. 82)	
	– Assessment (FAAHN p. 1318, AHN p. 82)	
	– Diagnostic tests (FAAHN p. 1318, AHN p. 82)	
	– Medical management (FAAHN p. 1318, AHN p. 82)	
	– Nursing interventions and patient teaching (FAAHN p. 1318, AHN p. 82)	
	☐ Acne vulgaris (FAAHN p. 1319, AHN p. 83)	
	– Etiology and pathophysiology (FAAHN p. 1319, AHN p. 83)	
	– Clinical manifestations (FAAHN p. 1319, AHN p. 83)	
	– Assessment (FAAHN p. 1319, AHN p. 83)	
	– Diagnostic tests (FAAHN p. 1319, AHN p. 83)	
	– Medical management (FAAHN p. 1319, AHN p. 83)	
	– Nursing interventions and patient teaching (FAAHN p. 1319, AHN p. 83)	
	– Prognosis (FAAHN p. 1320, AHN p. 84)	
	☐ Psoriasis (FAAHN p. 1320, AHN p. 84)	
	– Etiology and pathophysiology (FAAHN p. 1320, AHN p. 84)	
	– Clinical manifestations (FAAHN p. 1320, AHN p. 84)	
	– Assessment (FAAHN p. 1320, AHN p. 84)	
	– Diagnostic tests (FAAHN p. 1321, AHN p. 85)	

OBJECTIVES	CONTENT	TEACHING RESOURCES
	— Medical management (FAAHN p. 1321, AHN p. 85)	
	— Nursing interventions and patient teaching (FAAHN p. 1321, AHN p. 85)	
	— Prognosis (FAAHN p. 1321, AHN p. 85)	
	☐ Systemic lupus erythematosus (FAAHN p. 1321, AHN p. 85)	
	— Etiology and pathophysiology (FAAHN p. 1321, AHN p. 85)	
	— Clinical manifestations (FAAHN p. 1322, AHN p. 86)	
	— Diagnostic tests (FAAHN p. 1322, AHN p. 86)	
	— Medical management (FAAHN p. 1323, AHN p. 87)	
	— Nursing interventions and patient teaching (FAAHN p. 1323, AHN p. 87)	
	— Prognosis (FAAHN p. 1323, AHN p. 87)	

3.2 Homework/Assignments:

3.2 Instructor's Notes/Student Feedback:

Adult Health Nursing, 6th ed.

Christensen & Kockrow

LESSON 3.3

CRITICAL THINKING QUESTION

What elements must be included in the teaching plan for the mother of a child diagnosed with head lice?

Guidelines: The diagnosis of a parasitic infection in a family can be traumatic. There is often a social stigma concerning the hygiene of families in these situations. The cost of effective treatment can be a concern. The family must be educated concerning the mode of transmission, and the treatment plan and needed follow-up must be reviewed. The treatment plan needs to include availability of resources not only for the primary patient but also for all other members in the household and close contacts. The home environment will also require cleaning and treatment. Special treatment is required for toys belonging to the child.

OBJECTIVES	CONTENT	TEACHING RESOURCES
Identify the parasitic disorders of the skin.	■ Parasitic diseases of the skin (FAAHN p. 1323, AHN p. 87) ☐ Pediculosis (FAAHN p. 1323, AHN p. 87) – Etiology and pathophysiology (FAAHN p. 1323, AHN p. 87) – Clinical manifestations (FAAHN p. 1325, AHN p. 89) – Assessment (FAAHN p. 1325, AHN p. 89) – Diagnostic tests (FAAHN p. 1325, AHN p. 89) – Medical management (FAAHN p. 1325, AHN p. 89) – Nursing interventions and patient teaching (FAAHN p. 1325, AHN p. 89) – Prognosis (FAAHN p. 1325, AHN p. 89) ☐ Scabies (FAAHN p. 1325, AHN p. 89) – Etiology and pathophysiology (FAAHN p. 1325, AHN p. 89) – Clinical manifestations (FAAHN p. 1325, AHN p. 89) – Assessment (FAAHN p. 1326, AHN p. 90) – Diagnostic tests (FAAHN p. 1326, AHN p. 90)	▨ PPT 57 through 62, Ch. 43 FAAHN (Ch. 3 PPT 57 through 62 AHN) 🖉 EILR IC Ch. 43 images 12 through 14 FAAHN (Ch. 3 images 12 through 14 AHN) 🖉 EILR TB Ch. 43 questions 32, 38 FAAHN (Ch. 3 questions 32, 38 AHN) 📖 SG Parasites, Ch. 43 p. 337 FAAHN (Ch. 3 p. 25 AHN) **BOOK RESOURCES** Fig. 43-12 Eggs of pediculus attached to shafts of hair (FAAHN p. 1325) (Fig. 3-12 AHN p. 89) Fig. 43-13 Lice have six legs and are wingless (FAAHN p. 1325) (Fig. 3-13 AHN p. 89) Fig. 43-14 Scabies (FAAHN p. 1325) (Fig. 3-14 AHN p. 89) ▸ Discuss the transmission of parasitic skin disorders. ▸ Discuss populations at risk for parasitic skin disorders. What measures can be taken by members of the at-risk populations to reduce the possibility of infestation? ▸ Discuss the clinical manifestations of parasitic skin disorders. ▸ Discuss the psychosocial implications that can be encountered by the patient experiencing a parasitic skin disorder. *Class Activity Distribute note cards to the class. The cards are divided into three groups. The cards are labeled as clinical*

Adult Health Nursing, 6th ed.

Christensen & Kockrow

OBJECTIVES	CONTENT	TEACHING RESOURCES
	– Medical management (FAAHN p. 1326, AHN p. 90) – Nursing interventions and patient teaching (FAAHN0 p. 1326, AHN p. 90) – Prognosis (FAAHN p. 1326, AHN p. 90)	*manifestations, treatment, or nursing interventions for scabies and pediculosis. Each student is given a card to complete. After a brief time, the students are to group by disease process and share information.*
Describe the common tumors of the skin.	■ Tumors of the skin (FAAHN p. 1326, AHN p. 90) – Etiology, pathophysiology, and clinical manifestations (FAAHN p. 1326, AHN p. 90) – Assessment (FAAHN p. 1326, AHN p. 90) – Diagnostic tests (FAAHN p. 1326, AHN p. 90) – Medical management (FAAHN p. 1326, AHN p. 90) – Nursing interventions and patient teaching (FAAHN p. 1326, AHN p. 90) ☐ Keloids (FAAHN p. 1326, AHN p. 90) ☐ Angiomas (FAAHN p. 1327, AHN p. 91) ☐ Verruca (wart) (FAAHN p. 1327, AHN p. 91) ☐ Nevi (moles) (FAAHN p. 1327, AHN p. 91) ☐ Basal cell carcinoma (FAAHN p. 1327, AHN p. 91) ☐ Squamous cell carcinoma (FAAHN p. 1327, AHN p. 91) ☐ Malignant melanoma (FAAHN p. 1328, AHN p. 92) – Etiology and pathophysiology (FAAHN p. 1328, AHN p. 92) – Clinical manifestations (FAAHN p. 1328, AHN p. 92) – Assessment (FAAHN p. 1329, AHN p. 93)	PPT 63 through 70, Ch. 43 FAAHN (Ch. 3 PPT 63 through 70 AHN) EILR IC Ch. 43 images 15 through 18 FAAHN (Ch. 3 images 15 through 18 AHN) EILR TB Ch. 43 questions 9, 25, 28, 39 FAAHN (Ch. 3 questions 9, 25, 28, 39 AHN) SG Tumors, Ch. 43 p. 337 FAAHN (Ch. 3 p. 25 AHN) **BOOK RESOURCES** Fig. 43-15 Keloids (FAAHN p. 1327) (Fig. 3-15 AHN p. 91) Fig. 43-16 Basal cell carcinoma (FAAHN p. 1327) (Fig. 3-16 AHN p. 91) Fig. 43-17 Squamous cell carcinoma (FAAHN p. 1327) (Fig. 3-17 AHN p. 91) Evidence-Based Practice: Skin Cancer Prevention (FAAHN p. 1328) (AHN p. 92) Fig. 43-18 The ABCDs of melanoma (FAAHN p. 1329) (Fig. 3-18 AHN p. 93) ▸ Discuss the clinical manifestations of each type of common skin tumor. How do the prognoses differ among the types of skin malignancies? ▸ Discuss risk factors for the development of malignant skin conditions. ▸ Discuss behaviors that aid in the prevention of skin cancer development. *Class Activity Post a blank care plan form on the board for a nursing diagnosis related to an integumentary disorder. As a class, develop a nursing care plan for the patient diagnosed with a skin disorder.*

Mosby items and derived items © 2011 by Mosby, Inc., an affiliate of Elsevier Inc.
Some material was previously published.

Christensen & Kockrow

OBJECTIVES	CONTENT	TEACHING RESOURCES
	– Diagnostic tests (FAAHN p. 1329, AHN p. 93) – Medical management (FAAHN p. 1329, AHN p. 93) – Nursing interventions and patient teaching (FAAHN p. 1329, AHN p. 93) – Prognosis (FAAHN p. 1329, AHN p. 93)	
Identify the disorders associated with the appendages of the skin.	■ Disorders of the appendages (FAAHN p. 1330, AHN p. 94) ☐ Alopecia (FAAHN p. 1330, AHN p. 94) ☐ Hypertrichosis (hirsutism) (FAAHN p. 1330, AHN p. 94) ☐ Hypotrichosis (FAAHN p. 1330, AHN p. 94) ☐ Paronychia (FAAHN p. 1330, AHN p. 94)	PPT 71, 72, Ch. 43 FAAHN (Ch. 3 PPT 71, 72 AHN) SG Disorders of the Appendages, Ch. 43 p. 338 FAAHN (Ch. 3 p. 26 AHN) ▸ Discuss the appearances of disorders of the skin appendages. ▸ Discuss the psychosocial considerations when caring for a patient having disorders of the appendages. *Class Activity Distribute a note card to each student. Ask each to record anticipated feelings when faced with a disorder involving an appendage of the skin.*
State the pathophysiology involved in a burn injury.	☐ Burns (FAAHN p. 1330, AHN p. 94) – Etiology and pathophysiology (FAAHN p. 1330, AHN p. 94)	PPT 73, Ch. 43 FAAHN (Ch. 3 PPT 73 AHN) EILR TB Ch. 43 questions 10, 12, 14, 19 FAAHN (Ch. 3 questions 10, 12, 14, 19 AHN) SG Explanation of Burn Injury, Ch. 43 p. 339 FAAHN (Ch. 3 p. 27 AHN) **BOOK RESOURCES** Safety Alert! Prevention of Burns (FAAHN p. 1330) (AHN p. 94) Table 43-3 Causes and Factors Determining Depth of Burn Injury (FAAHN p. 1331) (Table 3-3 AHN p. 95) ▸ Discuss types of burns that may occur. ▸ Discuss the physiological process that takes place in the body after a burn. What are the most important nursing functions occurring during each of these stages?

ELSEVIER

OBJECTIVES	CONTENT	TEACHING RESOURCES
		Class Activity Ask each student to identify the types of burns that a patient can experience.
Identify the methods used to classify the extent of a burn injury.	– Assessment (FAAHN p. 1331, AHN p. 95)	PPT 74, 75, Ch. 43 FAAHN (Ch. 3 PPT 74, 75AHN)
		EILR IC Ch. 43 images 10 through 22 FAAHN (Ch. 3 images 10 through 22 AHN)
		SG Rule of Nines, Ch. 43 p. 339 FAAHN (Ch. 3 p. 27 AHN)
		BOOK RESOURCES
		Table 43-3 Causes and Factors Determining Depth of Burn Injury (FAAHN p. 1331) (Table 3-3 AHN p. 95)
		Fig. 43-19 Classification of burn depth (FAAHN p. 1332) (Fig. 3-19 AHN p. 96)
		Fig. 43-20 Superficial partial-thickness injury (FAAHN p. 1332) (Fig. 3-20 AHN p. 96)
		Fig. 43-21 Full-thickness thermal injury (FAAHN p. 1332) (Fig. 3-21 AHN p. 96)
		Fig. 43-22 Rule of nines (FAAHN p. 1332) (Fig. 3-22 AHN p. 96)
		Box 43-4 Classification of Severity of Burns (FAAHN p. 1333) (Box 3-4 AHN p. 97)
		▸ Discuss the differing prognosis for superficial, partial thickness, and full-thickness burns.
		▸ Discuss the differences between estimating the amount of body tissue involved for adults and children. Why are differing methods used depending upon the age of the patient?
		Class Activity Post multiple figure outlines around the room. Each figure should have a brief description of the location of the body burned. Assign the students the task of rotating to each station. At each station, ask the groups of students to estimate the percent of body area burned.

OBJECTIVES	CONTENT	TEACHING RESOURCES
Discuss the stages of burn care with appropriate nursing interventions.	☐ Burns (FAAHN p. 1330, AHN p. 94) – Etiology and pathophysiology (FAAHN p. 1330, AHN p. 94) – Clinical manifestations (FAAHN p. 1331, AHN p. 95) – Assessment (FAAHN p. 1331, AHN p. 95) – Diagnostic tests (FAAHN p. 1333, AHN p. 97) – Medical management (FAAHN p. 1333, AHN p. 97) – Patient teaching (FAAHN p. 1338, AHN p. 102) – Evaluation (FAAHN p. 1338, AHN p. 102) – Prognosis (FAAHN p. 1339, AHN p. 103)	▣ PPT 76 through 79, Ch. 43 FAAHN (Ch. 3 PPT 76 through 79 AHN) 🖅 EILR IC Ch. 43 images 23 through 25 FAAHN (Ch. 3 images 23 through 25 AHN) 🖅 EILR TB Ch. 43 questions 13, 15, 16, 23, 24, 36, 40, 41 FAAHN (Ch. 3 questions 13, 15, 16, 23, 24, 36, 40, 41 AHN) ▣ SG Stages of Burns, Ch. 43 p. 339 FAAHN (Ch. 3 p. 27 AHN) **BOOK RESOURCES** Box 43-5 Indications for Fluid Resusitation (FAAHN p. 1334) Box 3-5 AHN p. 98) Fig. 43-23 Endotrachael intubation for patient with severe edema 5 hours after a burn injury (FAAHN p. 1334) (Box 3-23 AHN p. 98) Box 43-6 Nursing Diagnoses for the Emergent Phase of Burns (FAAHN p. 1334) (Box 3-6 AHN p. 98) Fig. 43-24 Postburn *Pseudomonas* infection (FAAHN p. 1335) (Fig. 3-24 AHN p. 99) Fig. 43-25 Grid escharotomy used to alleviate circulatory and pulmonary constriction (FAAHN p. 1335) (Fig. 3-25 AHN p. 99) Patient Teaching: Skin Grafts (FAAHN p. 1336) (AHN p. 100) Table 43-4 Medications for burn therapy skin grafts (FAAHN p. 1337) (Table 3-4 AHN p. 101) Box 43-7 Nursing Diagnoses for the Acute Phase of Burns (FAAHN p. 1338) (Box 3-7 AHN p. 102) Box 43-8 Nursing Diagnoses for the Rehabilitation Phase of Burns (FAAHN p. 1338) (Box 3-8 AHN p. 102) Home Care Considerations: Burns (FAAHN p. 1338) (AHN p. 102) ▸ Discuss signs and symptoms of each major complication that can occur in a patient who has suffered from a burn. ▸ Discuss the management of burn complications.

OBJECTIVES	CONTENT	TEACHING RESOURCES
		Class Activity Using the descriptions listed in the above activity, ask each member of the class to select a complication associated with that person's burn. After the complication is selected, assign a nursing care plan that will require a modification of the nursing diagnoses, interventions, and rationale.
Discuss how to use the nursing process in caring for patients with skin disorders.	☐ Nursing process *for the patient with an integumentary disorder* (FAAHN p. 1339, AHN p. 103) — Assessment (FAAHN p. 1339, AHN p. 103) — Nursing diagnosis (FAAHN p. 1339, AHN p. 103) — Expected outcomes and planning (FAAHN p. 1340, AHN p. 104) — Implementation (FAAHN p. 1340, AHN p. 104) — Evaluation (FAAHN p. 1341, AHN p. 105)	PPT 80 Ch. 43 FAAHN (Ch. 3 PPT 80 AHN) EILR TB Ch. 43 question 6 FAAHN (Ch. 3 question 6 AHN) SG Stages of Burns Ch. 43 p. 339 FAAHN (Ch. 3 p. 27 AHN) **BOOK RESOURCES** Life Span Considerations, Older Adults: Effects of Aging on the Integumentary System (FAAHN p. 1339) (AHN p. 103) Home Care Considerations: Home Care Guidelines for Baths and Soaks (FAAHN p. 1340) (AHN p. 104) Complementary and Alternative Therapies: Integumentary Disorders (FAAHN p. 1341) (AHN p. 105) ▸ Discuss the role of the LPN/LVN in the care of an integumentary disorder. ▸ Discuss the elements of a productive patient interview. What types of questions should be avoided? What type of setting is most appropriate? *Class Activity Assign each student a nursing care plan to complete for the integumentary disorder of his/her choice. The plan should include a minimum of two nursing diagnoses. Each diagnosis should reflect at least three nursing interventions. Rationale should be included for each intervention.*

Identify general nursing interventions for the patient with a skin disorder.	☐ Nursing process *for the patient with an integumentary disorder* (FAAHN p. 1339, AHN p. 103) – Assessment (FAAHN p. 1339, AHN p. 103) – Nursing diagnosis (FAAHN p. 1339, AHN p. 103) – Expected outcomes and planning (FAAHN p. 1340, AHN p. 104) – Implementation (FAAHN p. 1340, AHN p. 104) – Evaluation (FAAHN p. 1341, AHN p. 105)	PPT 80, Ch. 43 FAAHN (Ch. 3 PPT 80 AHN) SG Stages of Burns Ch. 43 p. 339 FAAHN (Ch. 3 p. 27 AHN) **BOOK RESOURCES** Life Span Considerations, Older Adults: Effects of Aging on the Integumentary Ssytem (FAAHN p. 1339) (AHN p. 103) Home Care Considerations: Home Care Guidelines for Baths and Soaks (FAAHN p. 1340) (AHN p. 104) Complementary and Alternative Therapies: Integumentary Disorders (FAAHN p. 1341) (AHN p. 105)
Performance Evaluation		EILR TB Ch. 43 questions 1 through 41 FAAHN (Ch. 3 questions 1 through 41 AHN) EILR Open Book Quiz Ch. 43 questions 1 through 10 FAAHN (Ch. 3 questions 1 through 10 AHN) ESLR Review Questions for the NCLEX Examination Ch. 43 questions 1 through 10 FAAHN (Ch. 3 questions 1 through 10 AHN) SG Ch. 43 pp. 21 through 30 FAAHN (Ch. 3 pp. 333 through 342 AHN) **BOOK RESOURCES** Nursing Care Plan 43-1 The Patient with Herpes Zoster (FAAHN p. 1309) (NCP 3-1 AHN p. 73) NCP CTQ 1, 2 (FAAHN p. 1306) (AHN p. 73) Review Questions for the NCLEX Examination Ch. 43 questions 1 through 32 FAAHN (Ch. 3 questions 1 through 32 AHN)

3.3 Homework/Assignments:

3.3 Instructor's Notes/Student Feedback:

Mosby items and derived items © 2011 by Mosby, Inc., an affiliate of Elsevier Inc.
Some material was previously published.

Slide 1

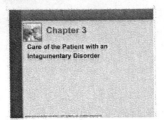

Slide 2

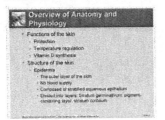

- The skin is vital to life. Its protective functions are needed for survival.

- The skin serves as the body's barrier from the outside. Protection is given from infection and injury.

- By assisting in thermoregulation, the skin also acts to maintain homeostasis within the body.

- As the skin serves its protective functions, it also receives messages via touch, pressure, and temperature. These messages are then relayed to the central nervous system for interpretation and action.

- Cholesterol compounds within the skin are changed to vitamin D with light exposure.

Slide 3

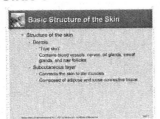

Slide 4

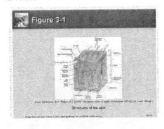

- This figure outlines the composition and locations of the skin structures.

- Placement of the skin's appendages and glands in relation to the skin's layers should be noted.

Christensen & Kockrow

Slide 5

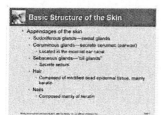

- There are approximately 3 million sweat glands in the body. They function to cool the body by excreting sweat.

- Sweat is composed of water, salts, urea, uric acid, ammonia, sugar, lactic acid, and ascorbic acid.

- Ceruminous glands secrete cerumen (earwax), which provides protection to the ears by keeping potential foreign bodies out.

- Sebaceous glands secrete oil. These oils provide lubrication and inhibit the growth of bacteria.

- What is the potential impact of impaired functioning of these glands?

- What is the function of the skin's glands in relation to patient age?

Slide 6

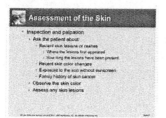

- The skin assessment aids in providing a clinical picture of the patient's health status.

- The nurse should question the patient to obtain a detailed health history.

- Review the elements needed for a successful patient interview and examination.

- What senses will the nurse employ to complete the skin assessment?

- The senses of touch, sight, and smell should be combined with palpation and inspection to complete a thorough assessment.

Slide 7

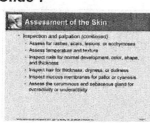

- At what point during the interaction should the skin assessment take place?

Slide 8

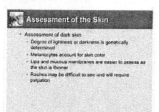

- The skin structures of the darker skinned individual are no different from those of a person with a fairer complexion.

Adult Health Nursing, 6th ed.

Christensen & Kockrow

Slide 9

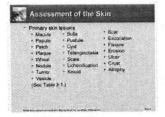

- Characteristics of specific lesions can be used in the diagnostic process.

- The specific location and pattern of lesions might indicate specific disorders.

- Review a few lesion types and associate with respective skin disorders.

Slide 10

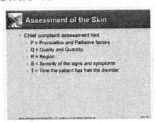

- Review questions that may be used to obtain additional information from the patient concerning the presence of skin lesions.

Slide 11

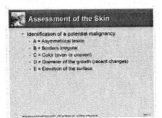

Slide 12

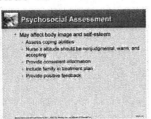

- The patient could experience significant psychosocial effects relating to dermatological conditions. There may be feelings of embarrassment and isolation.

- Social contacts might avoid the patient because of the appearance of the disorder or concerns about it being communicable.

- The dignity and privacy of the patient should be respected and promoted during the examination.

- Discuss the demeanor the nurse should employ during the skin examination.

Slide 13

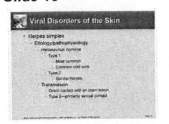

- Herpes simplex is a viral disorder, and it is a chronic condition.

- There is no cure. The goal is to manage symptoms.

- What is the impact a diagnosis of herpes simplex can have on the patient's long-term behaviors? How can herpes simplex influence a patient's relationships?

ELSEVIER

Adult Health Nursing, 6th ed.

Christensen & Kockrow

Slide 14

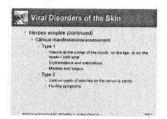

- What are some situations that might be associated with an outbreak of herpes simplex?

Slide 15

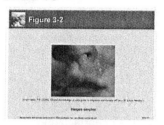

- Review the characteristic appearance of herpes simplex lesions. How do they differ from herpes zoster or impetigo?

Slide 16

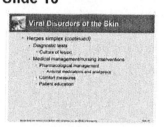

- Diagnosis of herpes is supported by an inspection of the lesions and the patient's history.

- The focus of medical management is the promotion of comfort and reduction of episode duration.

- Nursing management seeks to provide patient education, comfort measures, and emotional support.

- Discuss potential comfort measures that can be implemented.

Slide 17

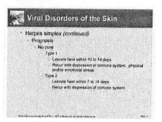

- Approximately 75% of all patients will experience a reoccurrence. Repeated outbreaks are usually milder and shorter in duration.

- The number of outbreaks is individualized with two thirds of infected individuals having between one and five occurrences per year.

- What is the emotional and physiological impact of future outbreaks?

Slide 18

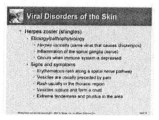

- What is the relationship between herpes zoster and chickenpox?

- Populations at risk for herpes zoster include the elderly, immunosuppressed patients, and HIV and AIDS sufferers.

- Why are these patients at risk for herpes zoster?

Slide 19

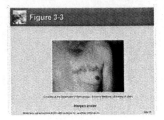

- The photograph of herpes zoster demonstrates the linear pattern of the lesions associated with this disorder.

Slide 20

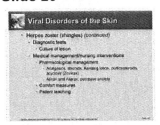

- In addition to culturing the lesion, the patient should have a complete physical examination and health history.

- Medical management is directed at controlling the pain and prevention of secondary complications. Review those measures that might be prescribed by the physician.

- Nursing management seeks to relieve symptoms such as pain, pruritus, and the prevention of secondary complications. Discuss nursing interventions that could be used to care for a patient during an initial outbreak of herpes simplex.

Slide 21

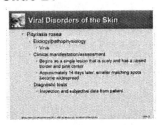

- There is no specific diagnostic test for this disorder. Subjective data and inspection of the skin is used to confirm diagnosis. Review the types of subjective data that might be obtained.

- Primary sites for the lesions include the chest, abdomen, back, and groin.

Slide 22

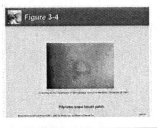

- Reinforce the characteristic appearance of rosea.

Slide 23

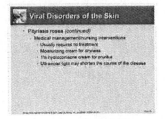

- Nursing interventions include symptomatic relief of the presenting symptoms such as pruritus. What measures may be implemented to promote comfort? What complications can occur if the patient begins to scratch lesions?

Christensen & Kockrow

Slide 24

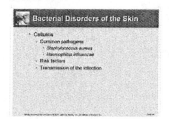

- Identify populations who are at risk for developing cellulitis. Why do these groups have a greater risk?
- What events may make a patient susceptible to developing cellulitis?

Slide 25

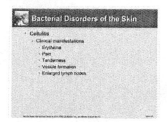

Slide 26

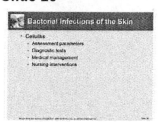

- When caring for the patient suspected of having cellulitis, what diagnostic tests can be anticipated?
- Identify two nursing interventions for the patient diagnosed with cellulitis.

Slide 27

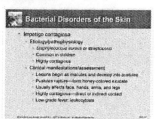

Slide 28

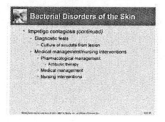

- The culture will definitively pinpoint the specific bacteria involved.
- Antibiotics of choice include erythromycin or cephalosporin.
- The crust must be removed and the area must be clean prior to application of topical medications. What methods could be used to safely remove the crust? How will the skin beneath the crust look?

Adult Health Nursing, 6th ed.
Christensen & Kockrow

Slide 29

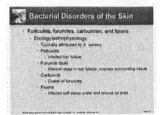

- Populations at risk for furuncles and carbuncles include those who are obese, have poor nutrition, are untreated for diabetes mellitus, or have poor hygiene. What is the commonality between these populations?

Slide 30

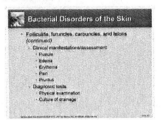

Slide 31

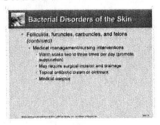

- Identify 2 nursing interventions for the patient diagnosed with folliculitis, furuncles, carbuncles or felons.

Slide 32

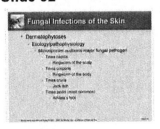

- Superficial fungal infections are known as dermatophytoses.

- The most common are tinea capitis, tinea corporis, tinea cruris, and tinea pedis.

- Tinea refers to the common disorder known as "ringworm." Ringworm is not a parasitic disorder. The name comes from its characteristic ring-shaped lesion and the location of infection.

Slide 33

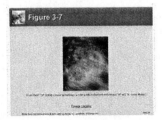

Slide 34

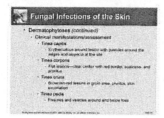

- Tinea capitis refers to ringworm of the scalp. The hair can break off at the scalp, and hair loss is typically not permanent.

- Tinea corporis refers to ringworm of the body. Outbreaks are typically in hairless areas.

- Tinea cruris is also known as "jock itch." These lesions migrate outward from the groin region. Tenderness and excoriation are common.

- Tinea pedis is also known as "athlete's foot." This infection is associated with more skin maceration than the other types of tinea.

- What is the mode of infection/transmission of each of the types of tinea infections?

- Does the appearance or treatment of tinea differ by location?

Slide 35

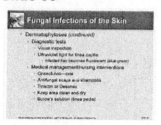

- What are some of the mistaken ideas that could accompany a diagnosis of tinea infection?

- Education should focus on correcting misconceptions and providing self-care information.

- Review elements of patient education.

Slide 36

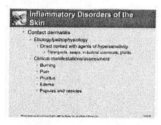

- The nursing assessment should include a complete review of the patient's history and activities.

- A recall log of activities for the 48-hour period preceding the onset of symptoms might assist in identifying the cause.

- What are some questions/prompts for the patient's review of the past 48 hours?

Slide 37

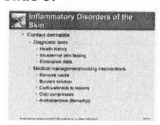

- Review the principles of implementing an elimination diet. How should this diet process be recorded?

- What are the nursing implications of intradermal testing?

- What is the therapeutic effect of the medication classifications that could be prescribed to manage dermatitis?

Adult Health Nursing, 6th ed.
Christensen & Kockrow

Slide 38

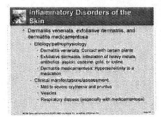

- Review the transmission of inflammatory skin disorders.
- What culprits are associated with inflammatory skin disorders?

Slide 39

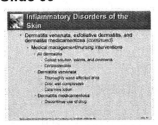

- What outcomes are desired with the medical/nursing management plans for these skin disorders?

Slide 40

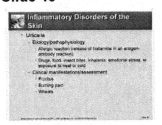

- The causes of allergic reactions include drugs, food, insect bites, inhalants, emotional stress, or exposure to heat and cold.
- Capillaries are dilated in response to the increase in histamine release.

Slide 41

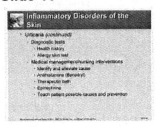

- What are the therapeutic effects associated with antihistamine and epinephrine therapies?
- What patient teaching should be included for these patients?

Slide 42

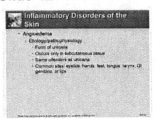

- How do urticaria and angioedema differ? How are they similar?

ELSEVIER

Mosby items and derived items © 2011, 2007 by Mosby, Inc., an affiliate of Elsevier Inc.
Some material was previously published.

Adult Health Nursing, 6th ed.
Christensen & Kockrow

Slide 43

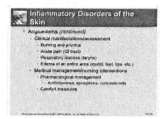

- Respiratory assessment is paramount to the assessment of a patient experiencing an allergic reaction. What respiratory behaviors warrant further interventions or medical care?

- Patients must be advised of the importance of wearing a Medic Alert bracelet.

Slide 44

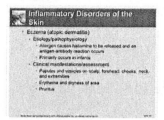

- Eczema is associated with allergies. Common allergies include eggs, chocolate, wheat, and orange juice.

- Subjective data associated with eczema patients include a family history of allergies, fussiness, irritability, and anorexia.

Slide 45

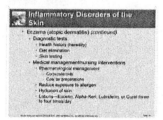

- Wet dressings are used to promote skin hydration.

- The discomfort of lesions is relieved with topical steroids. How do topical steroids work? List trade names of topical steroids that could be prescribed for eczema.

- Lotions are used after the onset of healing to increase skin moisture.

- The scaling appearance often results in stares from observers. Patients report feelings of embarrassment.

Slide 46

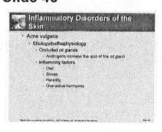

- Acne incidence is elevated during the teen years. This is associated with the increase of hormone levels.

- Studies have not supported hygiene as a cause of acne. What other misconceptions could be held about acne development or outbreaks?

Slide 47

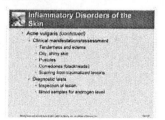

- Ask the class what causes a comedone to become black.

Slide 48

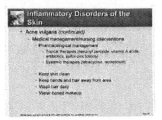

- Review the desired therapeutic effect of each of the medical treatments.
- Are there any special nursing implications associated with the commonly prescribed acne treatment medications?
- The emotional impact of acne on the patient cannot be discounted. What are interventions that should be implemented to provide emotional support?

Slide 49

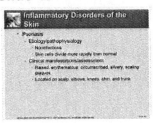

- Psoriasis can occur at any age. There are no specific predisposing factors.
- The characteristic rapid cell division can increase fourfold. It is this overproduction that results in the classic, raised scaling lesion appearance associated with the disorder.
- Identify at-risk populations. What behaviors make these populations at risk?
- What are preventive behaviors?

Slide 50

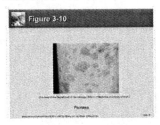

- What are the characteristics of the psoriasis lesions?

Slide 51

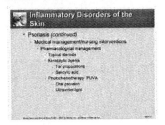

- There are no tests specific to the diagnosis of psoriasis.
- What are the desired therapeutic effects of the treatments employed for psoriasis?

Slide 52

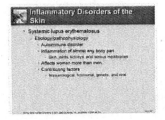

Slide 53

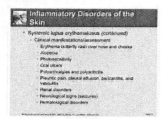

- What are the common clinical manifestations associated with lupus?
- What is the impact of each of the signs and symptoms?

Slide 54

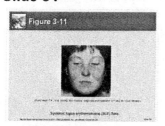

- Describe the characteristic butterfly rash.

Slide 55

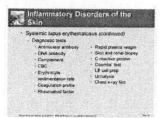

- Review the method of collection of each of the diagnostic tests.
- What findings for each of these tests are indicative of lupus?
- Are any special preparations needed for these tests?

Slide 56

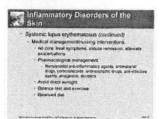

- What is the impact of a chronic disease with no cure?
- What are the psychological issues that could occur?
- What are the desired effects of the medication classifications used in the treatment of lupus?
- Review the nursing care plan for a patient diagnosed with lupus.

Slide 57

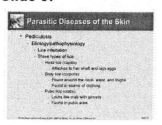

- What are the different types of lice?
- Identify common misconceptions concerning pediculosis.

ELSEVIER
Adult Health Nursing, 6th ed.
Christensen & Kockrow

Slide 58

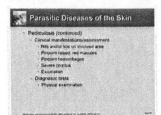

- What are screening techniques for suspected cases of lice?

Slide 59

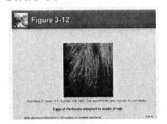

- What education must accompany the treatments prescribed to cure lice?
- What financial impact might a diagnosis of pediculosis carry?

Slide 60

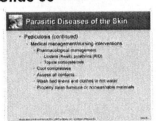

- What interventions can be taken to manage items that cannot be washed?
- Discuss the potential cost of managing a case of pediculosis in the home.

Slide 61

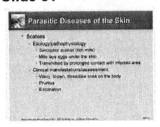

- What are the findings that support a diagnosis of scabies?
- Define at-risk populations.
- What are examples of opportunities for transmission?

Slide 62

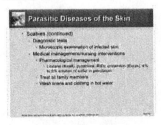

- What are the nursing implications for the treatment regimen for scabies?
- Discuss follow-up treatment needs.

ELSEVIER

Adult Health Nursing, 6th ed.
Christensen & Kockrow

Slide 63

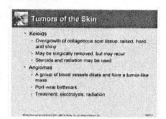

- Define at-risk populations for keloid formation.
- What are potential treatment options?

Slide 64

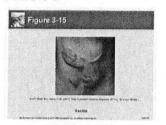

Slide 65

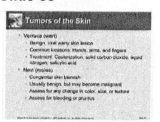

- What changes in warts or moles would warrant further investigation?

Slide 66

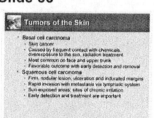

- Each type of skin cancer has a unique appearance.
- How does the prognosis differ between cancer types?

Slide 67

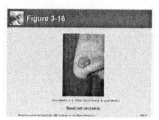

Slide 68

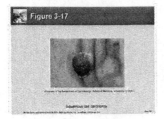

Slide 69

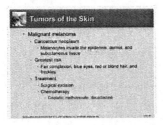

- How does malignant melanoma differ from basal cell and squamous cell carcinoma?
- Why are fair-skinned, blue-eyed people at higher risk for the development of malignant melanoma?

Slide 70

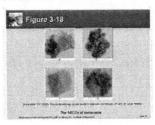

- Discuss "ABCD." What does each of the letters represent?

Slide 71

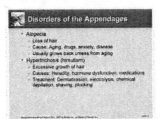

Slide 72

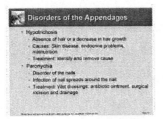

Slide 73

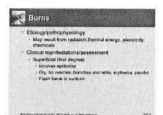

- Review each type of burn. What are examples of potential causes for each?

Slide 74

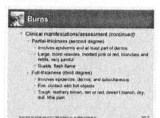

- For each burn type, what are the long-range implications regarding recovery prognosis?
- Develop nursing diagnoses for second- and third-degree burns.

Slide 75

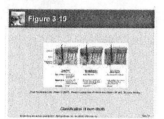

Slide 76

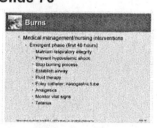

- What determines what phase of burn recovery is at hand?
- What complications are at highest risk during the acute phase? Discuss the signs and symptoms that signal complication development.

Slide 77

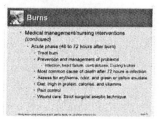

- What measures protect the patient from the development of complications during this phase?
- Discuss pain management during this phase of recovery. What route of analgesic therapy should be initiated? What are the nursing implications?

Adult Health Nursing, 6th ed.
Christensen & Kockrow

Slide 78

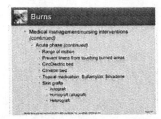

- Discuss the nutritional assessment that should begin during the acute phase. Include special nutritional challenges that will be encountered in a burn patient.

- What impact will positive nutritional outcomes have on the recovery of a burn patient?

Slide 79

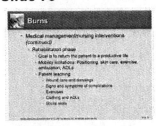

- What are the actual nursing interventions to include in the care plan of a burn patient?

Slide 80

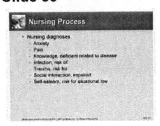

- Review goal setting for patients experiencing a burn.

- How will the outcomes for a burn patient be monitored?

ELSEVIER

Christensen & Kockrow

Mosby items and derived items © 2011, 2007 by Mosby, Inc., an affiliate of Elsevier Inc. Some material was previously published.

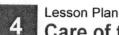

4 Care of the Patient with a Musculoskeletal Disorder

TEACHING FOCUS

In this chapter, the student will be introduced to the structure and function of the musculoskeletal system. Next, the student will explore the various laboratory and diagnostic examinations used in the study of this system. The student then will be introduced to disorders of the musculoskeletal system, followed by surgical interventions, skeletal fixation devices, and nonsurgical interventions. Finally, the student will have the opportunity to learn about various traumatic injuries.

MATERIALS AND RESOURCES

- ☐ Computer/overhead projector (all lessons)
- ☐ White/black board and marker/chalk (all lessons)
- ☐ Small, soft ball or pillow that can be tossed around the room (Lessons 4.1 and 4.5)
- ☐ Pictures of the skeleton, half with the anterior view and half with the posterior view (Lesson 4.1)
- ☐ Candy or fruit to use as a prize (Lesson 4.1)
- ☐ List of diagnostic tests (Lesson 4.1)
- ☐ Hip prosthetics for students to examine (borrow from the surgical department of a local hospital) (Lesson 4.2)
- ☐ Note cards, each with a different patient complaint related to a fracture (Lesson 4.4)

LESSON CHECKLIST

Preparations for this lesson include:

- Lecture
- Invite a guest speaker suffering from rheumatoid arthritis.
- Invite a physical therapist to discuss a possible exercise plan for a patient diagnosed with rheumatoid arthritis.
- Invite a patient education specialist, physical therapist, or utilization review staff member from a local hospital to talk with the class about the care of a patient who has undergone hip replacement.

KEY TERMS

ankylosis (FAAHN p. 1356, AHN p. 120)
arthrocentesis (FAAHN p. 1352, AHN p. 116)
arthrodesis (FAAHN p. 1369, AHN p. 133)
arthroplasty (FAAHN p. 1369, AHN p. 133)
bipolar hip replacement (hemiarthroplasty)
  (FAAHN p. 1375, AHN p. 139)
blanching test (FAAHN p. 1406, AHN p. 170)
callus (FAAHN p. 1380, AHN p. 144)
Colles' fracture (FAAHN p. 1378, AHN p. 142)
compartment syndrome (FAAHN p. 1384, AHN
  p. 148)
crepitus (FAAHN p. 1380, AHN p. 144)

fibromyalgia (FAAHN p. 1367, AHN p. 131)
kyphosis (FAAHN p. 1406, AHN p. 170)
lordosis (FAAHN p. 1406, AHN p. 170)
open reduction with internal fixation (ORIF)
  (FAAHN p. 1380, AHN p. 144)
paresthesia (FAAHN p. 1399, AHN p. 163)
scoliosis (FAAHN p. 1406, AHN p. 170)
sequestrum (FAAHN p. 1367, AHN p. 131)
subluxation (FAAHN p. 1398, AHN p. 162)
tophi (FAAHN p. 1363, AHN p. 127)
Volkmann's contracture (FAAHN p. 1385,
  AHN p. 149)

ADDITIONAL RESOURCES (AHN)

PPT Ch. 44, 1 through 78 FAAHN (Ch. 4, 1 through 78 AHN)
EILR IC images Ch. 44, 1 through 41 FAAHN (Ch. 4, 1 through 41 AHN)
EILR TB questions Ch. 44, 1 through 46 FAAHN (Ch. 4, 1 through 46 AHN)
EILR Open Book Quiz Ch. 44, 1 through 10 FAAHN (Ch. 4, 1 through 10 AHN)
ESLR Review Questions for the NCLEX® Examination Ch. 44, 44-01 through 44-10 FAAHN (Ch. 4, 04-01 through 04-10 AHN)

Adult Health Nursing, 6th ed.
Christensen & Kockrow

Legend

PPT
PowerPoint
Slides

EILR
EVOLVE Instructor
Learning Resources:
Image Collection, Test
Bank, Open Book Quizzes

ESLR
EVOLVE Student
Learning Resources:
Review Questions
for the NCLEX
Examination

SG
Study Guide

NCP CTQ
Nursing Care Plan
Critical Thinking
Question

Class Activities are indicated in ***bold italic***.

LESSON 4.1

PRETEST

1. The relationship between phosphorus and calcium is best described by which of the following statements?
   a. Calcium and phosphorus share a relationship of equality. Both are present in equal amounts in the blood stream.
   b. Calcium and phosphorus share an inverse relationship. Both minerals are elevated in the blood stream when both are elevated in the body's skeleton.
   c. Calcium and phosphorus share a negative relationship. Both minerals are decreased in the blood stream when they are elevated in the body's skeleton.
   d. Calcium and phosphorus share an inverse relationship. When calcium is elevated, phosphorus levels are reduced.

2. Risk factors for the development of osteoporosis include:
   a. obesity, European ancestry, and a diagnosis of rheumatoid arthritis.
   b. slender build, European ancestry, and cigarette smoking.
   c. menopause, African ancestry, and a diagnosis of gout.
   d. Asian ancestry, slender build, and a diagnosis of gout.

3. Rheumatoid arthritis and osteoarthritis differ in which of the following ways?
   a. Older patients are more frequently affected by rheumatoid arthritis than osteoarthritis.
   b. Rheumatoid arthritis is associated with obesity, whereas osteoarthritis is associated with patients having a slender build.
   c. Rheumatoid arthritis is more often treated with surgery than osteoarthritis.
   d. Rheumatoid arthritis is a systemic disorder, whereas the effects of osteoarthritis are limited to the body's joints.

4. When assigning a diagnosis of rheumatoid arthritis, the following diagnostic test results are present:
   a. an elevated RF and an elevated red blood cell count.
   b. an absence of anti-IgG antibodies and an elevated red blood cell count.
   c. a reduction in the white blood cell count and a low erythrocyte sedimentation rate.
   d. a reduced red blood cell count and an elevated RF.

5. When administering Tolmetin sodium to manage rheumatoid arthritis, the following nursing implications are indicated: Select all that apply.
   a. Monitor blood pressure.
   b. Give with food or milk.
   c. Give with an antacid.
   d. Avoid aspirin and aspirin products while taking this medication.
   e. Avoid driving during initial phases of therapy.

6. A patient diagnosed with osteoarthritis asks what type of exercise is beneficial to her condition. Based upon your understanding, you encourage:
   a. swimming.
   b. a combination of running and walking.
   c. aerobic dancing.
   d. stair climbing.

7. A 65-year-old male patient presents to the clinic. He has complaints of severe pain at night. The assessment reveals a reddened, edematous great toe. Tophi are noted along the rim of the left ear. Based upon your knowledge, you anticipate a diagnosis of:
   a. rheumatoid arthritis.
   b. osteoarthritis.
   c. osteoporosis.
   d. gout.

8. A 54-year-old male patient has a checkup with the physician. He has a 4-year history of osteoarthritis, non–insulin-dependent diabetes, and hypertension. The only medications he takes on a regular basis are NSAIDs for the management of his arthritis, Lantus to manage the diabetes, and vitamin supplements. Which of the following will be most closely monitored at this appointment given his health history?
   a. Rheumatoid factor
   b. Blood cell profile
   c. Blood pressure
   d. Heart rate

9. After undergoing an amputation of the lower left leg, the patient complains of discomfort in his left leg and foot. He requests pain medication for the sensation. The nurse's best course of action will be:
   a. medicate the patient for the complaints of pain.
   b. attempt to distract the patient from the situation.
   c. explain to the patient the discomfort he is reporting is not possible since his limb is missing.
   d. contact the physician concerning a possible consult with a psychologist.

10. When performing an assessment of a patient's capillary refill in the extremity that has been casted for a fracture, the following findings are normal:
    a. return to normal within 5 to 7 seconds.
    b. return to normal within 2 to 3 seconds.
    c. sluggish return to normal.
    d. no blanch is noted.

Answers:

1. d	2. b	3. d	4. d	5. b, e
6. a	7. d	8. c	9. a	10. b

BACKGROUND ASSESSMENT

Question: After being thrown from a motorcycle, a 31-year-old male suffered a compound fracture to the right ulna. After it is surgically reduced and stabilized, the physician prescribes intravenous antibiotics to be administered during the hospitalization. He also orders a home health nurse to visit the patient to continue the therapy after discharge for the next 3 weeks. The patient reports he does not feel this extra treatment is necessary because he is not sick. What are the reasons for the continued treatments?

Answer: A compound fracture involves a broken bone that extends out of the skin. This break in the integrity of the skin exposes the bone and surrounding tissue to a variety of bacteria and other toxins. Compound fractures increase the incidence of osteomyelitis, an infection and inflammation of the bone and a serious condition that can become chronic and result in pain, bone weakness, and pathological fractures. The treatments ordered are prophylactic in nature.

Question: A 41-year-old female patient seeks medical care after feeling ill for the past several months. Her symptoms include muscle pain, excessive fatigue, anxiety, and bouts of depression. She states she has seen two other physicians for the same disorder but no diagnosis has ever been made. The physician orders blood

Adult Health Nursing, 6th ed.

Mosby items and derived items © 2011 by Mosby, Inc., an affiliate of Elsevier Inc.   Christensen & Kockrow
Some material was previously published.

tests including a complete blood count, an electrolyte panel, and an erythrocyte sedimentation rate. A sleep study is also ordered. After the test results are reviewed, the physician diagnoses fibromyalgia syndrome. Despite being initially happy that a diagnosis was finally reached, the patient returns to the clinic reporting she continues to have difficulty sleeping. She asks for suggestions. How should the nurse respond?

Answer: The teaching focus should involve methods to promote a restful environment at bedtime. Reduce noise and odors. A pattern of going to bed at the same time each night is helpful. Advise the patient to avoid taking naps during the day and evening hours. Warm baths can promote feelings of relaxation and will be helpful to add to the evening routine. Adding exercise to the daily routine is also a positive means to promote rest and relaxation.

CRITICAL THINKING QUESTION

A 24-year-old female patient has been experiencing episodes of joint pain and fatigue. After being seen by her primary care physician, laboratory tests including an erythrocyte sedimentation rate, complete blood count, and rheumatoid factor are ordered to assess for rheumatoid arthritis. After you have explained where and when to have the tests performed, the patient states, "I am so glad these tests are finally being done. If they are all positive I will know I have arthritis." What factors will you include in your responses?

Guidelines: Although the patient's test results will provide valuable information to be used by her physician to make a diagnosis, rheumatoid arthritis does not have a definitive test. The diagnosis is made based upon the review of the patient's health history, assessment findings, and inferences made from a series of laboratory tests. The erythrocyte sedimentation rate (ESR) is increased in the presence of inflammation. This test is higher in rheumatoid arthritis sufferers. The rheumatoid factor (RF) is a titer that identifies an abnormal serum protein concentration. Although the majority of people having rheumatoid arthritis do possess this immunoglobulin, it is also associated with other disorders such as lupus. The complete blood cell count will provide an evaluation of the red blood cell count. Anemia (low red blood cell count) is present in chronic infections. Regardless of the test results, the patient requires emotional support for the probable diagnosis. She also needs education concerning the tests being ordered.

OBJECTIVES	CONTENT	TEACHING RESOURCES
List the five basic functions of the skeletal system.	■ Anatomy and physiology of the musculoskeletal system (FAAHN p. 1345, AHN p. 109) □ Functions of the skeletal system (FAAHN p. 1345, AHN p. 109) – Support (FAAHN p. 1345, AHN p. 109) – Protection (FAAHN p. 1345, AHN p. 109) – Movement (FAAHN p. 1346, AHN p. 110) – Mineral storage (FAAHN p. 1346, AHN p. 110) – Hematopoiesis (FAAHN p. 1346, AHN p. 110)	PPT 1 through 2, Ch. 44 FAAHN (Ch. 4 PPT 1 through 2 AHN) EILR Open Book Quiz Ch. 44 question 1 FAAHN (Ch. 4 question 1 AHN) SG Functions of the Musculoskeletal System, Ch. 44 p. 343 FAAHN (Ch. 4 p. 31 AHN) **BOOK RESOURCES** Fig. 44-1 Structure of a freely movable (diarthrotic) joint (FAAHN p. 1346) (Fig. 4-1 AHN p. 110) ▶ Discuss the impact dietary intake has on the health and composition of the skeletal system. ▶ Discuss the functions of the skeletal system. Review the impact on one's life if the skeletal system's functioning is impaired. ▶ Discuss the differences and similarities among gout, osteoarthritis, and rheumatoid arthritis. List the treatments for each.

OBJECTIVES	CONTENT	TEACHING RESOURCES
		Class Activity Pass an object such as a small ball. The student receiving the ball is asked to relate a fact about the skeletal system's function.
List the two divisions of the skeleton.	☐ Structure of bones (FAAHN p. 1346, AHN p. 110) ☐ Articulations (joints) (FAAHN p. 1346, AHN p. 110) ☐ Divisions of the skeleton (FAAHN p. 1346, AHN p. 110)	▣ PPT 5, Ch. 44 FAAHN (Ch. 4 PPT 5 AHN) ✎ EILR IC Ch. 44 images 1, 2 FAAHN (Ch. 4 images 1, 2 AHN) ✎ ESLR Review Questions for the NCLEX Examination Ch. 44 question 1 FAAHN (Ch. 4 question 1 AHN) 📖 SG Bones: Location and Skeletal Division Ch. 44 p. 343 FAAHN (Ch. 4 p. 31 AHN) **BOOK RESOURCES** Box 44-1 Main Parts of the Skeleton (FAAHN p. 1346) (Box 4-1 AHN p. 110) Fig. 44-2 Skeleton, anterior view (FAAHN p. 1347) (Fig. 4-2 AHN p. 111) Fig. 44-3 Skeleton, posterior view (FAAHN p. 1347) (Fig. 4-3 AHN p. 111) ▶ Discuss the possible types of joint movements. ▶ Discuss the manner in which the skeleton is divided. ▶ Discuss differences and similarities among ankylosing spondylitis and osteoarthritis. Discuss nursing interventions for each. *Class Activity Divide the students into groups. Each group will be assigned one of three categories. The categories will include synarthrosis, amphiarthrosis, and diarthrosis joints. Ask each group to discuss and determine which joints in the body best fit into the assigned category. After a brief time, bring the class back together and share the findings.*

OBJECTIVES	CONTENT	TEACHING RESOURCES
Describe the location of major bones of the skeleton.	☐ Divisions of the skeleton (FAAHN p. 1346, AHN p. 110)	PPT 3 through 6, Ch. 44 FAAHN (Ch. 4 PPT 3 through 6 AHN) EILR IC Ch. 44 images 2, 3 FAAHN (Ch. 4 images 2, 3 AHN) SG Bones: Location and Skeletal Division, Ch. 44 p. 343 FAAHN (Ch. 4 p. 31 AHN) **BOOK RESOURCES** Fig. 44-2 Skeleton, anterior view (FAAHN p. 1347) (Fig. 4-2 AHN p. 111) Fig. 44-3 Skeleton, posterior view (FAAHN p. 1347) (Fig. 4-3 AHN p. 111) ▸ Discuss the four classifications of bones in the body. *Class Activity Instruct each student to choose a partner. Provide each pair a picture of the skeleton. Half of the pairs will have the anterior view and the remaining groups will have the posterior view. Each group will be asked to label the body's bones. Allow only 5 to 10 minutes. Provide a small prize (candy or fruit) for the pair with the most correct answers.*
Describe the location of major muscles of the body.	– Muscle contraction (FAAHN p. 1349, AHN p. 113) – Skeletal muscle groups (FAAHN p. 1349, AHN p. 113)	PPT 8, 9, Ch. 44 FAAHN (Ch. 4 PPT 8, 9 AHN) EILR IC Ch. 44 images 5, 6 FAAHN (Ch. 4 images 5, 6 AHN) EILR TB Ch. 44 question 2 FAAHN (Ch. 4 question 2 AHN) SG Location of Muscles, Ch. 44 p. 344 FAAHN (Ch. 4 p. 32 AHN) **BOOK RESOURCES** Fig. 44-5 Anterior view of the body (FAAHN p. 1350) (Fig. 4-5 AHN p. 114) Fig. 44-6 Posterior view of the body (FAAHN p. 1350) (Fig. 4-6 AHN p. 114) ▸ Discuss the functions of muscles and tendons. What is the relationship between muscles and tendons? ▸ Discuss the physiological processes that allow muscles to respond to messages from the body.

OBJECTIVES	CONTENT	TEACHING RESOURCES
		*Class Activity **Lead a class discussion concerning the locations of the body's muscles.***
List the types of body movements.	– Muscle contraction (FAAHN p. 1349, AHN p. 113)	PPT 10, Ch. 44 FAAHN (Ch. 4 PPT 10 AHN) EILR TB Ch. 44 question 1 FAAHN (Ch. 4 question 1 AHN) SG Moveable Joints, Ch. 44 p. 345 FAAHN (Ch. 4 p. 33 AHN) **BOOK RESOURCES** Table 44-1 Principal Muscles of the Body (FAAHN p. 1348) (Table 4-1 AHN p. 112) Table 44-2 Muscles Grouped According to Function (FAAHN p. 1349) (Table 4-2 AHN p. 113) Box 44-2 Types of Body Movement (FAAHN p. 1349) (Box 4-2 AHN p. 113) Fig. 44-4 Extension of the lower arm and lower leg (FAAHN p. 1350) (Fig. 4-4 AHN p. 114) ▸ Discuss the factors that determine the force (strength) of muscle response. *Class Activity **Ask each student to stand up. Read each type of body movement. After each description is read, ask the students to demonstrate the different motions.***
Describe three vital functions muscles perform when they contract.	☐ Functions of the muscular system (FAAHN p. 1346, AHN p. 110) – Skeletal muscle structure (FAAHN p. 1347, AHN p. 111) – Nerve and blood supply (FAAHN p. 1347, AHN p. 111) – Muscle contraction (FAAHN p. 1349, AHN p. 113)	PPT 7, Ch. 44 FAAHN (Ch. 4 PPT 7 AHN) EILR IC Ch. 44 image 4 FAAHN (Ch. 4 image 4 AHN) EILR TB Ch. 44 question 46 FAAHN (Ch. 4 question 46 AHN) SG Functions, Ch. 44 p. 345 FAAHN (Ch. 4 p. 33 AHN) **BOOK RESOURCES** Table 44-1 Principal Muscles of the Body (FAAHN p. 1348) (Table 4-1 AHN p. 112) Table 44-2 Muscles Grouped According to Function (FAAHN p. 1349) (Table 4-2 AHN p. 113)

OBJECTIVES	CONTENT	TEACHING RESOURCES
		Box 44-2 Types of Body Movement (FAAHN p. 1349) (Box 4-2 AHN p. 113) Fig. 44-4 Extension of the lower arm and lower leg (FAAHN p. 1350) (Fig. 4-4 AHN p. 114) ▸ Discuss how muscles produce movement. ▸ Discuss the differences between voluntary and involuntary muscle activity. *Class Activity Ask each student to select a partner. Once paired, ask each group to select one body system. The students are to review the functions of the body system and the muscles located in the body system. Finally the students are asked to determine the types of muscle functions performed in their chosen system.*
List diagnostic procedures pertinent to musculoskeletal function.	■ Laboratory and diagnostic examinations (FAAHN p. 1349, AHN p. 113) ☐ Radiographic studies (FAAHN p. 1349, AHN p. 113) – Myelogram (FAAHN p. 1351, AHN p. 115) – Nuclear scanning (FAAHN p. 1351, AHN p. 115) – Magnetic resonance imaging (FAAHN p. 1351, AHN p. 115) – Computed tomography (FAAHN p. 1351, AHN p. 115) – Bone scan (FAAHN p. 1352, AHN p. 116) ☐ Endoscopic examination (FAAHN p. 1352, AHN p. 116) – Arthroscopy (FAAHN p. 1352, AHN p. 116) – Endoscopic spinal microsurgery (FAAHN p. 1352, AHN p. 116) ☐ Aspiration (FAAHN p. 1352, AHN p. 116) – Synovial fluid aspiration (FAAHN p. 1352, AHN p. 116)	PPT 11, 12, Ch. 44 FAAHN (Ch. 4 PPT 11, 12 AHN) EILR TB Ch. 44 question 3 FAAHN (Ch. 4 question 3 AHN) EILR Open Book Quiz Ch. 44 questions 2 through 5 FAAHN (Ch. 4 questions 2 through 5 AHN) ESLR Review Questions for the NCLEX Examination Ch. 44 questions 2, 3 FAAHN (Ch. 4 questions 2, 3 AHN) SG Diagnostic Procedures Ch. 44 p. 345 FAAHN (Ch. 4 p. 33 AHN) **BOOK RESOURCES** Table 44-3 Laboratory Tests for Musculoskeletal Disorders (FAAHN p. 1353) (Table 4-3 AHN p. 117) ▸ Discuss the nursing responsibilities when preparing patients for musculoskeletal laboratory testing. ▸ Discuss patient contraindications for diagnostic testing used to detect musculoskeletal disorders. ▸ Discuss and differentiate the diagnostic tests performed to evaluate the body's bones and the tests performed to evaluate the body's muscles. *Class Activity Divide students into small groups. Assign each group a different diagnostic test. Allow each group a period of time to develop a*

Adult Health Nursing, 6th ed.
Christensen & Kockrow

OBJECTIVES	CONTENT	TEACHING RESOURCES
	☐ Electrographic procedure (FAAHN p. 1353, AHN p. 117) – Electromyogram (FAAHN p. 1353, AHN p. 117) ☐ Laboratory tests (FAAHN p. 1353, AHN p. 117) ☐ Effects of bed rest on mineral content in bone (FAAHN p. 1353, AHN p. 117)	*brief overview of each of the tests. The overview should include why the test would be ordered, normal and abnormal findings, and nursing implications. The overview will then be presented to the class.*

4.1 Homework/Assignments:

4.1 Instructor's Notes/Student Feedback:

CRITICAL THINKING QUESTION

Osteoporosis tends to lead to fracture in older adults. What can a younger adult do that will prevent the progression of this disease and keep the body more mobile while aging?

Guidelines: The dietary intake of vitamin D and calcium are important, starting at an early age. Avoiding smoking and obesity prevents extra strain on the muscle and bones. Finally, daily exercise is important to keep weight-bearing joints more mobile.

OBJECTIVES	CONTENT	TEACHING RESOURCES
Compare the medical regimens for patients suffering from gouty arthritis, rheumatoid arthritis, and osteoarthritis.	■ Disorders of the musculoskeletal system (FAAHN p. 1353, AHN p. 117) ☐ Inflammatory disorders (FAAHN p. 1353, AHN p. 117) ☐ Arthritis (FAAHN p. 1353, AHN p. 117) – Rheumatoid arthritis (FAAHN p. 1354, AHN p. 118) – Ankylosing spondylitis (FAAHN p. 1359, AHN p. 123) – Osteoarthritis (degenerative joint disease) (FAAHN p. 1361, AHN p. 125) – Gout (gouty arthritis) (FAAHN p. 1363, AHN p. 127)	PPT 13 through 17, 22 through 26, Ch. 44 FAAHN (Ch. 4 PPT 13 through 17, 22 through 26 AHN) EILR IC Ch. 44 images 7 through 9 FAAHN (Ch. 4 images 7 through 9 AHN) EILR TB Ch. 44 questions 18 through 21, 31, 34 FAAHN (Ch. 4 questions 18 through 21, 31, 34 AHN) EILR Open Book Quiz Ch. 44 question 6 FAAHN (Ch. 4 question 6 AHN) ESLR Review Questions for the NCLEX Examination Ch. 44 questions 4 through 6 FAAHN (Ch. 4 questions 4 through 6 AHN) SG Arthritis, Ch. 44 p. 347 FAAHN (Ch. 4 p. 35 AHN) **BOOK RESOURCES** Table 44-4 Comparison of Rheumatoid Arthritis and Osteoarthritis (FAAHN p. 1354) (Table 4-4 AHN p. 118) Table 44-5 Medications for Rheumatoid Arthritis (FAAHN p. 1355) (Table 4-5 AHN p. 119) Fig. 44-7 Theumatoid arthritis of hands (FAAHN p. 1355) (Fig. 4-7 AHN p. 119) Box 44-3 Osteoarthritis (FAAHN p. 1361) (Box 4-3 AHN p. 125) Fig. 44-8 Joints most frequently involved in osteoarthritis (FAAHN p. 1361) (Fig. 4-8 AHN p. 125) Fig. 44-9 Heberden's nodes (FAAHN p. 1362) (Fig. 4-9 AHN p. 126) Complementary and Alternative Therapies: Musculoskeletal Disorders (FAAHN p. 1362) (AHN p. 126) ▸ Discuss the differences and similarities among gout, osteoarthritis, and rheumatoid arthritis.

OBJECTIVES	CONTENT	TEACHING RESOURCES
		▶ Discuss joints in the body most often affected by rheumatoid arthritis, osteoarthritis, and gout.
		Class Activity Invite a guest speaker suffering from rheumatoid arthritis. Ask the speaker to focus on the changes encountered in his life related to the disease.
Discuss the nursing interventions appropriate for rheumatoid arthritis.	– Rheumatoid arthritis (FAAHN p. 1354, AHN p. 118)	PPT 13 through 17, Ch. 44 FAAHN (Ch. 4 PPT 13 through 17 AHN)
		EILR IC Ch. 44 image 8 FAAHN (Ch. 4 image 8 AHN)
		EILR TB Ch. 44 question 19 FAAHN (Ch. 4 question 19 AHN)
		SG Nursing Interventions Ch. 44 p. 347 FAAHN (Ch. 4 p. 35 AHN)
		BOOK RESOURCES
		Table 44-4 Comparison of Rheumatoid Arthritis and Osteoarthritis (FAAHN p. 1354) (Table 4-4 AHN p. 118)
		Table 44-5 Medications for Rheumatoid Arthritis (FAAHN p. 1355) (Table 4-5 AHN p. 119)
		Fig. 44-7 Rheumatoid arthritis of hands (FAAHN p. 1355) (Fig. 4-7 AHN p. 119)
		▶ Discuss the population most commonly affected by rheumatoid arthritis.
		▶ Discuss the manner in which rheumatoid arthritis differs from osteoarthritis and gout.
		Class Activity Invite a physical therapist to speak with the class. Ask the therapist to review the elements that might be included in an exercise plan for a patient diagnosed with rheumatoid arthritis.
Describe the nursing interventions appropriate for degenerative joint disease (osteoarthritis).	– Ankylosing spondylitis (FAAHN p. 1359, AHN p. 123) – Osteoarthritis (degenerative joint disease) (FAAHN p. 1361, AHN p. 125)	PPT 18 through 23, Ch. 44 FAAHN (Ch. 4 PPT 18 through 23 AHN)
		EILR IC Ch. 44 images 8, 9 FAAHN (Ch. 4 images 8, 9 AHN)
		EILR TB Ch. 44 question 37 FAAHN (Ch. 4 question 37 AHN)
		SG Nursing Interventions, Ch. 44 p. 347 FAAHN (Ch. 4 p. 35 AHN)
		BOOK RESOURCES
		Box 44-3 Osteoarthritis (FAAHN p. 1361) (Box 4-3 AHN p. 125)

OBJECTIVES	CONTENT	TEACHING RESOURCES
		Fig. 44-9 Joints most frequently involved in osteoarthritis (FAAHN p. 1361) (Fig. 4-9 AHN p. 126)
		▶ Discuss differences and similarities between ankylosing spondylitis and osteoarthritis.
		▶ Discuss safe, effective exercise for the patient diagnosed with osteoarthritis.
		Class Activity Obtain x-ray films of adults at varying ages. Review the x-rays with the class to illustrate the changes in the adult skeleton that are consistent with the aging process.
List at least four healthy lifestyle measures a person can practice to reduce the risk of developing osteoporosis.	☐ Other musculoskeletal disorders (FAAHN p. 1364, AHN p. 128) ☐ Osteoporosis (FAAHN p. 1364, AHN p. 128) – Etiology and pathophysiology (FAAHN p. 1364, AHN p. 128) – Clinical manifestations (FAAHN p. 1364, AHN p. 128) – Assessment (FAAHN p. 1364, AHN p. 128) – Diagnostic tests (FAAHN p. 1364, AHN p. 128) – Medical management (FAAHN p. 1365, AHN p. 129) – Nursing interventions and patient teaching (FAAHN p. 1366, AHN p. 130) – Prognosis (FAAHN p. 1367, AHN p. 131) ☐ Osteomyelitis (FAAHN p. 1367, AHN p. 131) – Etiology and pathophysiology (FAAHN p. 1367, AHN p. 131) – Clinical manifestations (FAAHN p. 1367, AHN p. 131) – Assessment (FAAHN p. 1367, AHN p. 131) – Diagnostic tests (FAAHN p. 1367, AHN p. 131)	🖥 PPT 27 through 28, Ch. 44 FAAHN (Ch. 4 PPT 27 through 28 AHN) 📼 EILR IC Ch. 44 image 10 FAAHN (Ch. 4 image 10 AHN) 📼 EILR TB Ch. 44 questions 32, 33, 36, 38 FAAHN (Ch. 4 questions 32, 33, 36, 38 AHN) 📼 ESLR Review Questions for the NCLEX Examination Ch. 44 questions 7, 8 FAAHN (Ch. 4 questions 7, 8 AHN) 📓 SG Lifestyle Ch. 44 p. 348 FAAHN (Ch. 4 p. 36 AHN) **BOOK RESOURCES** Cultural Considerations: Osteoporosis (FAAHN p. 1364) (AHN p. 128) Fig. 44-10 A normal spine at 40 years and osteoporotic changes at ages 60 and 70 years. (FAAHN p. 1365) (Fig. 4-10 AHN p. 129) Patient Teaching: Dietary Needs in Osteoporosis (FAAHN p. 1366) (AHN p. 130) Table 44-7 Medications for Fibromyalgia Syndrome (FAAHN p. 1368) (Table 4-7 AHN p. 132) Patient Teaching: Sleep Hygiene (FAAHN p. 1369) (AHN p. 133) ▶ Discuss the risk factors associated with the development of osteoporosis. Which of these factors are modifiable? ▶ Discuss dietary prevention for osteoporosis. ▶ Discuss the manner in which rheumatoid arthritis differs from osteoarthritis and gout. List the nursing interventions for rheumatoid arthritis.

OBJECTIVES	CONTENT	TEACHING RESOURCES
	– Medical management (FAAHN p. 1367, AHN p. 131) – Nursing interventions and patient teaching (FAAHN p. 1367, AHN p. 131) – Prognosis (FAAHN p. 1367, AHN p. 131) ☐ Fibromyalgia syndrome (FAAHN p. 1367, AHN p. 131) – Etiology and pathophysiology (FAAHN p. 1367, AHN p. 131) – Clinical manifestations (FAAHN p. 1368, AHN p. 132) – Assessment (FAAHN p. 1368, AHN p. 132) – Diagnostic tests (FAAHN p. 1368, AHN p. 132) – Medical management (FAAHN p. 1368, AHN p. 132) – Nursing interventions (FAAHN p. 1368, AHN p. 132) – Prognosis (FAAHN p. 1369, AHN p. 133)	*Class Activity* Ask each student to record his/her diet for a period of 1 week. The following week ask each student to critically review the diet journals. Discuss as a class the degree of risk each student presents for the development of osteoporosis relating to calcium intake.

4.2 Homework/Assignments:

4.2 Instructor's Notes/Student Feedback:

LESSON 4.3

CRITICAL THINKING QUESTION

An elderly patient who was just admitted to the hospital with a fractured hip voices questions. She has never had problems and simply bent down to pick up something on the floor and heard a "popping" sound. She states she still does not understand how this could have caused a hip fracture. She reports the physician said something about a condition called osteoporosis. She asked how she could have "caught it," how can she "cure it," and what can she do to prevent further problems? Based upon your understanding of the disease process and treatment, how will you respond?

Guidelines: The patient will be advised that osteoporosis is a disease characterized by a loss of bone mass. The reduced bone mass promotes a fragility in the body's skeleton. Once the body's bones lose mass, it becomes possible for minor accidents and traumas as well as normal daily actions to result in bone fractures. Osteoporosis is not a communicable disease that can be "caught." There are a variety of risk factors associated with the development of the disease. Risk factors include white race, slender build, reduced dietary calcium intake, smoking, estrogen deficiency, inactivity, and caffeine intake. Because there is no cure for the disease, the goal is prevention and management for those diagnosed with the disease.

It is possible for even slight movements and falls to result in fractures. Treatment for the disorder includes calcium supplements, exercise, and reduction of high-risk behaviors.

OBJECTIVES	CONTENT	TEACHING RESOURCES
Describe the surgical intervention for arthritis of the hip and knee.	■ Surgical interventions for total knee or total hip replacement (FAAHN p. 1369, AHN p. 133) □ Knee arthroplasty (total knee replacement) (FAAHN p. 1369, AHN p. 133) □ Unicompartmental knee arthroplasty (FAAHN p. 1369, AHN p. 133) – Assessment (FAAHN p. 1370, AHN p. 134) – Diagnostic tests (FAAHN p. 1370, AHN p. 134) – Nursing interventions and patient teaching (FAAHN p. 1370, AHN p. 134) □ Hip arthroplasty (total hip replacement) (FAAHN p. 1371, AHN p. 135) – Assessment (FAAHN p. 1371, AHN p. 135) – Nursing interventions and patient teaching (FAAHN p. 1371, AHN p. 135)	▦ PPT 34 through 38, Ch. 44 FAAHN (Ch. 4 PPT 34 through 38 AHN) *e* EILR IC Ch. 44 images 11 through 21 FAAHN (Ch. 4 images 11 through 21 AHN) *e* EILR TB Ch. 44 questions 4, 40, 44 FAAHN (Ch. 4 questions 4, 40, 44 AHN) *e* EILR Open Book Quiz Ch. 44 question 7 FAAHN (Ch. 4 question 7 AHN) *e* ESLR Review Questions for the NCLEX Examination Ch. 44 questions 9, 10 FAAHN (Ch. 4 questions 9, 10 AHN) 📖 SG Surgery, Ch. 44 p. 348 FAAHN (Ch. 4 p. 36 AHN) **BOOK RESOURCES** Fig. 44-11 Tibian and femoral components of total knee prosthesis (FAAHN p. 1369) (Fig. 4-11 AHN p. 133) Fig. 44-12 Total joint replacements: knee (FAAHN p. 1369) (Fig. 4-12 AHN p. 133) ▸ Discuss the diagnostic tests that would be ordered for a patient scheduled to undergo surgical repair of a hip fracture. ▸ Discuss management of the hip fracture prior to surgical management.

OBJECTIVES	CONTENT	TEACHING RESOURCES
	☐ Fracture of the hip (FAAHN p. 1373, AHN p. 137) – Etiology and pathophysiology (FAAHN p. 1373, AHN p. 137) – Clinical manifestations (FAAHN p. 1374, AHN p. 138) – Assessment (FAAHN p. 1374, AHN p. 138) – Diagnostic tests (FAAHN p. 1375, AHN p. 139) – Medical management (FAAHN p. 1375, AHN p. 139) – Nursing interventions (FAAHN p. 1375, AHN p. 139) – Prognosis (FAAHN p. 1378, AHN p. 142)	*Class Activity Contact the surgical department of a local hospital. Ask to borrow hip prosthetics similar to those used in a hip replacement procedure. During class pass the equipment around. This will allow the students the opportunity to see and touch the materials used in the surgical intervention.*
Describe the nursing interventions for the patient undergoing a total hip or knee replacement.	■ Surgical interventions for total knee or total hip replacement (FAAHN p. 1369, AHN p. 133) ☐ Knee arthroplasty (total knee replacement) (FAAHN p. 1369, AHN p. 133) ☐ Hip arthroplasty (total hip replacement) (FAAHN p. 1371, AHN p. 135) – Assessment (FAAHN p. 1371, AHN p. 135) – Nursing interventions and patient teaching (FAAHN p. 1371, AHN p. 135)	PPT 34 through 38, Ch. 44 FAAHN (Ch. 4 PPT 34 through 38 AHN) EILR IC Ch. 44 images 11 through 21 FAAHN (Ch. 4 images 11 rthrough 21 AHN) EILR TB Ch. 44 questions 4, 6, 17, 40 FAAHN (Ch. 4 questions 4, 6, 17, 40 AHN) EILR Open Book Quiz Ch. 44 question 7 FAAHN (Ch. 4 question 7 AHN) SG Total Hip or Knee Replacement, Ch. 44 p. 348 FAAHN (Ch. 4 p. 36 AHN) **BOOK RESOURCES** Box 44-4 Nursing Interventions for the Patient Undergoing Total Knee Replacement (FAAHN p. 1370) (Box 4-4 AHN p. 134) Fig. 44-13 Continuous passive motion machine (FAAHN p. 1370) (Fig. 4-13 AHN p. 134) Fig. 44-14 Hip arthroplasty (total hip replacement) (FAAHN p. 1371) (Fig. 4-14 AHN p. 135)

Christensen & Kockrow

OBJECTIVES	CONTENT	TEACHING RESOURCES
		Fig. 44-15 Maintaining postoperative abduction after total hip replacement (FAAHN p. 1372) (Fig. 4-15 AHN p. 136) ▶ Discuss the complications that can occur in the postoperative period after a surgical hip replacement. ▶ Discuss patient teaching in preparation for discharge after a joint replacement surgery. *Class Activity Lead the class in a discussion concerning positions that patients must avoid after undergoing a total hip replacement. During the discussion, ask each student to demonstrate the positions that must be avoided.*
Discuss nursing interventions appropriate for a patient with a fractured hip after open reduction with internal fixation (ORIF) and bipolar hip prosthesis (hemiarthroplasty).	☐ Other fractures (FAAHN p. 1378, AHN p. 142) – Etiology and pathophysiology (FAAHN p. 1378, AHN p. 142) – Clinical manifestations (FAAHN p. 1380, AHN p. 144) – Assessment (FAAHN p. 1380, AHN p. 144) – Diagnostic tests (FAAHN p. 1381, AHN p. 145) – Medical management (FAAHN p. 1381, AHN p. 145) – Nursing interventions and patient teaching (FAAHN p. 1381, AHN p. 145) – Prognosis (FAAHN p. 1381, AHN p. 145) ☐ Fracture of the vertebrae (FAAHN p. 1381, AHN p. 145) – Etiology and pathophysiology (FAAHN p. 1381, AHN p. 145) – Clinical manifestations (FAAHN p. 1381, AHN p. 145) – Assessment (FAAHN p. 1381, AHN p. 145)	▨ PPT 39 through 44, Ch. 44 FAAHN (Ch. 4 PPT 39 through 44 AHN) 🄴 EILR IC Ch. 44 images 22 through 24 FAAHN (Ch. 4 images 22 through 24 AHN) 🄴 EILR TB Ch. 44 questions 24 through 26, 28, 29, 41 FAAHN (Ch. 4 questions 24 through 26, 28, 29, 41 AHN) 📖 SG Fractures, Ch. 44 p. 349 FAAHN (Ch. 4 p. 37 AHN) **BOOK RESOURCES** Life Span Considerations, Older Adults: Musculoskeletal Disorder (FAAHN p. 1373) (AHN p. 137) Health Promotion: Hip Fracture (FAAHN p. 1373) (AHN p. 137) Fig. 44-16 Fractures of the hip (FAAHN p. 1373) (Fig. 4-16 AHN p. 137) Fig. 44-17 Femur with location of various types of fractures (FAAHN p. 1374) (Fig. 4-17 AHN p. 138) Fig. 44-18 Anterior and posterior arterial blood supply to hip joint (FAAHN p. 1374) (Fig. 4-18 AHN p. 138) Fig. 44-19 Bipolar hip replacement (FAAHN p. 1374) (Fig. 4-19 AHN p. 138) Fig. 44-20 Nails and screws for fracture repair (FAAHN p. 1374) (Fig. 4-20 AHN p. 138)

ELSEVIER

OBJECTIVES	CONTENT	TEACHING RESOURCES
	– Diagnostic tests (FAAHN p. 1382, AHN p. 146) – Medical management (FAAHN p. 1382, AHN p. 146) – Nursing interventions and patient teaching (FAAHN p. 1382, AHN p. 146) – Prognosis (FAAHN p. 1383, AHN p. 147) ☐ Fracture of the pelvis (FAAHN p. 1383, AHN p. 147) – Etiology and pathophysiology (FAAHN p. 1383, AHN p. 147) – Clinical manifestations (FAAHN p. 1383, AHN p. 147) – Assessment (FAAHN p. 1383, AHN p. 147) – Diagnostic tests (FAAHN p. 1383, AHN p. 147) – Medical management (FAAHN p. 1384, AHN p. 148) – Nursing interventions and patient teaching (FAAHN p. 1384, AHN p. 148) – Prognosis (FAAIIN p. 1384, AHN p. 148)	Fig. 44-21 Instruction sheet for the patient with a bipolar hip replacement (hip prosthetic implant) (FAAHN p. 1376) (Fig. 4-21 AHN p. 140) Patient Teaching: Quadriceps Setting Exercises (FAAHN p. 1376) (AHN p. 140) Nursing Care Plan 14-1 The Patient with a Fractured Hip (FAAHN p. 1377) (AHN p. 141) Fig. 44-26 Compartment syndrome (FAAHN p. 1385) (Fig. 4-26 AHN p. 149) ▸ Discuss the use of a clinical pathway for the patient recovering from hip replacement surgery. ▸ Discuss the postoperative rehabilitation that is needed after surgery for hip replacement. *Class Activity Contact the local hospital. Invite a patient education staff member to speak to the class about the postoperative care of a patient who has hip replacement surgery. Other options for a speaker relating to this topic would include physical therapists or utilization review staff members.* *Class Activity Have students go to the lab and practice on each other as if the student has had a total hip replacement. Be sure to have students help the "patient" get out of bed and into a chair.*
Discuss the physiology of fracture healing (hematoma, granulation tissue, and callus formation).	☐ Other fractures (FAAHN p. 1378, AHN p. 142) – Etiology and pathophysiology (FAAHN p. 1378, AHN p. 142)	EILR TB Ch. 44 questions 9, 35 FAAHN (Ch. 4 questions 9, 35 AHN) EILR Open Book Quiz Ch. 44 question 10 FAAHN (Ch. 4 question 10 AHN) SG Fracture Healing, Ch. 44 p. 350 FAAHN (Ch. 4 p. 38 AHN) **BOOK RESOURCES** Fig. 44-22 Closed and open fractures (FAAHN p. 1378) (Fig. 4-22 AHN p. 142) Fig. 44-23 Common types of fractures (FAAHN p. 1379) (Fig. 4-23 AHN p. 143) Fig. 44-24 Bone fractures (FAAHN p. 1379) (Fig. 4-24 AHN p. 143)

Mosby items and derived items © 2011 by Mosby, Inc., an affiliate of Elsevier Inc.
Some material was previously published.

Christensen & Kockrow

OBJECTIVES	CONTENT	TEACHING RESOURCES
		Fig. 44-25 Halos (FAAHN p. 1382) (Fig. 4-25 AHN p. 146) ▸ Discuss the signs and symptoms of a fracture. ▸ Discuss the phases of bone healing. ▸ Discuss the comfort measures that can be provided to the patient who has experienced a fracture. *Class Activity Lead a class discussion in which potential causes of differing types of fractures are reviewed. Then have the students discuss how the bones actually heal.*

4.3 Homework/Assignments:

4.3 Instructor's Notes/Student Feedback:

Adult Health Nursing, 6th ed.
Christensen & Kockrow

LESSON 4.4

CRITICAL THINKING QUESTION

After being involved in a serious automobile accident, a 50-year-old man has been brought to the emergency room. The radiographic studies have been completed. The patient's physician has diagnosed a fractured right femur. After a closed reduction, the extremity was aligned. A long leg plaster cast was applied. The patient was then admitted to the hospital's orthopedic unit for overnight observation. What should be included in the nursing care during the first day after the cast has been applied? What information should be provided to the patient in preparation for discharge regarding cast care?

Guidelines: After the cast has been applied, it must be carefully handled. The nurse should only touch the fresh cast with the palms of the hands, thus avoiding the development of internal pressure points. The risk of pressure point development remains until the cast has dried (24 to 48 hours). The cast's drying may be facilitated by using a dryer on the low setting, exposing it to air, or placing it on cotton blankets.

The risk of edema is greatest during the initial period. Elevating the extremity on pillows will reduce this occurrence. Neurological assessments must be completed every 2 to 4 hours. These assessments include a review of the extremity's color, temperature, mobility, pulse, and sensation. Abnormal findings are cause for concern and are to be reported to the physician. An evaluation of pain is also needed. The characteristics of the pain need to be carefully monitored. Unrelieved pain could signal complications relating to pressure points or impaired circulation. Pain management is vital. Administer analgesics as prescribed.

Discharge teaching for the patient will include a discussion of nutritional needs, activity levels, signs and symptoms to report, potential complications, and general cast care.

OBJECTIVES	CONTENT	TEACHING RESOURCES
Describe the signs and symptoms of compartment syndrome.	☐ Complications of fractures (FAAHN p. 1384, AHN p. 148) ☐ Compartment syndrome (FAAHN p. 1384, AHN p. 148) – Assessment (FAAHN p. 1384, AHN p. 148) – Medical management (FAAHN p. 1384, AHN p. 148) – Nursing interventions (FAAHN p. 1384, AHN p. 148) – Prognosis (FAAHN p. 1385, AHN p. 149) ☐ Shock (FAAHN p. 1385, AHN p. 149) – Assessment (FAAHN p. 1385, AHN p. 149) – Medical management (FAAHN p. 1385, AHN p. 149) – Nursing interventions (FAAHN p. 1385, AHN p. 149) – Prognosis (FAAHN p. 1386, AHN p. 150)	▨ PPT 52, 53, Ch. 44 FAAHN (Ch. 4 PPT 52, 53 AHN) ▰ EILR IC Ch. 44 image 26 FAAHN (Ch. 4 image 26 AHN) ▰ EILR TB Ch. 44 questions 7, 23, 27, 39 FAAHN (Ch. 4 questions 7, 23, 27, 39 AHN) ▣ SG Fracture Complications, Ch. 44 p. 351 FAAHN (Ch. 4 p. 39 AHN) **BOOK RESOURCES** Fig. 44-27 External fixation apparatuses (FAAHN p. 1385) (Fig. 4-27 AHN p. 149) ▸ Discuss the signs and symptoms associated with compartment syndrome. ▸ Discuss the prognosis of the patient who develops compartment syndrome. What determines the long-range patient outcome? *Class Activity Develop note cards with a series of patient complaints. Gear the complaints toward the complications associated with fractures. This list would include compartment syndrome, fat embolus, shock, and osteomyelitis. Divide the students into groups of two. Assign each pair a*

OBJECTIVES	CONTENT	TEACHING RESOURCES
		complaint card. Instruct each group to role-play the patient reporting the signs and symptoms. After reviewing the clinical manifestations, each group is asked to determine the complication being reviewed.
List nursing interventions appropriate for a fat embolism.	☐ Fat embolism (FAAHN p. 1386, AHN p. 150) – Assessment (FAAHN p. 1386, AHN p. 150) – Diagnostic tests (FAAHN p. 1386, AHN p. 150) – Medical management (FAAHN p. 1386, AHN p. 150) – Nursing interventions (FAAHN p. 1386, AHN p. 150) – Prognosis (FAAHN p. 1386, AHN p. 150) ☐ Gas gangrene (FAAHN p. 1386, AHN p. 150) – Assessment (FAAHN p. 1386, AHN p. 150) – Medical management (FAAHN p. 1387, AHN p. 151) – Nursing interventions (FAAHN p. 1387, AHN p. 151) – Prognosis (FAAHN p. 1387, AHN p. 151) ☐ Thromboembolus (FAAHN p. 1387, AHN p. 151) – Etiology and pathophysiology (FAAHN p. 1387, AHN p. 151) – Clinical manifestations (FAAHN p. 1387, AHN p. 151) – Assessment (FAAHN p. 1387, AHN p. 151) – Diagnostic tests (FAAHN p. 1387, AHN p. 151) – Medical management (FAAHN p. 1387, AHN p. 151) – Nursing interventions (FAAHN p. 1387, AHN p. 151)	▣▬ PPT 55 through 58, Ch. 44 FAAHN (Ch. 4 PPT 55 through 58 AHN) ✎ EILR TB Ch. 44 questions 13, 14, 29 FAAHN (Ch. 4 questions 13, 14, 29 AHN) SG Fracture Complications, Ch. 44 p. 351 FAAHN (Ch. 4 p. 39 AHN) **BOOK RESOURCES** Safety Alert! Thromboembolus (FAAHN p. 1387) (AHN p. 151) ▸ Discuss the pathophysiology of a fat embolism. ▸ Discuss prioritization of the treatment interventions that are implemented when a fat embolism occurs. *Class Activity Divide students into groups of three or four. Ask each group to develop an NCLEX-style question for each of the complications of a fracture. Ask the group to provide rationales for the correct answers and explanations for why each of the wrong answers was not the best selection. After the groups are allowed to finish the task, collect the questions. Plan to use them as discussion points and group presentations at a later date.*

OBJECTIVES	CONTENT	TEACHING RESOURCES
	– Prognosis (FAAHN p. 1387, AHN p. 151)	
	☐ Delayed fracture healing (FAAHN p. 1388, AHN p. 152)	
	– Prognosis (FAAHN p. 1388, AHN p. 152)	
List at least two types of skin and skeletal traction.	■ Skeletal fixation devices (FAAHN p. 1388, AHN p. 152)	🖳 PPT 59 through 60, Ch. 44 FAAHN (Ch. 4 PPT 59 through 60 AHN)
	☐ External fixation devices (FAAHN p. 1388, AHN p. 152)	📖 EILR IC Ch. 44 images 31, 32 FAAHN (Ch. 4 images 31, 32 AHN)
	– Skeletal pin external fixation (FAAHN p. 1388, AHN p. 152)	📖 EILR TB Ch. 44 questions 15, 42, 43 FAAHN (Ch. 4 questions 15, 42, 43 AHN)
	■ Nonsurgical interventions for musculoskeletal disorders (FAAHN p. 1389, AHN p. 153)	📖 SG Traction, Ch. 44 p. 351 FAAHN (Ch. 4 p. 39 AHN)
	☐ Casts (FAAHN p. 1389, AHN p. 153)	**BOOK RESOURCES**
		Fig. 44-28 Spica casts (FAAIIN p. 1389) (Fig. 4-28 AHN p. 153)
	– Cast brace (FAAHN p. 1389, AHN p. 153)	Fig. 44-29 Short-leg walking cast with cast shoe (FAAHN p. 1390) (Fig. 4-29 AIIN p. 154)
	– Assessment (FAAHN p. 1389, AHN p. 153)	Fig. 44-30 Capillary refill assessment (FAAHN p. 1390) (Fig. 4-30 AHN p. 154)
	– Nursing interventions and patient teaching (FAAHN p. 1390, AHN p. 154)	Fig. 44-31 Traction (FAAHN p. 1392) (Fig. 4-31 AHN p. 156)
	☐ Cast removal (FAAHN p. 1392, AHN p. 156)	Skill 44-1 Care of the Patient in a Case (FAAHN pp. 1390-1392) (Skill 4-1 AHN pp. 154-156)
	☐ Traction (FAAHN p. 1392, AHN p. 156)	Box 44-6 Nursing Interventions for the Patient in Traction (FAAHN p. 1393) (Box 4-6 AHN p. 157)
	– Skeletal traction (FAAHN p. 1392, AHN p. 156)	Fig. 44-32 Three types of traction (FAAHN p. 1393) (Fig. 4-32 AHN p. 157)
	– Skin traction (FAAHN p. 1392, AHN p. 156)	Fig. 44-33 Crutch walking (FAAHN p. 1394) (Fig. 4-33 AHN p. 158)
	– Nursing interventions (FAAHN p. 1393, AHN p. 157)	Safety Alert! Crutch Safety (FAAHN p. 1394) (AHN p. 158)
	☐ Orthopedic devices (FAAHN p. 1393, AHN p. 157)	Fig. 44-34 Assisting the patient with crutch walking (FAAHN p. 1395) (Fig 4-34 AHN p. 159)
		Fig. 44-35 Quad cane (FAAHN p. 1395) (Fig. 4-35 AHN p. 159)
		Fig. 44-36 Patient using a walker(FAAHN p. 1395) (Fig. 4-36 AHN p. 159)

Christensen & Kockrow

OBJECTIVES	CONTENT	TEACHING RESOURCES
		Fig. 44-37 The Roll-A-Bout walker (FAAHN p. 1395) (Fig. 4-37 AHN p. 159)
		Fig. 44-38 Treatment of carpal tunnel syndrome (FAAHN p. 1399) (Fig. 4-38 AHN p. 163)
		Fig. 44-39 Sagittal section of vertebrae showing both normal and herniated disks (FAAHN p. 1400) (Fig. 4-39 AHN p. 164)
		▸ Discuss the nursing responsibilities for care of a patient in traction.
		▸ Discuss the differences between skeletal and skin traction.
		*Class Activity **Lead a group discussion to develop a nursing care plan for the patient in traction. Include three priority nursing diagnoses. Provide rationale for each of the nursing interventions.***
Compare methods for assessing circulation, nerve damage, and infection in a patient who has a traumatic insult to the musculoskeletal system.	■ Traumatic injuries (FAAHN p. 1396, AHN p. 160) □ Contusions (FAAHN p. 1396, AHN p. 160) – Etiology and pathophysiology/clinical manifestations (FAAHN p. 1396, AHN p. 160) – Medical management (FAAHN p. 1396, AHN p. 160) – Prognosis (FAAHN p. 1396, AHN p. 160) □ Sprains (FAAHN p. 1396, AHN p. 160) – Etiology and pathophysiology/clinical manifestations (FAAHN p. 1396, AHN p. 160) – Prognosis (FAAHN p. 1396, AHN p. 160) □ Whiplash (FAAHN p. 1396, AHN p. 160) – Etiology and pathophysiology/clinical manifestations (FAAHN p. 1396, AHN p. 160) – Assessment (FAAHN p. 1396, AHN p. 160) – Diagnostic tests (FAAHN p. 1396, AHN p. 160)	⊠ PPT 61 through 72, Ch. 44 FAAHN (Ch. 4 PPT 61 through 72 AHN) ▰ EILR IC Ch. 44 image 30 FAAHN (Ch. 4 image 30 AHN) ▰ EILR TB Ch. 44 questions 8, 10, 12, 16, 45 FAAHN (Ch. 4 questions 8, 10, 12, 16, 45 AHN) ▤ SG Data Collection, Ch. 44 p. 352 FAAHN (Ch. 4 p. 40 AHN) **BOOK RESOURCES** Box 44-5 Circulation Check (Neurovascular Assessment) (FAAHN p. 1375) (Box 4-5 AHN p. 139) ▸ Discuss the activities associated with the development of contusions, sprains, whiplash, and strains. How do these injuries differ? ▸ Discuss nursing care for the patient who has experienced a traumatic injury to the musculoskeletal system. *Class Activity **Ask each student to develop an NCLEX-style question involving sprains, strains, contusions, or whiplash. Collect the questions. Use the questions as a review for the material.***

OBJECTIVES	CONTENT	TEACHING RESOURCES
	– Medical management (FAAHN p. 1396, AHN p. 160)	
	– Nursing interventions (FAAHN p. 1397, AHN p. 161)	
	– Prognosis (FAAHN p. 1397, AHN p. 161)	
	☐ Ankle sprains (FAAHN p. 1397, AHN p. 161)	
	– Etiology and pathophysiology (FAAHN p. 1397, AHN p. 161)	
	– Clinical manifestations (FAAHN p. 1397, AHN p. 161)	
	– Assessment (FAAHN p. 1397, AHN p. 161)	
	– Diagnostic tests (FAAHN p. 1397, AHN p. 161)	
	– Medical management (FAAHN p. 1397, AHN p. 161)	
	– Nursing interventions (FAAHN p. 1397, AHN p. 161)	
	– Prognosis (FAAHN p. 1397, AHN p. 161)	
	☐ Strains (FAAHN p. 1397, AHN p. 161)	
	– Etiology and pathophysiology/ clinical manifestations (FAAHN p. 1397, AHN p. 161)	
	– Assessment (FAAHN p. 1397, AHN p. 161)	
	– Diagnostic tests (FAAHN p. 1397, AHN p. 161)	
	– Medical management (FAAHN p. 1397, AHN p. 161)	
	– Nursing interventions (FAAHN p. 1397, AHN p. 161)	
	– Prognosis (FAAHN p. 1397, AHN p. 161)	
	☐ Dislocations (FAAHN p. 1398, AHN p. 162)	
	– Etiology and pathophysiology (FAAHN p. 1398, AHN p. 162)	
	– Clinical manifestations (FAAHN p. 1398, AHN p. 162)	

Christensen & Kockrow

OBJECTIVES	CONTENT	TEACHING RESOURCES
	– Assessment (FAAHN p. 1398, AHN p. 162)	
	– Diagnostic tests (FAAHN p. 1398, AHN p. 162)	
	– Medical management (FAAHN p. 1398, AHN p. 162)	
	– Nursing interventions and patient teaching (FAAHN p. 1398, AHN p. 162)	
	– Prognosis (FAAHN p. 1399, AHN p. 163)	
	☐ Airbag injuries (FAAHN p. 1399, AHN p. 163)	
	☐ Carpal tunnel syndrome (FAAHN p. 1399, AHN p. 163)	
	– Etiology and pathophysiology (FAAHN p. 1399, AHN p. 163)	
	– Clinical manifestations (FAAHN p. 1399, AHN p. 163)	
	– Assessment (FAAHN p. 1399, AHN p. 163)	
	– Diagnostic tests (FAAHN p. 1399, AHN p. 163)	
	– Medical management (FAAHN p. 1400, AHN p. 164)	
	– Nursing interventions and patient teaching (FAAHN p. 1400, AHN p. 164)	
	– Prognosis (FAAHN p. 1400, AHN p. 164)	
	☐ Herniation of intervertebral disk (herniated nucleus pulposus) (FAAHN p. 1400, AHN p. 164)	
	– Etiology and pathophysiology (FAAHN p. 1400, AHN p. 164)	
	– Clinical manifestations (FAAHN p. 1400, AHN p. 164)	
	– Assessment (FAAHN p. 1401, AHN p. 165)	
	– Diagnostic tests (FAAHN p. 1401, AHN p. 165)	

OBJECTIVES	CONTENT	TEACHING RESOURCES
	– Medical management (FAAHN p. 1401, AHN p. 165)	
	– Nursing interventions and patient teaching (FAAHN p. 1401, AHN p. 165)	
	– Prognosis (FAAHN p. 1402, AHN p. 166)	

4.4 Homework/Assignments:

4.4 Instructor's Notes/Student Feedback:

Christensen & Kockrow

LESSON 4.5

CRITICAL THINKING QUESTION

A 40-year-old woman, who had a recent mastectomy, is discussing her pain with the nurse about the right pain control for her situation. What questions should the nurse ask the woman so the pain is described accurately?

Guidelines: The nurse might ask the woman where the pain is located, how the pain feels, the degree of pain, and how frequently the pain occurs. The nurse should document the pain on the patient's record, recommend interventions for pain control methods, and monitor the patient's response to those methods.

OBJECTIVES	CONTENT	TEACHING RESOURCES
List four nursing interventions appropriate for bone cancer.	☐ Tumors of the bone (FAAHN p. 1402, AHN p. 166) – Etiology and pathophysiology (FAAHN p. 1402, AHN p. 166) – Clinical manifestations (FAAHN p. 1402, AHN p. 166) – Assessment (FAAHN p. 1402, AHN p. 166) – Diagnostic tests (FAAHN p. 1402, AHN p. 166) – Medical management (FAAHN p. 1402, AHN p. 166) – Nursing interventions (FAAHN p. 1403, AHN p. 167) – Prognosis (FAAHN p. 1403, AHN p. 167)	PPT 73, 74, Ch. 44 FAAHN (Ch. 4 PPT 73, 74 AHN) Bone Cancer, Ch. 44 p. 352 FAAHN (Ch. 4 p. 40 AHN) ▶ Discuss populations at increased risk of developing bone cancer. ▶ Discuss the signs and symptoms of bone cancer. ▶ Discuss the anticipated diagnostic test results associated with bone cancer. ▶ Discuss the prognosis of bone cancer. *Class Activity Perform a test review of the content. Group the class into two or three teams. Ask questions of each team involving tumors of the bone. The group having the most correct answers will win.*
Describe the phenomenon of phantom pain.	☐ Amputation (FAAHN p. 1403, AHN p. 167) – Preoperative assessment (FAAHN p. 1403, AHN p. 167) – Diagnostic tests (FAAHN p. 1403, AHN p. 167) – Medical management (FAAHN p. 1403, AHN p. 167) – Postoperative assessment, nursing interventions, and patient teaching (FAAHN p. 1404, AHN p. 168) – Prognosis (FAAHN p. 1405, AHN p. 169)	PPT 75, 76, Ch. 44 FAAHN (Ch. 4 PPT 75, 76 AHN) EILR IC Ch. 44 image 40 FAAHN (Ch. 4 image 40 AHN) EILR TB Ch. 44 questions 5, 11 FAAHN (Ch. 4 questions 5, 11 AHN) SG Phantom Pain, Ch. 44 p. 353 FAAHN (Ch. 4 p. 41 AHN) **BOOK RESOURCES** Fig. 44-40 Correct method of bandaging amputation stump (FAAHN p. 1404) (Fig. 4-40 AHN p. 168) ▶ Discuss the medical reasons that necessitate surgical amputation.

Adult Health Nursing, 6th ed.
Christensen & Kockrow

OBJECTIVES	CONTENT	TEACHING RESOURCES
		▶ Discuss postoperative positioning for the patient who has had an amputation.
		*Class Activity **Assign each student a partner. Next, pass an object around the room. Ask a question about amputations to each pair when they have the object. After the pair provides a correct answer, they may sit down. Continue the game until the entire class is sitting.***
Describe the following conditions: lordosis, scoliosis, and kyphosis.	☐ Nursing process for musculoskeletal function (FAAHN p. 1405, AHN p. 169) — Assessment (FAAHN p. 1405, AHN p. 169) — Nursing diagnosis (FAAHN p. 1406, AHN p. 170) — Expected outcomes and planning (FAAHN p. 1406, AHN p. 170) — Implementation (FAAHN p. 1407, AHN p. 171) — Evaluation (FAAHN p. 1407, AHN p. 171)	▣▬ PPT 77, Ch. 44 FAAHN (Ch. 4 PPT 77 AHN) ▰ EILR IC Ch. 44 image 41 FAAHN (Ch. 4 image 41 AHN) ▰ EILR TB Ch. 44 question 30 FAAHN (Ch. 4 question 30 AHN) ▰ SG Medical Terminology Versus Patient Terminology, Ch. 44 p. 353 FAAHN (Ch. 4 p. 41 AHN) **BOOK RESOURCES** Fig. 44-41 Abnormal spinal curvatures (FAAHN p. 1406) (Fig. 4-41 AHN p. 170) ▶ Discuss the clinical manifestations associated with abnormal spinal curvatures. ▶ Discuss the psychological concerns that accompany the diagnosis and treatment of scoliosis. *Class Activity **Invite a school nurse to come to the class. Ask the school nurse to review the process used in screening children for scoliosis.***

OBJECTIVES	CONTENT	TEACHING RESOURCES
Performance Evaluation		EILR TB Ch. 44 questions 1 through 46 FAAHN (Ch. 4 questions 1 through 46 AHN) EILR Open Book Quiz Ch. 44 questions 1 through 10 FAAHN (Ch. 4 questions 1 through 10 AHN) ESLR Review Questions for the NCLEX Examination Ch. 44 questions 1 through 10 FAAHN (Ch. 4 questions 1 through 10 AHN) SG Ch. 44 pp. 343-356 FAAHN (Ch. 4 pp. 31-44 AHN) **BOOK RESOURCES** Review Questions for the NCLEX Examination Ch. 10 questions 1 through 25 FAAHN (Ch. 10 questions 1 through 25 AHN)

4.5 Homework/Assignments:

4.5 Instructor's Notes/Student Feedback:

Adult Health Nursing, 6th ed.
Christensen & Kockrow

Slide 1

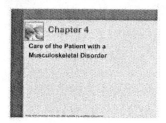

Slide 2

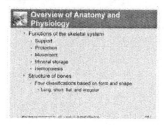

- The skeletal system performs five vital functions in the body. These functions include support, protection, movement, mineral storage, and hemopoiesis.

- Review the minerals that play a role in the functioning of the skeletal system.

- How does the body compensate for alterations in dietary intake of these minerals?

Slide 3

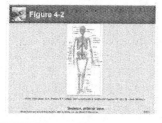

- Review the types of bones discussed in the previous slide. What are specific examples of each of the different types of bones in the skeleton?

Slide 4

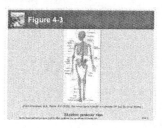

Slide 5

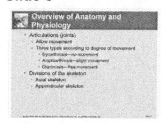

- What are examples of each of the joint types?

- Provide examples of bones in the axial skeleton.

- What are some of the bones in the appendicular skeleton?

Slide 6

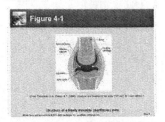

Slide 7

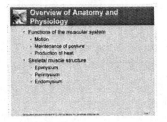

- Contraction and relaxation provides the motion needed for muscular movement.
- Review how tendons and ligaments differ.
- How do muscles provide posture for the body?
- Approximately 85% of the body's heat is produced by the muscles. What processes are responsible for this vital function?

Slide 8

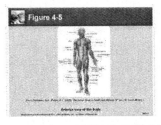

- The body contains more than 600 muscles.

Slide 9

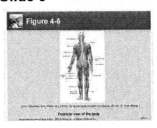

- Nearly 40% to 50% of the body's weight is due to its muscles.

Slide 10

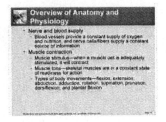

- Nutrition and oxygenation are chief requirements for muscle health. Optimal muscle health is needed to maintain the constant state of readiness of the body for action and reaction.
- How will disease processes of the muscles impact the body's ability to move?

Slide 11

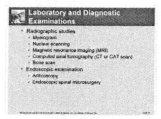

- Radiographic studies are the most common type of diagnostic testing done for the musculoskeletal system.

- What special precautions and nursing implications are needed for patients undergoing radiographic studies?

- How is arthroscopy both diagnostic and therapeutic in nature?

Slide 12

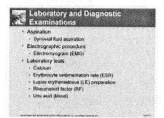

- Needle aspiration is used to obtain body fluids from joint cavities. Review the nursing interventions when caring for a patient having this type of examination.

- When caring for a patient undergoing diagnostic musculoskeletal testing, what education should be provided to the patient?

Slide 13

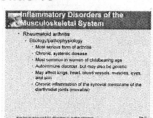

- An estimated 50 million Americans are victims of arthritis. Arthritis is a costly disease resulting in lost wages and health care expenses.

- Review the autoimmune reaction that is suspected when rheumatoid arthritis strikes.

Slide 14

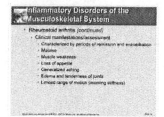

Slide 15

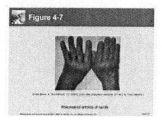

- Notice how the patient's fingers are affected by rheumatoid arthritis.

Adult Health Nursing, 6th ed.
Christensen & Kockrow

Slide 16

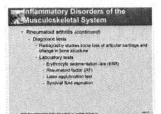

- A single definitive diagnostic tool for rheumatoid arthritis is not available. A diagnosis involves a complete physical examination and patient history.
- Review the anticipated findings in the erythrocyte sedimentation rate, Rheumatoid factor, latex agglutination test, and synovial fluid aspiration when a diagnosis of rheumatoid arthritis is confirmed.
- What other disorders could have similar diagnostic test results?

Slide 17

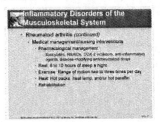

- Rheumatoid arthritis is a chronic disease with no known cure.
- "Quiet" exercise is recommended. What are examples of quiet exercise?
- What are the goals of disease management?
- Given the age of the most commonly stricken population and the absence of a complete cure, what are potential psychosocial implications for a family after a member is diagnosed with rheumatoid arthritis?

Slide 18

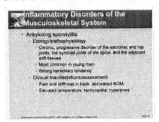

- Ankylosing spondylitis is a progressive inflammatory disorder. Although both men and women are affected, it is typically milder in women.
- How does ankylosing spondylitis differ from rheumatoid arthritis?

Slide 19

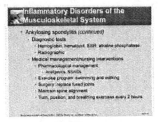

- Review the diagnostic tests used to confirm the presence of anklyosing spondylitis. What findings for each test are used in the confirmation process?

Slide 20

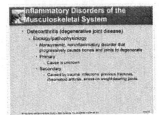

- Osteoarthritis is the most common type of arthritis. It is a chief cause of disability.
- What risk factors are associated with the development of osteoarthritis?
- Differentiate between the modifiable and nonmodifiable risk factors.
- What impact does aging have on the development of osteoarthritis?

Adult Health Nursing, 6th ed.

Mosby items and derived items © 2011, 2007 by Mosby, Inc., an affiliate of Elsevier Inc. Some material was previously published.

Christensen & Kockrow

Slide 21

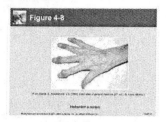

- Heberden's nodes are nodules on the distal sides of the fingers' joints.
- Explain how Heberden's nodes differ from Bouchard's nodes.

Slide 22

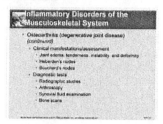

- There are no definitive tests available for osteoarthritis.
- What findings can be anticipated when a diagnosis of osteoarthritis is confirmed?
- Compare and contrast osteoarthritis and rheumatoid arthritis.

Slide 23

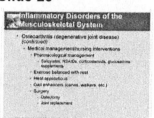

- What are the goals of disease management for osteoarthritis?
- What is the role of the nurse in the care of a patient diagnosed with osteoarthritis?

Slide 24

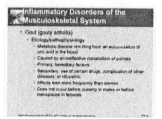

Slide 25

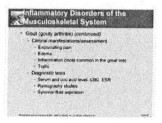

- Discuss the characteristics of the pain experienced by the patient having gout.
- What subjective data should be collected by the nurse from the patient suspected of having gout?

Slide 26

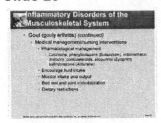

- Develop a list of foods that should be avoided by the patient diagnosed with gout.

- What is the importance of monitoring kidney function in the patient with gout?

- Purines are restricted in the patient with gout. What foods should be avoided?

Slide 27

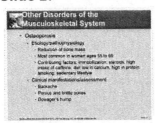

- Osteoporosis is a disorder in which the skeleton's function is impaired because of the loss of bone mass.

- Explore reasons that support the development of osteoporosis in high-risk populations. Why are women affected more often than men? How does immobility or a sedentary lifestyle influence the onset of osteoporosis?

Slide 28

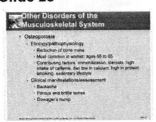

- What laboratory findings support a diagnosis of osteoporosis?

- Develop a list of calcium-rich foods.

- Review the nursing implications for the administration of Fosamax.

Slide 29

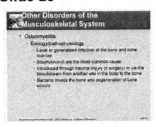

- What other organisms are associated with osteomyelitis?

- Identify patient populations at increased risk for the development of osteomyelitis. What behaviors or pathophysiology increase their risk of developing the infection?

Slide 30

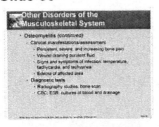

- What subjective data will be collected by the nurse?

- What objective data will be collected by the nurse?

- Review diagnostic findings supportive of a diagnosis of osteomyelitis.

Adult Health Nursing, 6th ed.

Christensen & Kockrow

Slide 31

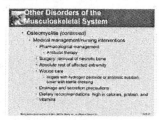

- The treatment regimen prescribed for osteomyelitis is lengthy.

- Parenteral antibiotics are needed for several weeks.

- What broad-spectrum antibiotics could be used to treat osteomyelitis?

- When planning patient education, what elements concerning safety should be included for the patient diagnosed with osteomyelitis?

Slide 32

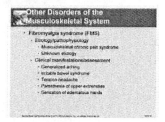

- Fibromyalgia syndrome is a disorder associated with chronic pain. The vague complaints often make diagnosis challenging.

- In what population is fibromyalgia syndrome most commonly seen?

Slide 33

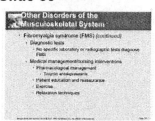

- Given the often lengthy period of illness that precedes a diagnosis, what are some psychological concerns that could be experienced by a patient suspected of having fibromyalgia syndrome?

- What is the impact of tricyclic antidepressants on the patient with fibromyalgia?

Slide 34

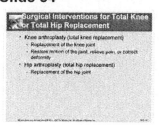

- What patients can be helped/treated by undergoing a hip or knee replacement?

Slide 35

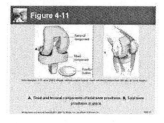

Slide 36

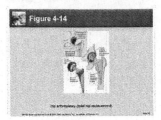

Slide 37

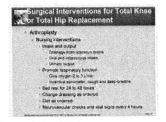

- What are the patient goals for the patient undergoing a total joint replacement?
- Outline the priorities for nursing care during the postoperative period following a total joint replacement.

Slide 38

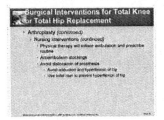

Slide 39

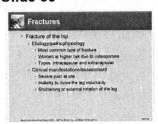

- The elderly are at risk for hip fractures. What factors associated with aging promote this population's increased risk?
- How can hip fractures in the elderly be prevented?
- Review the 7-Ps that must be reviewed when completing a neurological assessment in a patient suspected of having a fractured hip.
- How should abnormal findings in the "7-P" assessment be handled?

Slide 40

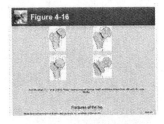

Slide 41

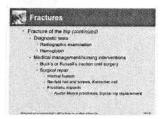

- In an effort to prevent further damage, the leg and hip must be kept as still as possible. Review the role of traction in the care of a patient who has suffered a fracture to the hip. How is this traction applied?
- What laboratory test results can be seen when evaluating the hemoglobin and blood glucose of a patient whose hip is fractured?

Slide 42

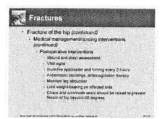

- What are the goals of nursing care for the patient who has undergone a total hip or knee replacement?
- Review the parameters for abnormal and normal findings in the postoperative period.

Slide 43

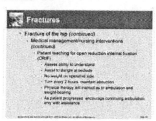

- List the potential complications associated with total hip and knee replacement surgeries.

Slide 44

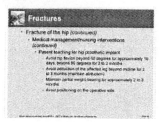

- Demonstrate positioning options for the patient who has had a total hip replacement surgery. Define abduction and adduction.
- What positions are contraindicated? Why? Review alternative positions that can be used by the patient.

Slide 45

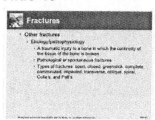

- Fractures occurring as a result of an injury or trauma are termed "spontaneous."
- Pathological fractures happen due to a disease process.
- Give examples of both spontaneous and pathological fractures.

Adult Health Nursing, 6th ed.

Christensen & Kockrow

Slide 46

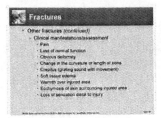

Slide 47

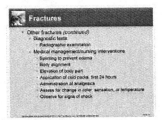

- Review the rationale for the interventions to manage a fracture.

Slide 48

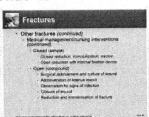

- An open fracture is one in which the bone has broken through the skin. A closed fracture has not protruded through the skin.

- When caring for a closed fracture, a cast can be employed to immobilize the fracture. Review the nursing responsibilities when caring for a newly casted extremity.

- An open fracture has a unique set of potential risk factors. What medical concerns are raised when an open fracture occurs?

Slide 49

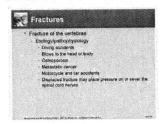

- Vertebral fractures happen due to a variety of causes. Injuries can involve the vertebral body, articulating processes, and lamina.

- What factors will determine if permanent paralysis will occur as a result of the injury?

Slide 50

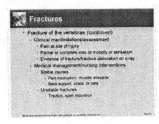

- The patient might or might not experience pain after a vertebral fracture. How can a lack of discomfort be explained?

- Assessment of neurological function is vital when caring for the patient who has suffered a vertebral fracture. What should be included in the neurological assessment?

- Review the medication therapy that will accompany the postinjury care of a patient who has experienced a vertebral fracture.

ELSEVIER

Adult Health Nursing, 6th ed.
Christensen & Kockrow

Slide 51

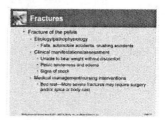

- A fracture of the pelvis may be accompanied with injuries to other parts of the body.

- What other body systems can be involved?

- Review signs and symptoms that indicate additional trauma to the area.

Slide 52

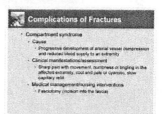

- Review the presence of compartments in the body's extremities.

- What prognosis accompanies the development of compartment syndrome?

- Identify factors that affect this prognosis.

Slide 53

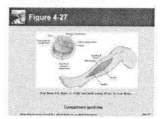

Slide 54

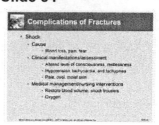

- Shock related to a bone fracture can occur for one of two reasons. Bone is vascular and can experience blood loss. Severed blood vessels from the injury can also cause significant blood loss followed by shock.

- Review the early and late clinical manifestations of shock.

- Prioritize the interventions associated with treatment and management of shock.

- What precautions should be taken during management of the patient experiencing shock?

Slide 55

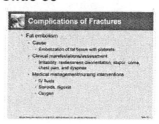

- Development of a fat embolism is rare.

- Identify at-risk populations for the occurrence of a fat embolism.

- In what time frame is the typical fat embolism seen in the patient?

- Prioritize care and treatment interventions for the management of a patient who has experienced a fat embolism.

ELSEVIER

Adult Health Nursing, 6th ed.

Mosby items and derived items © 2011, 2007 by Mosby, Inc., an affiliate of Elsevier Inc.
Some material was previously published.

Christensen & Kockrow

Slide 56

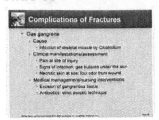

- How can a patient be exposed to the *Clostridium* toxin associated with gas gangrene?

Slide 57

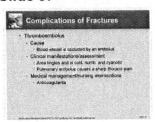

- A clot carried through the bloodstream from the site of formation to another site, resulting in an occluded vessel, is known as a thromboembolism.

- Identify fractures that are at higher risk for developing this complication.

- Demonstrate an assessment for the Homan's sign.

- What nursing implications accompany the administration of anticoagulation therapy?

- What diagnostic tests can be anticipated with the development of this complication?

Slide 58

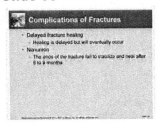

- Identify populations at an increased risk for delayed fracture healing or nonunion.

- Review the prognosis for these diseases.

Slide 59

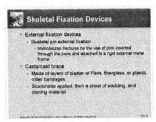

- Numerous options are available to manage fractures. What information will be used to determine the best option for an individual patient?

- When a cast is used to immobilize a fracture, what postapplication assessments will the nurse perform?

- How should a cast be cared for?

- Discuss care of the extremity after the cast is removed.

Slide 60

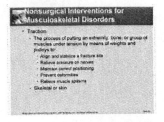

- Compare and contrast skeletal and skin traction.

Adult Health Nursing, 6th ed.

Christensen & Kockrow

Slide 61

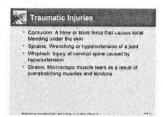

- Injuries to the musculoskeletal system's supportive structures result from a variety of actions including sports, exercise, and accidents.
- What types of activities would result in contusions, sprains, whiplash, and strains?
- What do sprains, whiplash, and strains have in common?

Slide 62

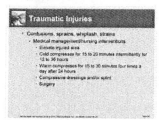

- The care given to contusions, sprains, whiplash, and strains is initially supportive in nature. What are the primary goals of treatment?
- Review the rationale for the use of cold and warm compresses. Why is cold therapy used initially?
- When does surgery become needed?

Slide 63

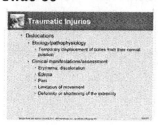

- Dislocations can result from the following: congenital causes, trauma, or disease processes.
- What are some of the more common locations affected by dislocations? What do these locations have in common?

Slide 64

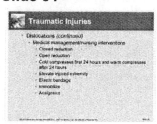

- Treatment of dislocations can be noninvasive or surgical.
- What are the primary goals of the nursing care for dislocations?
- Identify examples of analgesics that are to be used to treat dislocations.

Slide 65

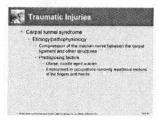

- Compression of the median nerve within the wrist results in a syndrome known as carpal tunnel. It is a painful disorder.
- Populations at risk for development of the disorder include obese, middle-aged women, occupations using repetitive wrist and hand movements, and pregnancy. Why do the people in these categories develop this disorder?

Adult Health Nursing, 6th ed.

Mosby items and derived items © 2011, 2007 by Mosby, Inc., an affiliate of Elsevier Inc.   Christensen & Kockrow
Some material was previously published.

Slide 66

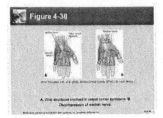

Slide 67

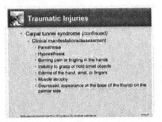

Slide 68

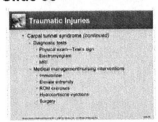

- The diagnosis of carpal tunnel includes an electromyogram and an MRI. What findings from these tests are indicative of carpal tunnel syndrome?

- What is the role of the nurse in the provision of care for the patient undergoing surgical management of carpal tunnel syndrome?

Slide 69

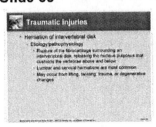

- Any portion of the spine can be affected with disk herniation. Herniation could occur suddenly or over time as a result of a disease process.

- Provide examples of disorders that could cause a herniation.

- Lumbar and cervical herniations are seen most frequently. What about their location predisposes for this condition?

Slide 70

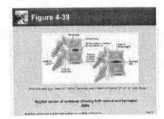

Adult Health Nursing, 6th ed.
Christensen & Kockrow

Slide 71

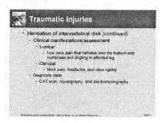

- When the patient seeks treatment for the herniated disk, pain is one of the common complaints. What questions should the nurse ask when gathering the health history relating to this situation?
- Diagnostic tests employed to diagnose a herniated disk include a CT scan, myelography, and electromyelography. What findings are supportive of a diagnosis of disk herniation?

Slide 72

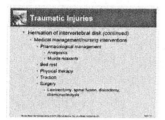

- Typically conservative management interventions are implemented in the care of the herniated disk. Rest, pharmacological therapies, and physical therapy are implemented first.
- What is the desired outcome of physical therapy?
- Discuss the medications prescribed in the management of herniated disks.

Slide 73

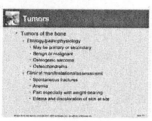

- Osteogenic sarcoma is a rapidly growing malignant tumor. The involved bones are usually the femur, tibia, and humerus. It is most commonly seen in males 10 to 25 years old.
- Osteochondroma is the most common benign tumor. Like osteogenic sarcoma, it is most commonly seen in the femur, tibia, and humerus. Again, males are the most commonly involved population.
- Why do spontaneous fractures accompany bone tumors?
- Review the etiology of anemia that can occur with a bone tumor.

Slide 74

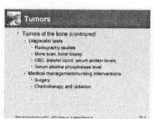

- When bone tumors are suspected, serum blood levels may be assessed. What findings are expected on complete blood counts, platelet counts, and serum protein levels when a diagnosis of a bone tumor is present?
- What factors will determine the treatment regimen employed?
- Discuss the prognosis that accompanies a diagnosis of bone cancer.

Slide 75

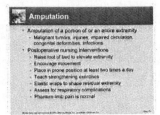

- Amputation is the removal of all or a portion of an extremity. The amputation can be traumatic or surgical.

- Amputation is done for differing purposes. It might be done to promote function, to treat a disease process, or for cosmetic functions.

- The loss of a body part is accompanied with psychological anguish. What concerns and feelings might be voiced by a patient who has had an amputation?

- What is the role of the nurse during the period preceding the amputation?

- Identify the role of the nurse in the postoperative period.

Slide 76

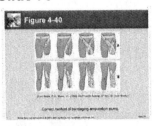

- Following an amputation, the extremity is usually wrapped using elastic bandages. What purpose does this serve? How long are the elastic bandages used?

Slide 77

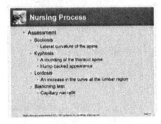

Slide 78

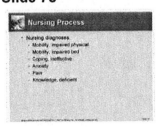

- When developing a care plan for the patient experiencing complications of the musculoskeletal system, potential nursing diagnoses involve mobility, coping, anxiety, pain, and knowledge deficit.

- What patient outcomes can accompany these diagnoses? How are they best evaluated?

5 Care of the Patient with a Gastrointestinal Disorder

TEACHING FOCUS

In this chapter, the student will be introduced to the structure and function of the gastrointestinal system. The student then will explore the diagnostic tools and the nursing interventions for patients with gastrointestinal disorders. The student will have the opportunity to investigate a variety of gastrointestinal disorders, along with nursing care of the gastric surgery patient.

MATERIALS AND RESOURCES

- ☐ Computer/overhead projector (all lessons)
- ☐ White/black board and marker/chalk (all lessons)
- ☐ Tennis ball (Lesson 5.4)

LESSON CHECKLIST

Preparations for this lesson include:

- Lecture
- Invite a cancer survivor who has had gastric surgery to speak to the class.
- Invite a patient educator or other professional from a local hospital to discuss the nurse's role in the care of the patient who has had a fecal diversion.

KEY TERMS

achalasia (FAAHN p. 1425, AHN p. 189)
achlorhydria (FAAHN p. 1416, AHN p. 180)
anastomosis (FAAHN p. 1425, AHN p. 189)
cachexia (FAAHN p. 1457, AHN p. 221)
carcinoembryonic antigen (CEA) (FAAHN p. 1457, AHN p. 221)
dehiscence (FAAHN p. 1436, AHN p. 200)
dysphagia (FAAHN p. 1424, AHN p. 188)
evisceration (FAAHN p. 1436, AHN p. 200)
exacerbations (FAAHN p. 1441, AHN p. 205)
hematemesis (FAAHN p. 1428, AHN p. 192)
intussusception (FAAHN p. 1418, AHN p. 182)

leukoplakia (FAAHN p. 1421, AHN p. 185)
lumen (FAAHN p. 1418, AHN p. 182)
melena (FAAHN p. 1428, AHN p. 192)
occult blood (FAAHN p. 1418, AHN p. 182)
paralytic (adynamic) ileus (FAAHN p. 1454, AHN p. 218)
pathognomonic (FAAHN p. 1419, AHN p. 183)
remissions (FAAHN p. 1441, AHN p. 205)
steatorrhea (FAAHN p. 1446, AHN p. 210)
stoma (FAAHN p. 1445, AHN p. 209)
tenesmus (FAAHN p. 1438, AHN p. 202)
volvulus (FAAHN p. 1454, AHN p. 218)

ADDITIONAL RESOURCES (AHN)

PPT Ch. 45, 1 through 69 FAAHN (Ch. 5, 1 through 69 AHN)
EILR IC images Ch. 45, 1 through 20 FAAHN (Ch. 5, 1 through 20 AHN)
EILR TB questions Ch. 45, 1 through 37 FAAHN (Ch. 5, 1 through 37 AHN)
EILR Open Book Quiz Ch. 45, 1 through 10 FAAHN (Ch. 5, 1 through 10 AHN)
ESLR Review Questions for the NCLEX® Examination Ch. 45, 45-01 through 45-10 FAAHN (Ch. 5, 05-01 through 05-10 AHN)

Legend

PPT
PowerPoint
Slides

EILR
EVOLVE Instructor
Learning Resources:
Image Collection, Test
Bank, Open Book Quizzes

ESLR
EVOLVE Student
Learning Resources:
Review Questions
for the NCLEX
Examination

SG
Study Guide

NCP CTQ
Nursing Care Plan
Critical Thinking
Question

Class Activities are indicated in **bold italic**.

LESSON 5.1

PRETEST

1. A 56-year-old patient who is undergoing chemotherapy reports to the clinic with thick white patches on her tongue and mucous membranes. The physician makes a diagnosis of *Candida albicans*. Based upon your knowledge, you anticipate the most likely treatment will include:
   a amoxicillin 500 mg QID.
   b. half-strength commercial mouthwash TID.
   c. nystatin vaginal tablets 100,000 units.
   d. full-strength hydrogen peroxide rinses QID.

2. A 43-year-old male is scheduled to undergo a colonoscopy. In preparation for the examination the teaching provided should include which of the following points?
   a. NPO 4 to 6 hours before the procedure.
   b. Continue normal dietary intake until the day of the procedure.
   c. Enemas or cathartics will be administered to reduce the residue in the bowel.
   d. The week prior to the procedure, the patient will need to begin a soft diet.

3. _____ is a diagnostic procedure that can also be used to remove polyps and coagulate sources of bleeding.
   a. Esophagogastroduodenoscopy
   b. Upper gastrointestinal study
   c. Bernstein test
   d. Sigmoidoscopy

4. A 32-year-old female presents to the clinic with complaints of heartburn, flatulence, dysphagia, and a sour taste in her mouth. After an examination you anticipate a diagnosis of:
   a. carcinoma of the esophagus.
   b. leukoplakia.
   c. gastroesophageal reflux disease.
   d. gastric ulcers.

5. A patient has recently been diagnosed with duodenal ulcers. The physician has prescribed Carafate to manage the condition. The patient asks you to explain the purpose of this medication. You understand this medication functions to:
   a. heal the ulcers by adhering to the proteins in the ulcer base.
   b. neutralize the acidity of the stomach contents.
   c. inhibit gastric acid secretion.
   d. block histamine receptors.

6. A 23-year-old female patient is being treated for gastric ulcers that have occurred as a result of the medications she takes to manage her arthritis. The physician has prescribed Cytotec (misoprostol). Based upon your knowledge of this medication, what is a chief nursing implication?
   a. This medication causes CNS depression, and alcohol ingestion must be avoided.
   b. Monitor serum electrolytes.
   c. Monitor liver enzyme levels.
   d. Ensure patient is using a reliable form of contraceptive.

7. A patient presents with complaints of hemorrhoids. He reports they have been a source of concern for the past 2 years. His physician has decided to perform surgery to treat the problem. Which of the following diagnoses would you expect to see on this patient's nursing care plan?
   a. Pain, related to edema
   b. Disturbed body image, related to loss of normal body image
   c. Imbalanced nutrition: less than body requirements, related to decreased oral intake
   d. Potential for complications related to reduced hemoglobin

Adult Health Nursing, 6th ed.
Christensen & Kockrow

8. A 43-year-old female patient has been diagnosed with peritonitis. Her recent health history includes childbirth via vaginal delivery, dental extraction, and appendicitis. She asks how she could have gotten this illness. Which of the following has placed her at greatest risk?
   a. Her age
   b. Recent childbirth
   c. Recent dental work
   d. Recent appendicitis

9. A 73-year-old male patient is being treated for colon cancer. The physician will be performing a proctocolectomy. The patient asks what this surgery entails. Based upon your knowledge, you understand this procedure involves:
   a. removal of anus, rectum, and colon.
   b. removal of a portion of the large intestine and anastomosis of the remaining segment.
   c. surgical formation of an opening of the ileum onto the surface of the abdomen, through which fecal matter is emptied.
   d. surgical formation of an opening onto the surface of the abdomen for the passage of urinary wastes.

10. A patient scheduled to undergo diagnostic testing of the intestines has been prescribed GoLYTELY. He asks what the medication will accomplish. Based upon your knowledge, you understand this medication will be used to:
    a. aid in the prevention of infection.
    b. cleanse the bowel.
    c. reduce peristalsis.
    d. increase peristalsis.

Answers:

1. c	2. c	3. a	4. c	5. a
6. d	7. a	8. d	9. a	10. b

BACKGROUND ASSESSMENT

Question: A 32-year-old male patient presents with complaints of mild tenderness in the lower abdomen. Assessment reveals a small, 2-inch bulge just below the umbilicus. After the examination, the physician makes the diagnosis of an umbilical hernia. The patient is nervous and asks what causes this to happen and how it will be managed. What should be included in your response to the patient?

Answer: The hernia was caused by a weakness in the abdominal wall in the umbilical area. There are risk factors that are associated with the development of abdominal hernias. These risk factors include obesity, multiple surgeries in the same area, poor nutrition, or infection. Management of hernias is usually conservative. As long as the hernia is reducible, conservative management is acceptable. A truss can be utilized on the abdomen. Elective surgery is also an option if the patient desires.

Question: A 54-year-old patient suspected of having polyps of the colon has been scheduled to have a barium enema. The procedure is completed as scheduled. The patient tolerated the test without difficulty. After the procedure, the physician has ordered milk of magnesia. Why has the physician ordered this medication? What are the nursing interventions after the procedure?

Answer: The milk of magnesia has been ordered to stimulate peristalsis and to promote evacuation of the barium from the bowel. The nurse's responsibilities in the care of this patient are to administer the prescribed medication, encourage fluids, and assess the abdomen and stool passed to ensure the barium is passed from the patient.

CRITICAL THINKING QUESTION

While caring for a patient suspected of having a parasitic infection, an order for a stool culture has been given by the physician. What steps will be needed to successfully obtain the specimen?

Guidelines: The stool will need to be collected and sent to the laboratory right after it is collected. The stool will need to be kept separate from any urine voided by the patient. Utilize a puritan hat, placed in the rear of the stool or commode, to collect the specimen. If an enema is used to obtain the specimen, only normal saline or tap water should be used. Any other substances can hinder the testing.

ELSEVIER

Adult Health Nursing, 6th ed.

Christensen & Kockrow

OBJECTIVES	CONTENT	TEACHING RESOURCES

List in sequence each of the component parts or segments of the alimentary canal, and identify the accessory organs of digestion.	■ Anatomy and Physiology of the Gastrointestinal System (FAAHN p. 1411, AHN p. 175)
	
	☐ Digestive system (FAAHN p. 1411, AHN p. 175)
	
	  – Organs of the digestive system and their functions (FAAHN p. 1412, AHN p. 176)
	
	☐ Accessory organs of digestion (FAAHN p. 1415, AHN p. 179)
	
	  – Liver (FAAHN p. 1415, AHN p. 179)
	
	  – Pancreas (FAAHN p. 1415, AHN p. 179)
	
	☐ Regulation of food intake (FAAHN p. 1416, AHN p. 180)
		PPT 1 through 4 Ch. 45 FAAHN (Ch. 5 PPT 1 through 4 AHN)
		
		EILR IC Ch. 45 images 1 through 4 FAAHN (Ch. 5 images 1 through 4 AHN)
		
		ESLR Review Questions for the NCLEX Examination Ch. 45 question 1 FAAHN (Ch. 5 question 1 AHN)
		
		SG Location of Digestive Organs Ch. 45 p. 357 FAAHN (Ch. 5 p. 45 AHN)
		
		BOOK RESOURCES
		
		Fig. 45-1 Location of digestive organs (FAAHN p. 1412) (Fig. 5-1 AHN p. 176)
		
		Box 45-1 Organs of the Digestive System (FAAHN p. 1413) (Box 5-1 AHN p. 177)
		
		Fig. 45-2 Stomach (FAAHN p. 1413) (Fig. 5-2 AHN p. 177)
		
		Fig. 45-3 Divisions of the large intestine (FAAHN p. 1414) (Fig. 5-3 AHN p. 178)
		
		Fig. 45-4 Gallbladder and bile ducts (FAAHN p. 1415) (Fig. 5-4 AHN p. 179)
		
		▶ Discuss a working definition of the alimentary canal. What is the role of the alimentary canal?
		
		▶ Discuss the role of the accessory organs. Identify the accessory organs.
		
		Class Activity Design a "live" alimentary canal. Assign each student a component of the alimentary canal. You can repeat the organs once a complete canal has been made. Group the students by individual canal. Ask the students to stand in order of their canal component.

Discuss the function of each digestive and accessory organ.	■ Anatomy and Physiology of the Gastrointestinal System (FAAHN p. 1411, AHN p. 175) ☐ Digestive system (FAAHN p. 1411, AHN p. 175) – Organs of the digestive system and their functions (FAAHN p. 1412, AHN p. 176) ☐ Accessory organs of digestion (FAAHN p. 1415, AHN p. 179)	PPT 2 through 4 Ch. 45 FAAHN (Ch. 5 PPT 2 through 4 AHN) EILR TB Ch. 45 question 1, 19 FAAHN (Ch. 5 question 1, 19 AHN) ESLR Review Questions for the NCLEX Examination Ch. 45 question 1 FAAHN (Ch. 5 question 1 AHN) SG Food's Journey Ch. 45 p. 358 FAAHN (Ch. 5 p. 46 AHN)

OBJECTIVES	CONTENT	TEACHING RESOURCES
	– Liver (FAAHN p. 1415, AHN p. 179) – Pancreas (FAAHN p. 1415, AHN p. 179) ☐ Regulation of food intake (FAAHN p. 1416, AHN p. 180)	▸ Discuss the function of each of the organs of digestion. How are these organs interrelated? How does their individual function impact the others? *Class Activity Utilize the "live" alimentary canal used in the previous activity. Instruct each of the students to review the functions of the assigned organ. Ask each chain to stand in the front of the class and present a fact relating to the function of the organ. To reinforce the location and sequence of the organs, require the students to present in order of their organ in the chain.*
Discuss the laboratory and diagnostic examinations and give the nursing interventions for patients with disorders of the gastrointestinal tract.	■ Laboratory and diagnostic examinations (FAAHN p. 1416, AHN p. 180) ☐ Upper gastrointestinal study (upper GI series, UGI) (FAAHN p. 1416, AHN p. 180) – Rationale (FAAHN p. 1416, AHN p. 180) – Nursing interventions (FAAHN p. 1416, AHN p. 180) ☐ Tube gastric analysis (FAAHN p. 1416, AHN p. 180) – Rationale (FAAHN p. 1416, AHN p. 180) – Nursing interventions (FAAHN p. 1416, AHN p. 180) ☐ Esophagogastroduodenoscopy (EGD, UGI Endoscopy, Gastroscopy) (FAAHN p. 1416, AHN p. 180) – Rationale (FAAHN p. 1416, AHN p. 180) – Nursing interventions (FAAHN p. 1416, AHN p. 180) ☐ Capsule endoscopy (FAAHN p. 1417, AHN p. 181) – Rationale (FAAHN p. 1417, AHN p. 181) – Nursing interventions (FAAHN p. 1417, AHN p. 181)	▦ PPT 5 Ch. 45 FAAHN (Ch. 5 PPT 5 AHN) *e* EILR IC Ch. 45 images 5, 6 FAAHN (Ch. 5 images 5, 6 AHN) *e* EILR TB Ch. 45 questions 5, 12, 13, 31, 35, 36, 37 FAAHN (Ch. 5 questions 5, 12, 13, 31, 35, 36, 37 AHN) *e* EILR Open Book Quiz Ch. 45 question 1, 2 FAAHN (Ch. 5 question 1, 2 AHN) *e* ESLR Review Questions for the NCLEX Examination Ch. 45 questions 2, 3 FAAHN (Ch. 5 questions 2, 3 AHN) ▣ SG Diagnostic Procedures Ch. 45 p. 358 FAAHN (Ch. 5 p. 46 AHN) **BOOK RESOURCES** Fig. 45-5 Fiberoptic endoscopy of the stomach (FAAHN p. 1416) (Fig. 5-5 AHN p. 180) Fig. 45-6 Capsule endoscopy (FAAHN p. 1417) (Fig. 5-6 AHN p. 181) Box 45-2 GoLYTELY Bowel Preparation (FAAHN p. 1419) (Box 5-2 AHN p. 183) Health Promotion Prevention or Early Detection of Esophageal Cancer (FAAHN p. 1424) (AHN p. 188) ▸ Discuss the responsibilities of the nurse in preparing the patient for the diagnostic examinations of the gastrointestinal tract. ▸ Discuss documentation that will accompany completion of patient teaching regarding

Christensen & Kockrow

OBJECTIVES	CONTENT	TEACHING RESOURCES
	☐ Barium swallow/gastrografin studies (FAAHN p. 1417, AHN p. 181)	diagnostic examinations of the gastrointestinal tract.
	– Rationale (FAAHN p. 1417, AHN p. 181)	*Class Activity Divide students into 11 groups or pairs. The size of the group will be determined by the class size. Assign each group a gastrointestinal diagnostic examination. The groups are responsible for reviewing the purpose and preparation of the assigned tests. Give students about 15 minutes to research their assigned exam. After being allowed to complete their investigation, the groups are to present findings to the entire class.*
	– Nursing interventions (FAAHN p. 1417, AHN p. 181)	
	☐ Esophageal function studies (Bernstein test) (FAAHN p. 1417, AHN p. 181)	
	– Rationale (FAAHN p. 1417, AHN p. 181)	
	– Nursing interventions (FAAHN p. 1417, AHN p. 181)	
	☐ Examination of stool for occult blood (FAAHN p. 1418, AHN p. 182)	
	– Rationale (FAAHN p. 1418, AHN p. 182)	
	– Nursing interventions (FAAHN p. 1418, AHN p. 182)	
	☐ Sigmoidoscopy (FAAHN p. 1418, AHN p. 182)	
	– Rationale (FAAHN p. 1418, AHN p. 182)	
	– Nursing interventions (FAAHN p. 1418, AHN p. 182)	
	☐ Barium enema study (lower GI series) (FAAHN p. 1418, AHN p. 182)	
	– Rationale (FAAHN p. 1418, AHN p. 182)	
	– Nursing interventions (FAAHN p. 1418, AHN p. 182)	
	☐ Colonoscopy (FAAHN p. 1418, AHN p. 182)	
	– Rationale (FAAHN p. 1418, AHN p. 182)	
	– Nursing interventions (FAAHN p. 1418, AHN p. 182)	
	☐ Stool culture (FAAHN p. 1419, AHN p. 183)	

Adult Health Nursing, 6th ed.

Christensen & Kockrow

OBJECTIVES	CONTENT	TEACHING RESOURCES
	− Rationale (FAAHN p. 1419, AHN p. 183)	
	− Nursing interventions (FAAHN p. 1419, AHN p. 183)	
	☐ Obstruction series (flat plate of the abdomen) (FAAHN p. 1419, AHN p. 183)	
	− Rationale (FAAHN p. 1419, AHN p. 183)	
	− Nursing interventions (FAAHN p. 1419, AHN p. 183)	

5.1 Homework/Assignments:

5.1 Instructor's Notes/Student Feedback:

ELSEVIER

LESSON 5.2

CRITICAL THINKING QUESTION

A 35-year-old male patient diagnosed with gastric ulcers has just finished seeing the doctor in the clinic in which you are employed. The patient has several questions about his medications, diet, and why he should not smoke. He reports the physician has prescribed Mylanta and Tagamet. He asks how these medications will work and how they should be taken. He states he just wants to "do the right thing" and get better. What information should be given to him concerning his prescribed treatments?

Guidelines: Mylanta is an antacid. It will be used to neutralize gastric acid. Tagamet is an H2 receptor. It is used to inhibit gastric acid secretion. These medications should not be taken together. They should be given at least 2 hours apart. This will promote optimal absorption of the medications. Research does not currently consider a bland diet beneficial. It is considered best to encourage small, frequent meals. The smaller meals will reduce the gastric motor activity. The diet should also reflect the elimination or reduction of caffeinated and decaffeinated coffee, tobacco, and alcohol. These substances also irritate the gastric mucosa. Smoking also acts as an irritant to the gastric mucosa. It will increase gastric motility and delay in mucosal healing.

OBJECTIVES	CONTENT	TEACHING RESOURCES
Explain the etiology/ pathophysiology, clinical manifestations, assessments, diagnostic tests, medical-surgical management, and nursing interventions for the patient with disorders of the mouth, esophagus, stomach, and intestines.	■ Disorders of the mouth (FAAHN p. 1419, AHN p. 183) □ Dental plaque and caries (FAAHN p. 1419, AHN p. 183) – Etiology and pathophysiology (FAAHN p. 1419, AHN p. 183) – Medical management (FAAHN p. 1419, AHN p. 183) – Nursing interventions and patient teaching (FAAHN p. 1419, AHN p. 183) – Prognosis (FAAHN p. 1420, AHN p. 184) □ Candidiasis (FAAHN p. 1420, AHN p. 184) – Etiology and pathophysiology (FAAHN p. 1420, AHN p. 184) – Clinical manifestations (FAAHN p. 1420, AHN p. 184) – Medical management (FAAHN p. 1420, AHN p. 184) – Nursing interventions (FAAHN p. 1420, AHN p. 184) – Prognosis (FAAHN p. 1420, AHN p. 184) □ Carcinoma of the oral cavity (FAAHN p. 1420, AHN p. 184) – Etiology and pathophysiology (FAAHN p. 1420, AHN p. 184)	PPT 6 through 50 Ch. 45 FAAHN (Ch. 5 PPT 6 through 50 AHN) EILR TB Ch. 45 questions 4, 6, 22, 27, 28, 29 FAAHN (Ch. 5 questions 4, 6, 22, 27, 28, 29 AHN) EILR Open Book Quiz Ch. 45 questions 1 through 9 FAAHN (Ch. 5 questions 1 through 9 AHN) ESLR Review Questions for the NCLEX Examination Ch. 45 questions 4 through 7, 27 through 30 FAAHN (Ch. 5 questions 4 through 7, 27 through 30 AHN) SG Disorders of the Mouth Ch. 45 p. 359 FAAHN (Ch. 5 p. 47 AHN) **BOOK RESOURCES** NCP CTQ 1 through 3 (FAAHN p. 1434) (AHN p. 198) Health Promotion Prevention or Early Detection of Esophageal Cancer (FAAHN p. 1424) (Ch. 5 AHN p. 188) Box 45-3 Nursing Interventions for the Patient Experiencing Esophageal Surgery (FAAHN p. 1426) (Box 45-3 AHN p. 190) Table 45-1 Medications for Gastrointestinal Disorders (FAAHN p. 1429) (Table 5-1 AHN p. 193)

OBJECTIVES	CONTENT	TEACHING RESOURCES
	– Clinical manifestations (FAAHN p. 1421, AHN p. 185)	Fig. 45-7 Types of gastric resections with anastomoses (FAAHN p. 1431) (Fig. 5-7 AHN p. 195)
	– Assessment (FAAHN p. 1421, AHN p. 185)	Fig. 45-8 Types of vagotomies (FAAHN p. 1432) (Fig. 5-8 AHN p. 196)
	– Diagnostic tests (FAAHN p. 1421, AHN p. 185)	Table 45-2 Purposes of Nasogastric Intubation (FAAHN p. 1433) (Table 5-2 AHN p. 197)
	– Medical management (FAAHN p. 1421, AHN p. 185)	Communication: Patient with a GI Bleed (FAAHN p. 1433) (AHN p. 197)
	– Nursing interventions and patient teaching (FAAHN p. 1422, AHN p. 186)	Nursing Care Plan 45-1 The Patient with Gastrointestinal Bleeding (FAAHN p. 1434) (NCP 5-1 AHN p. 198)
	– Prognosis (FAAHN p. 1422, AHN p. 186)	Home Care Considerations: Peptic Ulcer Disease (FAAHN p. 1435) (AHN p. 199)
	☐ Disorders of the esophagus (FAAHN p. 1422, AHN p. 186)	Complementary and Alternative Therapies: Irritable Bowel Syndrome (FAAHN p. 1441) (AHN p. 205)
	☐ Gastroesophageal reflux disease (FAAHN p. 1422, AHN p. 186)	Life Span Considerations, Older Adults: Gastrointestinal Disorders (FAAHN p. 1454) (AHN p. 218)
	– Etiology and pathophysiology (FAAHN p. 1422, AHN p. 186)	▸ Discuss the incidence of disorders of the mouth, esophagus, stomach, and intestines. What populations are at higher risk for the development of these disorders?
	– Clinical manifestations (FAAHN p. 1422, AHN p. 186)	
	– Assessment (FAAHN p. 1423, AHN p. 187)	▸ Discuss the impact disorders of the mouth and esophagus have on nutrition and overall health status.
	– Diagnostic tests (FAAHN p. 1423, AHN p. 187)	
	– Medical management (FAAHN p. 1423, AHN p. 187)	*Class Activity Lead a group discussion regarding the incidence of gastroesophageal reflux disease. During the discussion develop a care plan for the patient with this disorder.*
	– Nursing interventions and patient teaching (FAAHN p. 1423, AHN p. 187)	
	– Prognosis (FAAHN p. 1423, AHN p. 187)	
	☐ Carcinoma of the esophagus (FAAHN p. 1424, AHN p. 188)	
	– Etiology and pathophysiology (FAAHN p. 1424, AHN p. 188)	
	– Clinical manifestations (FAAHN p. 1424, AHN p. 188)	
	– Assessment (FAAHN p. 1424, AHN p. 188)	
	– Diagnostic tests (FAAHN p. 1424, AHN p. 188)	
	– Medical management (FAAHN p. 1424, AHN p. 188)	

Christensen & Kockrow

OBJECTIVES	CONTENT	TEACHING RESOURCES

	– Nursing interventions and patient teaching (FAAHN p. 1425, AHN p. 189)
	
	    – Prognosis (FAAHN p. 1425, AHN p. 189)
	
	  ☐ Achalasia (FAAHN p. 1425, AHN p. 189)
	
	    – Etiology and pathophysiology (FAAHN p. 1425, AHN p. 189)
	
	    – Clinical manifestations (FAAHN p. 1425, AHN p. 189)
	
	    – Assessment (FAAHN p. 1425, AHN p. 189)
	
	    – Diagnostic tests (FAAHN p. 1425, AHN p. 189)
	
	    – Medical management (FAAHN p. 1425, AHN p. 189)
	
	    – Nursing interventions and patient teaching (FAAHN p. 1426, AHN p. 190)
	
	    – Prognosis (FAAHN p. 1426, AHN p. 190)
	
	■ Disorders of the stomach (FAAHN p. 1426, AHN p. 190)
	
	  ☐ Gastritis (acute) (FAAHN p. 1426, AHN p. 190)
	
	    – Etiology and pathophysiology (FAAHN p. 1426 AHN p. 190)
	
	    – Clinical manifestations (FAAHN p. 1426, AHN p. 190)
	
	    – Assessment (FAAHN p. 1427, AHN p. 191)
	
	    – Diagnostic tests (FAAHN p. 1427, AHN p. 191)
	
	    – Medical management (FAAHN p. 1427, AHN p. 191)
	
	    – Nursing interventions and patient teaching (FAAHN p. 1427, AHN p. 191)
	
	    – Prognosis (FAAHN p. 1427, AHN p. 191)
	
	  ☐ Peptic ulcers (FAAHN p. 1427, AHN p. 191)	

Adult Health Nursing, 6th ed.
Christensen & Kockrow

OBJECTIVES	CONTENT	TEACHING RESOURCES
	☐ Gastric ulcers (FAAHN p. 1427, AHN p. 191)	
	☐ Physiologic stress ulcers (FAAHN p. 1428, AHN p. 192)	
	☐ Duodenal ulcers (FAAHN p. 1428, AHN p. 192)	
	– Etiology and pathophysiology (FAAHN p. 1428, AHN p. 192)	
	– Clinical manifestations (FAAHN p. 1428, AHN p. 192)	
	– Assessment (FAAHN p. 1428, AHN p. 192)	
	– Diagnostic tests (FAAHN p. 1428, AHN p. 192)	
	– Medical management (FAAHN p. 1429, AHN p. 193)	
	– Nursing interventions and patient teaching (FAAHN p. 1432, AHN p. 196)	
	– Prognosis for peptic ulcers (FAAHN p. 1436, AHN p. 200)	
	☐ Cancer of the stomach (FAAHN p. 1436, AHN p. 200)	
	– Etiology and pathophysiology (FAAHN p. 1436, AHN p. 200)	
	– Clinical manifestations (FAAHN p. 1436, AHN p. 200)	
	– Assessment (FAAHN p. 1436, AHN p. 200)	
	– Diagnostic tests (FAAHN p. 1436, AHN p. 200)	
	– Medical management (FAAHN p. 1436, AHN p. 200)	
	– Nursing interventions and patient teaching (FAAHN p. 1437, AHN p. 201)	
	– Prognosis (FAAHN p. 1437, AHN p. 201)	
	■ Disorders of the intestines (FAAHN p. 201, AHN p. 1437)	
	☐ Infections (FAAHN p. 1437, AHN p. 201)	
	– Etiology and pathophysiology (FAAHN p. 1437, AHN p. 201)	

Adult Health Nursing, 6th ed.
Christensen & Kockrow

OBJECTIVES	CONTENT	TEACHING RESOURCES
	– Clinical manifestations (FAAHN p. 1438, AHN p. 202)	
	– Assessment (FAAHN p. 1438, AHN p. 202)	
	– Diagnostic tests (FAAHN p. 1438, AHN p. 202)	
	– Medical management (FAAHN p. 1438, AHN p. 202)	
	– Nursing interventions and patient teaching (FAAHN p. 1439, AHN p. 203)	
	– Prognosis (FAAHN p. 1439, AHN p. 203)	
	☐ Irritable bowel syndrome (FAAHN p. 1439, AHN p. 203)	
	– Etiology and pathophysiology (FAAHN p. 1439, AHN p. 203)	
	– Clinical manifestations (FAAHN p. 1439, AHN p. 203)	
	– Assessment (FAAHN p. 1440, AHN p. 204)	
	– Diagnostic tests (FAAHN p. 1440, AHN p. 204)	
	– Medical management (FAAHN p. 1440, AHN p. 204)	
	– Nursing interventions and patient teaching (FAAHN p. 1440, AHN p. 204)	
	– Prognosis (FAAHN p. 1441, AHN p. 205)	
	☐ Inflammatory bowel disease (FAAHN p. 1441, AHN p. 205)	
	☐ Ulcerative colitis (FAAHN p. 1441, AHN p. 205)	
	– Etiology and pathophysiology (FAAHN p. 1441, AHN p. 205)	
	– Clinical manifestations (FAAHN p. 1442, AHN p. 206)	
	– Assessment (FAAHN p. 1442, AHN p. 206)	
	– Diagnostic tests (FAAHN p. 1443, AHN p. 207)	
	– Medical management (FAAHN p. 1443, AHN p. 207)	

ELSEVIER

Mosby items and derived items © 2011 by Mosby, Inc., an affiliate of Elsevier Inc.
Some material was previously published.

Adult Health Nursing, 6th ed.

Christensen & Kockrow

OBJECTIVES	CONTENT	TEACHING RESOURCES
	– Nursing interventions (FAAHN p. 1444, AHN p. 208)	
	– Patient teaching (FAAHN p. 1445, AHN p. 209)	
	– Prognosis (FAAHN p. 1445, AHN p. 209)	
	☐ Crohn's disease (FAAHN p. 1445, AHN p. 209)	
	– Etiology and pathophysiology (FAAHN p. 1445, AHN p. 209)	
	– Clinical manifestations (FAAHN p. 1446, AHN p. 210)	
	– Assessment (FAAHN p. 1446, AHN p. 210)	
	– Diagnostic tests (FAAHN p. 1446, AHN p. 210)	
	– Medical management (FAAHN p. 1446, AHN p. 210)	
	– Nursing interventions (FAAHN p. 1447, AHN p. 211)	
	– Nursing interventions and patient teaching (FAAHN p. 1448, AHN p. 212)	
	– Prognosis (FAAHN p. 1448, AHN p. 212)	
Identify nursing interventions for preoperative and postoperative care of the patient who requires gastric surgery.	☐ Duodenal ulcers (FAAHN p. 1428, AHN p. 192)	PPT 38 through 40, 50 Ch. 45 FAAHN (Ch. 5 PPT 38 through 40, 50 AHN)
	– Etiology and pathophysiology (FAAHN p. 1428, AHN p. 192)	EILR IC Ch. 45 images 7, 8 FAAHN (Ch. 5 images 7, 8 AHN)
	– Clinical manifestations (FAAHN p. 1428, AHN p. 192)	EILR TB Ch. 45 questions 7, 10, 18, 21 FAAHN (Ch. 5 questions 7, 10, 18, 21 AHN)
	– Assessment (FAAHN p. 1428, AHN p. 192)	SG Gastric Surgery Ch. 45 p. 361 FAAHN (Ch. 5 p. 49 AHN)
	– Diagnostic tests (FAAHN p. 1428, AHN p. 192)	**BOOK RESOURCES**
	– Medical management (FAAHN p. 1429, AHN p. 193)	Box 45-4 Surgical Interventions for Ulcerative Colitis (FAAHN p. 1443) (Box 5-4 AHN p. 207)
	– Nursing interventions and patient teaching (FAAHN p. 1432, AHN p. 196)	▸ Discuss the potential postoperative complications associated with gastric surgery.
	– Prognosis for peptic ulcers (FAAHN p. 1436, AHN p. 200)	▸ Discuss the differing types of surgical procedures available to treat gastric disorders.

OBJECTIVES	CONTENT	TEACHING RESOURCES
	☐ Cancer of the stomach (FAAHN p. 1436, AHN p. 200)	*Class Activity Invite a cancer survivor who has had gastric surgery to speak to the class. The focus of the speaker should be on the surgical experience and postoperative care received. To aid the speaker in developing the speech, ask the class to develop one or two questions and turn them in. These questions can be given to the speaker prior to the seminar.*
	– Etiology and pathophysiology (FAAHN p. 1436, AHN p. 200)	
	– Clinical manifestations (FAAHN p. 1436, AHN p. 200)	
	– Assessment (FAAHN p. 1436, AHN p. 200)	
	– Diagnostic tests (FAAHN p. 1436, AHN p. 200)	
	– Medical management (FAAHN p. 1436, AHN p. 200)	
	– Nursing interventions and patient teaching (FAAHN p. 1437, AHN p. 201)	
	– Prognosis (FAAHN p. 1437, AHN p. 201)	

5.2 Homework/Assignments:

5.2 Instructor's Notes/Student Feedback:

ELSEVIER

Adult Health Nursing, 6th ed.
Christensen & Kockrow

LESSON 5.3

CRITICAL THINKING QUESTION

While working in a physician's office, you collect data from a 47-year-old patient presenting for her annual physical examination. During the session, the patient says a neighbor has recently been diagnosed with colon cancer. She reports the diagnosis was made so late, there is little hope of survival. The patient asks if she is at risk for developing this type of cancer. What information should be provided concerning the risk factors for the development of colon cancer? What preventive screening is recommended?

Guidelines: Colon cancer occurs in both men and women with the same frequency. The development of the cancer increases in people over age 60. The exact cause is unknown. There are identified risk factors: ulcerative colitis, diverticulosis, and the presence of polyps. Preventive measures include diet. Diets high in fiber and low in fat are considered healthy for the intestines. Cruciferous vegetables can also provide some degree of protection. The American Cancer Society recommends annual digital rectal examinations and occult blood screening beginning at age 50. Flexible sigmoidoscopy testing should be done every 5 years. At-risk patients might require more frequent exams. Detailed screening examinations, such as a colonoscopy, are recommended every 10 years after age 50.

OBJECTIVES	CONTENT	TEACHING RESOURCES
Compare and contrast the inflammatory bowel diseases of ulcerative colitis and Crohn's disease including etiology and pathophysiology, clinical manifestations, medical management, and nursing interventions.	☐ Inflammatory bowel disease (FAAHN p. 1441, AHN p. 205) ☐ Ulcerative colitis (FAAHN p. 1441, AHN p. 205) – Etiology and pathophysiology (FAAHN p. 1441, AHN p. 205) – Clinical manifestations (FAAHN p. 1442, AHN p. 206) – Assessment (FAAHN p. 1442, AHN p. 206) – Diagnostic tests (FAAHN p. 1443, AHN p. 207) – Medical management (FAAHN p. 1443, AHN p. 207) – Nursing interventions (FAAHN p. 1444, AHN p. 208) – Patient teaching (FAAHN p. 1445, AHN p. 209) – Prognosis (FAAHN p. 1445, AHN p. 209) ☐ Crohn's disease (FAAHN p. 1445, AHN p. 209) – Etiology and pathophysiology (FAAHN p. 1445, AHN p. 209) – Clinical manifestations (FAAHN p. 1446, AHN p. 210)	☒ PPT 36 through 43 Ch. 45 FAAHN (Ch. 5 PPT 36 through 43 AHN) 🔲 EILR IC Ch. 45 image 11 FAAHN (Ch. 5 image 11 AHN) 🔲 EILR TB Ch. 45 questions 2, 3, 8, 9, 11, 14, 23 through 26, 32 FAAHN (Ch. 5 questions 2, 3, 8, 9, 11, 14, 23 through 26, 32 AHN) 🔲 EILR Open Book Quiz Ch. 45 question 9 FAAHN (Ch. 5 question 9 AHN) 🔲 ESLR Review Questions for the NCLEX Examination Ch. 45 questions 9, 10 FAAHN (Ch. 5 questions 9, 10 AHN) 🔲 SG Intestinal Disorders, Ch. 45 p. 362 FAAHN (Ch. 5 p. 50 AHN) **BOOK RESOURCES** Table 45-2 Purposes of Nasogastric Intubation (FAAHN p. 1433) (Table 5-2 AHN p. 197) Box 45-4 Surgical Interventions for Ulcerative Colitis (FAAHN p. 1443) (Box 5-4 AHN p. 207) Box 45-5 Postoperative Nursing Interventions for Ulcerative Colitis (FAAHN p. 1445) (Box 5-5 AHN p. 209) ▸ Discuss the physiological differences between ulcerative colitis and Crohn's

ELSEVIER

OBJECTIVES	CONTENT	TEACHING RESOURCES
	– Assessment (FAAHN p. 1446, AHN p. 210) – Diagnostic tests (FAAHN p. 1446, AHN p. 210) – Medical management (FAAHN p. 1446, AHN p. 210) – Nursing interventions (FAAHN p. 1447, AHN p. 211) – Nursing interventions and patient teaching (FAAHN p. 1448, AHN p. 212) – Prognosis (FAAHN p. 1448, AHN p. 212)	disease. ▶ Discuss the treatment options for ulcerative colitis and Crohn's disease. ***Class Activity** Lead a class discussion on Crohn's disease and ulcerative colitis. During the discussion, develop a chart to highlight the differences between the diseases.*
Identify five nursing interventions for the patient with a stoma for fecal diversion.	☐ Ulcerative colitis (FAAHN p. 1441, AHN p. 205) – Etiology and pathophysiology (FAAHN p. 1441, AHN p. 205) – Clinical manifestations (FAAHN p. 1442, AHN p. 206) – Assessment (FAAHN p. 1442, AHN p. 206) – Diagnostic tests (FAAHN p. 1443, AHN p. 207) – Medical management (FAAHN p. 1443, AHN p. 207) – Nursing interventions (FAAHN p. 1444, AHN p. 208) – Patient teaching (FAAHN p. 1445, AHN p. 209) – Prognosis (FAAHN p. 1445, AHN p. 209)	🖥 PPT 38 through 40 Ch. 45 FAAHN (Ch. 5 PPT 38 through 40 AHN) 💾 EILR IC Ch. 45 images 9, 10, 12 through 14 FAAHN (Ch. 5 images 9, 10, 12 through 14 AHN) 💾 EILR TB Ch. 45 questions 16, 17, 20 FAAHN (Ch. 5 questions 16, 17, 20 AHN) 📖 SG Fecal Diversion Ch. 45 p. 362 FAAHN (Ch. 5 p. 50 AHN) **BOOK RESOURCES** Fig. 45-9 Kock pouch (FAAHN p. 1444) (Fig. 5-9 AHN p. 208) Fig. 45-10 Ileostomy with absence of resected bowel (FAAHN p. 1444) (Fig. 5-10 AHN p. 208) Box 45-5 Postoperative Nursing Interventions for Ulcerative Colitis (FAAHN p. 1445) (Box 5-5 AHN p. 209) ▶ Discuss the psychological implications for the patient undergoing surgical interventions for fecal diversion. ▶ Discuss the nursing assessment of the patient experiencing fecal diversion. ***Class Activity** Invite a guest speaker to the class to discuss the nursing role in the care of the patient who has had fecal diversion. The local hospitals might be able to provide a patient educator for the discussion.*

OBJECTIVES	CONTENT	TEACHING RESOURCES
Discuss the etiology/ pathophysiology, clinical manifestations, assessment, diagnostic tests, medical management, and nursing interventions for the patient with acute abdominal inflammations (appendicitis, diverticulitis, and peritonitis).	☐ Acute abdominal inflammations (FAAHN p. 1448, AHN p. 212) ☐ Appendicitis (FAAHN p. 1448, AHN p. 212) – Etiology and pathophysiology (FAAHN p. 1448, AHN p. 212) – Clinical manifestations (FAAHN p. 1448, AHN p. 212) – Assessment (FAAHN p. 1448, AHN p. 212) – Diagnostic tests (FAAHN p. 1448, AHN p. 212) – Medical management (FAAHN p. 1448, AHN p. 212) – Nursing interventions and patient teaching (FAAHN p. 1448, AHN p. 212) – Prognosis (FAAHN p. 1449, AHN p. 213) ☐ Diverticular disease of the colon (FAAHN p. 1449, AHN p. 213) – Etiology and pathophysiology (FAAHN p. 1449, AHN p. 213) – Clinical manifestations (FAAHN p. 1449, AHN p. 213) – Assessment (FAAHN p. 1450, AHN p. 214) – Diagnostic tests (FAAHN p. 1450, AHN p. 214) – Medical management (FAAHN p. 1450, AHN p. 214) – Nursing interventions and patient teaching (FAAHN p. 1451, AHN p. 215) – Prognosis (FAAHN p. 1451, AHN p. 215) ☐ Peritonitis (FAAHN p. 1451, AHN p. 215) – Etiology and pathophysiology (FAAHN p. 1451, AHN p. 215)	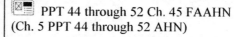 PPT 44 through 52 Ch. 45 FAAHN (Ch. 5 PPT 44 through 52 AHN) EILR TB Ch. 45 questions 2, 3, 8, 9, 11, 14, 23 through 26, 32 FAAHN (Ch. 5 questions 2, 3, 8, 9, 11, 14, 23 through 26, 32 AHN) SG Acute Abdominal Inflammations Ch. 45 p. 363 FAAHN (Ch. 5 p. 51 AHN) **BOOK RESOURCES** Safety Alert! Appendicitis (FAAHN p. 1449) (AHN p. 213) Fig. 45-11 Diverticulosis (FAAHN p. 1449) (Fig. 5-11 AHN p. 213) Fig. 45-12 Hartmann's pouch (FAAHN p. 1450) (Fig. 5-12 AHN p. 214) Fig. 45-13 Double-barrel transverse colostomy (FAAHN p. 1450) (Fig. 5-13 AHN p. 214) Fig. 45-14 Transverse loop colostomy with rod or butterfly (FAAHN p. 1451) (Fig. 5-14 AHN p. 215) ▸ Discuss the clinical manifestations of the patient experiencing appendicitis. ▸ Discuss the nursing care and management of the patient in pain due to appendicitis (preoperatively). *Class Activity Divide the students into three groups. Have the first group list the diagnostic tests for appendicitis, the next group list tests for diverticular disease, and the last group list tests for peritonitis. Are there similarities and/or differences among the tests?*

OBJECTIVES	CONTENT	TEACHING RESOURCES
	– Clinical manifestations (FAAHN p. 1451, AHN p. 215)	
	– Assessment (FAAHN p. 1451, AHN p. 215)	
	– Diagnostic tests (FAAHN p. 1452, AHN p. 216)	
	– Medical management (FAAHN p. 1452, AHN p. 216)	
	– Nursing interventions and patient teaching (FAAHN p. 1452, AHN p. 216)	
	– Prognosis (FAAHN p. 1452, AHN p. 216)	

5.3 Homework/Assignments:

5.3 Instructor's Notes/Student Feedback:

LESSON 5.4

CRITICAL THINKING QUESTION

A patient presents to the emergency room with complaints of lower abdominal pain, nausea, an elevated temperature of 101.1, and hypoactive bowel sounds. Appendicitis is suspected. What diagnostic tests are anticipated? What nursing measures can be implemented to promote comfort prior to surgery?

Guidelines: The diagnostic tests used to determine appendicitis include a white blood cell count, abdominal CT scan, and ultrasound. The patient should be kept NPO as surgery is imminent. Ice can be applied to the lower abdomen to promote comfort. This will also reduce the inflammatory process. Heat cannot be used because it could promote rupture of the appendicitis. Analgesic therapy is avoided as it would mask symptoms. Emotional support is important to both the patient and family.

OBJECTIVES	CONTENT	TEACHING RESOURCES
Discuss the etiology/ pathophysiology, clinical manifestations, assessment, diagnostic tests, medical management, and nursing interventions for the patient with external hernias and hiatal hernia.	☐ Hernias (FAAHN p. 1452, AHN p. 216) ☐ External hernias (FAAHN p. 1452, AHN p. 216) – Etiology and pathophysiology (FAAHN p. 1452, AHN p. 216) – Assessment (FAAHN p. 1452, AHN p. 216) – Diagnostic tests (FAAHN p. 1453, AHN p. 217) – Medical management (FAAHN p. 1453, AHN p. 217) – Nursing interventions and patient teaching (FAAHN p. 1453, AHN p. 217) ☐ Hiatal hernia (FAAHN p. 1453, AHN p. 217) – Medical management (FAAHN p. 1454, AHN p. 218) – Nursing interventions (FAAHN p. 1454, AHN p. 218) – Prognosis (FAAHN p. 1454, AHN p. 218)	PPT 53 through 58 Ch. 45 FAAHN (Ch. 5 PPT 53 through 58 AHN) SG Hernias Ch. 45 p. 364 FAAHN (Ch. 5 p. 52 AHN) **BOOK RESOURCES** Fig. 45-15 Hiatal hernia (FAAHN p. 1453) (Fig. 5-15 AHN p. 217) Life Span Considerations, Older Adults: Gastrointestinal Disorders (FAAHN p. 1454) (AHN p. 218) Fig. 45-16 Nissen fundoplication for hiatal hernia (FAAHN p. 1454) (Fig. 5-16 AHN p. 218) ▸ Discuss the different types of hernias (location and reducibility). ▸ Discuss the patient teaching that should be provided concerning signs and symptoms of complications. *Class Activity Ask each student to develop two NCLEX-style questions concerning hernias. After the questions are completed, divide the students into groups of four. Allow the students to use the groups' total questions to do a quick review of the topic.*
Differentiate between mechanical and nonmechanical intestinal obstruction including	☐ Intestinal obstruction (FAAHN p. 1454, AHN p. 218) – Etiology and pathophysiology (FAAHN p. 1454, AHN p. 218)	PPT 59 through 61 Ch. 45 FAAHN (Ch. 5 PPT 59 through 61 AHN) SG Intestinal Obstructions Ch. 45 p. 365 FAAHN (Ch. 5 p. 53 AHN)

Mosby items and derived items © 2011 by Mosby, Inc., an affiliate of Elsevier Inc.
Some material was previously published.

Adult Health Nursing, 6th ed.
Christensen & Kockrow

OBJECTIVES	CONTENT	TEACHING RESOURCES
causes, medical management, and nursing interventions.	– Clinical manifestations (FAAHN p. 1455, AHN p. 219) – Assessment (FAAHN p. 1455, AHN p. 219) – Diagnostic tests (FAAHN p. 1455, AHN p. 219) – Medical management (FAAHN p. 1455, AHN p. 219) – Nursing interventions and patient teaching (FAAHN p. 1456, AHN p. 220) – Prognosis (FAAHN p. 1456, AHN p. 220)	**BOOK RESOURCES** Fig. 45-17 Intestinal obstructions (FAAHN p. 1455) (Fig. 5-17 AHN p. 219) ▶ Discuss causes of mechanical obstruction. ▶ Discuss the physiological implications of an intestinal obstruction. *Class Activity Group the students in pairs. To promote maximum class interaction, pair students with someone from another part of the class. Pass a tennis ball around. As each pair receives the ball, ask a question concerning intestinal obstructions. Together, the students can develop an answer to the question. Topics for questions include clinical manifestations, diagnosis, nursing care, medical management, and prognosis.*
Describe the etiology/ pathophysiology, clinical manifestations, assessment, diagnostic tests, medical management, surgical procedures, and nursing interventions for the patient with colorectal cancer.	□ Colorectal cancer (FAAHN p. 1456, AHN p. 220) – Etiology and pathophysiology (FAAHN p. 1456, AHN p. 220) – Clinical manifestations (FAAHN p. 1457, AHN p. 221) – Assessment (FAAHN p. 1457, AHN p. 221) – Diagnostic tests (FAAHN p. 1457, AHN p. 221) – Medical management (FAAHN p. 1457, AHN p. 221) – Nursing interventions and patient teaching (FAAHN p. 1458, AHN p. 222) – Prognosis (FAAHN p. 1460, AHN p. 224) □ Hemorrhoids (FAAHN p. 1460, AHN p. 224) – Etiology and pathophysiology (FAAHN p. 1460, AHN p. 224) – Clinical manifestations (FAAHN p. 1460, AHN p. 224) – Assessment (FAAHN p. 1460, AHN p. 224)	PPT 62 through 68 Ch. 45 FAAHN (Ch. 5 PPT 62 through 68 AHN) SG Cancer Ch. 45 p. 366 FAAHN (Ch. 5 p. 54 AHN) **BOOK RESOURCES** Health Promotion: Screening for Colorectal Cancer (FAAHN p. 1457) (AHN p. 221) Fig. 45-18 Bowel resection (FAAHN p. 1458) (Fig. 5-18 AHN p. 222) Fig. 45-19 Descending or sigmoid colostomy (FAAHN p. 1458) (Fig. 5-19 AHN p. 222) Fig. 45-20 Rubber band ligation of an internal hemorrhoid (FAAHN p. 1460) (Fig. 5-20 AHN p. 224) Cultural Considerations: Gastrointestinal Disorders (FAAHN p. 1463) (AHN p. 227) ▶ Discuss the recommended screening for colorectal cancer. ▶ Discuss populations at risk for the development of colorectal cancer. *Class Activity Divide the class into groups. Groups will include etiology, clinical manifestations, diagnostic tests, medical management, and nursing interventions. Ask each group to research the information on its topic. Require each group to put together a short (5- to 10-minute) presentation to the class.*

OBJECTIVES	CONTENT	TEACHING RESOURCES
	– Medical management (FAAHN p. 1460, AHN p. 224) – Nursing interventions and patient teaching (FAAHN p. 1461, AHN p. 225) – Prognosis (FAAHN p. 1462, AHN p. 226) ☐ Anal fissure and fistula (FAAHN p. 1462, AHN p. 226) – Prognosis (FAAHN p. 1462, AHN p. 226) ☐ Nursing process for the patient with a gastrointestinal disorder (FAAHN p. 1463, AHN p. 227) – Assessment (FAAHN p. 1463, AHN p. 227) – Nursing diagnoses (FAAHN p. 1463, AHN p. 227) – Expected outcomes and planning (FAAHN p. 1463, AHN p. 227) – Implementation (FAAHN p. 1463, AHN p. 227) – Evaluation (FAAHN p. 1464, AHN p. 228)	
Explain the etiologies, medical management, and nursing interventions for the patient with fecal incontinence.	☐ Fecal incontinence (FAAHN p. 1462, AHN p. 226) – Etiology and pathophysiology (FAAHN p. 1462, AHN p. 226) – Medical management and nursing interventions (FAAHN p. 1462, AHN p. 226) – Patient teaching (FAAHN p. 1462, AHN p. 226)	▶ Discuss populations at increased risk for fecal incontinence. ▶ Discuss the use of biofeedback training for the management of fecal incontinence. *Class Activity Divide students into small groups of three or four students. Instruct students to work on developing a bowel training program for an individual experiencing fecal incontinence. After allowing time for the groups to work together on the assigned task, allow time for the groups to share their work. What are the positive elements in the student's bowel training programs?*

Performance Evaluation		EILR TB Ch. 45 questions 1 through 37 FAAHN (Ch. 5 questions 1 through 37 AHN)
		EILR Open Book Quiz Ch. 45 questions 1 through 10 FAAHN (Ch. 5 questions 1 through 10 AHN)
		ESLR Review Questions for the NCLEX Examination Ch. 45 questions 1 through 10 FAAHN (Ch. 5 questions 1 through 10 AHN)
		SG Ch. 44 pp. 357 through 368 FAAHN (Ch. 5 pp. 45 through 56 AHN)
		BOOK RESOURCES
		Nursing Care Plan 45-1 The Patient with Gastrointestinal Bleeding (FAAHN p. 1434) (NCP 5-1 AHN p. 198)
		NCP CTQ 1 through 3 (FAAHN p. 1434) (AHN p. 198)
		Review Questions for the NCLEX Examination Ch. 5 questions 1 through 30 FAAHN (Ch. 5 questions 1 through 30 AHN)

5.4 Homework/Assignments:

5.4 Instructor's Notes/Student Feedback:

Slide 1

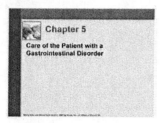

Slide 2

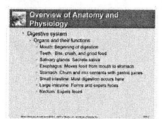

- It is a well understood fact that the digestive system functions to process the foods and nutrients taken into the body.

- Along its journey, the food becomes involved with a group of supportive organs known as accessory organs. What function do accessory organs serve for the digestive system?

Slide 3

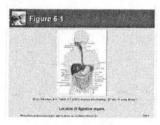

- The digestive process begins in the mouth. From the time the food enters the mouth, the chemical digestive process begins.

- Review the chemicals and enzymes secreted in the process of digestion. Where do these substances enter the alimentary canal? What is their source?

- The fundamental purpose of dietary intake is to nourish the body. At what point do the nutritional sources begin to be absorbed by the body? What processes facilitate this to occur?

Slide 4

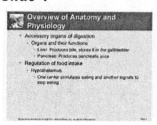

- Discuss the sequence of the digestive process. Be sure to note the function of each of the organs in the steps.

Christensen & Kockrow

Slide 5

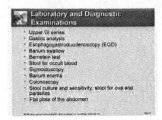

- The majority of diagnostic exams associated with the digestive system are used to visualize the areas of concern.

- When a patient is scheduled for a diagnostic exam, what are the responsibilities of the nurse? What responsibilities are associated with the physician? How do these scopes of practice/responsibility differ?

- For each of the diagnostic tests listed, what preparation is required? Review the documentation that is necessary concerning the preparation. What are the nursing responsibilities after each of the procedures?

Slide 6

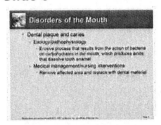

- Dental decay is a phenomenon having a profound impact on the health of Americans. It is estimated 95% of Americans will experience dental decay during their lives.

- What factors are associated with dental decay? Identify steps to prevent dental decay.

- What is the impact of dental decay on the patient's health status?

Slide 7

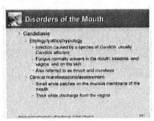

- Candidiasis is a fungal infection.

- List factors that can contribute to the development of a candidiasis infection.

Slide 8

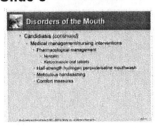

- When caring for a patient having a candidiasis infection, what are the nursing responsibilities? Please include care, assessment, and health teaching.

Slide 9

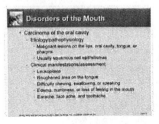

- In the United States, 2% to 4% of cancers are oral in nature.

- Unfortunately, the number of young people suffering from oral cancers continues to grow. What factors can be attributed to this occurrence?

- The mortality rate of oral cancers involves the high degree of metastasis seen in them. Discuss the causes associated with the mortality rates of oral cancer.

- Differentiate between early and late signs and symptoms associated with oral cancer.

Slide 10

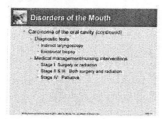

- Expound on the manner in which the diagnostic examinations differ with the type of suspected oral malignancy being evaluated.
- Identify factors that determine what type of medical management options will be utilized.

Slide 11

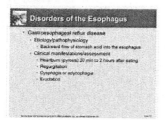

- Gastroesophageal reflux disease is commonly referred to as GERD.
- GERD is the reflux of stomach acid into the esophagus. What factors are associated with the development of this manifestation?
- Discuss attributes that impact the severity of the disorder.

Slide 12

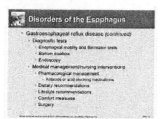

- Discuss the rationale for the prescribed nursing actions.
- Are there any dietary modifications that can be used to alleviate symptoms?
- Outline the mode of action for the medications commonly used to manage GERD.

Slide 13

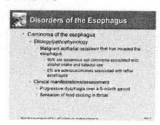

- Review risk factors for the development of carcinoma of the esophagus.

Slide 14

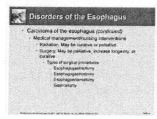

- The patient having oral or esophageal cancer has both psychological and physiological needs. What are the nursing responsibilities in the plan of care for these patients?

ELSEVIER

Adult Health Nursing, 6th ed.
Christensen & Kockrow

Slide 15

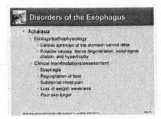

- What are the results of achalasia? What is the underlying cause of the disorder?

- Review at-risk populations.

- Explain the reason for the signs and symptoms that occur with the disorder.

- Separate and identify the early and late clinical manifestations.

Slide 16

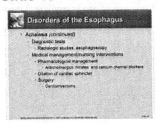

- The chief diagnostic studies used for achalasia involve radiologic studies or esophagoscopy. What findings are indicative of this condition?

Slide 17

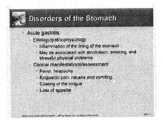

Slide 18

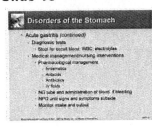

- Review the common names of medications commonly used in the management of acute gastritis.

- Develop appropriate nursing diagnoses for the patient with acute gastritis.

Slide 19

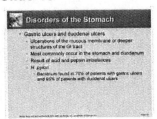

- What variables are implicated in the development of a gastric ulcer?

- H. pylori has been associated with gastric ulcer occurrence. What is H. pylori? How do individuals become infected with the bacterium?

Adult Health Nursing, 6th ed.

Christensen & Kockrow

Slide 20

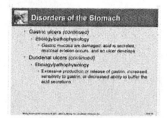

- Discuss stress ulcers. How do they develop?

Slide 21

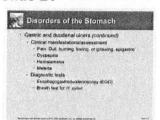

- Explain the underlying cause for the signs and symptoms experienced by the patient suffering from a gastric ulcer.

Slide 22

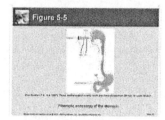

- Discuss the use of fiberoptic endoscopy of the stomach to diagnose gastrointestinal disorders.

Slide 23

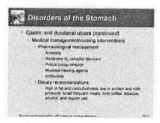

- Develop teaching plans for the patient with a gastric or duodenal ulcer.

- What are the nursing responsibilities for the patient with an ulcer?

- What are the goals of treatment for patients experiencing gastric and duodenal ulcers?

Slide 24

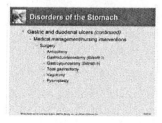

- Surgical intervention is needed for approximately 20% of patients having ulcers. The decision to perform surgery is determined by the patient's unique health status.

- What events may necessitate a patient having surgery to treat gastric ulcers?

- Outline the differences between the surgical procedures that might be used in the treatment of patients diagnosed with ulcers.

Christensen & Kockrow

Slide 25

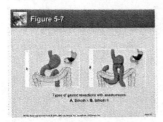

Slide 26

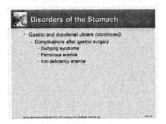

- At what point in the postoperative process are the complications of dumping syndrome, pernicious anemia, and iron deficiency most likely to occur?

- What impact do these complications have on the patient's health status?

- How are the potential complications prevented and managed?

Slide 27

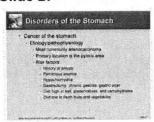

- Although the rates of gastric cancer are declining in the United States, it still remains a cause of concern.

- Studies have identified risk factors for the development of gastric cancer. Why do patients experiencing these circumstances have a higher risk of gastric cancer development?

Slide 28

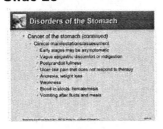

- The patient suffering from gastric cancer may be asymptomatic initially.

- What signs and symptoms are seen early in the development of the disease? What signs and symptoms are considered late?

- Anemia can also accompany gastric cancer. Why does the patient experience anemia?

Slide 29

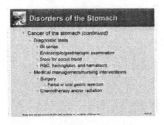

- What findings are typically found to support a diagnosis of gastric cancer?

- After a diagnosis of gastric cancer is found, what treatment options are available?

- What is the role of the nurse when caring for the patient experiencing gastric cancer?

Adult Health Nursing, 6th ed.
Christensen & Kockrow

Slide 30

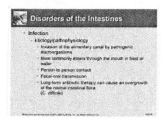

- There are numerous means for the intestinal tract to be exposed to infectious matter. With so many available avenues to become infected, how does the body resist these infections?
- List some of the potential pathogens that can affect the intestinal tract.

Slide 31

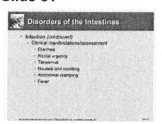

- The typical patient experiencing an intestinal infection will present with complaints of nausea, vomiting, and diarrhea. These symptoms are common and might accompany other disorders. To aid the physician in making a diagnosis, what additional data should the nurse attempt to collect from the patient?

Slide 32

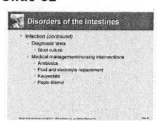

- When collecting a stool specimen, what education should be given to the patient? How should the stool be handled after collection?
- What are the nursing responsibilities/implications in the treatment plan?

Slide 33

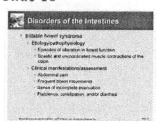

- Irritable bowel syndrome (IBS) is a common disorder possibly affecting 20% of the population.
- What causes IBS?

Slide 34

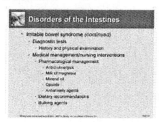

- The diagnosis of IBS is often made by taking a history and performing a physical examination. What elements in the patient's health history should be reviewed?
- Treatment for IBS includes diet and bulking agents. Review the dietary recommendations for the patient diagnosed with IBS. What effect do bulking agents have on the bowel?
- Review the desired mode of action and desired outcomes for the classifications of medications prescribed to treat IBS.
- In addition to the traditional medication therapy, alternative therapies are being used to treat the disorder. Discuss their use.

Christensen & Kockrow

Slide 35

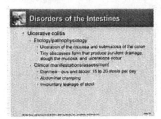

- Ulcerative colitis is a chronic inflammatory bowel disease.
- What portion of the bowel is involved in ulcerative colitis?
- Discuss the progression of the disease.

Slide 36

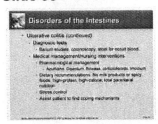

- Review the factors that are utilized to determine the course of treatment.
- Medications prescribed for the management of ulcerative colitis include sulfasalazine, non-sulfa drugs, corticosteroids, and antidiarrheal agents. How do these medications work?

Slide 37

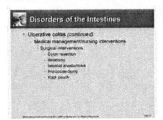

- Surgical interventions might be used to manage ulcerative colitis if the condition does not respond to traditional therapies.
- Review the surgical interventions that could be used to treat ulcerative colitis.
- What are the nursing assessment responsibilities during the postoperative phase?

Slide 38

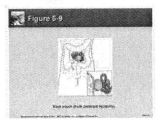

Slide 39

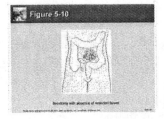

Adult Health Nursing, 6th ed.
Christensen & Kockrow

Slide 40

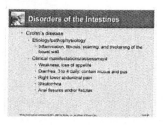

- Crohn's disease is an inflammatory bowel disease with an increasing incidence in the United States.
- What factors might be associated with this increase?
- Identify the population affected most by Crohn's disease.
- Review the progression of the disease.
- The disease is associated with significant changes in bowel habits. What type of bowel function is characteristic of Crohn's disease?

Slide 41

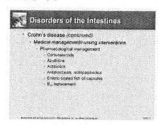

- Once a diagnosis of Crohn's disease is made, a plan of treatment is devised. What factors play a role in the determination of the plan of care?
- Medications are used to treat Crohn's disease. What mode of action does each of medication classification have?

Slide 42

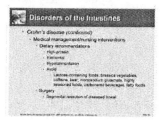

- Dietary management is a central part of the patient's treatment plan. Review the dietary modifications that might be recommended to the patient with Crohn's disease.
- What role does each of the elements of the dietary plan have in the management of this condition?

Slide 43

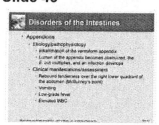

- Appendicitis occurs when the vermiform appendix becomes inflamed. What is the vermiform appendix? What is its physiological purpose? Where is it located?
- How should the assessment be performed for the patient who is suspected of having appendicitis?

Slide 44

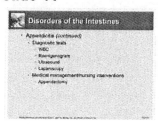

- Once a patient presents with the clinical signs and symptoms indicative of appendicitis, diagnostic tests are performed to establish additional supportive data.
- What findings on the white blood cell count will support a diagnosis of appendicitis?
- When a diagnosis of appendicitis is confirmed, surgery will be performed. What measures/interventions are contraindicated? Why?

ELSEVIER

Adult Health Nursing, 6th ed.

Christensen & Kockrow

Slide 45

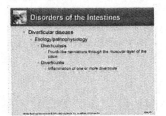

- Review the clinical process that accompanies diverticulosis/diverticulitis.

Slide 46

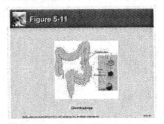

Slide 47

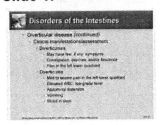

- Differing symptoms are associated with diverticulosis and diverticulitis. Why do these clinical presentations differ?

Slide 48

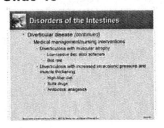

- The treatment of diverticulosis and diverticulitis can include medication, dietary modification, and surgery.

- Review factors that could be used to determine the best course of treatment.

Slide 49

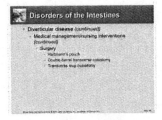

- What nursing diagnoses can be utilized in the plan of care for the patient diagnosed with diverticulosis or diverticulitis?

ELSEVIER

Mosby items and derived items © 2011, 2007 by Mosby, Inc., an affiliate of Elsevier Inc.
Some material was previously published.

Adult Health Nursing, 6th ed.
Christensen & Kockrow

Slide 50

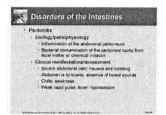

- Peritonitis is a serious infection in the abdominal peritoneum. What factors might be associated with the development of this condition?

Slide 51

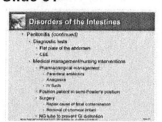

- The treatment of peritonitis is aggressive. What patient teaching should be provided concerning the disease, its management, and its prognosis?

Slide 52

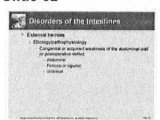

- The protrusion of a viscus through an abdominal opening, or weakened area in which it is usually contained, results in a hernia.
- Identify populations at risk for the development of hernias. Which of their attributes place them at increased risk?

Slide 53

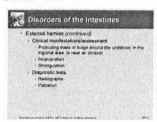

- Define reducible, incarcerated, and strangulated hernias.
- What medical concerns accompany incarcerated and strangulated hernias?

Slide 54

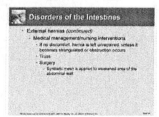

- Discuss assessment of the patient presenting with a hernia.
- Review the signs and symptoms signaling a complication with the hernia.

ELSEVIER

Adult Health Nursing, 6th ed.

Christensen & Kockrow

Slide 55

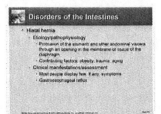

- What complications may result with a hiatal hernia?

Slide 56

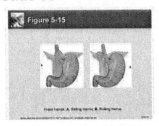

- A hiatal hernia could be sliding or rolling. How do they differ?

Slide 57

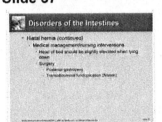

- What nursing diagnoses would be appropriate for inclusion in a care plan for the patient diagnosed with a hiatal hernia?

- When caring for the patient with a hiatal hernia, what should be included in the teaching plan for the patient?

Slide 58

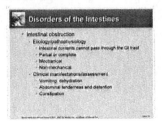

- Intestinal obstruction is a serious medical complication. It could be mechanical or non-mechanical.

- What are possible causes of mechanical obstructions? Non-mechanical obstructions?

- Why is the development of an intestinal obstruction serious? What are the clinical implications associated with an intestinal obstruction?

- The clinical manifestations of an intestinal obstruction vary with location and onset. What are early signs and symptoms associated with an intestinal obstruction?

Slide 59

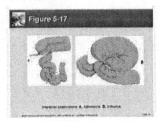

ELSEVIER
Mosby items and derived items © 2011, 2007 by Mosby, Inc., an affiliate of Elsevier Inc.
Some material was previously published.

Adult Health Nursing, 6th ed.
Christensen & Kockrow

Slide 60

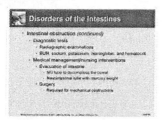

- Radiographic studies provide a visualization of the abdomen and bowel. What findings are present with x-ray studies that support a diagnosis of intestinal obstruction?

- How are electrolyte levels impacted when an intestinal obstruction is located?

- What nursing assessments are required when caring for the patient with an intestinal obstruction?

Slide 61

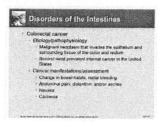

- Colon cancer equally affects men and women. An estimated 70% of colon cancers are found in the sigmoid, rectal, cecum, and ascending colon.

- Studies have pinpointed risk factors associated with the development of colon cancer. Review the risk factors.

- Review the signs and symptoms of colon cancer. Differentiate between early and late manifestations.

Slide 62

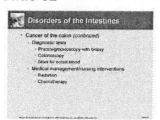

- Early diagnosis of colon cancer is key in preventing death.

- What preventative tests are available to detect colon cancer? Review the medical recommendations for preventive screening.

- In the event colon cancer is suspected, what diagnostic test findings are indicative of the disease?

Slide 63

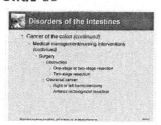

- When the medical management of colon cancer includes surgical intervention, a number of options are available. Compare and contrast the surgical interventions used in the treatment plan.

- What are the nursing responsibilities during the postoperative period?

- What is the prognosis for colon cancer? What determines the patient's prognosis?

Slide 64

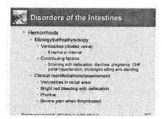

ELSEVIER

Mosby items and derived items © 2011, 2007 by Mosby, Inc., an affiliate of Elsevier Inc.
Some material was previously published.

Adult Health Nursing, 6th ed.
Christensen & Kockrow

Slide 65

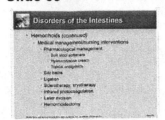

- In most cases, hemorrhoids respond to conservative management. Discuss the desired outcomes of each of the treatment options.

Slide 66

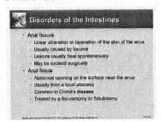

- What are examples of patients who have fissures?

Slide 67

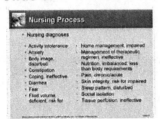

- Disorders of the digestive system are often invasive and far-reaching. There is immeasurable impact on the patients affected. Review the provided nursing diagnoses. Which of the digestive disorders do they most pertain to?

Slide 68

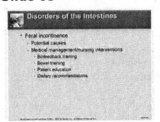

- Discuss the steps that should be included in a bowel training plan.

ELSEVIER

Adult Health Nursing, 6th ed.
Christensen & Kockrow

Lesson Plan

6 Care of the Patient with a Gallbladder, Liver, Biliary Tract, or Exocrine Pancreatic Disorder

TEACHING FOCUS

In this chapter, the student will be introduced to the care of the patient with a gallbladder, liver, biliary tract, or exocrine pancreatic disorder. The student will have the opportunity to learn the etiology, pathophysiology, clinical manifestations, assessment, diagnostic tests, medical management, and nursing interventions for patients with these disorders. The student will explore in detail viral hepatitis, liver transplantation, cirrhosis of the liver, and cholecystitis/cholelithiasis.

MATERIALS AND RESOURCES

- ☐ Computer/overhead projector (Lessons 6.1 and 6.2)
- ☐ White/black board and marker/chalk (Lessons 6.1 and 6.2)
- ☐ List of diagnostic tests used to evaluate disorders of the gallbladder, liver, biliary tract, and exocrine pancreas (Lesson 6.1)
- ☐ List of ways to medically manage cirrhosis of the liver.
- ☐ Nursing care plan that can be used for a patient diagnosed with cirrhosis of the liver (Lesson 6.1)
- ☐ Chart listing signs associated with early and later stage jaundice (Lesson 6.1).
- ☐ List of signs and symptoms associated with liver abscesses (Lesson 6.1).
- ☐ List of side effects and nursing implications associated with each medication used to treat pancreatic and cancer of the pancreas (Lesson 6.1).
- ☐ Chart with six columns listing the six types of viral hepatitis and rows listing etiology, clinical manifestations, diagnostic tests, management, and prognosis (Lesson 6.2)
- ☐ Chart listing signs and symptoms associated with viral hepatitis (Lesson 6.2).
- ☐ List of factors used to determine which surgical procedure may used to treat cholecystitis/cholelithiasis (Lesson 6.2).

LESSON CHECKLIST

Preparations for this lesson include:

- Lecture
- Invite a representative of a cancer care organization to speak about the problems encountered with a diagnosis of carcinoma of the liver and pancreas.
- Invite a representative from a local hospital to discuss the protocols for organ donation.

KEY TERMS

ascites (FAAHN p. 1472, AHN p. 236)
asterixis (FAAHN p. 1476, AHN p. 240)
esophageal varices (FAAHN p. 1474, AHN |p. 238)
flatulence (FAAHN p. 1485, AHN p. 249)
hepatic encephalopathy (FAAHN p. 1476, AHN p. 240)
hepatitis (FAAHN p. 1470, AHN p. 234)

jaundice (FAAHN p. 1473, AHN p. 237)
occlusion (FAAHN p. 1489, AHN p. 253)
paracentesis (FAAHN p. 1473, AHN p. 237)
parenchyma (FAAHN p. 1472, AHN p. 236)
spider telangiectases (FAAHN p. 1472, AHN p. 236)
steatorrhea (FAAHN p. 1475, AHN p. 249)

ADDITIONAL RESOURCES (AHN)

PPT Ch. 46, 1 through 44FAAHN (Ch. 6, 1 through 44 AHN)
EILR IC images Ch. 46, 1 through 9 FAAHN (Ch. 6, 1 through 9 AHN)
EILR TB questions Ch. 46, 1 through 41 FAAHN (Ch. 6, 1 through 41 AHN)
EILR Open Book Quiz Ch. 46, 1 through 10 FAAHN (Ch.6, 1 through 10 AHN)
ESLR Review Questions for the NCLEX® Examination Ch. 46, 46-01 through 46-10 FAAHN (Ch. 6, 06-01 through 06-10 AHN)

Legend

PPT
PowerPoint
Slides

EILR
EVOLVE Instructor
Learning Resources:
Image Collection, Test
Bank, Open Book Quizzes

ESLR
EVOLVE Student
Learning Resources:
Review Questions
for the NCLEX
Examination

SG
Study Guide

NCP CTQ
Nursing Care Plan
Critical Thinking
Question

Class Activities are indicated in **bold italic**.

LESSON 6.1

PRETEST

1. The patient who is undergoing an oral cholecystography test can expect which of the following medication regimens before the procedure?
   a. The nurse will administer iodine via piggyback IV just before the procedure.
   b. The nurse has no medication responsibilities for the test because the medications will be administered by the radiology technician.
   c. There are no preparatory medications given for this test.
   d. The patient will begin to take iopanoic acid tablets after the last evening meal.

2. A review of an indirect bilirubin test is 0.2 mg/dL. These results indicate:
   a. normal indirect bilirubin values.
   b. an elevation in the indirect bilirubin levels.
   c. a slight decrease in indirect bilirubin levels.
   d. a markedly reduced indirect bilirubin level.

3. A patient presents with complaints of abdominal pain that radiates to the back. Diagnostic tests are ordered to determine if the cause is pancreatitis. Which of the following results support the diagnosis of pancreatitis?
   a. Reduced serum amylase and lipase
   b. Leukocytosis, decreased hematocrit, and hypercalcemia
   c. Leukocytosis, reduced serum amylase and lipase
   d. Leukocytosis, hypoalbuminemia, and hyperglycemia

4. The patient diagnosed with cirrhosis should be advised to avoid which of the following medications?
   a. Acetaminophen
   b. Iron supplements
   c. Calcium supplements
   d. Vitamin supplements

5. A patient diagnosed with hepatitis A asks how she could have contracted the disease. She should be advised that:
   a. this type of hepatitis can be transmitted via contaminated with fecal material.
   b. the cause of this type of hepatitis is unknown.
   c. hepatitis A can be transmitted via blood transfusions.
   d. she was probably infected by sexual contact with an infected individual.

6. The mother of a 16-year-old patient asks you about vaccinating her daughter against hepatitis B. Based upon your knowledge, you say:
   a. she is too old to be vaccinated; it should have been done during her early childhood.
   b. she can begin the three-shot series at any age.
   c. she can begin the four-shot series at any age.
   d. the teen is not at any risk for becoming infected and should not be vaccinated at this time.

7. While you are working at the clinic, a patient presents with complaints of nausea and vomiting. She reports experiencing localized right upper quadrant pain. Which of the following conditions is associated with these clinical manifestations?
   a. Pancreatic cancer
   b. Cholelithiasis
   c. Hepatitis G
   d. Pancreatitis

8. A patient who was admitted with biliary pain is requesting an analgesic. He reports morphine has been effective when he was hospitalized for another unrelated health crisis. What actions should the nurse take?
   a. The patient should be advised that morphine is not administered in biliary pain because it can mask important clinical manifestations.
   b. The physician should be advised of the patient's preference of analgesic.
   c. The patient should be advised that morphine is not administered for biliary pain because it can cause further discomforts due to spasms of the sphincter of Oddi.
   d. Medications to reduce biliary pain are limited due to the risk of addiction. Alternative pain relief therapies should be initiated.

9. The physician orders neomycin for a patient diagnosed with cirrhosis. Which of the following statements best explains the rationale for its use?
   a. Neomycin is used to reduce the ammonia levels and reduce hepatic encephalopathy.
   b. Neomycin, an antibiotic, is used to prevent infection.
   c. Neomycin will be used to bind with the bile acids in the GI tract and reduce the levels of bile acids.
   d. This medication will be used to manage bleeding esophageal varices.

10. Older adults often demonstrate altered responses to medications such as anticonvulsants, psychotropics, and oral anticoagulants. These changes can result due to:
    a. the older adult's reduced vascular elasticity, which reduces the rate of medication metabolism.
    b. the older adult's reduced cardiovascular functioning limiting the blood transport of the medications.
    c. the decrease in protein synthesis altering drug metabolism in the older adult.
    d. the fact that there are fewer liver cells in the older adult, limiting the surface area available to aid in drug metabolism.

Answers:

1. d	2. a	3. d	4. a	5. a
6. b	7. b	8. c	9. a	10. c

BACKGROUND ASSESSMENT

Question: A patient reports to the clinic with complaints of malaise, aching muscles, nausea, and diarrhea. Diagnostic testing indicates that the patient has contracted hepatitis A. The patient becomes tearful and asks how he could have contracted this disease. He states he has never used IV drugs or had unprotected sex. What information should be provided this patient?

Answer: The patient's misconceptions concerning hepatitis A will need to be corrected first. He should be advised that hepatitis A is not related to IV drug use or unprotected sex. Hepatitis A is transmitted via the oral-fecal route. The culprit is typically water or food contaminated with feces. It is the most common of the viral hepatitis infections. Teaching topics include mode of transmission, appropriate personal hygiene, precautions to be taken by the patient and his family, diet, and prescriptive therapies. The prognosis is good for the patient diagnosed with hepatitis A.

Question: A 45-year-old female reports to the emergency room. She states she is concerned she might be having a heart attack. She has complaints of pain in her upper right epigastric region. The pain is radiating around her midtorso to the right scapular area. She states she has been experiencing nausea and vomiting as well. The patient's heart rate and respiratory rate are elevated above normal. The patient's recall of her dietary intake for the past several hours includes a hamburger, French fries, and a chocolate milk shake. What is the suspected biliary disorder? What diagnostic tests will be ordered to confirm the diagnosis?

ELSEVIER

Answer: The patient appears to be experiencing an acute episode of cholecystitis. Diagnostic tests that will be ordered to confirm the diagnosis include fecal studies, serum bilirubin tests, gallbladder ultrasound, HIDA scan, and an oral cholecystogram.

CRITICAL THINKING QUESTION

A 45-year-old man has been diagnosed with late-stage cirrhosis. His history includes alcoholism. His assessment includes dyspepsia, altered bowel habits, weight loss, and ascites. He voices concern about his "fat" stomach. He asks how he can look so fat in his abdominal region while he is unable to eat. He asks what can be done to lose the weight.

Guidelines: This candidate needs a great deal of patient education. Ascites is a complication associated with the later stages of cirrhosis. It is an accumulation of fluid and albumin in the peritoneal cavity. It is the result of the increased venous pressure in the portal circulation. A diet will not cure ascites. Management may include intake and output monitoring. There may be dietary restrictions of fluid and sodium. Diuretics may be prescribed to promote diuresis. If these less invasive methods do not reduce fluid accumulation, it may be necessary to remove the fluid by using a shunt or paracentesis.

OBJECTIVES	CONTENT	TEACHING RESOURCES
Discuss nursing interventions for the diagnostic examinations of patients with disorders of the gallbladder, liver, biliary tract, and exocrine pancreas.	■ Laboratory and diagnostic examinations in the assessment of the hepatobiliary and pancreatic systems (FAAHN p. 1467, AHN p. 231) □ Serum bilirubin test (FAAHN p. 1467, AHN p. 231) – Rationale (FAAHN p. 1467, AHN p. 231) – Nursing interventions (FAAHN p. 1467, AHN p. 231) □ Liver enzyme tests (FAAHN p. 1467, AHN p. 231) – Rationale (FAAHN p. 1468, AHN p. 232) – Nursing interventions (FAAHN p. 1468, AHN p. 232) □ Serum protein test (FAAHN p. 1468, AHN p. 232) – Rationale (FAAHN p. 1468, AHN p. 232) – Nursing interventions (FAAHN p. 1468, AHN p. 232) □ Oral cholecystography (FAAHN p. 1468, AHN p. 232) – Rationale (FAAHN p. 1468, AHN p. 232)	⊠ PPT 2, 3, Ch. 46 FAAHN (Ch. 6 PPT 2, 3 AHN) 🖭 EILR IC Ch. 46 image 1 FAAHN (Ch. 6 image 1 AHN) 🖭 EILR TB Ch. 46 questions 1 through 4, 7, 9, 17, 23, 30, 36 FAAHN (Ch. 6 questions 1 through 4, 7, 9, 17, 23, 30, 36 AHN) 🖭 EILR Open Book Quiz Ch. 46 questions 1 through 4, 9 FAAHN (Ch. 6 questions 1 through 4 , 9 AHN) 🖭 ESLR Review Questions for the NCLEX Examination Ch. 46 questions 2, 4, 5 FAAHN (Ch. 6 questions 2, 4, 5 AHN) 📕 SG Nursing Interventions, Ch. 43 p. 369 FAAHN (Ch. 6 p. 57 AHN) **BOOK RESOURCES** Fig. 46-1 Endoscopic retrograde cholangiopancreatography (ERCP) (FAAHN p. 1471) (Fig. 6-1 AHN p. 235) ▸ Discuss the nursing responsibilities associated with preparing the patient for diagnostic examinations and evaluations for disorders of the gallbladder, liver, biliary tract, and exocrine pancreas. ▸ Discuss the normal values associated with healthy functioning of the gallbladder, liver, biliary tract, and exocrine pancreas. *Class Activity Divide the class into four groups. Assign each group a diagnostic test used to*

ELSEVIER
Mosby items and derived items © 2011 by Mosby, Inc., an affiliate of Elsevier Inc.
Some material was previously published.

Adult Health Nursing, 6th ed.
Christensen & Kockrow

OBJECTIVES	CONTENT	TEACHING RESOURCES
	– Nursing interventions (FAAHN p. 1468, AHN p. 232)	*evaluate disorders of the gallbladder, liver, biliary tract, and exocrine pancreas. Instruct each group to develop three to five questions concerning its assigned test. These questions can be combined and used as a review for the entire class.*
	☐ Intravenous cholangiography (FAAHN p. 1468, AHN p. 232)	
	– Rationale (FAAHN p. 1468, AHN p. 232)	
	☐ Operative cholangiography (FAAHN p. 1468, AHN p. 232)	
	☐ T-tube cholangiography (postoperative cholangiography) (FAAHN p. 1469, AHN p. 233)	
	– Rationale (FAAHN p. 1469, AHN p. 233)	
	– Nursing interventions (FAAHN p. 1469, AHN p. 233)	
	☐ Ultrasonography (echogram) of the liver, gallbladder, and biliary system (FAAHN p. 1469, AHN p. 233)	
	– Rationale (FAAHN p. 1469, AHN p. 233)	
	– Nursing interventions (FAAHN p. 1469, AHN p. 233)	
	☐ Gallbladder scanning (hepatobiliary scintigraphy imaging, HIDA scanning) (FAAHN p. 1469, AHN p. 233)	
	– Rationale (FAAHN p. 1469, AHN p. 233)	
	– Nursing interventions (FAAHN p. 1469, AHN p. 233)	
	☐ Needle liver biopsy (FAAHN p. 1469, AHN p. 233)	
	– Rationale (FAAHN p. 1469, AHN p. 233)	
	– Nursing interventions (FAAHN p. 1469, AHN p. 233)	
	☐ Radioisotope liver scanning (FAAHN p. 1470, AHN p. 234)	

OBJECTIVES	CONTENT	TEACHING RESOURCES
	– Rationale (FAAHN p. 1470, AHN p. 234)	
	– Nursing interventions (FAAHN p. 1470, AHN p. 234)	
	☐ Serum ammonia test (FAAHN p. 1470, AHN p. 234)	
	– Rationale (FAAHN p. 1470, AHN p. 234)	
	– Nursing interventions (FAAHN p. 1470, AHN p. 234)	
	☐ Hepatitis virus studies (hepatitis-associated antigen [HAA]) (FAAHN p. 1470, AHN p. 234)	
	– Rationale (FAAHN p. 1470, AHN p. 234)	
	– Nursing interventions (FAAHN p. 1470, AHN p. 234)	
	☐ Serum amylase test (FAAHN p. 1470, AHN p. 234)	
	– Rationale (FAAHN p. 1470, AHN p. 234)	
	– Nursing interventions (FAAHN p. 1470, AHN p. 234)	
	☐ Urine amylase test (FAAHN p. 1470, AHN p. 234)	
	– Rationale (FAAHN p. 1470, AHN p. 234)	
	– Nursing interventions (FAAHN p. 1470, AHN p. 234)	
	☐ Serum lipase test (FAAHN p. 1471, AHN p. 235)	
	– Rationale (FAAHN p. 1471, AHN p. 235)	
	– Nursing interventions (FAAHN p. 1471, AHN p. 235)	

OBJECTIVES	CONTENT	TEACHING RESOURCES
	☐ Ultrasonography of the pancreas (FAAHN p. 1471, AHN p. 235)	
	– Rationale (FAAHN p. 1471, AHN p. 235)	
	– Nursing interventions (FAAHN p. 1471, AHN p. 235)	
	☐ Computed tomography (CT) of the abdomen (FAAHN p. 1471, AHN p. 235)	
	– Rationale (FAAHN p. 1471, AHN p. 235)	
	– Nursing interventions (FAAHN p. 1471, AHN p. 235)	
	☐ Endoscopic retrograde cholangiopancreatography (ERCP) of the pancreatic duct (FAAHN p. 1471, AHN p. 235)	
	– Rationale (FAAHN p. 1471, AHN p. 235)	
	– Nursing interventions (FAAHN p. 1471, AHN p. 235)	

Explain the etiology, pathophysiology, clinical manifestations, assessment, diagnostic tests, medical management, and nursing interventions for the patient with cirrhosis of the liver, carcinoma of the liver, hepatitis, liver abscesses, cholecystitis, cholelithiasis, pancreatitis, and cancer of the pancreas.	■ Disorders of the liver, biliary tract, gallbladder, and exocrine pancreas (FAAHN p. 1472, AHN p. 236)
	
	☐ Cirrhosis (FAAHN p. 1472, AHN p. 236)
	
	   – Etiology and pathophysiology (FAAHN p. 1472, AHN p. 236)
	
	   – Clinical manifestations (FAAHN p. 1472, AHN p. 236)
	
	   – Assessment (FAAHN p. 1473, AHN p. 237)
	
	   – Diagnostic tests (FAAHN p. 1473, AHN p. 237)
	
	   – Medical management (FAAHN p. 1473, AHN p. 237)
		⊠ PPT 7 through 15, Ch. 46 FAAHN (Ch. 6 PPT 7 through 15 AHN)
		
		🅔 EILR IC Ch. 46 image 2 FAAHN (Ch. 6 image 2 AHN)
		
		🅔 EILR TB Ch. 46 questions 8, 11, 12, 21, 24, 25, 31 through 34, 37 FAAHN (Ch. 6 questions 8, 11, 12, 21, 24, 25, 31 through 34, 37 AHN)
		
		🅔 EILR Open Book Quiz Ch. 46 questions 5, 7 FAAHN (Ch. 6 questions 5, 7 AHN)
		
		🅔 ESLR Review Questions for the NCLEX Examination Ch. 46 question 10 FAAHN (Ch. 6 question 10 AHN)
		
		📗 SG Cirrhosis, Ch. 46 p. 373 FAAHN (Ch. 6 p. 61 AHN)
		
		📗 SG Liver, Pancreas, and Gallbladder, Ch. 46 p. 374 FAAHN (Ch. 6 p. 62 AHN)

Adult Health Nursing, 6th ed.
Christensen & Kockrow

OBJECTIVES	CONTENT	TEACHING RESOURCES
	– Nursing interventions and patient teaching (FAAHN p. 1476, AHN p. 240) ☐ Liver cancer (FAAHN p. 1477, AHN p. 241) – Etiology and pathophysiology (FAAHN p. 1477, AHN p. 241) – Clinical manifestations/ diagnostic tests (FAAHN p. 1478, AHN p. 242) – Medical management and nursing interventions (FAAHN p. 1478, AHN p. 242) – Prognosis (FAAHN p. 1479, AHN p. 243) ☐ Hepatitis (FAAHN p. 1479, AHN p. 243) – Etiology and pathophysiology (FAAHN p. 1479, AHN p. 243) – Clinical manifestations (FAAHN p. 1480, AHN p. 244) – Assessment (FAAHN p. 1480, AHN p. 244) – Diagnostic tests (FAAHN p. 1480, AHN p. 244) – Medical management (FAAHN p. 1480, AHN p. 244) – Nursing interventions and patient teaching (FAAHN p. 1482, AHN p. 246) – Prognosis (FAAHN p. 1483, AHN p. 247) ☐ Liver abcesses (FAAHN p. 1483, AHN p. 247) – Etiology and pathophysiology (FAAHN p. 1483, AHN p. 247) – Clinical manifestations (FAAHN p. 1483, AHN p. 247)	**BOOK RESOURCES** Fig. 46-2 Systemic clinical manifestations of liver cirrhosis (FAAHN p. 1474) (Fig. 6-2 AHN p. 238) ▸ Discuss the sequencing of events anticipated during the development of cirrhosis of the liver. ▸ Discuss the psychosocial care needed by the patient with a diagnosis of carcinoma of the liver. *Class Activity **Without mentioning names or relation, ask students to share with the class if they know someone who has developed cirrhosis, how it first manifested itself, and if/how the disease is being managed medically.***

Adult Health Nursing, 6th ed.

Christensen & Kockrow

OBJECTIVES	CONTENT	TEACHING RESOURCES

	– Assessment (FAAHN p. 1483, AHN p. 247)
	
	    – Diagnostic tests (FAAHN p. 1483, AHN p. 247)
	
	    – Medical management (FAAHN p. 1483, AHN p. 247)
	
	    – Nursing interventions and patient teaching (FAAHN p. 1483, AHN p. 247)
	
	    – Prognosis (FAAHN p. 1484, AHN p. 248)
	
	☐ Cholecystitis and cholelithiasis (FAAHN p. 1484, AHN p. 248)
	
	    – Etiology and pathophysiology (FAAHN p. 1484, AHN p. 248)
	
	    – Clinical manifestations (FAAHN p. 1485, AHN p. 249)
	
	    – Assessment (FAAHN p. 1485, AHN p. 249)
	
	    – Diagnostic tests (FAAHN p. 1485, AHN p. 249)
	
	    – Medical management (FAAHN p. 1485, AHN p. 249)
	
	    – Nursing interventions and patient teaching (FAAHN p. 1487, AHN p. 251)
	
	    – Prognosis (FAAHN p. 1488, AHN p. 252)
	
	☐ Pancreatitis (FAAHN p. 1489, AHN p. 253)
	
	    – Etiology and pathophysiology (FAAHN p. 1489, AHN p. 253)
	
	    – Clinical manifestations (FAAHN p. 1489, AHN p. 253)	

Christensen & Kockrow

OBJECTIVES	CONTENT	TEACHING RESOURCES
	– Assessment (FAAHN p. 1489, AHN p. 253)	
	– Diagnostic tests (FAAHN p. 1489, AHN p. 253)	
	– Medical management (FAAHN p. 1490, AHN p. 254)	
	– Nursing interventions and patient teaching (FAAHN p. 1490, AHN p. 254)	
	– Prognosis (FAAHN p. 1491, AHN p. 255)	
	☐ Cancer of the pancreas (FAAHN p. 1491, AHN p. 255)	
	– Etiology and pathophysiology (FAAHN p. 1492, AHN p. 256)	
	– Clinical manifestations (FAAHN p. 1492, AHN p. 256)	
	– Assessment (FAAHN p. 1492, AHN p. 256)	
	– Diagnostic tests (FAAHN p. 1492, AHN p. 256)	
	– Medical management (FAAHN p. 1492, AHN p. 256)	
	– Nursing interventions and patient teaching (FAAHN p. 1493, AHN p. 257)	
	– Prognosis (FAAHN p. 1493, AHN p. 257)	

OBJECTIVES	CONTENT	TEACHING RESOURCES
Discuss specific complications and patient teaching content for the patient with cirrhosis of the liver.	– Medical management (FAAHN p. 1473, AHN p. 237) – Nursing interventions and patient teaching (FAAHN p. 1496, AHN p. 240) – Prognosis (FAAHN p. 1497, AHN p. 241)	PPT 7 through 15, Ch. 46 FAAHN (Ch. 6 PPT 7 through 15 AHN) EILR IC Ch. 46 images 3 through 5 FAAHN (Ch. 6 images 3 through 5 AHN) EILR TB Ch. 46 questions 13 through 15, 26, 40, 41 FAAHN (Ch. 6 questions 13 through 15, 26, 40, 41 AHN) EILR Open Book Quiz Ch. 46 question 6 FAAHN (Ch. 6 question 6 AHN) ESLR Review Questions for the NCLEX Examination Ch. 46 questions 7, 8 FAAHN (Ch. 6 questions 7, 8 AHN) SG Cirrhosis, Ch. 46 p. 373 FAAHN (Ch. 6 p. 61 AHN) **BOOK RESOURCES** Fig. 46-3 LeVeen continuous peritoneal jugular shunt (FAAHN p. 1474) (Fig. 6-3 AHN p. 238) Fig. 46-4 Esophogeal tamponade accomposhed with Sengstaken-Blakemore tube (FAAHN p. 1475) (Fig. 6-4 AHN p. 239) Home Care Considerations: Cirrhosis of the Liver (FAAHN p. 1477) (AHN p. 241) Nursing Care Plan 46-1 The Patient with Cirrhosis of the Liver (FAAHN p. 1478) (NCP 6-1 AHN p. 242) NCP CTQ 1, 2 (FAAHN p. 1478) (AHN p. 242) ▸ Discuss the typical prognosis for the patient diagnosed with cirrhosis of the liver. *Class Activity Develop a nursing care plan that can be used for the patient diagnosed with cirrhosis of the liver.*
Define jaundice, and describe signs and symptoms that may occur with jaundice.	– Assessment (FAAHN p. 1480, AHN p. 244)	PPT 8, 24, 25, 29, 34, 38, 41, Ch. 46 FAAHN (Ch. 6 PPT 8, 24, 25, 29, 34, 38, 41 AHN) EILR TB Ch. 46 question 38 FAAHN (Ch. 6 question 38 AHN) ESLR Review Questions for the NCLEX Examination Ch. 46 question 1 FAAHN (Ch. 6 question 1 AHN)

Christensen & Kockrow

OBJECTIVES	CONTENT	TEACHING RESOURCES
		SG Signs and Symptoms, Ch. 46 p. 371 FAAHN (Ch. 6 p. 59 AHN) **BOOK RESOURCES** Fig. 46-5 Severe jaundice (FAAHN p. 1480) (Fig. 6-5 AHN p. 244) ▸ Discuss the pathophysiology that is responsible for the appearance of jaundice. ▸ Discuss the locations to best assess for jaundice. *Class Activity On the board, have students list the objective data in two columns related to jaundice: early stage and later stage.*

6.1 Homework/Assignments:

6.1 Instructor's Notes/Student Feedback:

LESSON 6.2

CRITICAL THINKING QUESTION

After repeated episodes of cholecystitis, a patient and physician agree that surgical intervention is necessary. The surgery is performed without difficulty. Later that evening, the patient voices concerns about when he will be discharged. What factors will determine his physical and cognitive readiness to be sent home? What information will be included in the patient's discharge education?

Guidelines: Some patients who have had a laparoscopic cholecystectomy are able to be discharged several hours after surgery. Most patients spend a night in the hospital for observation.

Before discharge, the patient needs to exhibit stable vital signs, and the laparoscopic puncture sites must be intact and absent of bile drainage. The patient must eat, ambulate, and void without problems. Patient education topics include care of the incision, signs and symptoms to report, and follow-up care plans.

OBJECTIVES	CONTENT	TEACHING RESOURCES
State the six types of viral hepatitis, including their modes of transmission.	☐ Hepatitis (FAAHN p. 1479, AHN p. 243) – Etiology and pathophysiology (FAAHN p. 1479, AHN p. 243) – Clinical manifestations (FAAHN p. 1480, AHN p. 244) – Assessment (FAAHN p. 1480, AHN p. 244) – Diagnostic tests (FAAHN p. 1480, AHN p. 244) – Medical management (FAAHN p. 1480, AHN p. 244) – Nursing interventions and patient teaching (FAAHN p. 1482, AHN p. 246) – Prognosis (FAAHN p. 1483, AHN p. 247)	▨ PPT 20 through 27, Ch. 46 FAAHN (Ch. 6 PPT 20 through 27 AHN) 🔋 EILR TB Ch. 46 questions 10, 19, 20 FAAHN (Ch. 6 questions 10, 19, 20 AHN) 🔋 EILR Open Book Quiz Ch. 46 question 8 FAAHN (Ch. 6 question 8 AHN) 🔋 ESLR Review Questions for the NCLEX Examination Ch. 46 questions 6, 9 FAAHN (Ch. 6 questions 6, 9 AHN) ▦ SG Viral Hepatitis, Ch. 46 p. 371 FAAHN (Ch. 6 p. 59 AHN) **BOOK RESOURCES** Box 46-1 Modes of Transmission of the Six Types of Viral Hepatitis (FAAHN p. 1480) (Box 6-1 AHN p. 244) ▸ Discuss the similarities and differences between the six types of viral hepatitis. ▸ Discuss populations at risk for contracting the three most common types of viral hepatitis. *Class Activity Develop a chart listing each of the six types of viral hepatitis across the top columns. Along the side, list etiology, clinical manifestations, diagnostic tests, management, and prognosis. Invite class participation to complete the chart. Once completed, the chart can be a study tool for the students.*
List the subjective and objective data for the patient with viral hepatitis.	– Assessment (FAAHN p. 1480, AHN p. 244)	▨ PPT 20 through 27, Ch. 46 FAAHN (Ch. 6 PPT 20 through 27 AHN) EILR TB Ch. 46 questions 22, 42 FAAHN (Ch. 6 questions 22, 42 AHN) ▦ SG Viral Hepatitis, Ch. 46 p. 371 FAAHN (Ch. 6 p. 59 AHN)

ELSEVIER

Mosby items and derived items © 2011 by Mosby, Inc., an affiliate of Elsevier Inc.
Some material was previously published.

Adult Health Nursing, 6th ed.

Christensen & Kockrow

OBJECTIVES	CONTENT	TEACHING RESOURCES
		▸ Discuss the nursing assessment of the patient diagnosed with viral hepatitis. ***Class Activity On the board, have students list the objective data and subjective data in two columns related to viral hepatitis.***
Discuss the indicators for liver transplantation and the immunosuppressant drugs to reduce rejection.	– Medical management (FAAHN p. 1480, AHN p. 244)	⚡ EILR TB Ch. 46 questions 27 through 39 FAAHN (Ch. 6 questions 27 through 39 AHN) 📗 SG Liver Transplantation, Ch. 46 p. 376 FAAHN (Ch. 6 p. 64 AHN) ▸ Discuss the patients who are suitable candidates for liver transplantation. ▸ Discuss the lifelong implications associated with a liver transplant. ***Class Activity Invite a representative from the local hospital to discuss protocols for organ donation.***

Discuss the two methods of surgical treatment for cholecystitis/ cholelithiasis.	☐ Cholecystitis and cholelithiasis (FAAHN p. 1484, AHN p. 248)
	
	  – Medical management (FAAHN p. 1485, AHN p. 249)
	
	☐ Nursing process for patients with gallbladder, liver, biliary tract, or exocrine pancreatic disorder (FAAHN p. 1493, AHN p. 257)
	
	  – Assessment (FAAHN p. 1494, AHN p. 258)
	
	  – Nursing diagnosis (FAAHN p. 1494, AHN p. 258)
	
	  – Expected outcomes and planning (FAAHN p. 1494, AHN p. 258)
	
	  – Implementation (FAAHN p. 1494, AHN p. 258)
	
	  – Evaluation (FAAHN p. 1494, AHN p. 258)
		🖳 PPT 31 through 36, Ch. 46 FAAHN (Ch. 6 PPT 31 through 36 AHN)
		
		⚡ EILR IC Ch. 46 images 6 through 9 FAAHN (Ch. 6 images 6 through 9 AHN)
		
		⚡ EILR TB Ch. 46 questions 5, 6, 16, 18, 35 FAAHN (Ch. 6 questions 5, 6, 16, 18, 35 AHN)
		
		⚡ EILR Open Book Quiz Ch. 46 question 10 FAAHN (Ch. 6 question 10 AHN)
		
		⚡ ESLR Review Questions for the NCLEX Examination Ch. 46 question 5 FAAHN (Ch. 6 question 5 AHN)
		
		📗 SG Liver, Pancreas, and Gallbladder, Ch. 46 p. 374 FAAHN (Ch. 6 p. 62 AHN)
		
		BOOK RESOURCES
		
		Box 46-2 Definitions (FAAHN p. 1484) (Box 6-2 AHN p. 248)
		
		Fig. 46-6 Common sites of gallstones (FAAHN p. 1484) (Fig. 6-6 AHN p. 248)
		
		Complementary and Alternative Therapies: Gallbladder, Biliary, and Pancreatic Disorders (FAAHN p. 1485, AHN p. 249)
		
		Fig. 46-7 Endoscopic sphincterotomy (FAAHN p. 1486) (Fig. 6-7 AHN p. 250)
		
		Fig. 46-8 T-tube in common bile duct (FAAHN p. 1486) (Fig. 6-8 AHN p. 250)

OBJECTIVES	CONTENT	TEACHING RESOURCES
		Life Span Considerations: Older adults Gallbladder, Liver, Biliary Tract, or Exocrine Pancreatic Disorder (FAAHN p. 1489) (AHN p. 253) Table 46-1 Medications for Disorders of the Gallbladder, Liver, Biliary Tract, and Exocrine Pancreas (FAAHN p. 1491) (Table 6-1 AHN p. 255) ▸ Discuss the similarities between the methods of surgical treatment for cholecystitis/cholelithiasis. Class Activity ***On the board, have the students list the factors that determine which of the surgical procedures will be used on a patient to manage cholecystitis/cholelithiasis.***
Performance Evaluation		EILR TB Ch. 46 questions 1 through 41 FAAHN (Ch. 6 questions 1 through 41 AHN) EILR Open Book Quiz Ch. 46 questions 1 through 10 FAAHN (Ch. 6 questions 1 through 10 AHN) ESLR Review Questions for the NCLEX Examination Ch. 46 questions 1 through 10 FAAHN (Ch. 6 questions 1 through 10 AHN) SG Ch. 46 pp. 369 through 380 FAAHN (Ch. 6 pp. 57 through 68 AHN) **BOOK RESOURCES** Nursing Care Plan 46-1 The Patient with Cirrhosis of the Liver (FAAHN p. 1478) (NCP 6-1 AHN p. 242) NCP CTQ 1-2 (FAAHN p. 1478) (AHN p. 242) Review Questions for the NCLEX Examination Ch. 46 questions 1 through 29 FAAHN (Ch. 6 questions 1 through 29 AHN)

6.2 Homework/Assignments:

6.2 Instructor's Notes/Student Feedback:

Mosby items and derived items © 2011 by Mosby, Inc., an affiliate of Elsevier Inc.
Some material was previously published.

6 **Care of the Patient with a Gallbladder, Liver, Biliary Tract, or Exocrine Pancreatic Disorder**

Slide 1

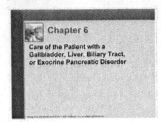

- The exocrine organs of digestion are those whose functions aid the body in digesting nutrients.

Slide 2

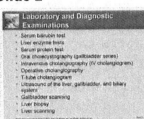

- When the body becomes jaundiced, a yellow skin discoloration results. When visualization of jaundice results, the total serum bilirubin exceeds 2.5 mg/dL.

- What types of information can be gleaned from the bilirubin values?

The results provide information for diagnosis and evaluation of liver disease, biliary obstruction, erythroblastosis fetalis, and hemolytic anemia.

- What is the rationale for assessing liver enzymes? Why do their levels change with liver disease?

Injury and diseases promote the release of intracellular enzymes into the bloodstream.

Slide 3

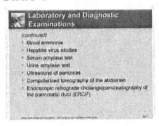

- What nursing assessments must be performed before each of the listed diagnostic tests?

Slide 4

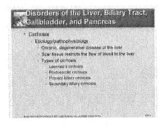

- Cirrhosis is the fourth leading cause of death in the United States for adults between 40 and 60.

- During its progression, cirrhosis causes the degeneration of liver tissue, which results in the formation of fibrous tissue and fat infiltration of the lobules. These events cause the reduction of blood flow, further compounding the problem.

- There are different types of cirrhosis. Discuss the different types of cirrhosis and their causes.

Adult Health Nursing, 6th ed.
Christensen & Kockrow

Slide 5

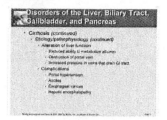

- As cirrhosis continues to progress, there are resulting complications. These complications include portal hypertension, ascites, esophageal varices, and hepatic encephalopathy. What is the underlying cause of each of these?

Slide 6

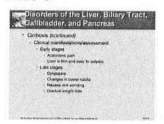

- When providing care to a patient diagnosed with cirrhosis, what nursing interventions are appropriate?

Slide 7

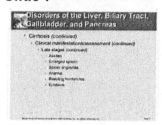

- As cirrhosis continues the physiological destruction of the liver, there is an increase in the severity of clinical manifestations. What factors should be assessed for the patient?

Slide 8

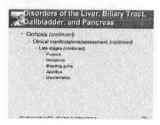

- What teaching should be provided to the patient concerning cirrhosis?

Slide 9

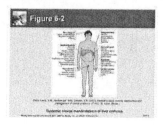

ELSEVIER

Mosby items and derived items © 2011, 2007 by Mosby, Inc., an affiliate of Elsevier Inc.
Some material was previously published.

Adult Health Nursing, 6th ed.
Christensen & Kockrow

Slide 10

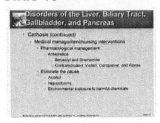

- The removal of the underlying causes of liver damage can aid in the prevention of additional damage to the structure.

- What is a commonly taken over-the-counter hepatotoxin?

- Antiemetics can be administered to reduce nausea and vomiting. What nursing assessments and diagnostic monitoring must accompany the administration of these medications?

Slide 11

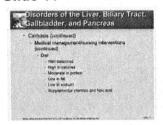

- Diet management is vital in the treatment of cirrhosis. Ideally the diet should include between 2,500 and 3,000 calories per day.

- What are the goals of dietary modifications?

Diet therapy is aimed at correcting malnutrition and promoting regeneration of the functional liver tissue and compensating for the liver's deficits.

- What are the caloric needs of the patient diagnosed with cirrhosis?

Slide 12

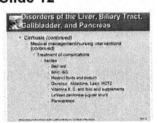

- The severity of ascites will determine the medical management employed.

- At the very least, intake and output will be monitored.

- Diuretics can be prescribed. Review the mode of action for diuretics.

- If the ascites is severe, a paracentesis can be done. What nursing care should be performed before and after the procedure?

Slide 13

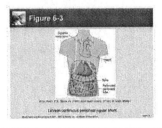

- The LeVeen shunt allows for continuous shunting of ascitic fluid from the abdominal cavity via a one-way, pressure-sensitive valve into a silicone tube and empties into the superior vena cava.

- What complications are associated with the use of the LeVeen shunt?

- *Congestive heart failure, leakage of ascitic fluid, infection at the insertion site, peritonitis, septicemia, and shunt thrombosis.*

Slide 14

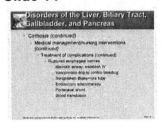

- Esophageal varices occur because of portal hypertension. What is the primary goal of esophageal varices management?

The avoidance of further bleeding and hemorrhage.

- What actions can result in bleeding or hemorrhage of the varices?

Slide 15

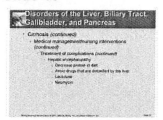

- Hepatic encephalopathy is a type of brain damage caused by ammonia intoxication.

- What clinical manifestations can accompany this complication?

- In an effort to restrict protein and reduce ammonia formation in the intestines, dietary management might be needed. What foods would be appropriate for the diet of a patient experiencing hepatic encephalopathy? What foods should be avoided?

Slide 16

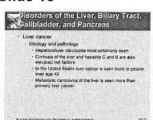

- Increases in liver cancer in the United States are tied to an increased incidence of hepatitis C.

Slide 17

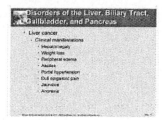

Slide 18

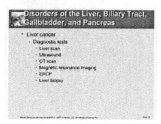

- Diagnosing liver cancer can be difficult.

Slide 19

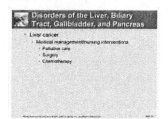

- The prognosis for cancer of the liver is poor. What is the typical life expectancy for the patient with liver cancer?

- What nursing diagnoses would be appropriate for the patient diagnosed with liver cancer?

ELSEVIER

Mosby items and derived items © 2011, 2007 by Mosby, Inc., an affiliate of Elsevier Inc.
Some material was previously published.

Adult Health Nursing, 6th ed.
Christensen & Kockrow

Slide 20

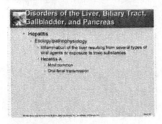

- Hepatitis A is the most common type of hepatitis. It is estimated that up to 50% of people in the United States are infected by the time they reach adulthood.

- What reporting is required of patients diagnosed with viral hepatitis?

- Identify situations in which a person could become infected with hepatitis A.

- List interventions to aid in the prevention of hepatitis A.

Slide 21

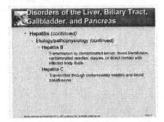

- Hepatitis B was formerly known as serum hepatitis.

- Hepatitis B is associated with a long incubation period.

Slide 22

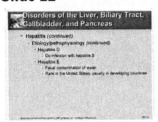

- Hepatitis D is also known as delta virus. It causes hepatitis as a co-infection with hepatitis B. It can progress to cirrhosis and chronic hepatitis.

- Hepatitis E is also referred to as enteric non-A non-B hepatitis.

Slide 23

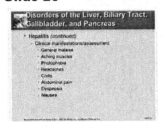

- Provide a brief summation of the differences in the incubation periods for the types of hepatitis.

- The signs and symptoms of viral hepatitis vary greatly among patients.

Slide 24

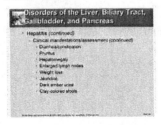

- Two common clinical manifestations associated with hepatitis are pruritus and jaundice. What is the underlying cause of each of these symptoms?

Christensen & Kockrow

Slide 25

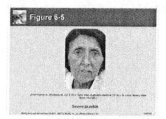

- Review the key locations to assess the patient for jaundice.

Slide 26

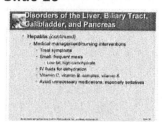

- Management of the patient diagnosed with hepatitis is directed toward supportive therapy for the signs and symptoms and prevention of disease spread to others.

- Dietary management includes vitamin B, vitamin B–complex, and vitamin K. What is the rationale for these supplements for the patient with hepatitis?

Slide 27

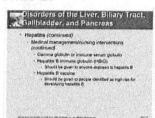

- Gamma globulin or immune serum globulin is a treatment geared toward patients who have been exposed to hepatitis B. When and how should these therapies be administered?

- Discuss the administration of the hepatitis B vaccine. Who are appropriate candidates for this medication?

- What is the prognosis for the patient who has been diagnosed with hepatitis?

Slide 28

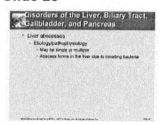

- Liver abscesses can form if a bacterial infection can become colonized. What are potential sources of this infection?

Slide 29

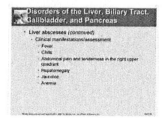

- Patients having liver abscesses present with vague signs and symptoms. The most common complaints include fever, pain, and upper right quadrant tenderness.

- What nursing diagnoses would be appropriate for this patient?

Christensen & Kockrow

Slide 30

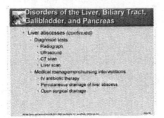

- The prognosis for the patient with liver abscesses has improved over the past several years. What can be attributed to the improvements in clinical outcomes?

Slide 31

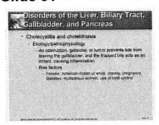

- In the United States, more than 500,000 patients are hospitalized with biliary system disorders.

Slide 32

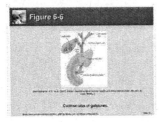

- What are potential complications associated with this condition?

Slide 33

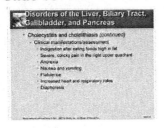

- The onset of symptoms might be sudden or demonstrated in a chronic manner with recurrent episodes of milder attacks.

- The clinical manifestations can cause the patient to believe he or she is experiencing a heart attack.

- Chronic attacks can be associated with the ingestion of a high-fat meal. Why does an elevated fat intake act as a catalyst for the attack?

Slide 34

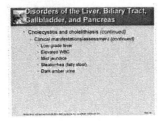

- Objective data collected might reflect an elevated leukocyte count, clay-colored stools, and amber-colored urine. Review the pathology responsible for these findings.

ELSEVIER

Adult Health Nursing, 6th ed.
Christensen & Kockrow

Slide 35

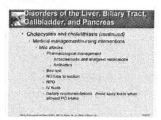

- Management for mild attacks is typically conservative in nature.
- Conservative management seeks to rest the GI tract and the gallbladder.
- Pharmacological management includes antispasmodics, analgesics, and antibiotics.
- What is the rationale for each of the drug types prescribed?
- Review the rationale for the avoidance of morphine administration for patients experiencing biliary pain.

Slide 36

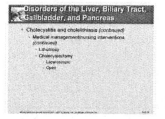

- Lithotripsy and surgical management seek to break up or remove offending stones.
- What pre-procedure/preoperative patient education is needed for these patients?
- What are the nursing responsibilities for the postprocedure care of these patients?

Slide 37

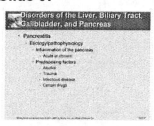

- Pancreatitis is in inflammation of the pancreas. It can be acute or chronic. Discuss the pathophysiologic processes of this disorder.

Slide 38

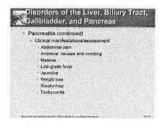

- Patients having pancreatitis might express symptoms along a vast continuum. The most common is abdominal pain that radiates to the back. What is the root cause of the pain?
- What diagnostic tests can be used to support a diagnosis of pancreatitis?

Slide 39

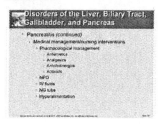

- Unless the cause of pancreatitis is related to biliary tract disease, the management of the disease is medical.
- Foods and fluid are restricted. What is the rationale for this intervention?
- Parenteral anticholinergics may also be indicated. What is the rationale for the administration of this classification of medication?
- Dietary management for chronic pancreatitis might be initiated. What would characteristics of this diet be?

ELSEVIER

Christensen & Kockrow

Slide 40

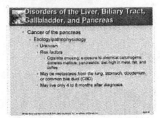

- Pancreatic cancer is the fourth leading cause of cancer death in the United States and Canada.

- To what can the high death rate be attributed?

Slide 41

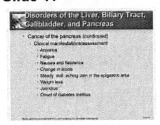

- In addition to the assessment of physical signs and symptoms, the patient's occupation should be investigated. What occupations would place a worker at higher risk of pancreatic cancer?

Slide 42

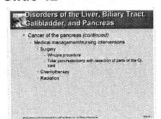

- Review the diagnostic tests used to identify pancreatic cancer.

- What prognosis is associated with pancreatic cancer?

Slide 43

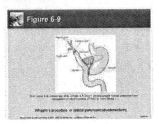

Slide 44

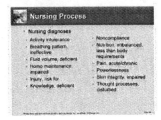

7 | Lesson Plan
Care of the Patient with a Blood or Lymphatic Disorder

TEACHING FOCUS

In this chapter, the student will be introduced to the care of the patient with a blood or lymphatic disorder. The student will begin by exploring the anatomy and physiology of blood and the lymphatic system and structures. The student will then have the opportunity to learn about the common diagnostic tests for blood and lymph disorders. Next, the student will explore the types of anemia, disorders of coagulation, shock, leukemia, and other disorders of the blood or lymphatic system.

MATERIALS AND RESOURCES

- ☐ Computer/overhead projector (Lessons 7.1 and 7.2)
- ☐ White/black board and marker/chalk (Lessons 7.1 and 7.2)
- ☐ Thread and glue (Lesson 7.1)
- ☐ Kits from a medical lab technology program, including lancets and pipettes (Lesson 7.1)
- ☐ Unlabeled diagram of the organs of the lymphatic system (Lesson 7.1)
- ☐ Small prizes, such as fruit or pencils (Lesson 7.1)
- ☐ Nursing care plan sheets (Lesson 7.2)

LESSON CHECKLIST

Preparations for this lesson include:

- Lecture
- Invite a member of the medical lab of a local hospital to bring a copy of the sheet used to report leukocyte differential results and speak to the class about how it is used.
- Invite a representative of a medical technician program to speak with the class and determine the blood types of a few student volunteers.
- Contact a local hospital or hospice to invite a professional to speak with the class about the care of patients living with leukemia.
- Invite a professional to speak with the class about the care of patients living with multiple myeloma, malignant lymphoma, or Hodgkin's disease.

KEY TERMS

anemia (FAAHN p. 1505, AHN p. 269)
aplasia (FAAHN p. 1509, AHN p. 273)
disseminated intravascular coagulation (DIC) (FAAHN p. 1525, AHN p. 289)
erythrocytosis (FAAHN p. 1515, AHN p. 279)
erythropoiesis (FAAHN p. 1499, AHN p. 263)
hemarthrosis (FAAHN p. 1523, AHN p. 287)
hemophilia A (FAAHN p. 1523, AHN p. 287)
heterozygous (FAAHN p. 1513, AHN p. 277)
homozygous (FAAHN p. 1512, AHN p. 276)
idiopathic (FAAHN p. 1509, AHN p. 273)
leukemia (FAAHN p. 1518, AHN p. 282)
leukopenia (FAAHN p. 1517, AHN p. 281)

lymphangitis (FAAHN p. 1528, AHN p. 292)
lymphedema (FAAHN p. 1529, AHN p. 293)
multiple myeloma (FAAHN p. 1527, AHN p. 291)
myeloproliferative (FAAHN p. 1515, AHN p. 279)
pancytopenic (FAAHN p. 1509, AHN p. 273)
pernicious (FAAHN p. 1508, AHN p. 272)
Reed-Sternberg cell (FAAHN p. 1530, AHN p. 294)
thrombocytopenia (FAAHN p. 1522, AHN p. 286)

ADDITIONAL RESOURCES (AHN)

PPT Ch. 47, 1 through 64 FAAHN (Ch. 7, 1 through 64 AHN)
EILR IC images Ch. 47, 1 through 5 FAAHN (Ch. 7, 1 through 5 AHN)
EILR TB questions Ch. 47, 1 through 40 FAAHN (Ch. 7, 1 through 40 AHN)
EILR Open Book Quiz Ch. 47, 1 through 10 FAAHN (Ch. 7, 1 through 10 AHN)
ESLR Review Questions for the NCLEX® Examination Ch. 47, 47-01 through 47-10 FAAHN (Ch. 7, 47-01 through 47-10 AHN)

ELSEVIER

Legend

PPT
PowerPoint
Slides

EILR
EVOLVE Instructor
Learning Resources:
Image Collection, Test
Bank, Open Book Quizzes

ESLR
EVOLVE Student
Learning Resources:
Review Questions
for the NCLEX
Examination

SG
Study Guide

NCP CTQ
Nursing Care Plan
Critical Thinking
Question

Class Activities are indicated in **bold italic**.

LESSON 7.1

PRETEST

1 The _____ are the main component of blood.
   a. platelets
   b. erythrocytes
   c. leukocytes
   d. neutrophils

2. The normal hemoglobin level in men is:
   a. 14 to 18 g/dL.
   b. 12 to 16 g/dL.
   c. 16 to 18 g/dL.
   d. 18 to 20 g/dL.

3. Which of the white blood cells plays a role in allergic reactions?
   a. Basophils
   b. Monocytes
   c. Eosinophils
   d. Neutrophils

4. When providing care to a patient who has suffered a large burn to the neck and chest, a WBC with differential test is ordered. Which of the following factors would most likely be noted?
   a. The monocyte level will be elevated.
   b. The erythrocyte sedimentation rate will be reduced.
   c. The hemoglobin level will be reduced.
   d. The neutrophil levels will be elevated.

5. The blood type _____ is often referred to as the universal recipient.
   a. AB
   b. B
   c. O
   d. A

6. Which mother will be a candidate for the administration of RhoGAM after the birth of a baby?
   a. The mother is O positive and the baby is O positive.
   b. The mother is AB positive and the baby is A positive.
   c. The mother is A negative the baby is AB negative.
   d. The mother is A negative and the baby is O positive.

7. When caring for a patient diagnosed with iron deficiency anemia, the nurse's responsibilities include patient education concerning dietary intake. What foods should be included in the diet?
   a. Strawberries, cantaloupe, and legumes
   b. Liver, citrus fruit, and cottage cheese
   d. Eggs, shellfish, and broccoli
   d. Whole-grain breads, nuts, and dried fruit

ELSEVIER

8. A patient is hospitalized with a diagnosis of lymphedema. When developing the plan of care, which of these interventions would be most appropriate?
    a. Reduced sodium intake
    b. Antiviral medication therapy
    c. Intravenous fluid replacement
    d. Restrictions in dietary protein

9. After the staging process, a patient being treated for Hodgkin's disease has been identified as being in stage II. Which of the following best describes her level of disease process?
    a. Diffuse and disseminated involvement of one or more extralymphatic tissues
    b. Two or more abnormal lymph nodes on the same side of the diaphragm
    c. Abnormal lymph node regions on both sides of the diaphragm
    d. Regional extranodal sites located

10. Which of the following statements is correct concerning the administration of oral iron therapy?
    a. If a dose is missed, do not double the next dose to catch up.
    b. Enteric-coated iron is an acceptable option for patients who have difficulty taking pills.
    c. Patients experiencing gastrointestinal upset when taking iron pills should take the pills accompanied with an antacid preparation.
    d. When diluting liquid iron preparations, use water, not juice.

Answers:

1. b	2. a	3. c	4. c	5. a
6. d	7. d	8. d	9. b	10. a

BACKGROUND ASSESSMENT

Question: A patient reports to the doctor that he is feeling tired all the time, despite how much rest he is getting. After a review of other potential health problems, a complete blood cell count is ordered. What is being measured? What condition is suspected? How will it be managed?

Answer: The patient is being evaluated for anemia. The complete blood cell count will be used to measure his hemoglobin. It is hemoglobin that carries the oxygen in his body. If it is diagnosed, he can be treated with iron supplements and dietary improvements.

Question: After evaluating a patient for an upper respiratory infection, the physician orders laboratory testing. The patient is diagnosed with "strep throat." What alterations are expected in the complete blood cell count?

Answer: The complete blood cell count with differential will be used to assess the patient's white blood cell count. The body's white blood cells are produced in response to infection. Different types of white blood cells are employed in different manners. The total white blood cell count will most likely be elevated. The neutrophils will usually reflect an elevation.

CRITICAL THINKING QUESTION

A patient who has undergone surgery has been found to need a blood transfusion. After completing the testing process, it has been determined the patient is O positive. Based upon your knowledge of the blood groups, what does this mean concerning the patient's blood characteristics?

Guidelines: This patient's blood is absent of both A or B antigens. The blood of this individual contains both anti-A and anti-B antibodies. This type of blood is compatible not only with other people with type O but with those having A and B. It is known as the universal donor blood.

OBJECTIVES	CONTENT	TEACHING RESOURCES

Describe the components of blood.	■ Anatomy and physiology of the hematological and lymphatic systems (FAAHN p. 1498, AHN p. 262)
	
	☐ Characteristics of blood (FAAHN p. 1498, AHN p. 262)
	
	  – Red blood cells (FAAHN p. 1499, AHN p. 263)
	
	  – White blood cells (FAAHN p. 1501, AHN p. 265)
	
	  – Thrombocytes (platelets) (FAAHN p. 1502, AHN p. 266)
	
	  – Hemostasis (FAAHN p. 1502, AHN p. 266)
	
	  – Blood types (groups) (FAAHN p. 1502, AHN p. 266)
	
	  – Rh factor (FAAHN p. 1503, AHN p. 267)
		PPT 1 through 8 Ch. 47 FAAHN (Ch. 7 PPT 1 through 8 AHN)
		
		EILR IC Ch. 47 image 1 FAAHN (Ch. 7 image 1 AHN)
		
		EILR TB Ch. 47 questions 3 through 5, 8, 35, 36, 40 FAAHN (Ch. 7 questions 3 through 5, 8, 35, 36, 40 AHN)
		
		SG Components of Blood, Ch. 47 p. 381 FAAHN (Ch. 7 p. 69 AHN)
		
		BOOK RESOURCES
		
		Fig. 47-1 Human blood cells (FAAHN p. 1499) (Fig. 7-1 AHN p. 263)
		
		▸ Discuss different categories of cells that compose the blood.
		
		▸ Discuss the critical functions of blood in the body.
		
		Class Activity Divide the class into three groups. Ask each group to illustrate one type of blood cell. After completion, use the drawings to compare and contrast the appearance of each classification of cells.

Differentiate between the functions of erythrocytes, leukocytes, and thrombocytes.	☐ Characteristics of blood (FAAHN p. 1498, AHN p. 262)
	
	  – Red blood cells (FAAHN p. 1499, AHN p. 263)
	
	  – White blood cells (FAAHN p. 1501, AHN p. 265)
	
	  – Thrombocytes (platelets) (FAAHN p. 1502, AHN p. 266)
	
	  – Hemostasis (FAAHN p. 1502, AHN p. 266)
	
	  – Blood types (groups) (FAAHN p. 1502, AHN p. 266)
	
	  – Rh factor (FAAHN p. 1503, AHN p. 267)
		PPT 3 Ch. 47 FAAHN (Ch. 7 PPT 3 AHN)
		
		EILR TB Ch. 47 questions 1, 35 FAAHN (Ch. 7 questions 1, 35 AHN)
		
		SG Components of Blood, Ch. 47 p. 381 FAAHN (Ch. 7 p. 69 AHN)
		
		BOOK RESOURCES
		
		Table 47-1 Diagnostic Blood Studies (FAAHN pp. 1499-1500) (Table 7-1 AHN pp. 263-264)
		
		▸ Discuss the different appearances of the types of blood cells.
		
		▸ Discuss the functions of each of the classifications of blood cells.
		
		Class Activity Beginning in the front row of the classroom, ask the students to begin

Christensen & Kockrow

OBJECTIVES	CONTENT	TEACHING RESOURCES
		counting off 1-2-3. Then repeat. After each student has been assigned a number, divide the students by numbered groups. Assign each number a type of blood cell. Instruct each group to write down three factors about its assigned cell type. After completion, the students will return to their normal seating area and share factors with their seatmates who were in different groups.
Discuss the several factors necessary for the formation of erythrocytes.	− Red blood cells (FAAHN p. 1499, AHN p. 263)	EILR TB Ch. 47 question 31, FAAHN (Ch. 7 question 31 AHN) SG Components of Blood, Ch. 47 p. 381 FAAHN (Ch. 7 p. 69 AHN) **BOOK REFERENCES** Review Questions for the NCLEX Examination Ch. 47 question 26 FAAHN (Ch. 7 question 26 AHN) ▸ Discuss the role of erythropoietin in the blood stream. ▸ Discuss the laboratory tests used to determine the level of red blood cells. *Class Activity Instruct each student to develop at least two short NCLEX-style questions concerning the formation of erythrocytes. After the questions are completed, collect them to use in a short class review of the content.*

OBJECTIVES	CONTENT	TEACHING RESOURCES

Define the white blood cell differential.	– White blood cells (FAAHN p. 1501, AHN p. 265)	EILR TB Ch. 47 questions 2, 6, 9, 10FAAHN (Ch. 7 questions 2, 6, 9 AHN)
		
		  ESLR Review Questions for the NCLEX Examination Ch. 47 question 1 FAAHN (Ch. 7 question 1AHN)
		
		  SG Components of Blood, Ch. 47 p. 381 FAAHN (Ch. 7 p. 69 AHN)
		
		 ▶ Discuss the cell types monitored in a leukocyte differential.
		
		 ▶ Discuss what can be determined when a leukocyte differential is performed.
		
		 Class Activity Contact a local hospital. Ask for a copy of the sheet used to report the leukocyte differential results. Ask a member of the medical lab to come to the class to explain its use.

Describe the blood clotting process.	– Thrombocytes (platelets) (FAAHN p. 1502, AHN p. 266)
	
	 – Hemostasis (FAAHN p. 1502, AHN p. 266)
		PPT 5 through 6 Ch. 47 FAAHN (Ch. 7 PPT 5 through 6 AHN)
		
		  EILR IC Ch. 47 image 2 FAAHN (Ch. 7 image 2 AHN)
		
		  SG Blood Clotting, Ch. 47 p. 282 FAAHN (Ch. 7 p. 70 AHN)
		
		 BOOK RESOURCES
		
		 Fig. 47-2 Blood clotting (FAAHN p. 1502) (Fig. 7-2 AHN p. 266)
		
		 ▶ Discuss the actions that take place during hemostasis.
		
		 ▶ Discuss the laboratory tests that can be utilized to monitor the hemostasis abilities of the body.
		
		 Class Activity Give the students thread and glue and have each student simulate clot formation with these objects. (Allow the glue to partially harden prior to adding more glue. The thread should be crossed in a fairly small interval vertically and horizontally so the glue eventually covers the area as a clot would cover a wound).

ELSEVIER

Adult Health Nursing, 6th ed.

Christensen & Kockrow

OBJECTIVES	CONTENT	TEACHING RESOURCES
List the names of the basic blood groups.	– Blood types (groups) (FAAHN p. 1502, AHN p. 266) – Rh factor (FAAHN p. 1503, AHN p. 267)	☒▬ PPT 7 through 8 Ch. 47 FAAHN (Ch. 7 PPT 7 through 8 AHN) ▰ EILR IC Ch. 47 image 3 FAAHN (Ch. 7 image 3 AHN) ▰ SG Blood Groups, Ch. 47 p. 382 FAAHN (Ch. 7 p. 70 AHN) **BOOK RESOURCES** Fig. 47-3 Results of different combinations of donor and recipient blood (FAAHN p. 1503) (Fig. 7-3 AHN p. 267) ▸ Discuss the types of blood that exist. ▸ Discuss the compatibility concerns when administering a blood transfusion. *Class Activity Obtain kits from a medical lab technology program. Allow students to use lancets and pipettes to perform experiments to determine the blood types of a few student volunteers.* *Note: You might feel more comfortable asking a representative of a medical technician program to attend the session to assist with the process.*

Christensen & Kockrow

OBJECTIVES	CONTENT	TEACHING RESOURCES
Describe the generalized functions of the lymphatic system, and list the primary lymphatic structures.	☐ Lymphatic system (FAAHN p. 1503, AHN p. 267) – Lymph and lymph vessels (FAAHN p. 1503, AHN p. 267) – Lymphatic tissue (FAAHN p. 1504, AHN p. 268)	▨▤ PPT 9 through 12 Ch. 47 FAAHN (Ch. 7 PPT 9 through 12 AHN) 🔁 EILR IC Ch. 47 image 4 FAAHN (Ch. 7 image 4 AHN) 📕SG SG Organs of the Lymphatic System, Ch. 47 p. 383 FAAHN (Ch. 7 p. 71 AHN) **BOOK RESOURCES** Fig. 47-4 Principal organs of the lymphatic system (FAAHN p. 1504) (Fig. 7-4 AHN p. 268) Review Questions for the NCLEX Examination Ch. 47 question 3 FAAHN (Ch. 7 question 3 AHN) ▸ Discuss the roles of the lymphatic system. ▸ Discuss the structures that are part of the lymphatic system. *Class Activity **Distribute an unlabeled diagram of the organs of the lymphatic system. Instruct the students to label the principal organs in the system.*** ***Note: It might be helpful to do this at the beginning of the lecture to assess students' level of knowledge.***
List common diagnostic tests for evaluation of blood and lymph disorders, and discuss the significance of the results.	■ Anatomy and Physiology of the Hematological and Lymphatic Systems (FAAHN p. 1498, AHN p. 262) ☐ Laboratory and diagnostic tests (FAAHN p. 1505, AHN p. 269) – Complete blood count (FAAHN p. 1505, AHN p. 269) – Erythrocyte indexes (FAAHN p. 1505, AHN p. 269) – Peripheral smear (FAAHN p. 1505, AHN p. 269) – Schilling test and megaloblastic anemia profile (FAAHN p. 1505, AHN p. 269)	▨▤ PPT 13 Ch. 47 FAAHN (Ch. 7 PPT 13 AHN) 🔁 EILR TB Ch. 47 questions 7, 9 FAAHN (Ch. 7 questions 7, 9 AHN) 🔁 ESLR Review Questions for the NCLEX Examination Ch. 47 question 3 FAAHN (Ch. 7 question 3 AHN) 📕SG SG Diagnostic Tests, Ch. 47 p. 384 FAAHN (Ch. 7 p. 72 AHN) **BOOK RESOURCES** Review Questions for the NCLEX Examination Ch. 47 questions 2, 7, 8, 25, 32 FAAHN (Ch. 7 questions 2, 7, 8, 25, 32 AHN) ▸ Discuss the nursing implications associated with monitoring laboratory results.

OBJECTIVES	CONTENT	TEACHING RESOURCES
	– Gastric analysis (FAAHN p. 1505, AHN p. 269) – Radiological studies (FAAHN p. 1505, AHN p. 269) – Bone marrow aspiration or biopsy (FAAHN p. 1505, AHN p. 269)	▸ Discuss the normal and abnormal values associated with more commonly used diagnostic tests. *Class Activity Divide students into teams of four students. Ask the teams questions concerning common diagnostic tests. For each correct answer the team reports, add a point. After a short time, tally the points. The team having the most points will win. Provide a small prize, such as fruit or pencils.*

7.1 Homework/Assignments:

7.1 Instructor's Notes/Student Feedback:

LESSON 7.2

CRITICAL THINKING QUESTION

After undergoing elective surgery, a patient has reported to the clinic with complaints of weakness, fatigue, and shortness of breath. After assessing the patient the physician diagnoses the patient with iron deficiency anemia. Based upon your knowledge, how has the patient most likely become affected with this disorder? What other conditions/events could predispose a patient to iron deficiency anemia? What treatments will be used to manage this condition? In general, what prognosis is associated with the disorder?

Guidelines: Iron deficiency anemia results when the body's red blood cells contain reduced levels of hemoglobin. Conditions that put a patient at an increased risk of developing the disorder include weight loss, surgery, inadequate dietary intake, malabsorption of iron, and blood loss. Management of this condition will include dietary and pharmacological therapies. A diet rich in iron is indicated, and oral iron supplements will be prescribed. The physician could choose to order intramuscular administration of iron should the blood count levels indicate the need. The prognosis for iron deficiency anemia is good. After treatment, the patient should be fine.

OBJECTIVES	CONTENT	TEACHING RESOURCES
Compare and contrast the different types of anemia in terms of etiology and pathophysiology, clinical manifestations, assessment, diagnostic tests, medical management, nursing interventions, patient teaching, and prognosis.	☐ Disorders associated with erythrocytes (FAAHN p. 1505, AHN p. 269) ☐ Anemia (FAAHN p. 1505, AHN p. 269) – Etiology and pathophysiology (FAAHN p. 1505, AHN p. 269) – Clinical manifestations (FAAHN p. 1506, AHN p. 270) – Assessment (FAAHN p. 1506, AHN p. 270) – Diagnostic tests (FAAHN p. 1506, AHN p. 270) – Medical management (FAAHN p. 1506, AHN p. 270) – Nursing interventions and patient teaching (FAAHN p. 1506, AHN p. 270) – Hypovolemic anemia (blood loss anemia) (FAAHN p. 1507, AHN p. 271) – Pernicious anemia (FAAHN p. 1508, AHN p. 272) – Aplastic anemia (FAAHN p. 1509, AHN p. 273)	PPT 14 through 36 Ch. 47 FAAHN (Ch. 7 PPT 14 through 36 AHN) EILR TB Ch. 47 questions 12, 15, 16 through 18, 24, 32, 34, 39 FAAHN (Ch. 7 questions 12, 15 through 18, 24, 32, 34, 39 AHN) EILR Open Book Quiz Ch. 47 questions 1 through 3, FAAHN (Ch. 7 questions 1 through 3, AHN) ESLR Review Questions for the NCLEX Examination Ch. 47 questions 4 through 6 FAAHN (Ch. 7 questions 4 through 6 AHN) SG Anemia, Ch. 47 p. 386 FAAHN (Ch. 7 p. 74 AHN) **BOOK RESOURCES** Cultural Considerations: Jehovah's Witness Opposition to Blood Transfusion (FAAHN p. 1506) (AHN p. 270) Safety Alert! Aplastic Anemia (FAAHN p. 1511) (AHN p. 275) Box 47-1 Causes of Iron Deficiency Anemia (FAAHN p. 1512) (Box 7-1 AHN p. 276) Box 47-2 Food Sources of Nutrients Needed for Erythropoiesis (FAAHN p. 1513) (Box 7-2 AHN p. 277)

ELSEVIER

OBJECTIVES	CONTENT	TEACHING RESOURCES
	– Iron deficiency anemia (FAAHN p. 1511, AHN p. 275) – Sickle cell anemia (FAAHN p. 1512, AHN p. 276) – Polycythemia (erythrocytosis) (FAAHN p. 1515, AHN p. 279) ☐ Disorders associated with leukocytes (FAAHN p. 1517, AHN p. 281) ☐ Agranulocytosis (FAAHN p. 1517, AHN p. 281) – Etiology and pathophysiology (FAAHN p. 1517, AHN p. 281) – Clinical manifestations (FAAHN p. 1517, AHN p. 281) – Assessment (FAAHN p. 1517, AHN p. 281) – Diagnostic tests (FAAHN p. 1517, AHN p. 281) – Medical management (FAAHN p. 1517, AHN p. 281) – Nursing interventions and patient teaching (FAAHN p. 1517, AHN p. 281)	Health Promotion: Iron Administration (FAAHN p. 1513) (AHN p. 277) Review Questions for the NCLEX Examination Ch. 47 questions 11 through 13, 15, 17 through 20, 29, 34 FAAHN (Ch. 7 questions 11 through 13, 15, 17 through 20, 29, 34AHN) ▸ Discuss the differing etiologies associated with the different types of anemia. ▸ Discuss the dietary management that can be implemented to manage iron deficiency anemia. *Class Activity Allow the students to break into small groups of three or four students. Assign each group a different type of anemia. Instruct each group to modify a short care plan relating to the care and treatment for patients who are diagnosed with the assigned type of anemia.*
List six signs and symptoms associated with hypovolemic shock.	– Hypovolemic anemia (blood loss anemia) (FAAHN p. 1507, AHN p. 271)	PPT 19 through 21 Ch. 47 FAAHN (Ch. 7 PPT 19 through 21 AHN) EILR TB Ch. 47 questions 11, 33, 37 FAAHN (Ch. 7 questions 11, 33, 37 AHN) SG Hypovolemic Shock, Ch. 47 p. 389 FAAHN (Ch. 7 p. 77 AHN) **BOOK RESOURCES** Review Questions for the NCLEX Examination Ch. 47 questions 30, 33 FAAHN (Ch. 7 questions 30, 33 AHN) ▸ Discuss the signs and symptoms associated with hypovolemic shock. ▸ Discuss the potential causes of hypovolemic shock.

Christensen & Kockrow

OBJECTIVES	CONTENT	TEACHING RESOURCES
		Class Activity Instruct each student to develop two NCLEX- style questions concerning hypovolemic shock. After completion, instruct students to select a partner. Instruct the pairs to share the information developed with each other.
Discuss important aspects that should be presented in patient teaching and home care planning for the patient with pernicious anemia.	– Pernicious anemia (FAAHN p. 1508, AHN p. 272)	⊠▰ PPT 22 through 25 Ch. 47 FAAHN (Ch. 7 PPT 22 through 25 AHN) 🖺 EILR Open Book Quiz Ch. 47 questions 4 through 8 FAAHN (Ch. 7 questions 4 through 8 AHN) 🗐 SG Anemia, Ch. 47 p. 386 FAAHN (Ch. 7 p. 74 AHN) **BOOK RESOURCES** Review Questions for the NCLEX Examination Ch. 47 question 14 FAAHN (Ch. 7 question 14 AHN) ▸ Discuss the therapies employed to manage pernicious anemia. ▸ Discuss the causes of pernicious anemia. *Class Activity Divide the class into small groups of three or four students. Instruct students to modify care plans for the patient diagnosed with pernicious anemia.*

ELSEVIER

Mosby items and derived items © 2011 by Mosby, Inc., an affiliate of Elsevier Inc.
Some material was previously published.

Adult Health Nursing, 6th ed.
Christensen & Kockrow

OBJECTIVES	CONTENT	TEACHING RESOURCES
Discuss the etiology/ pathophysiology, clinical manifestations, assessment, diagnostic tests, medical management, nursing interventions, patient teaching, and prognosis for patients with acute and chronic leukemia.	☐ Leukemia (FAAHN p. 1518, AHN p. 282) – Etiology and pathophysiology (FAAHN p. 1518, AHN p. 282) – Classification (FAAHN p. 1518, AHN p. 282) – Clinical manifestations (FAAHN p. 1518, AHN p. 282) – Diagnostic tests (FAAHN p. 1518, AHN p. 282) – Assessment (FAAHN p. 1519, AHN p. 283) – Medical management (FAAHN p. 1519, AHN p. 283) – Nursing interventions and patient teaching (FAAHN p. 1520, AHN p. 284)	PPT 39 through 40 Ch. 47 FAAHN (Ch. 7 PPT 39 through 40 AHN) EILR TB Ch. 47 questions 14, 28, 30, 38 FAAHN (Ch. 7 questions 14, 28, 30, 38 AHN) ESLR Review Questions for the NCLEX Examination Ch. 47 question 7 FAAHN (Ch. 7 question 7 AHN) SG Prognosis Ch. 47 p. 390 FAAHN (Ch. 7 p. 78 AHN) **BOOK RESOURCES** Table 47-1 Medications for Blood and Lymphatic Disorders (FAAHN p. 1519) (Table 7-1 AHN p. 283) Nursing Care Plan 47-1 The Patient with Leukemia (FAAHN p. 1521) (NCP 7-1 AHN p. 285) NCP CTQ 1 through 3 (FAAHN p. 1521) (AHN p. 285) Review Questions for the NCLEX Examination Ch. 47 questions 9, 31 FAAHN (Ch. 7 questions 9, 31 AHN) ▶ Discuss the populations most frequently diagnosed with leukemia. ▶ Discuss the treatment options available for the care of the patient diagnosed with leukemia. ***Class Activity** **Invite a guest speaker to the class to discuss patients living with leukemia. A local hospital or hospice would be a good referral site to locate the speaker.***

OBJECTIVES	CONTENT	TEACHING RESOURCES
Compare and contrast the disorders of coagulation (thrombocytopenia, hemophilia, disseminated intravascular coagulation in terms of etiology and pathophysiology, clinical manifestations, assessment, diagnostic tests, medical management, nursing interventions, patient teaching, and prognosis.	□ Coagulation disorders (FAAHN p. 1520, AHN p. 284) – Etiology and pathophysiology (FAAHN p. 1520, AHN p. 284) – Clinical manifestations (FAAHN p. 1521, AHN p. 285) – Assessment (FAAHN p. 1521, AHN p. 285) – Diagnostic tests (FAAHN p. 1521, AHN p. 285) – Medical management (FAAHN p. 1522, AHN p. 286) – Nursing interventions (FAAHN p. 1522, AHN p. 286) □ Platelet disorders (FAAHN p. 1522, AHN p. 286) □ Thrombocytopenia (FAAHN p. 1522, AHN p. 286) – Etiology and pathophysiology (FAAHN p. 1522, AHN p. 286) – Clinical manifestations (FAAHN p. 1522, AHN p. 286) – Assessment (FAAHN p. 1522, AHN p. 286) – Diagnostic tests (FAAHN p. 1522, AHN p. 286) – Medical management (FAAHN p. 1522, AHN p. 286) – Nursing interventions and patient teaching (FAAHN p. 1523, AHN p. 287) □ Clotting factor defects (FAAHN p.1523 AHN p. 287) □ Hemophilia (FAAHN p. 1523, AHN p. 287) – Etiology and pathophysiology (FAAHN p. 1523, AHN p. 287) – Clinical manifestations (FAAHN p. 1523, AHN p. 287) – Assessment (FAAHN p. 1524, AHN p. 288)	▣ PPT 41 through 48 Ch. 47 FAAHN (Ch. 7 PPT 41 through 48 AHN) 🔲 EILR TB Ch. 47 questions 20, 21, 25 through 27, 29 FAAHN (Ch. 7 question 20, 21, 25 through 27, 29 AHN) 🔲 EILR Open Book Quiz Ch. 47 question 9 FAAHN (Ch. 7 question 9 AHN) 🔲 ESLR Review Questions for the NCLEX Examination Ch. 47 questions 8, 10 FAAHN (Ch. 7 questions 8, 10 AHN) 📖 SG Coagulation Disorders, Ch. 47 p. 388 FAAHN (Ch. 7 p. 76 AHN) **BOOK RESOURCES** Box 47-3 Medications with Thrombocytopenic Effects (FAAHN p. 1522) (Box 7-3 AHN p. 286) Home Care Considerations: Hemophilia (FAAHN p. 1525) (AHN p. 289) Box 47-4 Precipitating Causes of Disseminated Intravascular Coagulation (FAAHN p. 1526) (Box 7-4 AHN p. 290) Review Questions for the NCLEX Examination Ch. 47 questions 16, 23, 24, 27, 28 FAAHN (Ch. 7 questions 16, 23, 24, 27, 28 AHN) ▶ Discuss the impact of clotting disorders on the patient's ability to carry out normal activities of daily living. ▶ Discuss diagnostic testing used to assess for disorders of coagulation. *Class Activity Allow students to divide into three groups. Assign each group one of the following disorders: thrombocytopenia, hemophilia, and DIC. After the groups are formed, instruct the students to subdivide into smaller groups. The smaller subgroups will be assigned pathophysiology, clinical manifestations, and treatment options. After the final groups are set, allow a short time for each group to*

Adult Health Nursing, 6th ed.

Christensen & Kockrow

OBJECTIVES	CONTENT	TEACHING RESOURCES
	– Diagnostic tests (FAAHN p. 1524, AHN p. 288)	*review its assigned topic. Then bring the larger groups back together to share their findings.*
	– Medical management (FAAHN p. 1524, AHN p. 288)	***Note: If this activity is done before the lecture, it will be a useful review of the content.***
	– Nursing interventions and patient teaching (FAAHN p. 1524, AHN p. 288)	
	– Prognosis (FAAHN p. 1525, AHN p. 289)	
	☐ Von Willebrand's disease (FAAHN p. 1525, AHN p. 289)	
	– Etiology and pathophysiology (FAAHN p. 1525, AHN p. 289)	
	– Prognosis (FAAHN p. 1525, AHN p. 289)	
	☐ Disseminated intravascular coagulation (FAAHN p. 1525, AHN p. 289)	
	– Etiology and pathophysiology (FAAHN p. 1525, AHN p. 289)	
	– Clinical manifestations (FAAHN p. 1525, AHN p. 289)	
	– Assessment (FAAHN p. 1525, AHN p. 289)	
	– Diagnostic tests (FAAHN p. 1526, AHN p. 290)	
	– Medical management (FAAHN p. 1526, AHN p. 290)	
	– Nursing interventions and patient teaching (FAAHN p. 1526, AHN p. 290)	
	– Prognosis (FAAHN p. 1527, AHN p. 291)	

Christensen & Kockrow

| Discuss the etiology/ pathophysiology, clinical manifestations, assessment, diagnostic tests, medical management, nursing interventions, patient teaching, and prognosis for patients with multiple myeloma, malignant lymphoma, and Hodgkin's lymphoma. | ☐ Plasma cell disorder (FAAHN p. 1527, AHN p. 291)

☐ Multiple myeloma (FAAHN p. 1527, AHN p. 291)

– Etiology and pathophysiology (FAAHN p. 1527, AHN p. 291)

– Clinical manifestations (FAAHN p. 1527, AHN p. 291)

– Assessment (FAAHN p. 1527, AHN p. 291)

– Diagnostic tests (FAAHN p. 1527, AHN p. 291)

– Medical management (FAAHN p. 1528, AHN p. 292)

– Nursing interventions and patient teaching (FAAHN p. 1528, AHN p. 292)

– Prognosis (FAAHN p. 1528, AHN p. 292)

☐ Lymphatic disorders (FAAHN p. 1528, AHN p. 292)

☐ Lymphangitis (FAAHN p. 1528 AHN p. 292)

– Etiology and pathophysiology (FAAHN p. 1528, AHN p. 292)

– Clinical manifestations (FAAHN p. 1528, AHN p. 292)

– Medical management (FAAHN p. 1529, AHN p. 293)

– Nursing interventions (FAAHN p. 1529, AHN p. 293)

– Prognosis (FAAHN p. 1529, AHN p. 293)

☐ Lymphedema (FAAHN p. 1529, AHN p. 293)

– Etiology and pathophysiology (FAAHN p. 1529, AHN p. 293)

– Clinical manifestations (FAAHN p. 1529, AHN p. 293)

– Assessment and diagnostic test (FAAHN p. 1529, AHN p. 293) | PPT 49 through 52, and 55 through 63 Ch. 47 FAAHN (Ch. 7 PPT 49 through 52, and 55 through 63 AHN)

EILR IC Ch. 47 image 5 FAAHN (Ch. 7 image 5 AHN)

EILR TB Ch. 47 question 13, 22, 23 FAAHN (Ch. 7 question 13, 22, 23 AHN)

EILR Open Book Quiz Ch. 47 question 10 FAAHN (Ch. 7 question 10 AHN)

ESLR Review Questions for the NCLEX Examination Ch. 47 question 9 FAAHN (Ch. 7 question 9 AHN)

SG Multiple Myeloma, Ch. 47 p. 390; Hodgkin's or Non-Hodgkin's Disease, Ch. 47 p. 391 FAAHN (Ch. 7 pp. 78-79 AHN)

BOOK RESOURCES

Box 47-5 Clinical Staging System for Hodgkin's Disease (FAAHN p. 1530) (Box 7-5 AHN p. 294)

Fig. 47-5 Nodal involvement by stage in Hodgkin's disease (FAAHN p. 1531) (Fig. 7-5 AHN p. 295)

Communication: Patient with Hodgkin's Lymphoma (FAAHN p. 1532) (AHN p. 296)

Review Questions for the NCLEX Examination Ch. 47 questions 10, 21, 22 FAAHN (Ch. 7 questions 10, 21, 22 AHN)

▸ Discuss populations at risk for the development of multiple myeloma, malignant lymphoma, and Hodgkin's disease.

▸ Discuss the process of staging for both Hodgkin's and non-Hodgkin's disease.

Class Activity Invite a guest to speak to the class concerning patients living with multiple myeloma, malignant lymphoma, or Hodgkin's disease. |

    − Medical management (FAAHN
       p. 1529, AHN p. 293)

    − Nursing interventions and patient
       teaching (FAAHN p. 1529, AHN
       p. 293)

    − Prognosis (FAAHN p. 1529,
       AHN p. 293)

☐ Hodgkin's lymphoma (FAAHN
   p. 1529, AHN p. 293)

    − Etiology and pathophysiology
       (FAAHN p. 1529, AHN p. 293)

    − Clinical manifestations (FAAHN
       p. 1530, AHN p. 294)

    − Assessment (FAAHN p. 1530,
       AHN p. 294)

    − Diagnostic tests (FAAHN p.
       1530, AHN p. 294)

    − Medical management (FAAHN
       p. 1531, AHN p. 295)

    − Nursing interventions and patient
       teaching (FAAHN p. 1532, AHN
       p. 296)

    − Prognosis (FAAHN p. 1533,
       AHN p. 297)

☐ Non-Hodgkin's lymphoma
   (FAAHN p. 1533, AHN p. 297)

    − Etiology and pathophysiology
       (FAAHN p. 1533, AHN p. 297)

    − Clinical manifestations (FAAHN
       p. 1533, AHN p. 297)

    − Assessment (FAAHN p. 1533,
       AHN p. 297)

    − Diagnostic tests (FAAHN p.
       1533, AHN p. 297)

    − Medical management (FAAHN
       p. 1533, AHN p. 297)

    − Nursing interventions and patient
       teaching (FAAHN p. 1534, AHN
       p. 298)

    − Prognosis (FAAHN p. 1534,
       AHN p. 298)

Christensen & Kockrow

Discuss the primary goal of nursing interventions for the patient with lymphedema.	☐ Lymphedema (FAAHN p. 1529, AHN p. 293) – Etiology and pathophysiology (FAAHN p. 1529, AHN p. 293) – Clinical manifestations (FAAHN p. 1529, AHN p. 293) – Assessment and diagnostic test (FAAHN p. 1529, AHN p. 293) – Medical management (FAAHN p. 1529, AHN p. 293) – Nursing interventions and patient teaching (FAAHN p. 1529, AHN p. 293) – Prognosis (FAAHN p. 1529, AHN p. 293)	⊠▪ PPT 53, 54, and 55 Ch. 47 FAAHN (Ch. 7 PPT 53, 54, AHN) 📖 SG Lymphedema Ch. 47 p. 391 FAAHN (Ch. 7 p. 79 AHN) ▸ Discuss the cause of lymphedema. ▸ Discuss the treatment options for the patient diagnosed with lymphedema. *Class Activity Provide nursing care plan sheets for the students. Allow the students to work in pairs. Instruct the students to modify two nursing diagnoses and accompanying interventions for the patient diagnosed with lymphedema.*
Apply the nursing process to the care of the patient with disorders of the hematological and lymphatic systems.	☐ Nursing process for the patient with a blood or lymphatic disorder (FAAHN p. 1534, AHN p. 298) – Assessment (FAAHN p. 1534, AHN p. 298) – Nursing diagnosis (FAAHN p. 1534, AHN p. 298) – Expected outcomes and planning (FAAHN p. 1535, AHN p. 299) – Implementation (FAAHN p. 1535, AHN p. 299) – Evaluation (FAAHN p. 1535, AHN p. 299)	⊠▪ PPT 64 Ch. 47 FAAHN (Ch. 7 PPT 64 AHN) 📖 SG Nursing Process, Ch. 47 p. 386 FAAHN (Ch. 7 p. 74 AHN) **BOOK RESOURCES** Life Span Considerations, Older Adults: Blood or Lymphatic Disorder (FAAHN p. 1534) (AHN p. 298) ▸ Discuss the priorities for the care of the patient diagnosed with a hematological or lymphatic disorder. ▸ Discuss the referrals that might be needed by the patient diagnosed with a hematological or lymphatic disorder. *Class Activity Instruct the students to write a short list of the educational and support needs for the patient diagnosed with a lymphatic or hematological disorder. After 10 minutes has passed, ask student volunteers to share their thoughts.*

ELSEVIER

Adult Health Nursing, 6th ed.

Christensen & Kockrow

Performance Evaluation		EILR TB Ch. 47 questions 1 through 40 FAAHN (Ch. 7 questions 1 through 40 AHN)
		EILR Open Book Quiz Ch. 47 questions 1 through 10 FAAHN (Ch. 7 questions 1 through 10 AHN)
		ESLR Review Questions for the NCLEX Examination Ch. 47 questions 1 through 10FAAHN (Ch. 7 questions 1 through 10 AHN)
		SG Ch. 47 pp. 381 through 394 FAAHN (Ch. 7 pp. 69 through 82 AHN)
		BOOK RESOURCES
		Nursing Care Plan 47-1 The Patient with Leukemia (FAAHN p. 1521) (NCP 7-1 AHN p. 285)
		NCP CTQ 1-3 (FAAHN p. 1521) (AHN p. 285)
		Review Questions for the NCLEX Examination Ch. 47 questions 1 through 34 FAAHN (Ch. 7 questions 1 through 34 AHN)

7.2 Homework/Assignments:

7.2 Instructor's Notes/Student Feedback:

ELSEVIER

Adult Health Nursing, 6th ed.
Christensen & Kockrow

Slide 1

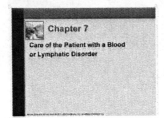

Slide 2

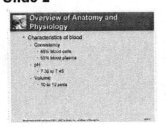

- Blood is the necessary life force in the human body.

- In ancient times it had a mystical allure.

- What are the primary functions of blood?

Slide 3

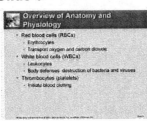

- The three primary types of blood cells are the red blood cells, white blood cells, and platelets.

- Red blood cells give the blood its red coloring.

- What is the relationship between the red blood cell and hemoglobin?

- What is the normal red blood cell count in the body? What testing processes measure the key properties of the red blood cells?

- White blood cells are colorless cells whose main functions involve defense of the body. What are the categories of the white blood cells?

- What laboratory tests are used to measure the white blood cell levels?

- The smallest blood cells are the platelets.

Slide 4

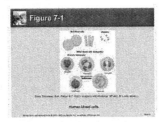

Christensen & Kockrow

Slide 5

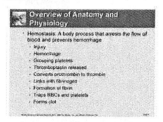

- Hemostasis is vital to the maintenance of the blood supply. If altered significantly, death will result.
- Identify and explain the actions that take place in the process of hemostasis.

Slide 6

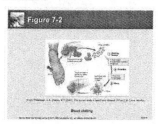

- The onset of injury immediately initiates the process of blood clotting. Although the process appears lengthy, it occurs instantly in the healthy individual.
- What analogies can be used to describe this process?

Slide 7

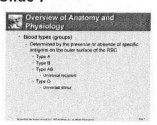

- At birth, the blood type is already determined by the type of antigens on the outer portion of the blood cell. A person with type B blood has no anti–B antibodies but instead has B antigens.
- How many students know their blood types?
- Draw a diagram to demonstrate the genetic determination of blood types.

Slide 8

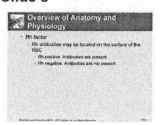

- The majority of the population is Rh positive. The assessment and monitoring of Rh factor is very important during pregnancy.
- Discuss the use of RhoGAM.

Slide 9

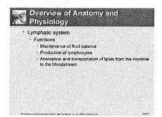

Christensen & Kockrow

Slide 10

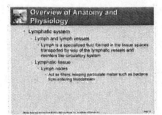

- The lymphatic system is composed of the lymph, nodes, and tissue.
- When and how are lymph nodes assessed? Where are they located? What is indicated when they are enlarged?

Slide 11

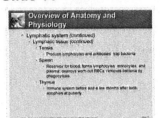

- The tonsils are two small, kidney-shaped organs in the rear of the throat. Their function is to trap bacteria. How does their function correspond with one of the leading causes of illness in children?

Slide 12

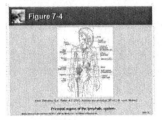

Slide 13

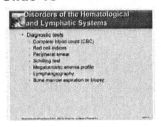

- Potential alterations in immunity can cause extreme physiological distress. Discuss the listed diagnostic examinations. When are they used?

Slide 14

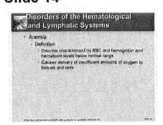

- Hemoglobin is the oxygen-carrying component in the blood cells. What are the normal values of the body's hemoglobin levels? Do the values for men and women differ?

ELSEVIER

Adult Health Nursing, 6th ed.
Christensen & Kockrow

Slide 15

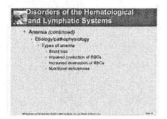

- Anemia has several potential causes. Discuss how the body compensates for the reduced hemoglobin levels.

Slide 16

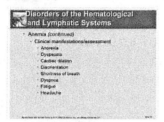

- The manifestations associated with anemia can vary between individuals. At what level do signs and symptoms become apparent?

- Why does the patient experience shortness of breath, fatigue, and headaches?

Slide 17

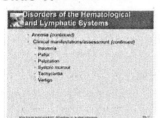

- What assessments can be used to identify a patient whose anemia is a long-term condition?

Slide 18

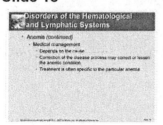

- The physiological impact on the patient experiencing anemia can be great. What are nursing interventions that can be instituted to assist the client during this phase?

- What education should be provided the patient?

- Some religions do not permit the administration of blood transfusions. What is the role of the nurse when confronted with this dilemma?

Slide 19

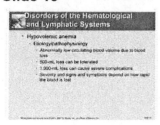

- Hypovolemic anemia can occur as a result of surgery or trauma. Initially the body does compensate, but as the losses continue, the body's organs become affected.

- How much circulating blood does the average adult have?

- How is the volume of circulating blood related to the body's hemoglobin level?

ELSEVIER

Adult Health Nursing, 6th ed.

Christensen & Kockrow

Slide 20

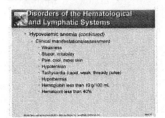

- When the body is no longer able to compensate for the loss in blood value, outward signs and symptoms become observable. The nursing assessment can identify the presence of pain. Why might pain occur with hypovolemic anemia?

Slide 21

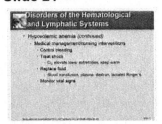

- Identification of the problem in a timely manner is key to instituting treatment. When are sudden changes in blood volume able to be detected in blood studies? If there is delay, why does this happen?

Slide 22

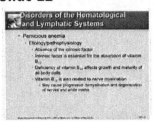

- Pernicious anemia is a serious disease. If not correctly managed, it will result in death.

- The condition is due to a lack of intrinsic factor. The intrinsic factor is produced by the gastric cells in the body.

- Who is at risk for the development of this disease? Why is this population at an increased risk?

Slide 23

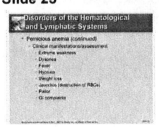

- Excessive weakness is reported overwhelmingly. What is the underlying cause of this fatigue?

- When collecting data from the patient who has presented with the clinical manifestations associated with pernicious anemia, what questions should be asked?

Slide 24

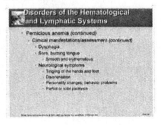

- After completing a systems assessment, laboratory testing will be ordered to support the diagnosis of pernicious anemia.

- What tests can be anticipated?

Christensen & Kockrow

Slide 25

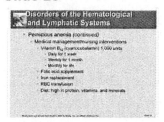

- The treatment/management of pernicious anemia involves lifelong medication.
- What information should the nurse provide to the patient?

Slide 26

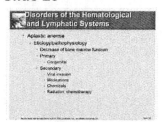

- There are two classifications of aplastic anemia. In up to 30% of the cases, it is genetic and is present at the time of birth. Many more cases are not tied to any particular cause. Autoimmune involvement is suspected in these diagnoses.

Slide 27

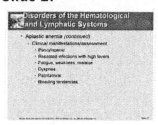

- The incidence of aplastic anemia is rare. An estimated 4 in 1 million people are affected.
- The mortality rate is high. What can the majority of aplastic anemia–related deaths be attributed to?

Slide 28

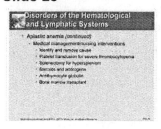

- When a patient presents with the clinical manifestations associated with the development of aplastic anemia, what diagnostic tests will be ordered to confirm the diagnosis?
- What results will signal a positive finding?

Slide 29

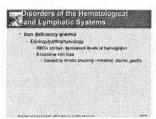

Christensen & Kockrow

Slide 30

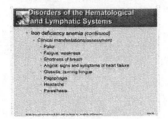

- The clinical manifestations of iron deficiency anemia are a result of the reduced oxygenation of the body's red blood cells.

- When collecting data from the patient, what questions should the nurse include?

Slide 31

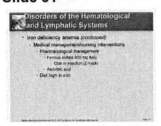

- A complete blood cell count can be ordered to determine the presence of iron deficiency anemia.

- Treatment will include both dietary modifications and pharmacological therapies. What information should be provided to the patient about taking iron supplements?

- What dietary education will be indicated?

Slide 32

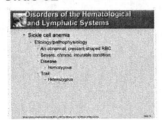

- Sickle cell anemia is the most common genetic order in the United States.

- Review the genetic transmission of this disorder.

Slide 33

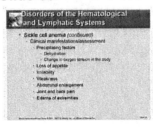

- In most cases, the patient who has sickle cell anemia is free of clinical manifestations between birth and the first 10 to 12 weeks. What phenomenon will explain the delay in the onset of symptoms?

Slide 34

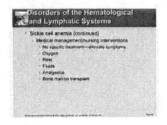

- Most people having sickle cell anemia experience periods of remissions and exacerbations. When the condition "flares up," treatment is needed.

- What is the nurse's role in providing care to the patient with sickle cell anemia?

- What are primary concerns during a sickle cell crisis?

ELSEVIER

Adult Health Nursing, 6th ed.
Christensen & Kockrow

Mosby items and derived items © 2011, 2007 by Mosby, Inc., an affiliate of Elsevier Inc.
Some material was previously published.

Slide 35

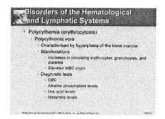

- What populations are most often diagnosed with polycythemia vera?
- Patients with polycythemia vera are at an increased risk for infarctions to vital organs. What pathology best explains this complication?

Slide 36

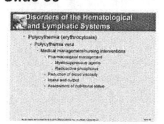

- Identify two nursing diagnoses for the patient diagnosed with polycythemia vera.

Slide 37

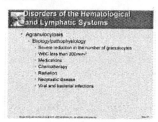

- Agranulocytosis is a severe condition that can result in death.
- How do the identified causes act as a catalyst for the disease?

Slide 38

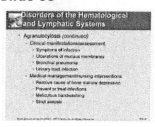

- When a patient presents with clinical manifestations consistent with agranulocytosis, what diagnostic tests can be anticipated? If the condition is present, what will the test results show?
- What are two nursing diagnoses applicable to this patient population?

Slide 39

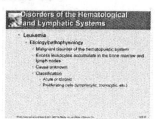

- The exact cause of leukemia is not known. There are, however, strongly supported theories to explain its cause. What are some of these theories?
- Identify populations who are at greatest risk for the development of leukemia.

Adult Health Nursing, 6th ed.
Christensen & Kockrow

Slide 40

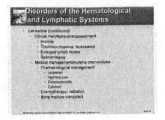

- Patients diagnosed with leukemia can present a variety of differing signs and symptoms. What questions should be asked by the nurse to facilitate the health intake assessment?

- What prognosis is associated with leukemia?

Slide 41

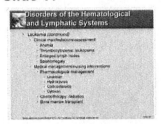

- Thrombocytopenia occurs when the number of healthy circulating platelets is significantly reduced.

- What conditions/factors can be attributed to a diagnosis of thrombocytopenia?

- When collecting data from the patient, what questions will assist in gathering subjective data to aid in the diagnostic process?

Slide 42

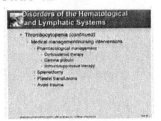

- Diagnostic tests used to confirm the presence of thrombocytopenia include complete blood counts and bone marrow studies.

- What nursing implications are associated with these tests?

- When medication therapies are initiated, explain how they will work to manage this disorder.

Slide 43

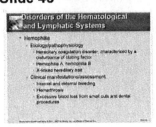

- Hemophilia is an inherited disorder. Explain the genetic transmission of the disorder.

Slide 44

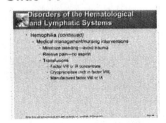

- Small, seemingly minor injuries can become life-threatening in the hemophiliac. What activities of daily living can become serious for the hemophiliac patient?

- What are the responsibilities of the nurse in providing care to this patient?

Slide 45

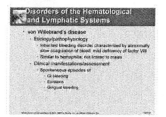

- von Willebrand's disease is a disorder of coagulation. How does this disease differ from hemophilia? How are the disorders similar?

Slide 46

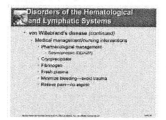

Slide 47

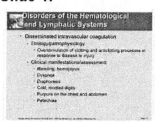

- What are examples of situations that can lead to the development of DIC?

- In addition to the outwardly obvious clinical manifestations, what subjective signs might exist in the patient?

Slide 48

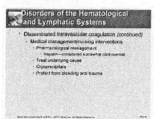

- Despite the overwhelming blood loss that results with the onset of DIC, treatment involves the administration of heparin and fibrinolytic inhibitors. How will these medications act to correct the disease process?

Slide 49

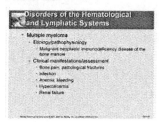

- Neoplastic plasma cells invade the bone marrow of the patient diagnosed with multiple myeloma.

- The loss of bone tissue causes the onset of bone pain and fractures.

- What populations are at the highest risk for the development of multiple myeloma?

ELSEVIER

Adult Health Nursing, 6th ed.

Christensen & Kockrow

Slide 50

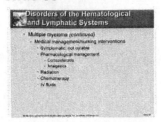

- The disorder is managed with symptomatic therapies.
- In addition to the pharmacologic measures, what nursing interventions should be initiated to provide care to this population?
- Review the prognosis of the patient with multiple myeloma.

Slide 51

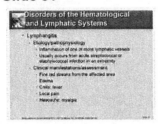

- What nursing diagnoses are appropriate for this patient population?
- Lymphangitis is a disorder that has a good prognosis after treatment.

Slide 52

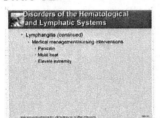

Slide 53

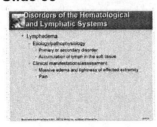

- The onset of lymphedema is a painful disorder in which there is an accumulation of lymph in the soft tissue.
- What causes this buildup of lymph and subsequent edema?

Slide 54

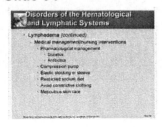

- Identify the goals of treatment for the patient diagnosed with lymphedema.
- Outline important points for patient education relating to the diagnosis of lymphedema.

Adult Health Nursing, 6th ed.
Christensen & Kockrow

Slide 55

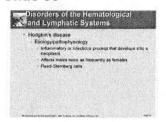

- What characteristics do people affected with Hodgkin's disease share?
- How do non-Hodgkin's and Hodgkin's lymphoma differ?

Slide 56

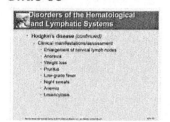

Slide 57

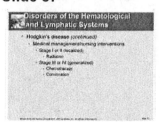

- A staging process is also used in Hodgkin's disease. Staging is used to determine the needed treatment plan.
- What are the goals of treatment?
- What is the prognosis for patients diagnosed with Hodgkin's disease?

Slide 58

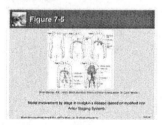

Slide 59

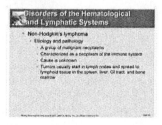

- NHL is the most common hematological cancer. Its rate of occurrence is increasing.
- What groups of patients are at a higher risk for the development of non-Hodgkin's lymphoma?
- What populations are associated with the development of non-Hodgkin's lymphoma? What theories are supported concerning the underlying cause for the disease?

Christensen & Kockrow

Slide 60

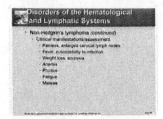

- After a review of the patient's health history, diagnostic tests will be ordered to confirm a diagnosis. What tests can be anticipated? What results will accompany a positive diagnosis?

Slide 61

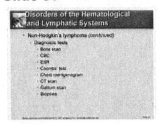

Slide 62

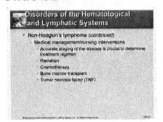

- After a diagnosis is confirmed, the disease will be staged. Staging serves to identify the advancement of the disease. Treatment options are based upon the stage of the disease process.

- Discuss the four stages of the disease.

Slide 63

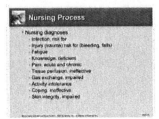

8 Care of the Patient with a Cardiovascular or a Peripheral Vascular Disorder

TEACHING FOCUS

In this chapter, the student will be introduced to the care of the patient with a cardiovascular or peripheral vascular disorder. The student will begin by exploring the structure and function of the heart. Next, the student will have the opportunity to learn the risk factors for cardiovascular disease and the diagnostic tests used to evaluate cardiovascular function. Finally, the student will explore the various cardiovascular and peripheral vascular disorders, including their etiology and pathophysiology, clinical manifestations, assessment, diagnostic tests, medical management, nursing interventions, and prognoses.

MATERIALS AND RESOURCES

- ☐ Computer/overhead projector (all lessons)
- ☐ White/black board and marker/chalk (all lessons)
- ☐ Copies of a diagram of the heart and major blood vessels in anterior view (Lesson 8.1)
- ☐ Three-dimensional model of a heart (Lesson 8.1)
- ☐ Several stethoscopes (Lesson 8.1)
- ☐ Small prizes such as fruit or pencils (Lesson 8.1)
- ☐ Copies of a list of the modifiable and nonmodifiable risk factors for the development of cardiovascular disease (Lesson 8.2)
- ☐ Several cardiac tracings (Lesson 8.2)
- ☐ Partially completed nursing care plan forms (Lesson 8.2)
- ☐ Ten to 15 short-answer questions about pulmonary edema (Lesson 8.2)
- ☐ Blank nursing care plans (Lesson 8.3)
- ☐ Sphygmomanometer (Lesson 8.3)
- ☐ Five short-answer questions about hypertension (Lesson 8.3)
- ☐ A series of questions on index cards relating to the etiology, diagnosis, clinical manifestations, care, and treatment of the patient diagnosed with thrombophlebitis (Lesson 8.4)

LESSON CHECKLIST

Preparations for this lesson include:
- Lecture
- Contact a meat packing company or small grocery store to request an animal heart.
- Contact the anatomy department at a college or university to request a dissected animal heart.
- Contact an acute care facility and request a tour of the facility's cardiac rehabilitation center.
- Contact a local cardiologist's office and request a speaker on the topic of cardiac transplantation.

KEY TERMS

aneurysm (FAAHN p. 1595, AHN p. 359)
angina pectoris (FAAHN p. 1557, AHN p. 321)
arteriosclerosis (FAAHN p. 1591, AHN p. 355)
atherosclerosis (FAAHN p. 1556, AHN p. 320)
bradycardia (FAAHN p. 1551, AHN p. 315)
B-type natriuretic peptide (BNP) (FAAHN p. 1547, AHN p. 311)
cardioversion (FAAHN p. 1546, AHN p. 310)
coronary artery disease (CAD) (FAAHN p. 1556, AHN p. 320)
defibrillation (FAAHN p. 1553, AHN p. 317)
dysrhythmia (FAAHN p. 1550, AHN p. 314)
embolus (FAAHN p. 1562, AHN p. 326)
endarterectomy (FAAHN p. 1594, AHN p. 358)
heart failure (FAAHN p. 1568, AHN p. 332)

hypoxemia (FAAHN p. 1546, AHN p. 310)
intermittent claudication (FAAHN p. 1585, AHN p. 349)
ischemia (FAAHN p. 1557, AHN p. 321)
myocardial infarction (MI) (FAAHN p. 1562, AHN p. 326)
occlusion (FAAHN p. 1562, AHN p. 326)
orthopnea (FAAHN p. 1570, AHN p. 334)
peripheral FAAHN p. 1584, AHN p. 348)
pleural effusion (FAAHN p. 1569, AHN p. 333)
polycythemia (FAAHN p. 1546, AHN p. 310)
pulmonary edema (FAAHN p. 1576, AHN p. 340)
tachycardia (FAAHN p. 1550, AHN p. 314)

ELSEVIER

Adult Health Nursing, 6th ed.

Mosby items and derived items © 2011 by Mosby, Inc., an affiliate of Elsevier Inc.
Some material was previously published.

Christensen & Kockrow

ADDITIONAL RESOURCES (AHN)

PPT Ch. 48, 1 through 83 FAAHN (Ch. 8, 1 through 83 AHN)

EILR IC images Ch. 48, 1 through 25 FAAHN (Ch. 8, 1 through 25 AHN)

EILR TB questions Ch. 48, 1 through 52 FAAHN (Ch. 8, 1 through 52 AHN)

EILR Open Book Quiz Ch. 48, 1 through 10 FAAHN (Ch. 8, 1 through 10 AHN)

ESLR Review Questions for the NCLEX® Examination Ch. 48, 48-01 through 48-10 FAAHN (Ch. 8, 08-01 through 08-10 AHN)

Legend

| **PPT**
PowerPoint
Slides | **EILR**
EVOLVE Instructor
Learning Resources:
Image Collection, Test
Bank, Open Book Quizzes | **ESLR**
EVOLVE Student
Learning Resources:
Review Questions
for the NCLEX
Examination | **SG**
Study Guide | **NCP CTQ**
Nursing Care Plan
Critical Thinking
Question |

Class Activities are indicated in **bold italic**.

LESSON 8.1

PRETEST

1. A patient reports being diagnosed with a murmur. Which of the following phenomena can be used to explain what might be the cause of this occurrence?
   a. Inappropriate closure of the ventricular lock
   b. The entrance of the blood into partially contracted chambers
   c. Ineffective closure of the valves
   d. Inadequate levels of blood as it leaves the atria

2. Which of the heart's chambers is the thickest and most muscular?
   a. Right atrium
   b. Right ventricle
   c. Left atrium
   d. Left ventricle

3. When preparing the patient for an electrocardiogram, which of the following configurations is correct for electrode placement?
   a. 6 electrodes on the chest and 4 on the limbs
   b. 8 electrodes on the chest and 4 on the limbs
   c. 5 electrodes on the chest and 4 on the limbs
   d. 6 electrodes on the chest and 6 on the limbs

4. The homocysteine test has been completed on your patient. Which of the following values, if noted, will be within normal limits?
   a. Less than 3 umol/L
   b. 8 Umol/L
   c. 23 Umol/L
   d. 25 to 32 Umol/L

5. Which of the following risk factors is considered nonmodifiable?
   a. Age
   b. Dietary intake
   c. Hyperlipidemia
   d. Sedentary lifestyle

Christensen & Kockrow

6. After completing a serum assessment of the LDL, which of the following is considered an optimal reading?
   a. Not in excess of 175 mg/dL
   b. 150 mg/dL to 174 mg/dL
   c. 125 mg/dL to 149 mg/dL
   d. Below 100 mg/dL

7. A beta-adrenergic blocker has been prescribed to manage a patient diagnosed with persistent sinus tachycardia. Which of the following medications can be anticipated?
   a. Digoxin (Lanoxin)
   b. Procainamide (Pronestyl)
   c. Verapamil (Calan)
   d. Propranolol (Inderal)

8. You are preparing to administer digoxin. Which of the assessments will need to be completed prior to administration?
   a. Assess apical pulse
   b. Monitor blood pressure
   c. Monitor for sleep disturbances
   d. Monitor for visual disturbances

9. A patient diagnosed with coronary artery disease has questions concerning the best diet for managing her condition. Which of the following diets would be most helpful?
   a. High protein, low fat
   b. 2 g sodium, low cholesterol, 1500 calories, fluid restriction
   c. 4 g sodium, restricted potassium, moderate fat, high protein
   d. Low protein, low fat, high phosphorus

10. A patient diagnosed with an elevated LDL plans to make dietary changes to her daily intake. Which of the following will be most therapeutic?
    a. 10 to 20 g of soluble fiber daily, including foods such as wheat bread and beans
    b. 20 to 30 mg of soluble fiber daily, including foods such as bran and broccoli
    c. 20 to 30 g of soluble fiber daily, including foods such as bran, beans, and peas
    d. 10 to 20 mg of insoluble fiber daily, including foods such as bran, beans, and wheat bread

Answers:

1. c	2. d	3. a	4. b	5. a
6. d	7. d	8. a	9. b	10. c

BACKGROUND ASSESSMENT

Question: You are caring for a 45-year-old patient who is being seen at the clinic for a routine physical examination. During the exam, the patient states he is becoming increasingly concerned about developing a cardiovascular disorder as he grows older. He asks why heart disease becomes more prevalent with aging. What information should be given to the patient?

Answer: During the aging process, the tissue and musculature changes seen in the body are also taking place in the heart. The aging heart begins to pump with reduced efficiency and strength. This loss of strength in contraction reduces perfusion in the body. The loss of elasticity in the vessels contributes to hypertension and circulatory impairments.

Question: During a routine physical examination, a patient, age 35, voices concern about the likelihood of developing heart disease. The patient reports her father was recently diagnosed with coronary artery disease and has a history of hypertension. She states both of her maternal grandparents died of heart-related disorders before age 65. Based upon her concerns, what information should be provided the patient?

Answer: The patient has one obvious risk factor: heredity. Further assessment would be needed to determine the presence of additional risk factors. Any modifiable factors for which the patient is at risk will need additional information presented to her concerning the implications of the behavior as well as counseling on modifying behaviors.

Christensen & Kockrow

CRITICAL THINKING QUESTION

Although the heart is one large organ, it acts as two independently functioning pumps. The interrelationship between these pumps is needed for human survival. Can you compare and contrast the roles of these unique pumps?

Guidelines: Each side of the heart has the commonality of function. Each acts as a pump. The left side of the heart is responsible for getting oxygenated blood from the lungs. This oxygenated blood is provided to the body by the left side's pumping actions. The right side of the body is responsible for pulmonary circulation. This blood has been utilized by the body and now requires oxygenation in the lungs. It travels from the right atrium to the right ventricle and is sent to the lungs. Once oxygenated, it is presented to the left side of the heart to repeat the circulation process.

OBJECTIVES	CONTENT	TEACHING RESOURCES
Discuss the location, size, and position of the heart.	■ Anatomy and physiology of the cardiovascular system (FAAHN p. 1540, AHN p. 304) □ Heart (FAAHN p. 1540, AHN p. 304) – Heart wall (FAAHN p. 1540, AHN p. 304) – Heart chambers (FAAHN p. 1540, AHN p. 304) – Heart valves (FAAHN p. 1541, AHN p. 305) – Electrical conduction system (FAAHN p. 1541, AHN p. 305) – Cardiac cycle (FAAHN p. 1542, AHN p. 306) □ Blood vessels (FAAHN p. 1542, AHN p. 306)	PPT 1 through 4, Ch. 48 FAAHN (Ch. 8 PPT 1 through 4 AHN) EILR IC Ch. 48 image 1 FAAHN (Ch. 8 image 1 AHN) EILR TB Ch. 48 question 49 FAAHN (Ch. 8 question 49 AHN) SG Tracing a Drop of Blood, Ch. 48 p. 395 FAAHN (Ch. 8 p. 83AHN) **BOOK RESOURCES** Fig. 48-1 Heart and major blood vessels viewed from front (anterior) (FAAHN p. 1540) (Fig. 8-1 AHN p. 304) Fig. 48-2 Interior of the heart (FAAHN p. 1541) (Fig. 8-2 AHN p. 305) ▸ Discuss the heart's size and shape in relation to the rest of the body's organs. ▸ Discuss the structural composition of the heart. *Class Activity Distribute copies of drawings of the heart and major blood vessels (use an anterior view). Request that the students attempt to label as many of the structures as possible in a limited period of time.*
Identify the chambers of the heart.	– Heart chambers (FAAHN p. 1540, AHN p. 304)	PPT 4, Ch. 48 FAAHN (Ch. 8 PPT 4 AHN) EILR IC Ch. 48 image 2 FAAHN (Ch. 8 image 2 AHN) SG Tracing a Drop of Blood, Ch. 48 p. 395 FAAHN (Ch. 8 p. 83 AHN)

OBJECTIVES	CONTENT	TEACHING RESOURCES
		BOOK RESOURCES Review Questions for the NCLEX Examination Ch. 48 questions 5, 6 FAAHN (Ch. 8 question 5, 6 AHN) ▸ Discuss the composition of the heart's chambers. ▸ Discuss the functions of the heart's ventricles.. *Class Activity* **Contact a meat packing company. Ask for an animal heart. (Another option might be a small grocery store that processes deer.) Take the heart to class and allow the students to visualize the structural composition of the heart.**
Identify the valves of the heart and their locations.	– Heart valves (FAAHN p. 1541, AHN p. 305)	PPT 4 through 5, Ch. 48 FAAHN (Ch. 8 PPT 4 through 5 AHN) SG Tracing a Drop of Blood, Ch. 48 p. 395 FAAHN (Ch. 8 p. 83 AHN) **BOOK RESOURCES** Review Questions for the NCLEX Examination Ch. 48 questions 3, 4 FAAHN (Ch. 8 question 3, 4 AHN) ▸ Discuss the different valves in the heart. ▸ Discuss the structural composition of the heart's valves. *Class Activity* **Obtain a 3D model of a heart. Bring the heart to class and allow the students the opportunity to explore the heart's structure.**
Discuss the electrical conduction system that causes the cardiac muscle fibers to contract.	– Electrical conduction system (FAAHN p. 1541, AHN p. 305)	PPT 6, 7, Ch. 48 FAAHN (Ch. 8 PPT 6, 7 AHN) EILR IC Ch. 48 image 3 FAAHN (Ch. 8 image 3 AHN) ESLR Review Questions for the NCLEX Examination Ch. 48 question 1 FAAHN (Ch. 8 question 1 AHN) SG Impulse Pattern, Ch. 48 p. 396 FAAHN (Ch. 8 p. 84 AHN) **BOOK RESOURCES** Fig. 48-3 Conduction system of the heart (FAAHN p. 1542) (Fig. 8-3 AHN p. 306)

OBJECTIVES	CONTENT	TEACHING RESOURCES
		Fig. 48-4 Blood flow during systole (FAAHN p. 1542) (Fig. 8-4 AHN p. 306)
		Fig. 48-5 Blood flow during diastole (FAAHN p. 1543) (Fig. 8-5 AHN p. 307)
		▶ Discuss the concept of automaticity.
		▶ Discuss stimuli that can impact the function of the heart's ability to contract.
		Class Activity Contact the anatomy department at a college or university. Ask to have access to a dissected animal heart. Allow students to see the muscle fibers under the microscope.
		Note: This will aid in understanding the structural components of the muscle fibers.
Explain what produces the two main heart sounds.	– Cardiac cycle (FAAHN p. 1542, AHN p. 306)	PPT 8 through 10, Ch. 48 FAAHN (Ch. 8 PPT 8 through 10 AHN)
		SG Tracing a Drop of Blood, Ch. 48 p. 395 FAAHN (Ch. 8 p. 83 AHN)
		▶ Discuss the actions that cause the characteristic "lubb/dubb" heart sounds.
		▶ Discuss what might be occurring if a "swishing" is heard.
		Class Activity Bring several stethoscopes to class. Allow students to hear the heart sounds of several peers. While the student is listening, discuss the activity that is causing the sounds being heard.
Trace the path of blood through the coronary circulation.	■ Circulation (FAAHN p. 1543, AHN p. 307)	PPT 11 through 14, Ch. 48 FAAHN (Ch. 8 PPT 11 through 14 AHN)
	☐ Coronary blood supply (FAAHN p. 1543, AHN p. 307)	EILR IC Ch. 48 images 4 through 6 FAAHN (Ch. 8 images 4 through 6 AHN)
	☐ Systemic circulation (FAAHN p. 1543, AHN p. 307)	EILR TB Ch. 48 question 50 FAAHN (Ch. 8 question 50 AHN)
	☐ Pulmonary circulation (FAAHN p .1544, AHN p. 308)	ESLR Review Questions for the NCLEX Examination Ch. 48 question 2 FAAHN (Ch. 8 question 2AHN)
		SG Coronary Circulation, Ch. 48 p. 396 FAAHN (Ch. 8 p. 84 AHN)

ELSEVIER

Mosby items and derived items © 2011 by Mosby, Inc., an affiliate of Elsevier Inc.
Some material was previously published.

Adult Health Nursing, 6th ed.

Christensen & Kockrow

OBJECTIVES	CONTENT	TEACHING RESOURCES
		BOOK RESOURCES Review Questions for the NCLEX Examination Ch. 48 questions 1, 2 FAAHN (Ch. 8 questions 1, 2 AHN) Fig. 48-6 Arterial coronary circulation (anterior) (FAAHN p. 1543) (Fig. 8-6 AHN p. 307) ▶ Discuss the path and concepts of systemic circulation and pulmonary circulation. *Class Activity Instruct each student to count off beginning with number 1 and ending with number 13. Continue the process as the number of students allows. Assign each student a location in the path of the circulation of blood. Challenge each group to learn in order the step-by-step locations in the path of blood during pulmonary circulation. Provide a small prize to the winning team.*

8.1 Homework/Assignments:

8.1 Instructor's Notes/Student Feedback:

Christensen & Kockrow

LESSON 8.2

CRITICAL THINKING QUESTION

A patient has been hospitalized for the management of angina pectoris. After being successfully treated, the physician has ordered the patient to be discharged. The patient will be sent home with prescriptions for nitroglycerine, verapamil, and aspirin. The patient reports being concerned about being sent home. He states that he does not feel safe alone at home with such a serious illness. What information should be provided the patient? What is the role of the nurse in this interaction?

Guidelines: At this time, the patient is in need of both emotional support and education. The nurse will need to act as a source of information as well as offer empathy for the patient during this frightening time. It might be necessary to review the cause of the angina. Angina results when the heart muscle does not obtain the needed oxygenated blood supply. Emphasis will need to be placed on avoiding triggering factors. Triggers for angina can include exposure to intense cold, strenuous exercise, smoking, heavy meals, and emotional stress. It is important to ensure that the patient has an understanding of the medications prescribed. The aspirin and verapamil are ordered on a daily schedule. Their focus is to reduce the workload of the heart. The nitroglycerine is used to reduce an angina episode. It is important to reinforce information concerning the proper storage and route of administration of the nitroglycerin. Finally, the patient will need information concerning signs and symptoms to report and when to seek medical intervention.

OBJECTIVES	CONTENT	TEACHING RESOURCES
List diagnostic tests used to evaluate cardiovascular function.	■ Laboratory and diagnostic tests (FAAHN p. 1544, AHN p. 308) □ Diagnostic imaging (FAAHN p. 1544, AHN p. 308) □ Cardiac catheterization and angiography (FAAHN p. 1544, AHN p. 308) □ Electrocardiography (FAAHN p. 1544, AHN p. 308) □ Cardiac monitors (FAAHN p. 1545, AHN p. 309) □ Thallium scanning (FAAHN p. 1546, AHN p. 310) □ Laboratory tests (FAAHN p. 1546, AHN p. 310)	PPT 15, 16, Ch. 48 FAAHN (Ch. 8 PPT 15, 16 AHN) EILR IC Ch. 48 images 7 through 9 FAAHN (Ch. 8 images 7 through 9 AHN) EILR TB Ch. 48 questions 12, 22, 41 FAAHN (Ch. 8 questions 12, 22, 41 AHN) EILR Open Book Quiz Ch. 48 questions 1 through 5 FAAHN (Ch. 8 questions 1 through 5 AHN) ESLR Review Questions for the NCLEX Examination Ch. 48 questions 3, 4 FAAHN (Ch. 8 questions 3, 4 AHN) SG Abnormalities, Ch. 48 p. 399 FAAHN (Ch. 8 p. 87 AHN) **BOOK RESOURCES** Review Questions for the NCLEX Examination Ch. 48 questions 19, 23, 24, 26, 27 FAAHN (Ch. 8 question 19, 23, 24, 26, 27 AHN) Fig. 48-7 Normal electrocardiographic (ECG) deflections (FAAHN p. 1545) (Fig. 8-7 AHN p. 309) ▶ Discuss the diagnostic tests that will require written consent prior to completion. ▶ Discuss the nursing implications for each of the diagnostic tests presented.

OBJECTIVES	CONTENT	TEACHING RESOURCES
		Class Activity Pair students. One student will be the patient and the other will act as the nurse. Assign each student a diagnostic test. Instruct each student to role-play the interaction and teaching that will be needed for each of the tests.
For coronary artery disease, compare nonmodifiable risk factors in coronary artery disease (CAD) with factors that are modifiable in lifestyle and health management.	■ Disorders of the cardiovascular system (FAAHN p. 1547, AHN p. 311) □ Normal aging patterns (FAAHN p. 1548, AHN p. 312) □ Risk factors (FAAHN p. 1548, AHN p. 312) – Nonmodifiable factors (FAAHN p. 1548, AHN p. 312) – Modifiable factors (FAAHN p. 1548, AHN p. 312)	PPT 17, 18, Ch. 48 FAAHN (Ch. 8 PPT 17, 18 AHN) EILR TB Ch. 48 questions 1, 42 FAAHN (Ch. 8 questions 1, 42 AHN) ESLR Review Questions for the NCLEX Examination Ch. 48 questions 5, 6 FAAHN (Ch. 8 questions 5, 6 AHN) SG Risk Factors, Ch. 48 p. 398 FAAHN (Ch. 8 p. 86 AHN) **BOOK RESOURCES** Review Questions for the NCLEX Examination Ch. 48 question 21 FAAHN (Ch. 8 question 21 AHN) Life Span Considerations, Older Adults: Cardiac Disease (FAAHN p. 1548) (AHN p. 312) Box 48-1 Cholesterol Numbers: What Do They Mean? (FAAHN p. 1549) (Box 8-1 AHN p. 313) ▶ Discuss the differences between modifiable and nonmodifiable risk factors. ▶ Discuss the interventions that can be used to reduce the risks associated with hyperlipidemia. *Class Activity Prepare a listing of the modifiable and nonmodifiable risk factors for the development of cardiovascular disease. Distribute the list to the students. Ask students to review and record their risk factors. Determine the level of risk for the students.* *Note: It might be helpful to determine if those students with elevated risk are aware of the implications of their own personal degree of risk.*
Describe five cardiac dysrhythmias.	□ Cardiac dysrhythmias (FAAHN p. 1550, AHN p. 314) – Types of cardiac dysrhythmias (FAAHN p. 1550, AHN p. 314)	PPT 19, Ch. 48 FAAHN (Ch. 8 PPT 19 AHN) EILR TB Ch. 48 question 29 FAAHN (Ch. 8 question 29 AHN)

Christensen & Kockrow

OBJECTIVES	CONTENT	TEACHING RESOURCES
	– Assessment (FAAHN p. 1553, AHN p. 317) – Diagnostic tests (FAAHN p. 1553, AHN p. 317) – Medical management (FAAHN p. 1553, AHN p. 317) – Nursing interventions and patient teaching (FAAHN p. 1553, AHN p. 317) ☐ Cardiac arrest (FAAHN p. 1555, AHN p. 319) – Artificial cardiac pacemakers (FAAHN p. 1555, AHN p. 319) – Nursing interventions and patient teaching (FAAHN p. 1556, AHN p. 320) – Prognosis (FAAHN p. 1556, AHN p. 320)	▣ EILR Open Book Quiz Ch. 48 question 4 FAAHN (Ch. 8 question 4 AHN) ▣ ESLR Review Questions for the NCLEX Examination Ch. 48 questions 7, 8 FAAHN (Ch. 8 questions 7, 8 AHN) ▣ SG Cardiac Dysrhythmias, Ch. 48 p. 400 FAAHN (Ch. 8 p. 88 AHN) **BOOK RESOURCES** Fig. 48-8 Ventricular pacing (FAAHN p. 1551) (Fig. 8-8 AHN p. 315) Fig. 48-9 A dual-chamber, rate-responsive pacemaker (FAAHN p. 1551) (Fig. 8-9 AHN p. 315) Table 48-1 Medications for Cardiac Dysrhythmias (FAAHN pp. 1554-1555) (Table 8-1 AHN pp. 318-319) ▸ Discuss the clinical manifestations associated with cardiac dysrhythmias. ▸ Discuss treatment interventions for cardiac dysrhythmias. *Class Activity Obtain several cardiac tracings. Bring them to class. Divide the students into groups of three or four people. Distribute the strips between the groups, and instruct the students to determine if they are able to identify the type of dysrhythmia presented.*
Compare the etiology and pathophysiology, clinical manifestations, assessment, diagnostic tests, medical management, nursing interventions, and prognosis for patients with angina pectoris, myocardial infarction, or heart failure.	■ Disorders of the heart (FAAHN p. 1556, AHN p. 320) ☐ Coronary atherosclerotic heart disease (FAAHN p. 1556, AHN p. 320) ☐ Angina pectoris (FAAHN p. 1557, AHN p. 321) – Etiology and pathophysiology(FAAHN p. 1557, AHN p. 321) – Clinical manifestations (FAAHN p. 1557, AHN p. 321) – Assessment (FAAHN p. 1558, AHN p. 322) – Diagnostic tests (FAAHN p. 1558, AHN p. 322)	▣ PPT 21 through 37, Ch. 48 FAAHN (Ch. 8 PPT 21 through 37 AHN) ▣ EILR IC Ch. 48 images 11 through 18 FAAHN (Ch. 8 images 11 through 18 AHN) ▣ EILR TB Ch. 48 questions 2, 4, 6, 7, 9, 10, 14, 17 through 19, 21, 26, 30, 43, 51 FAAHN (Ch. 8 questions 2, 4, 6, 7, 9, 10, 14, 17 through 19, 21, 26, 30, 43, 51 AHN) ▣ EILR Open Book Quiz Ch. 48 questions 6, 7 FAAHN (Ch. 8 questions 6, 7 AHN) ▣ ESLR Review Questions for the NCLEX Examination Ch. 48 questions 9, 10 FAAHN (Ch. 8 questions 9, 10 AHN) ▣ SG Angina Pectoris, Myocardial Infarction, and Heart Failure , Ch. 48 p. 400 FAAHN (Ch. 8 p. 88 AHN)

Adult Health Nursing, 6th ed.

Christensen & Kockrow

OBJECTIVES	CONTENT	TEACHING RESOURCES
	– Medical management (FAAHN p. 1558, AHN p. 322) – Nursing interventions and patient teaching (FAAHN p. 1560, AHN p. 324) – Prognosis (FAAHN p. 1561, AHN p. 325) ☐ Myocardial infarction (FAAHN p. 1562, AHN p. 326) – Etiology and pathophysiology(FAAHN p. 1562, AHN p. 326) – Clinical manifestations (FAAHN p. 1563, AHN p. 327) – Assessment (FAAHN p. 1563, AHN p. 327) – Diagnostic tests (FAAHN p. 1564, AHN p. 328) – Medical management (FAAHN p. 1564, AHN p. 328) – Nursing interventions and patient teaching (FAAHN p. 1566, AHN p. 330) – Prognosis (FAAHN p. 1568, AHN p. 332) ☐ Heart failure (FAAHN p. 1568, AHN p. 332) – Etiology and pathophysiology(FAAHN p. 1568, AHN p. 332) – Clinical manifestations (FAAHN p. 1570, AHN p. 334) – Assessment (FAAHN p. 1570, AHN p. 334) – Diagnostic tests (FAAHN p. 1570, AHN p. 334) – Medical management (FAAHN p. 1571, AHN p. 335) – Nursing interventions (FAAHN p. 1572, AHN p. 336) – Prognosis (FAAHN p. 1576, AHN p. 340)	**BOOK RESOURCES** Review Questions for the NCLEX Examination Ch. 48 questions 8, 11, 13, 15 through 18, 20, 22, 25, 28, 29, 31, 32, 37 FAAHN (Ch. 8 questions 8, 11, 13, 15 through 18, 20, 22, 25, 28, 29, 31, 32, 37 AHN) Fig. 48-10 Progressive development of coronary atheroscleorsis (FAAHN p. 1557) (Fig. 8-10 AHN p. 321) Cultural Considerations: Cardiovascular Disorder (FAAHN p. 1557) (AHN p. 321) ▸ Discuss populations at an increased risk of angina pectoris, myocardial infarction, or heart failure. ▸ Discuss the relationship between the onset of angina pectoris and the event of myocardial infarction. *Class Activity Divide the students into three groups. The groups will be assigned angina pectoris, myocardial infarction, and heart failure. Now, further subdivide the groups. Each group will have subgroups responsible for etiology/pathophysiology, diagnostic tests, clinical manifestations, and management. Instruct students to investigate the information needed to provide a 3-minute report to their larger group on the assigned subtopic.*

OBJECTIVES	CONTENT	TEACHING RESOURCES
Specify patient teaching for patients with cardiac dysrhythmias, angina pectoris, myocardial infarction, heart failure, and valvular heart disease.	☐ Cardiac dysrhythmias (FAAHN p. 1550, AHN p. 314) – Medical management (FAAHN p. 1553, AHN p. 317) – Nursing interventions and patient teaching (FAAHN p. 1553, AHN p. 317) ☐ Angina pectoris (FAAHN p. 1557, AHN p. 321) – Medical management (FAAHN p. 1558, AHN p. 322) – Nursing interventions and patient teaching (FAAHN p. 1560, AHN p. 324) – Prognosis (FAAHN p. 1561, AHN p. 325) ☐ Myocardial infarction (FAAHN p. 1562, AHN p. 326) – Medical management (FAAHN p. 1564, AHN p. 328) – Nursing interventions and patient teaching (FAAHN p. 1566, AHN p. 330) – Prognosis (FAAHN p. 1568, AHN p. 332) ☐ Heart failure (FAAHN p. 1568, AHN p. 332) – Medical management (FAAHN p. 1571, AHN p. 335) – Nursing interventions (FAAHN p. 1572, AHN p. 336) – Prognosis (FAAHN p. 1576, AHN p. 340) ☐ Valvular heart disease (FAAHN p. 1576, AHN p. 340) – Medical management (FAAHN p. 1577, AHN p. 341) – Nursing interventions and patient teaching (FAAHN p. 1578, AHN p. 342) – Prognosis (FAAHN p. 1578, AHN p. 342)	PPT 19, 23 through 37, 41 through 43, Ch. 48 FAAHN (Ch. 8 PPT 19, 23 through 37, 41 through 43AHN) EILR IC Ch. 48 image 1 FAAHN (Ch. 8 image 1 AHN) EILR TB Ch. 48 questions 4 through 6, 9, 10, 17, 18, 31, 34, 35, 41 FAAHN (Ch. 8 questions 4 through 6, 9, 10, 17, 18, 31, 34, 35, 41AHN) EILR Open Book Quiz Ch. 48 question 9 FAAHN (Ch. 8 question 9 AHN) SG Patient Teaching, Ch. 48 p. 403 FAAHN (Ch. 8 p. 91AHN) **BOOK RESOURCES** Table 48-1 Medications for Cardiac Dysrhythmias (FAAHN p. 1554) (Table 8-1 AHN p. 318) Fig. 48-11 Sites to which ischemic myocardial pain may be referred (FAAHN p. 1558) (Fig. 8-11 AHN p. 322) Fig. 48-12 A Saphenous vein (FAAHN p. 1559) (Fig. 8-12 AHN p. 323) Fig. 48-13 Coronary artery bypass graft (FAAHN p. 1559) (Fig. 8-13 AHN p. 323) Fig. 48-14 Percutaneous transluminal coronary angioplasty (PTCA) (FAAHN p. 1560) (Fig. 8-14 AHN p. 324) Fig. 48-15 Palmaz-Schatz stent (FAAHN p. 1560) (Fig. 8-15 AHN p. 324) Communication: Methods to Decrease Angina Pectoris Attacks (FAAHN p. 1561) (AHN p. 325) Patient Teaching: Angina Pectoris (FAAHN p. 1562) (AHN p. 326) Fig. 48-16 Four common locations where myocardial infarctions occur (FAAHN p. 1562) (Fig. 8-16 AHN p. 326) Table 48-3 Coronary Artery Disorders (FAAHN p. 1563) (Table 8-3 AHN p. 327) Table 48-4 Medications for Myocardial Infarction Table (FAAHN p. 1565) (Table 8-4 AHN p. 329) Health Promotion: Myocardial Infarction (FAAHN p. 1568) (AHN p. 332)

Adult Health Nursing, 6th ed.
Christensen & Kockrow

OBJECTIVES	CONTENT	TEACHING RESOURCES
		Home Care Considerations: Exercise Program after Myocardial Infarction (FAAHN p. 1568) (AHN p.332)
		Box 48-2 Classifying and Staging Heart Failure (FAAHN p. 1569) (Box 8-2 AHN p. 333)
		Fig. 48-17 Scale for pitting edema depth (FAAHN p. 1570) (Fig. 8-17 AHN p. 334)
		Box 48-3 Signs and Symptoms of Heart Failure (FAAHN p. 1570) (Box 8-3 AHN p. 334)
		Table 48-7 Medications for Heart Failure (FAAHN pp. 1572-1573) (Table 8-7 AHN pp. 336-337)
		Patient Teaching: Heart Failure (FAAHN p. 1575) (AHN p. 339)
		Box 48-4 Guidelines for Nursing Interventions for the Patient with Heart Failure (FAAHN p. 1575) (Box 8-4 AHN p. 339)
		Complementary and Alternative Therapies: Cardiovascular and Peripheral Vascular Disorders (FAAHN p. 1592) (AHN p. 356)
		▸ Discuss the priorities for care management in the patient diagnosed with cardiac dysrhythmias, angina pectoris, myocardial infarction, heart failure, and valvular heart disease.
		Class Activity *Distribute partially blank nursing care plan forms to each student. Allow the students to work in pairs. Instruct each pair to modify a nursing care plan for an assigned diagnosis.*
Discuss the purposes of cardiac rehabilitation.	☐ Myocardial infarction (FAAHN p. 1562, AHN p. 326) – Nursing interventions and patient teaching (FAAHN p. 1566, AHN p. 330) – Prognosis (FAAHN p. 1568, AHN p. 332)	🖳 PPT 26 through 32, Ch. 48 FAAHN (Ch. 8 PPT 26 through 32 AHN) 📓 SG Cardiac Rehabilitation, Ch. 48 p. 409 FAAHN (Ch. 8 p. 97 AHN) ▸ Discuss the scope/purposes of cardiac rehabilitation. ▸ Discuss the time frame of a normal cardiac rehabilitation. **Class Activity** *Contact a local, acute care facility. Arrange a tour of the facility's cardiac rehab center.* *Note: The tour itself will not take much time; perhaps it is possible to obtain a*

Adult Health Nursing, 6th ed.
Christensen & Kockrow

OBJECTIVES	CONTENT	TEACHING RESOURCES
		classroom to provide lecture content before or after the tour.
Discuss the etiology and pathophysiology, clinical manifestations, assessment, diagnostic tests, medical management, nursing interventions, and prognosis for the patient with pulmonary edema.	☐ Pulmonary edema (FAAHN p. 1576, AHN p. 340) – Etiology and pathophysiology(FAAHN p. 1576, AHN p. 340) – Clinical manifestations (FAAHN p. 1576, AHN p. 340) – Assessment (FAAHN p. 1576, AHN p. 340) – Diagnostic tests (FAAHN p. 1576, AHN p. 340) – Medical management (FAAHN p. 1576, AHN p. 340) – Nursing interventions (FAAHN p. 1576, AHN p. 340) – Prognosis (FAAHN p. 1576, AHN p. 340)	⊠ PPT 38 through 40, Ch. 48 FAAHN (Ch. 8 PPT 38 through 40) ▰ EILR TB Ch. 48 questions 24, 25, 27, 39, 40 FAAHN (Ch. 8 questions 24, 25, 27, 39, 40 AHN) ▰ SG Pulmonary Edema, Ch. 48 p. 401 FAAHN (Ch. 8 p. 89 AHN) **BOOK RESOURCES** Table 48-5 Cardiogenic Shock (FAAHN p. 1566) (Table 8-5 AHN p. 330) Box 48-5 Signs and Symptoms of Pulmonary Edema (FAAHN p. 1576) (Box 8-5 p. 340 AHN) ▸ Discuss the pathophysiology of pulmonary edema. ▸ Discuss the nursing assessment that is needed when providing care to the patient experiencing pulmonary edema. *Class Activity Develop 10 to 15 short-answer questions concerning pulmonary edema. Use the questions to provide a topical review to the class.*
Compare and contrast the etiology and pathophysiology, clinical manifestations, assessment, diagnostic tests, medical management, nursing interventions, and prognosis for the patient with rheumatic heart disease, pericarditis, or endocarditis.	☐ Inflammatory heart disorders (FAAHN p. 1578, AHN p. 342) ☐ Rheumatic heart disease (FAAHN p. 1578, AHN p. 342) – Etiology and pathophysiology(FAAHN p. 1578, AHN p. 342) – Clinical manifestations (FAAHN p. 1579, AHN p. 343) – Assessment (FAAHN p. 1579, AHN p. 343) – Diagnostic tests (FAAHN p. 1579, AHN p. 343) – Medical management (FAAHN p. 1579, AHN p. 343) – Nursing interventions and patient teaching (FAAHN p. 1579, AHN p. 343)	⊠ PPT 41 through 53, Ch. 48 FAAHN (Ch. 8 PPT 41 through 53) ▰ EILR TB Ch. 48 questions 11, 13, 28 FAAHN (Ch. 8 questions 11, 13, 28 AHN) ▰ SG Rheumatic Heart Disease, Pericarditis, and Endocarditis Ch. 48 p. 401 FAAHN (Ch. 8 p. 89 AHN) **BOOK RESOURCES** Review Questions for the NCLEX Examination Ch. 48 questions 9, 12 FAAHN (Ch. 8 questions 9, 12 AHN) ▸ Discuss the underlying causes associated with the development of rheumatic heart disease, pericarditis, and endocarditis. ▸ Discuss the treatment options available for rheumatic heart disease, pericarditis, and endocarditis. *Class Activity Instruct each student to develop three NCLEX-style questions*

OBJECTIVES	CONTENT	TEACHING RESOURCES
	– Prognosis (FAAHN p. 1579, AHN p. 343) ☐ Pericarditis (FAAHN p. 1579, AHN p. 343) – Etiology and pathophysiology(FAAHN p. 1579, AHN p. 343) – Clinical manifestations (FAAHN p. 1580, AHN p. 344) – Assessment (FAAHN p. 1580, AHN p. 344) – Diagnostic tests (FAAHN p. 1580, AHN p. 344) – Medical management (FAAHN p. 1580, AHN p. 344) – Nursing interventions (FAAHN p. 1580, AHN p. 344) – Prognosis (FAAHN p. 1581, AHN p. 345) ☐ Endocarditis (FAAHN p. 1581, AHN p. 345) – Etiology and pathophysiology(FAAHN p. 1581, AHN p. 345) – Clinical manifestations (FAAHN p. 1581, AHN p. 345) – Assessment (FAAHN p. 1581, AHN p. 345) – Diagnostic tests (FAAHN p. 1581, AHN p. 345) – Medical management (FAAHN p. 1581, AHN p. 345) – Nursing interventions and patient teaching (FAAHN p. 1582, AHN p. 346) – Prognosis (FAAHN p. 1582, AHN p. 346) ☐ Myocarditis (FAAHN p. 1582 AHN p. 346)	*concerning any one of the three disorders above. Instruct each student to pair with a student who selected a different disorder. Allow 5 minutes for the pairs to share developed information.*

Mosby items and derived items © 2011 by Mosby, Inc., an affiliate of Elsevier Inc.
Some material was previously published.

Adult Health Nursing, 6th ed.
Christensen & Kockrow

8.2 Homework/Assignments:

8.2 Instructor's Notes/Student Feedback:

LESSON 8.3

CRITICAL THINKING QUESTION

While seeing the physician about an allergy, a 62-year-old African American male patient is found to have an elevated blood pressure. The initial blood pressure reading was 147/96. The physician requested that the patient return for readings 48 hours later. At that time, the blood pressure was 145/99. The physician diagnosed the patient with hypertension and has prescribed Cardizem. What risk factors does the patient present? What are topics for educating the patient? Does the patient have primary, secondary, or malignant hypertension?

Guidelines: The risk factors evident are the patient's advancing age, race, and gender. The hypertension appears to be primary in nature. Education will be needed to ensure the patient begins the prescribed treatment regimen. The topics of education include dietary management and modification, the importance of exercise and weight control, and information concerning the prescribed medication.

OBJECTIVES	CONTENT	TEACHING RESOURCES
Identify 10 conditions that can result in the complication of secondary cardiomyopathy.	☐ Cardiomyopathy (FAAHN p. 1582, AHN p. 346) – Etiology and pathophysiology(FAAHN p. 1582, AHN p. 346) – Clinical manifestations (FAAHN p. 1583, AHN p. 347) – Diagnostic tests (FAAHN p. 1583, AHN p. 347)	PPT 54 through 56, Ch. 48 FAAHN (Ch. 8 PPT 54 through 56 43AHN) EILR TB Ch. 48 question 23 FAAHN (Ch. 8 question 23 AHN) SG Secondary Cardiomyopathy, Ch. 48 p. 403 FAAHN (Ch. 8 p. 91 AHN) ▸ Discuss the cause of cardiomyopathy. ▸ Discuss the clinical manifestations of cardiomyopathy. *Class Activity⎸Divide the class into five groups. Assign students to the following groups: etiology, clinical manifestations, diagnostic tests, medical management, and nursing care. Instruct each group to develop two NCLEX-style questions concerning its assigned topic. Next, allow the groups to quiz each other.*
Discuss the indications and contraindications for cardiac transplant.	– Medical management (FAAHN p. 1583, AHN p. 347) – Nursing interventions and patient teaching (FAAHN p. 1584, AHN p. 348) – Prognosis (FAAHN p. 1584, AHN p. 348)	PPT 54 through 56, Ch. 48 FAAHN (Ch. 8 PPT 54 through 56) EILR TB Ch. 48 question 39 FAAHN (Ch. 8 question 39 AHN) SG Cardiac Transplantation, Ch. 48 p. 404 FAAHN (Ch. 8 p. 92 AHN) **BOOK RESOURCES** Box 48-6 Indications and Contraindications for Cardiac Transplantation (FAAHN p. 1583) (Box 8-6 AHN p. 347) ▸ Discuss the indications for cardiac transplantation. ▸ Discuss the prognosis for patients after undergoing a cardiac transplantation.

Christensen & Kockrow

OBJECTIVES	CONTENT	TEACHING RESOURCES
		***Class Activity** Contact a local cardiologist's office. Request information to locate a speaker for the class involving cardiac transplantation.*
Describe the effects of aging on the peripheral vascular system.	■ Disorders of the peripheral vascular system (FAAHN p. 1584, AHN p. 348) □ Normal aging patterns (FAAHN p. 1584, AHN p. 348)	SG Aging, Ch. 48 p. 405 FAAHN (Ch. 8 p. 93 AHN) ▸ Discuss the changes in the peripheral vascular system associated with aging. ▸ Discuss the occurrence of comorbid conditions associated with aging that impact the peripheral vascular system. ***Class Activity** Ask each student to select a modifiable risk factor. Next, ask the students to write down all of the interventions that can be used to improve and reduce the risk. Allow students who selected the same risk factor time to compare notes.*
Identify risk factors associated with peripheral vascular disorders.	□ Risk factors (FAAHN p. 1584, AHN p. 348) – Nonmodifiable factors (FAAHN p. 1584, AHN p. 348) – Modifiable factors (FAAHN p. 1585, AHN p. 349) □ Assessment (FAAHN p. 1585, AHN p. 349) – Arterial assessment (FAAHN p. 1585, AHN p. 349) – Venous assessment (FAAHN p. 1586, AHN p. 350) – Diagnostic tests (FAAHN p. 1586, AHN p. 350)	PPT 57 through 59 Ch. 48 FAAHN (Ch. 8 PPT 57 through 59 AHN) EILR TB Ch. 48 question 8 FAAHN (Ch. 8 question 8 AHN) SG Risk Factors, Ch. 48 p. 398 FAAHN (Ch. 8 p. 86 AHN) **BOOK RESOURCES** Box 48-7 Capillary Refill Time (FAAHN p. 1585) (Box 8-7 AHN p. 349) ▸ Discuss the risk factors associated with peripheral vascular disorders. ▸ Discuss the manner in which a patient could reduce/alter the modifiable risk factors. ***Class Activity** Solicit student volunteers. Demonstrate the assessment of capillary refill time. After completion, demonstrate the documentation of the findings. If time permits, allow students to perform the assessment on each other.*

OBJECTIVES	CONTENT	TEACHING RESOURCES
Compare and contrast signs and symptoms associated with arterial and venous disorders.	☐ Arterial disorders (FAAHN p. 1591, AHN p. 355) ☐ Arteriosclerosis and atherosclerosis (FAAHN p. 1591, AHN p. 355) ☐ Peripheral arterial disease of the lower extremities (FAAHN p. 1591, AHN p. 355) – Etiology and pathophysiology(FAAHN p. 1591, AHN p. 355) – Clinical manifestations (FAAHN p. 1591, AHN p. 355) – Assessment (FAAHN p. 1591, AHN p. 355) – Diagnostic tests (FAAHN p. 1592, AHN p. 356) – Medical management (FAAHN p. 1592, AHN p. 356) – Nursing interventions and patient teaching (FAAHN p. 1593, AHN p. 357) – Prognosis (FAAHN p. 1593, AHN p. 357) ☐ Arterial embolism (FAAHN p. 1593, AHN p. 357) – Etiology and pathophysiology(FAAHN p. 1593, AHN p. 357) – Clinical manifestations (FAAHN p. 1593, AHN p. 357) – Assessment (FAAHN p. 1593, AHN p. 357) – Diagnostic tests (FAAHN p. 1593, AHN p. 357) – Medical management (FAAHN p. 1594, AHN p. 358) – Nursing interventions and patient teaching (FAAHN p. 1594, AHN p. 358) – Prognosis (FAAHN p. 1594, AHN p. 359)	⊠▤ PPT 60 through 82, Ch. 48 FAAHN (Ch. 8 PPT 60 through 82) 🅔 EILR IC Ch. 48 image 10 FAAHN (Ch. 8 image 10 AHN) 🅔 EILR TB Ch. 48 questions 15, 16 FAAHN (Ch. 8 questions 15, 16 AHN) 📓 SG Arterial and Venous Disorders, Ch. 48 p. 405 FAAHN (Ch. 8 p. 93 AHN) **BOOK RESOURCES** Table 48-7 Medications for Heart Failure (FAAHN p. 1572) (Table 8-7 AHN p. 336) Fig. 48-18 Common anatomic locations of atheroscleortic lesions of the abdominal aorta and lower extremities (FAAHN p. 1591) (Fig. 8-18 AHN p. 355) Fig. 48-19 A Femoral-popliteal bypass graft around an occluded superficial femoral artery (FAAHN p. 1593) (Fig. 8-19 AHN p. 357) ▸ Discuss the clinical manifestations associated with arterial and venous disorders. ▸ Discuss the Etiology and pathophysiology of arterial and venous disorders. *Class Activity **Divide the class into two groups. One group will be assigned to venous disorders and the other arterial disorders. Instruct each group to develop a list about the characteristics of its assigned disorder. Bring both groups together and allow the students to "debate" or discuss the differences.***

Adult Health Nursing, 6th ed.

Mosby items and derived items © 2011 by Mosby, Inc., an affiliate of Elsevier Inc.
Some material was previously published.

Christensen & Kockrow

OBJECTIVES	CONTENT	TEACHING RESOURCES

Discuss nursing interventions for arterial and venous disorders.	☐ Arterial disorders (FAAHN p. 1591, AHN p. 355)
	
	☐ Arteriosclerosis and atherosclerosis (FAAHN p. 1591, AHN p. 355)
	
	☐ Hypertension (FAAHN p. 1587, AHN p. 351)
	
	  – Nursing interventions and patient teaching (FAAHN p. 1590, AHN p. 354)
	
	☐ Peripheral arterial disease of the lower extremities (FAAHN p. 1591, AHN p. 355)
	
	  – Nursing interventions and patient teaching (FAAHN p. 1593, AHN p. 357)
	
	☐ Arterial embolism (FAAHN p. 1593, AHN p. 357)
	
	  – Nursing interventions and patient teaching (FAAHN p. 1594, AHN p. 358)
	
	☐ Arterial aneurysm (FAAHN p. 1595, AHN p. 359)
	
	  – Nursing interventions and patient teaching (FAAHN p. 1596, AHN p. 360)
	
	☐ Thromboangiitis obliterans (Buerger's disease) (FAAHN p. 1596, AHN p. 360)
	
	  – Nursing interventions and patient teaching (FAAHN p. 1597, AHN p. 361)
	
	☐ Raynaud's disease (FAAHN p. 1597, AHN p. 361)
	
	  – Nursing interventions and patient teaching (FAAHN p. 1598, AHN p. 362)
	
	☐ Venous disorders (FAAHN p. 1598, AHN p. 362)
	
	☐ Thrombophlebitis (FAAHN p. 1598, AHN p. 362)
		PPT 60 through 82 Ch. 48 FAAHN (Ch. 8 PPT 60 through 82)
		
		EILR IC Ch. 48 image 19 FAAHN (Ch. 8 image 19 AHN)
		
		EILR TB Ch. 48 questions 8, 15, 16, 44, 46, FAAHN (Ch. 8 questions 8, 15, 16, 44, 46 AHN)
		
		SG Nursing Interventions, Ch. 48 p. 405 FAAHN (Ch. 8 p. 93 AHN)
		
		BOOK RESOURCES
		
		Review Questions for the NCLEX Examination Ch. 48 questions 7, 14, 20, 30 FAAHN (Ch. 8 questions 7, 14, 20, 30 AHN)
		
		▸ Discuss the data collection by the nurse for arterial and venous disorders.
		
		▸ Discuss the scope of nursing practice as it relates to the care of patients diagnosed with arterial and venous disorders.
		
		Class Activity Provide a blank nursing care plan to each member of the class. Instruct each student to develop two nursing diagnoses for both the arterial and venous disorders. After the diagnoses have been formulated, allow students a few minutes to compare notes with a partner.

OBJECTIVES	CONTENT	TEACHING RESOURCES
	– Nursing interventions and patient teaching (FAAHN p. 1600, AHN p. 364) ☐ Varicose veins (FAAHN p. 1601, AHN p. 365) – Nursing interventions and patient teaching (FAAHN p. 1601, AHN p. 365) ☐ Venous stasis ulcers (FAAHN p. 1602, AHN p. 366) – Nursing interventions and patient teaching (FAAHN p. 1603, AHN p. 367)	
Compare essential (primary) hypertension, secondary hypertension, and malignant hypertension.	☐ Hypertension (FAAHN p. 1587, AHN p. 351) – Etiology and pathophysiology(FAAHN p. 1587, AHN p. 351) – Essential (primary) hypertension (FAAHN p. 1588, AHN p. 352) – Secondary hypertension (FAAHN p. 1588, AHN p. 352) – Malignant hypertension (FAAHN p. 1589, AHN p. 353)	PPT 61, 62, Ch. 48 FAAHN (Ch. 8 PPT 61, 62) EILR TB Ch. 48 question 20 FAAHN (Ch. 8 question 20 AHN) SG Hypertension, Ch. 48 p. 406 FAAHN (Ch. 8 p. 94 AHN) **BOOK RESOURCES** Box 48-8 Risk Factors for Essential Hypertension (FAAHN p. 1588) (Box 8-8 AHN p. 352) Table 48-11 Causes of Secondary Hypertension (FAAHN p. 1588) (Table 8-11 AHN p. 352) ▸ Discuss the parameters of the blood pressure reading that meet the criteria for a diagnosis of hypertension. ▸ Discuss the risk factors associated with the development of hypertension. *Class Activity Provide a "mini blood pressure clinic." Allow students to check the blood pressures of other class members. If time allows, invite the other nursing faculty members to have their readings assessed.*

OBJECTIVES	CONTENT	TEACHING RESOURCES
Discuss the etiology and pathophysiology, clinical manifestations, assessment, diagnostic tests, medical management, and nursing interventions for the patient with hypertension.	☐ Hypertension (FAAHN p. 1587, AHN p. 351) – Etiology and pathophysiology(FAAHN p. 1587, AHN p. 351) – Clinical manifestations (FAAHN p. 1589, AHN p. 353) – Assessment (FAAHN p. 1589, AHN p. 353) – Diagnostic tests (FAAHN p. 1589, AHN p. 353) – Medical management (FAAHN p. 1589, AHN p. 353) – Nursing interventions and patient teaching (FAAHN p. 1590, AHN p. 354)	⊠▤ PPT 62, Ch. 48 FAAHN (Ch. 8 PPT 62) ▰ EILR TB Ch. 48 questions 5, 6 FAAHN (Ch. 8 questions 5, 6 AHN) ▧ SG Hypertension, Ch. 48 p. 406 FAAHN (Ch. 8 p. 94 AHN) **BOOK RESOURCES** Review Questions for the NCLEX Examination Ch. 48 question 10 FAAHN (Ch. 8 question 10 AHN) Box 48-8 Risk Factors for Essential Hypertension (FAAHN p. 1588) (Box 8-8 AHN p. 352) Table 48-11 Causes of Secondary Hypertension (FAAHN p. 1588) (Table 8-11 AHN p. 352) ▸ Discuss the diagnostic tests that are utilized when a diagnosis of hypertension is suspected. ▸ Discuss the medication regimen associated with a diagnosis of hypertension. *Class Activity Develop five questions concerning hypertension. The best formats for the questions are short answer. Divide the class into three or four teams and have each team present questions to the other teams. Award points to the team who accurately answers the question first. The team who has correctly answered the most questions at the end of the game will win.*

OBJECTIVES	CONTENT	TEACHING RESOURCES
Discuss the importance of patient education for hypertension.	– Nursing interventions and patient teaching (FAAHN p. 1590, AHN p. 354)	PPT 62, Ch. 48 FAAHN (Ch. 8 PPT 62) EILR IC Ch. 48 image 1 FAAHN (Ch. 8 image 1 AHN) SG Hypertension, Ch. 48 p. 406 FAAHN (Ch. 8 p. 94 AHN) **BOOK RESOURCES** Box 48-9 Measures to Increase Compliance with Antihypertensive Therapy (FAAHN p. 1590) (Box 8-9 AHN p. 354) ▸ Discuss importance of diet for the patient diagnosed with hypertension. ▸ Discuss the need for follow-up care for the hypertensive patient. *Class Activity Assign each student a partner. One student will act as the nurse and the other will role-play the patient diagnosed with hypertension. The "nurse" will provide education for the patient.*

8.3 Homework/Assignments:

8.3 Instructor's Notes/Student Feedback:

Christensen & Kockrow

LESSON 8.4

CRITICAL THINKING QUESTION

Two days after undergoing a hysterectomy, a 32-year-old patient asks the nurse for pain medication for a cramp-like discomfort in her left calf. An assessment of the extremity reveals the area is warm, reddened, and has darker red streaks in the upper calf. There is a positive Homan's sign. What actions should the nurse take next? What is the anticipated diagnosis? What testing will be performed? Why has this patient developed this complication?

Guidelines: The patient is demonstrating symptoms consistent with thrombophlebitis. The nurse's next actions will be notification of the physician concerning the assessment findings and documentation. Testing that can be ordered to finalize the diagnosis include venous Doppler, duplex scanning, venogram, and a serum D-dimer test. Thrombophlebitis can occur in a number of populations. Individuals at risk include the elderly, postoperative patients, and patients who have had a myocardial infarction.

OBJECTIVES	CONTENT	TEACHING RESOURCES
Compare and contrast the etiology and pathophysiology, clinical manifestations, assessment, diagnostic tests, medical management, nursing interventions, and prognosis for patients with arterial aneurysm, Buerger's disease, and Raynaud's disease.	□ Arterial aneurysm (FAAHN p. 1595, AHN p. 359) – Etiology and pathophysiology(FAAHN p. 1595, AHN p. 359) – Clinical manifestations (FAAHN p. 1595, AHN p. 359) – Assessment (FAAHN p. 1595, AHN p. 359) – Diagnostic tests (FAAHN p. 1595, AHN p. 359) – Medical management (FAAHN p. 1595, AHN p. 359) – Nursing interventions and patient teaching (FAAHN p. 1596, AHN p. 360) – Prognosis (FAAHN p. 1596, AHN p. 360) □ Thromboangiitis obliterans (Buerger's disease) (FAAHN p. 1596, AHN p. 360) – Etiology and pathophysiology (FAAHN p. 1596, AHN p. 360) – Clinical manifestations (FAAHN p. 1596, AHN p. 360) – Assessment (FAAHN p. 1597, AHN p. 361) – Diagnostic tests (FAAHN p. 1597, AHN p. 361) – Medical management (FAAHN p. 1597, AHN p. 361)	▨ PPT 67 through 73, Ch. 48 FAAHN (Ch. 8 PPT 67 through 73) ▨ EILR IC Ch. 48 images 21, 22 FAAHN (Ch. 8 images 21, 22 AHN) ▨ EILR TB Ch. 48 questions 8, 36, 44, FAAHN (Ch. 8 questions 8, 36, 44, AHN) ▨ SG Arterial Aneurysm, Buerger's disease, and Raynaud's Disease Ch. 48 p. 407 FAAHN (Ch. 8 p. 95 AHN) **BOOK RESOURCES** Fig. 48-20 Types of aneurysms (FAAHN p. 1595) (Fig. 8-20 AHN p. 359) Fig. 48-21 Surgical repair of an abdominal aortic aneurysm (FAAHN p. 1596) (Fig. 8-21 AHN p. 360) Fig. 48-22 Replacement of aortolliac aneurysm with a bifurcated synthetic graft (FAAHN p. 1596) (Fig. 8-22 AHN p. 360) ▸ Discuss the treatment options to manage an arterial aneurysm. ▸ Discuss the etiology of Buerger's disease. *Class Activity Ask a question concerning arterial aneurysms, Buerger's disease, or Raynaud's disease. If the student gets the answer correct, he/she is allowed to sit down. The questions continue until all students are seated or time constraints require the questions to end.*

OBJECTIVES	CONTENT	TEACHING RESOURCES
	– Nursing interventions and patient teaching (FAAHN p. 1597, AHN p. 361) – Prognosis (FAAHN p. 1597, AHN p. 361) ☐ Raynaud's disease (FAAHN p. 1597, AHN p. 361) – Etiology and pathophysiology(FAAHN p. 1597, AHN p. 361) – Clinical manifestations (FAAHN p. 1597, AHN p. 361) – Assessment (FAAHN p. 1597, AHN p. 361) – Diagnostic tests (FAAHN p. 1597, AHN p. 361) – Medical management (FAAHN p. 1598, AHN p. 362) – Nursing interventions and patient teaching (FAAHN p. 1598, AHN p. 362) – Prognosis (FAAHN p. 1598, AHN p. 362)	
Discuss the etiology and pathophysiology, clinical manifestations, assessment, diagnostic tests, medical management, nursing interventions, and prognosis for patients with thrombophlebitis, varicose veins, and stasis ulcer.	☐ Thrombophlebitis (FAAHN p. 1598, AHN p. 362) – Etiology and pathophysiology (FAAHN p. 1598, AHN p. 362) – Clinical manifestations (FAAHN p. 1598, AHN p. 362) – Assessment (FAAHN p. 1598, AHN p. 362) – Diagnostic tests (FAAHN p. 1599, AHN p. 363) – Medical management (FAAHN p. 1599, AHN p. 363) – Nursing interventions and patient teaching (FAAHN p. 1600, AHN p. 364) – Prognosis (FAAHN p. 1601, AHN p. 365) ☐ Varicose veins (FAAHN p. 1601, AHN p. 365) – Etiology and pathophysiology (FAAHN p. 1601, AHN p. 365)	▨ PPT 74 through 82, Ch. 48 FAAHN (Ch. 8 PPT 74 through 82) 🖉 EILR IC Ch. 48 images 23 through 25 FAAHN (Ch. 8 images 23 through 25 AHN) 🖉 EILR TB Ch. 48 questions 32, 33, 37, 45, 47, 48 FAAHN (Ch. 8 questions 32, 33, 37, 45, 47, 48 AHN) 🖉 EILR Open Book Quiz Ch. 48 question 10 FAAHN (Ch. 8 question 10 AHN) 📓 SG Thrombophlebitis, Ch. 48 p. 408 FAAHN (Ch. 8 p. 96 AHN) **BOOK RESOURCES** Fig. 48-23 Deep-vein thrombophlebitis (FAAHN p. 1599) (Fig. 8-23 AHN p. 363) Fig 48-24 Venous leg ulcer (FAAHN p. 1602) (Fig 8-24 AHN p. 366) Fig. 48-25 Nurse applying paste boot (FAAHN p. 1603) (Fig 8-25 AHN p. 367)

OBJECTIVES	CONTENT	TEACHING RESOURCES
	– Clinical manifestations (FAAHN p. 1601, AHN p. 365) – Assessment (FAAHN p. 1601, AHN p. 365) – Diagnostic tests (FAAHN p. 1601, AHN p. 365) – Medical management (FAAHN p. 1601, AHN p. 365) – Nursing interventions and patient teaching (FAAHN p. 1601, AHN p. 365) – Prognosis (FAAHN p. 1602, AHN p. 366) ☐ Venous stasis ulcers (FAAHN p. 1602, AHN p. 366) – Etiology and pathophysiology (FAAHN p. 1602, AHN p. 366) – Clinical manifestations (FAAHN p. 1602, AHN p. 366) – Assessment (FAAHN p. 1602, AHN p. 366) – Diagnostic tests (FAAHN p. 1602, AHN p. 366) – Medical management (FAAHN p. 1602, AHN p. 366) – Nursing interventions and patient teaching (FAAHN p. 1603, AHN p. 367) – Prognosis (FAAHN p. 1603, AHN p. 367)	▶ Discuss populations at risk for thrombophlebitis. ▶ Discuss the clinical manifestations associated with thrombophlebitis. ***Class Activity** Bring students to the nursing lab. Recruit student volunteers and demonstrate the assessment of a client for thrombophlebitis.*
Discuss appropriate patient education for thrombophlebitis.	– Nursing interventions and patient teaching (FAAHN p. 1603, AHN p. 367) – Prognosis (FAAHN p. 1603, AHN p. 367) ☐ Nursing process for patients with a cardiovascular disorder (FAAHN p. 1603, AHN p. 367) – Assessment (FAAHN p. 1604, AHN p. 368) – Nursing diagnosis (FAAHN p. 1604, AHN p. 368) – Expected outcomes and planning (FAAHN p. 1604, AHN p. 368)	▦ PPT 76, 77, 83, Ch. 48 FAAHN (Ch. 8 PPT 76, 77, 83) ▦ SG Thrombophlebitis, Ch. 48 p. 408 FAAHN (Ch. 8 p. 96 AHN) ▶ Discuss appropriate nursing diagnoses for the care of the patient diagnosed with thrombophlebitis. ▶ Discuss the goals of education for the patient diagnosed with thrombophlebitis. ***Class Activity** Develop a series of questions on index cards relating to the etiology, diagnosis, clinical manifestations, care, and treatment of the patient diagnosed with thrombophlebitis.*

Christensen & Kockrow

OBJECTIVES	CONTENT	TEACHING RESOURCES
	– Implementation (FAAHN p. 1604, AHN p. 368) – Evaluation (FAAHN p. 1605, AHN p. 369)	*These questions will need to be "patient focused," reflecting the type of question a health care provider would expect a patient to ask concerning his/her diagnosis. Now, group students into pairs. One member of the pair will act as the patient and the other, the nurse.* *Give each pair a question to use in role-play. If time allows, students can trade cards and role-play another question for the nurse to answer.*
Performance Evaluation		▱ EILR TB Ch. 48 questions 1 through 52 FAAHN (Ch. 8 questions 1 through 52 AHN) ▱ EILR Open Book Quiz Ch. 48 questions 1 through 10 FAAHN (Ch. 8 questions 1 through 10 AHN) ▱ ESLR Review Questions for the NCLEX Examination Ch. 48 questions 1 through 10 FAAHN (Ch. 8 questions 1 through 10 AHN) ▱ SG Ch. 48 pp. 395-412 FAAHN (Ch. 8 pp. 83-100 AHN) **BOOK RESOURCES** Nursing Care Plan 48-1 The Patient with Heart Failure (FAAHN p. 1574) (NCP 8-1 AHN p. 338) ▱ NCP CTQ 1 through 3 (FAAHN p. 1575) (AHN p. 339) Review Questions for the NCLEX Examination Ch. 48 questions 1 through 37 FAAHN (Ch. 8 questions 1 through 37 AHN)

8.4 Homework/Assignments:

8.4 Instructor's Notes/Student Feedback:

Mosby items and derived items © 2011 by Mosby, Inc., an affiliate of Elsevier Inc.
Some material was previously published.

Adult Health Nursing, 6th ed.

Christensen & Kockrow

8

Care of the Patient with a Cardiovascular or a Peripheral Vascular Disorder

Slide 1

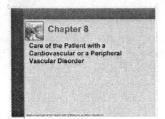

Slide 2

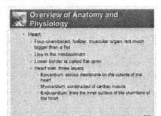

- The cardiovascular system has the awe-inspiring responsibility of providing sustenance to all of the cells and systems within the body.

- What phrases can be used to describe the functions of the cardiovascular system?

Slide 3

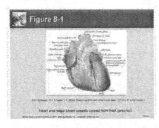

- The heart carries 1,000 gallons of blood each day. With each heartbeat, blood is circulated throughout the body.

- How many times per day do you estimate the heart beats?

Slide 4

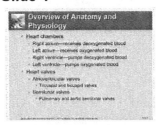

- A structure known as the septum divides the heart into halves. Each half functions as a unique and separate pumping station.

- The ventricles are separated by valves. What role is played by the valves?

Slide 5

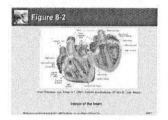

Slide 6

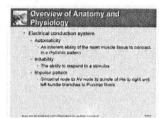

- A muscle, the heart performs by contracting in a rhythmic manner. Failure to contract as designed will result in illness or death.

- What factors may influence the ability of the heart to demonstrate synchronicity between the contracting structures?

Slide 7

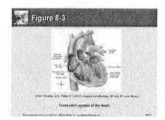

Slide 8

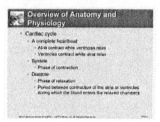

- When the heart is functioning as designed, there is coordination between contraction of the atria and ventricles. With each heartbeat cycle, there are the characteristic "lubb and dubb" sounds.

- What actions are responsible for these tones?

- What explanations could explain a heartbeat cycle without these tones or with modifications in these tones?

Slide 9

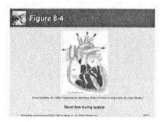

- During systole, there is relaxation of the ventricles during which the atria contract. Where does the blood distributed by the contraction travel?

Slide 10

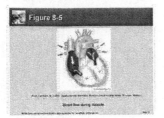

- A complicated network is responsible for carrying blood to and from the heart in the body.
- To what could this vast network be compared?

Slide 11

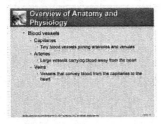

Slide 12

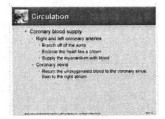

Slide 13

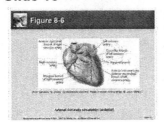

Slide 14

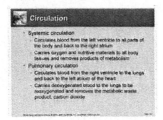

Adult Health Nursing, 6th ed.
Christensen & Kockrow

Slide 15

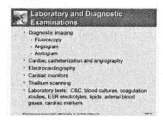

- Diagnostic studies of a cardiovascular disorder can be divided into categories: visualization, assessment of conduction, and serum values.

- Describe the use of imaging in providing diagnostic information about the heart.

- Which of the tests listed will require a signed consent from the patient?

Slide 16

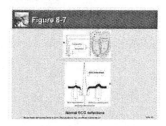

- An electrocardiogram involves the use of electrodes to assess cardiac impulses with the heart's conduction.

- Identify the three distinct waves in the electrocardiogram.

- Discuss placement of the electrodes during the test.

Slide 17

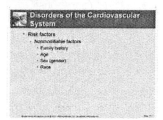

- Risk factors leading to the increased incidence of cardiovascular disease have been studied.

- Nonmodifiable risk factors are those which cannot be changed by patient intervention.

- Why does aging influence the onset of cardiovascular disease?

- Compare and contrast the risk factors of men and women.

Slide 18

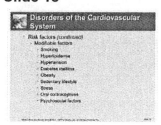

- Modifiable factors are those in which the patient can make life adjustments to reduce the incidence of heart disease.

- Assess the risk factors for the students in the class.

Slide 19

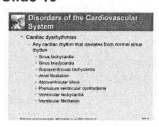

- The deviation from the normal sinus rhythm can cause physiological manifestations that are individualized by types.

- Review the characteristics of each of the identified dysrhythmias.

Christensen & Kockrow

Slide 20

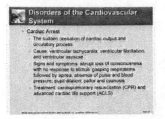

- When cardiac arrest occurs, immediate intervention is needed to revive the individual and to prevent permanent damage to the body's organs.

- The initiation of CPR involves the establishment and maintenance of the critical ABCs.

- What do the ABCs stand for?

- How much time can elapse between cardiac arrest and resuscitation before damage to vital organs and the accompanying loss of function result? Outline the parameters of ACLS.

Slide 21

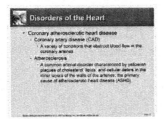

- Coronary artery disease is a growing health concern in the United States.

- What factors are associated with its development?

- What influence does race and ethnicity have on the development of coronary artery disease?

Slide 22

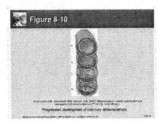

- The arteries of the heart can be likened to hoses. It is the responsibility of these hoses to carry blood and nutrients to areas of the body.

- Certain behaviors and groups of people can experience a narrowing in the pipes. See the figure illustrated. Each subsequent artery represents a reduction in diameter, thus increasing the level of compromise to the body.

Slide 23

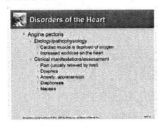

- The presence of angina can be a wakeup call to millions. The onset of the characteristic discomfort is an indication the body is unable to successfully supply the heart with oxygen and blood.

- The onset of an angina attack should be followed by seeking medical care.

- What factors can be associated with an episode of angina?

Slide 24

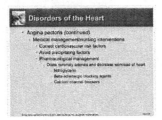

- When a patient presents with an episode of suspected angina, what data should be collected by the nurse? What subjective data might the patient report?

- What diagnostic tests will be ordered to determine the cause of the patient's complaints?

ELSEVIER

Christensen & Kockrow

Slide 25

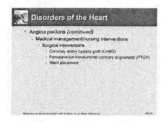

- At times, surgical intervention can be indicated in conjunction with or in lieu of pharmacological therapies. What patients are candidates for the procedures?

- Discuss the education that is needed for the patient undergoing CABG or PTCA.

Slide 26

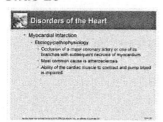

- A myocardial infarction can result from atherosclerosis, an embolus, or a thrombus. The loss of blood flow results in ischemia and damage to the affected tissues.

- What factors will determine the degree of damage or loss of function experienced by the patient?

Slide 27

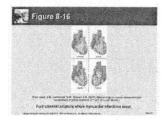

Slide 28

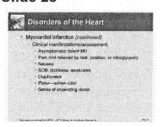

- The onset of discomfort is often met with denial by the patient. What types of explanations do patients frequently use to "explain away" the manifestations?

- Once the patient enters the health care system, prompt, accurate assessment by the team is vital to the patient's survival.

- What manifestations can be anticipated in the patient's vital signs?

Slide 29

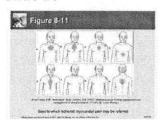

Slide 30

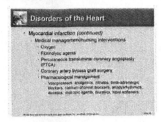

- The immediate priority for the management of care is to reduce cardiac ischemia and limit damage.

- What outcomes will be desired by the therapies?

- The role of the nurse in the care of a patient after a myocardial infarction is important. Describe nursing interventions and assessments that will be performed.

Slide 31

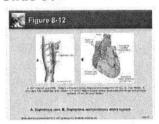

- Physicians can determine surgical intervention is needed to manage ASHD or CAD. Surgeons can use grafts to bypass occluded arteries and provide blood flow to the heart. Graft surgeries have an anticipated lifespan. How long can grafts from the saphenous vein be expected to last?

Slide 32

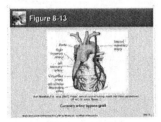

Slide 33

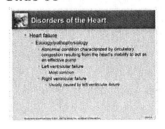

- Cardiac insufficiency results when the heart is no longer able to adequately provide perfusion to the entire body.

- This condition was once known as congestive heart failure. This term is now considered somewhat antiquated. Why has this term been replaced in the medical community?

- Heart failure can result from chronic neurohormonal conditions or result from other medical conditions. What are examples of medical conditions associated with the development of heart failure?

Slide 34

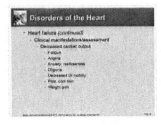

- In addition to the objective clinical manifestations, the nurse is also responsible for assessing subjective patient reports. What questions can the nurse ask to facilitate the exchange of information?

ELSEVIER
Christensen & Kockrow

Slide 35

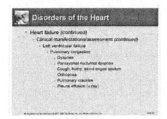

- The left side of the heart is responsible for pumping oxygenated blood to the body. When the left side of the heart is unable to meet the body's demands, decreased cardiac output results.

- What are the implications of untreated left-sided heart failure?

Slide 36

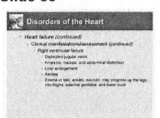

- Right ventricular failure most commonly results from effects of the failing left ventricle. What additional causes can be associated with the right-sided failure?

Slide 37

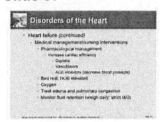

- Diagnosis of heart failure uses the presenting clinical manifestations and confirming tests. Chest radiographs, electrocardiograms, and echocardiography can be used. What findings will support a heart failure diagnosis?

- Laboratory testing is also common. What serum tests can be anticipated?

- What prognosis is associated with the diagnosis of heart failure?

Slide 38

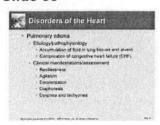

- Pulmonary edema is an acute and life-threatening event. It is caused by left-sided heart failure. The affected patient can literally drown in his/her own secretions.

Slide 39

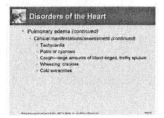

- When pulmonary edema is suspected, what diagnostic tests can be used to confirm diagnosis?

Christensen & Kockrow

Slide 40

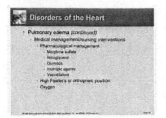

- The goals of management seek to increase oxygenation, improve cardiac output and reduce congestion.

- What will occur if the condition continues to progress unchecked?

- What nursing diagnoses would be appropriate for the care of the patient diagnosed with pulmonary edema?

- Discuss nursing implications/considerations for the medications that may be administered to the patient diagnosed with pulmonary edema.

- What manifestations will indicate that the medication therapies are having the desired effects?

Slide 41

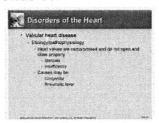

- Heart valves have the job of maintaining the direction of the blood flow through the right and left atrium and ventricles.

- How do the heart valves know when to open and close?

- Identify the names of the heart valves and their locations.

Slide 42

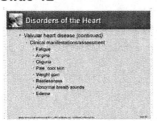

- Dysfunction of the valves can occur due to stenosis or a history of valvular heart disease.

- What can cause stenosis of the valves?

- Discuss populations at risk for the development of valvular heart disease.

Slide 43

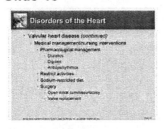

- Diagnostic tests used to confirm the presence of valvular heart disease include radiographs, ECG, echocardiogram, and cardiac catheterization.

- Initial management options focus on noninvasive interventions such as medications, diet, and activity restrictions. When these treatment modalities are no longer helpful, surgical intervention might be indicated.

- Outline the types of surgical intervention that can be undertaken.

Slide 44

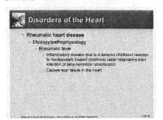

- Rheumatic heart disease occurs after an individual has had rheumatic fever. The time span between the two disorders can be many years.

- Since the 1980s, rheumatic fever has become increasingly uncommon in the United States. To what can this decline be attributed?

Slide 45

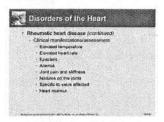

- Explain the changes in the heart's valves in response to the disease process.

- There is no specific diagnostic test. Diagnosis is made by combining the clinical manifestations with supportive data from the test results. Tests include scanning studies and laboratory tests. An echocardiogram and ECG can be ordered.

- What laboratory tests can be ordered?

Slide 46

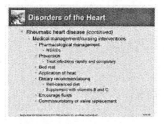

- The best cure for rheumatic heart disease is prevention. This can be accomplished by successful treatment of the originating disease process.

- If the disease results, treatment is largely supportive.

- What is the role of the nurse in providing care to the patient diagnosed with rheumatic heart disease?

- What is the prognosis for the patient diagnosed with rheumatic heart disease?

Slide 47

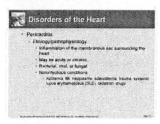

- Inflammation of the pericardium of the heart results in thickening and constriction of the structure.

- What alterations in functioning of the heart result from this process?

Slide 48

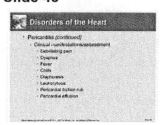

- An accurate assessment of the patient presenting with clinical manifestations of pericarditis is important. Both the subjective and objective data will need to be reported.

- What questions concerning the characteristics and precipitating the pain's onset are indicated? Provide examples of questions that can be used by the nurse to obtain additional information.

Slide 49

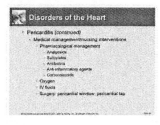

- If caught early, pericarditis can have a fair prognosis. As the disease progresses, there are increasing complications and death can result.

- Prompt diagnosis and treatment will determine the patient's final outcomes.

- What diagnostic tests are used to support the diagnosis of pericarditis?

- When is surgical intervention indicated?

ELSEVIER

Adult Health Nursing, 6th ed.

Christensen & Kockrow

Slide 50

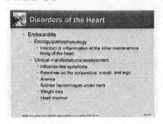

- Endocarditis can involve the innermost part of the heart or the heart's valves.
- The disease process is classified by the cause.
- What events might precede the onset of endocarditis?
- What populations are at an increased risk for the development of the disorder?
- Discuss changes in populations previously at increased risk for the development of endocarditis. Why have these changes occurred?

Slide 51

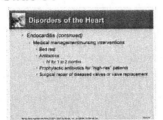

- Endocarditis can present in a rapid, acute manner, or it could be a slower onset.
- When the presentation does occur, diagnostic tests are indicated to pinpoint the cause to begin treatment.
- Diagnostic tests used are ECG, chest radiography, complete blood count, erythrocyte sedimentation rate, and blood cultures. What results will support an endocarditis diagnosis?
- What prognosis is associated with endocarditis?

Slide 52

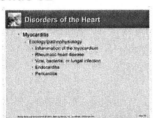

- A variety of causes can be to blame for the development of myocarditis. The clinical manifestations can also vary. The signs and symptoms presented will differ based upon the site of cardiac involvement.
- Identify clinical manifestations that can be associated with endocarditis.
- Why do dysrhythmias result with this disease process?

Slide 53

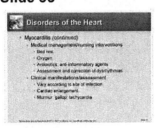

- The management of myocarditis is symptomatic.
- What prognosis can be anticipated? Are there long-range complications with this disorder?

Slide 54

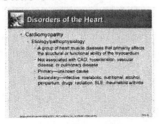

- Cardiomyopathy is classified by cause. It can be primary or secondary.
- Primary cardiomyopathy is a disease of the heart muscle with an unknown underlying cause. It is further subdivided by the type of damage.
- These subdivisions are dilated cardiomyopathy, hypertrophic cardiomyopathy, and restrictive cardiomyopathy. Explain the differences among the types.

ELSEVIER

Adult Health Nursing, 6th ed.

Christensen & Kockrow

Slide 55

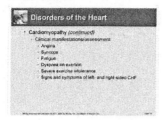

- The signs and symptoms are similar to those seen in heart failure. Why does this similarity exist?
- The most common symptom is severe exercise intolerance.

Slide 56

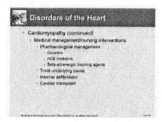

- Diagnosis is based upon both the clinical presentation and the results from supportive diagnostic tests.
- What diagnostic tests can be anticipated? What results will support a cardiomyopathy diagnosis?
- What actions are desired from the medication classifications used in the management of cardiomyopathy?
- When the condition is no longer able to respond to conventional treatment options, a heart transplant could be considered. If transplantation is being considered, which patients are viewed as suitable candidates? Which candidates are not eligible for a heart transplant?

Slide 57

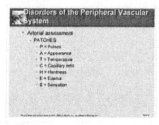

- Arterial blood circulation refers to the blood being transported from the heart to the body. What signs and symptoms are associated with insufficiencies?

Slide 58

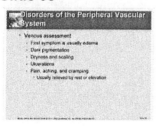

- Venous circulation involves the transportation of blood from the body's tissues en route to the lungs. This excess fluid remains in the tissues and manifests as characteristic edema.
- Another common symptom involves changes in skin appearance. What pathophysiology is responsible for this?
- What differences exist between arterial and peripheral disorders?

Adult Health Nursing, 6th ed.
Christensen & Kockrow

Slide 59

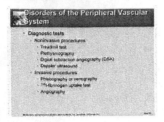

- Numerous tests are available to evaluate peripheral vascular status.

- The treadmill test is used to evaluate blood flow in the extremities after exercise. What education will need to be provided to the patient prior to the completion of the test?

- A Doppler ultrasound can be used to evaluate the blood flow in blood vessels. What types of disorders can be detected by using this test?

- Invasive tests include the phlebography, ^{125}I-fibrinogen uptake test, angiography, D-dimer, and duplex scanning tests. What responsibilities does the nurse have before an invasive test is performed?

Slide 60

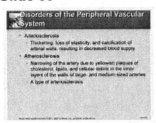

- The terms "arteriosclerosis" and "atherosclerosis" are often used interchangeably. Despite similarities, there are differences. Pinpoint the differences between the two conditions. What similarities do they have?

Slide 61

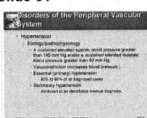

- A diagnosis of hypertension requires elevations in readings that meet the set criteria and are taken at different times.

- Risks for the development of hypertension exist for individuals who have what is termed as "prehypertension."

- Prehypertension is defined as a systolic blood pressure reading of 120 to 139 mm Hg or 80 to 89 mm Hg diastolic. The risk for the development of hypertension by these individuals doubles.

- Explain what encompasses the systolic reading. What is meant by the diastolic reading?

Slide 62

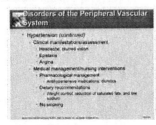

- There are two types of hypertension. Primary hypertension is most common. There is no exact cause for its development. What theories are available to explain this type?

- Secondary hypertension is identified with a specific medical diagnosis.

- Discuss the concept of malignant hypertension.

- What risk factors are associated with the development of hypertension?

- What is the long-range picture for the individual with hypertension?

Slide 63

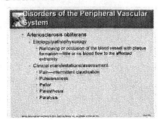

- When performing an assessment of the patient suspected of having arteriosclerosis, what questions should the nurse ask to collect data?

- What diagnostic tests will be employed to support the diagnosis?

Adult Health Nursing, 6th ed.

Christensen & Kockrow

Slide 64

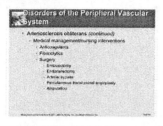

- The goals of treatment focus on the prevention of total arterial occlusion.

- Pharmacological agents used include anticoagulants, fibrinolytics, and vasodilators.

- What is the mode of action that aids in the management of this disease?

- When administering these medications, what are the nursing implications?

Slide 65

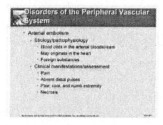

- The presence of arterial emboli is a potentially life-threatening condition.

- When the emboli lodge in the vessels, pain is a chief symptom. What is the cause of the pain?

- Data collection is necessary to make a timely diagnosis. What questions will the nurse need to ask to facilitate the collection of data?

Slide 66

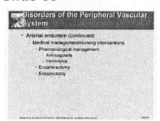

- Diagnostic testing will include Doppler ultrasonography and angiography testing.

- Once a diagnosis is made, management will include medications and possibly surgery.

- Identify nursing diagnoses applicable for the care of the patient experiencing arterial emboli.

Slide 67

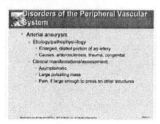

- Although aneurysms can occur in any vessel, there are vessels having an increased incidence of the phenomena. What sites are more commonly associated with the development of an aneurysm?

Slide 68

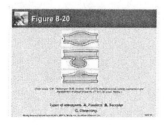

Christensen & Kockrow

Slide 69

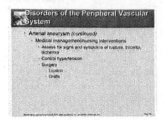

- Although aneurysms are largely asymptomatic, diagnostic tests are available to aid in the diagnostic process. What diagnostic tests will be anticipated if an aneurysm is suspected?

Slide 70

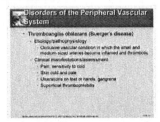

- The cause of thromboangiitis obliterans is not completely understood.
- What population is most likely to be affected by this disorder?
- What is the possible relationship between tobacco use and this disease?

Slide 71

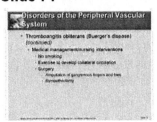

- When providing care to the patient diagnosed with thromboangiitis obliterans, what is the role of the nurse?
- Discuss the prognosis of the patient diagnosed with thromboangiitis obliterans.

Slide 72

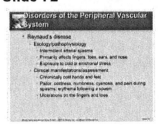

- The intermittent episodes of Raynaud's disease result from attacks of ischemia. The cause is unknown.
- The condition may be primary or associated with other diseases including scleroderma, rheumatoid arthritis, systemic lupus erythematosus, drug intoxication, and occupational trauma.
- What populations are more likely to develop this condition?

Slide 73

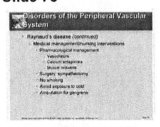

- Diagnosis of Raynaud's disease includes a cold stimulation test. What is involved in a cold stimulation test?
- The goals of therapy are geared at prevention. Pharmacological interventions often include calcium channel blockers. How do these medications work?
- What education will assist the patient to avoid episodes?

ELSEVIER

Adult Health Nursing, 6th ed.

Christensen & Kockrow

Slide 74

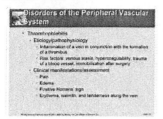

Slide 75

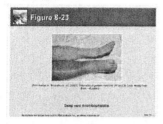

- The assessment of extremities affected by thrombophlebitis requires close observation.

- What observations can be charted in the permanent medical record?

Slide 76

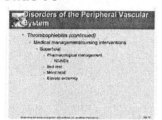

- Thrombophlebitis can be superficial or deep. How do these types differ?

- What diagnostic tests will be used to confirm the presence of thrombophlebitis?

Slide 77

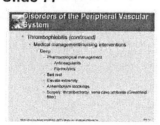

- Anticoagulant therapies are often prescribed to manage thrombophlebitis. When given, what are patient safety considerations? Discuss the role of the nurse.

Slide 78

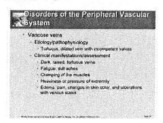

- Varicose veins impact approximately 15% of the population. What gender is most likely affected? Identify factors that can promote this problem.

- Varicose veins may be primary or secondary. Compare and contrast these types.

Christensen & Kockrow

Slide 79

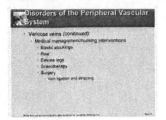

- The management of milder varicose veins employs special stockings, rest, and leg elevation. Surgical intervention might be indicated in more serious presentations.

- Outline the safety precautions that are indicated when elastic stockings or bandages are used for these patients.

Slide 80

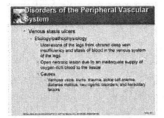

Slide 81

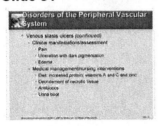

- Venous stasis ulcers present a challenge to manage. The reduced blood flow to the area makes healing prolonged. Further, the populations most likely affected frequently have comorbid conditions adding to this dilemma.

- Diet therapies are useful. What specific foods will promote healing?

- Discuss the types of debridement.

Slide 82

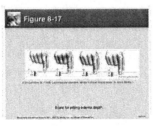

- An assessment of edema is needed for both cardiovascular and peripheral vascular disorders.

- How is edema documented?

Slide 83

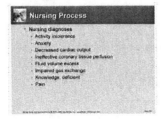

9 Lesson Plan
Care of the Patient with a Respiratory Disorder

TEACHING FOCUS

In this chapter, the student will be introduced to the care of the patient with a respiratory disorder. The student will begin by exploring the structure and function of the respiratory system. Next, the student will have the opportunity to learn about the diagnostic examinations of the respiratory system, the significance of various breath sounds, and the meanings of the blood gas values. Finally, the student will explore a variety of respiratory disorders, including their etiology and pathophysiology, clinical manifestations, assessment, diagnostic tests, medical management, nursing interventions, and prognoses.

MATERIALS AND RESOURCES

- ☐ Computer/overhead projector (all lessons)
- ☐ White/black board and marker/chalk (all lessons)
- ☐ Obtain an ambu-bag (Lesson 9.1).
- ☐ Copies of an unlabeled diagram of the respiratory system (Lesson 9.1)
- ☐ Three to five hypoxia scenarios written on note cards (Lesson 9.1)
- ☐ Several dual-head stethoscopes (Lesson 9.1)
- ☐ Three to five diagnostic test scenarios written on note cards (Lesson 9.1).
- ☐ Two blank index cards for each student (Lesson 9.1)
- ☐ Four nursing diagnoses for a patient who has had a laryngectomy (Lesson 9.2)
- ☐ Blank nursing care plan forms for each student (Lesson 9.3)
- ☐ Write the names of medications used to treat tuberculosis on index cards. Place one medication name per each card (Lesson 9.3).
- ☐ Closed-chest drainage equipment in the nursing lab (Lesson 9.3)
- ☐ Four role-play scenarios focusing on patients diagnosed with chronic obstructive pulmonary disease (COPD), including emphysema, chronic bronchitis, asthma, and bronchiectasis (Lesson 9.4)
- ☐ Two blank index cards for each student (Lesson 9.4)
- ☐ Oxygen-delivery equipment (Lesson 9.4)
- ☐ Blank nursing care plan forms for each student (Lesson 9.4)

LESSON CHECKLIST

Preparations for this lesson include:
- Lecture
- Contact a local chapter of the American Cancer Society or American Heart Association to borrow a "Smoking Joe" model.
- Arrange for the class to visit the nursing laboratory.
- Contact a meat packing plant or slaughter house and request the lungs of an animal.
- Contact a local hospital or your school's respiratory therapy program to request a speaker to discuss the role of the respiratory therapist in the care of lower airway disorders.
- Obtain the frequency of tuberculosis and information about the system of reporting it within your county from the local board of health.

KEY TERMS

adventitious (FAAHN p. 1615, AHN p. 379)
atelectasis (FAAHN p. 1646, AHN p. 410)
bronchoscopy (FAAHN p. 1617, AHN p. 381)
cor pulmonale (FAAHN p. 1657, AHN p. 421)
coryza (FAAHN p. 1627, AHN p. 391)
crackles (FAAHN p. 1615, AHN p. 379)
cyanosis (FAAHN p. 1624, AHN p. 388)
dyspnea (FAAHN p. 1614, AHN p. 378)
embolism (FAAHN p. 1652, AHN p. 416)
empyema (FAAHN p. 1644, AHN p. 408)

epistaxis (FAAHN p. 1620, AHN p. 384)
exacerbation (FAAHN p. 1660, AHN p. 424)
extrinsic (FAAHN p. 1662, AHN p. 426)
hypercapnia (FAAHN p. 1660, AHN p. 424)
hypoventilation (FAAHN p. 1646, AHN p. 410)
hypoxia (FAAHN p. 1615, AHN p. 379)
intrinsic (FAAHN p. 1662, AHN p. 426)
orthopnea (FAAHN p. 1615, AHN p. 379)
pleural friction rub (FAAHN p. 1615, AHN p. 379)

Christensen & Kockrow

pneumothorax (FAAHN p. 1647, AHN p. 411)
sibilant wheeze (FAAHN p. 1615, AHN p. 379)
sonorous wheeze (FAAHN p. 1615, AHN p. 379)

stertorous (FAAHN p. 1621, AHN p. 385)
tachypnea (FAAHN p. 1646, AHN p. 410)
thoracentesis (FAAHN p. 1614, AHN p. 378)
virulent (FAAHN p. 1634, AHN p. 398)

ADDITIONAL RESOURCES (AHN)

PPT Ch. 49, 1 through 79 FAAHN (Ch. 9, 1 through 79 AHN)
EILR IC images Ch. 49, 1 through 16 FAAHN (Ch. 9, 1 through 16 AHN)
EILR TB questions Ch. 49, 1 through 36 FAAHN (Ch. 9, 1 through 36 AHN)
EILR Open Book Quiz Ch. 43, 1 through 10 FAAHN (Ch. 3, 1 through 10 AHN)
ESLR Review Questions for the NCLEX® Examination Ch. 49, 49-01 through 49-10 FAAHN (Ch. 9, 09-01 through 09-10 AHN)

Legend

PPT	**EILR**	**ESLR**	**SG**	**NCP CTQ**
PowerPoint Slides	EVOLVE Instructor Learning Resources: Image Collection, Test Bank, Open Book Quizzes	EVOLVE Student Learning Resources: Review Questions for the NCLEX Examination	Study Guide	Nursing Care Plan Critical Thinking Question

Class Activities are indicated in **bold italic**.

LESSON 9.1

PRETEST

1. When performing a thoracentesis, the maximum amount of fluid that can be removed within a 30-minute period of time is:
   a. 1300 mL.
   b. 1000 mL.
   c. 2000 mL.
   d. 1500 mL.

2. While performing an assessment of lung sounds, brief intermittent, bubbling sounds are heard at the end of inspiration. Based upon your knowledge, you recognize these sounds as:
   a. pleural friction rubbing.
   b. sibilant wheezes.
   c. medium crackles.
   d. coarse crackles.

3. When performing an assessment of the respiratory system, you hear sonorous wheezes. To which of the following causes can these sounds be attributed?
   a. Caused by mucus or pus in the small airways and alveoli
   b. Associated with diseases in the bronchioles
   c. Caused by a narrowing in the bronchioles
   d. Caused by the transportation of air through the tracheobronchial passages

4. When comparing the characteristics of inhaled air and exhaled air, which of the following statements is most correct?
   a. Inhaled air contains about 20% oxygen and exhaled air has only about 10% oxygen.
   b. Inhaled air contains about 16% oxygen and exhaled air has about 16% oxygen.
   c. Exhaled air contains about 16% oxygen and 3.5 % carbon dioxide.
   d. Exhaled air contains about 15% oxygen and 10% carbon dioxide.

Mosby items and derived items © 2011 by Mosby, Inc., an affiliate of Elsevier Inc.
Some material was previously published.

Christensen & Kockrow

5. The _____ function(s) to assist with the determination or evaluation of carbon dioxide, oxygen, and acids.
   a. Chemoreceptors
   b. Visceral pleura
   c. Parietal pleura
   d. Hyoid

6. The physician has ordered a sputum specimen from the patient. Which of the following information is accurate regarding obtaining a sputum specimen?
   a. A hypotonic saline mist can be used to aid in obtaining the specimen.
   b. Obtain the sputum specimen before initiating antibiotic therapy.
   c. Collect the specimen after meals.
   d. The patient should avoid drinking any water 1 hour prior to obtaining the specimen.

7. When caring for a patient having respiratory acidosis, which of the following statements concerning the mode of compensation by the body is correct?
   a. Lungs retain CO_2 to lower the pH.
   b. The kidneys will retain increased amounts of HCO_3 to increase pH.
   c. The kidneys will begin to reduce the amounts of stored HCO_3 to increase pH.
   d. The lungs will "blow off" CO_2 to raise pH.

8. The most common causative agent of tonsillitis is:
   a. *Haemophilus influenzae*
   b. Staphylococcus
   c. Group B streptococci
   d. Group A streptococci

9. When administering corticosteroids for the care of a chronic respiratory disorder, which of the following information should be included during patient education?
   a. Do not discontinue medicine abruptly.
   b. The patient will require routine monitoring of kidney function.
   c. Take the medication on an empty stomach.
   d. The patient will require routine monitoring of liver function.

10. Which of the following statements about the cultural and ethnic considerations associated with tuberculosis is correct?
   a. The incidence of tuberculosis in whites is only slightly higher than that of nonwhites.
   b. In the United States, tuberculosis occurs in urban middle class and middle-aged citizens.
   c. The incidence of tuberculosis among immigrants from southeastern Asia and Haiti is similar to those of their home countries.
   d. There is a low incidence of tuberculosis in foreign-born individuals from Latin America and Africa.

Answers:

1. a	2. c	3. d	4. c	5. a
6. b	7. b	8. c	9. a	10. c

BACKGROUND ASSESSMENT

Question: A 10-year-old patient presents with complaints of body aches, chills, and sore throat. The assessment reveals enlarged cervical lymph nodes, reddened throat, and an elevation in body temperature to 101.4. Based upon your knowledge, what diagnosis can be anticipated? What diagnostic tests might be ordered? If confirmed, what will be included in the initial course of disease management? If surgical management is deemed appropriate, when will it be considered?

Answer: The patient could have acute follicular tonsillitis. This disease is commonly seen in school-aged children. It is caused most often by group B streptococci. It can be diagnosed by clinical picture, complete blood count, and a throat culture. The initial course of management will be conservative. This will consist of antipyretics, antibiotics, and rest. If this is a recurrent problem, surgical intervention could be warranted. If decided upon, surgery will take place 4 to 6 weeks after the attack has resolved.

ELSEVIER

Christensen & Kockrow

Question: You are assigned to care for a patient whose daughter is planning to have her placed in a long-term care facility. While you are discussing the plans for transfer, the daughter asks why her mother has been given tests for tuberculosis, and vaccines for influenza and pneumonia. What information concerning the rationale for the administration of the tests and vaccines should be given to the daughter?

Answer: The residents of long-term care facilities are at an increased risk for the development of respiratory illness. This is due in part to their close living arrangements. The typical resident of a long-term care facility is older and often has multiple health concerns. All of these factors combined are cause for concern. In an attempt to screen for tuberculosis, prospective residents of long-term care facilities are routinely screened prior to placement. The administration of flu and pneumonia vaccines is used to proactively prevent the transmission of the illnesses and reduce risk to the facility as a whole.

CRITICAL THINKING QUESTION

The patient has been diagnosed with an excessive amount of pleural fluid. The physician has ordered a thoracentesis to be performed. The patient is nervous and asks what will be done. Discuss the information that will need to be provided the patient. During the procedure, what are the nurse's responsibilities?

Guidelines: The patient will need to understand his responsibilities regarding positioning during the examination. The thoracentesis will involve the removal of pleural fluids from the chest using a needle aspiration technique. During the procedure, the patient will be sitting on the bed with the head elevated to 30 degrees. He will need to rest his head and arms on the overbed table. During the procedure, the nurse will be needed to assist with positioning and providing emotional support.

OBJECTIVES	CONTENT	TEACHING RESOURCES
Differentiate between external and internal respiration.	■ Anatomy and physiology of the respiratory system (FAAHN p. 1610, AHN p. 374)	▣ PPT 2 through 9, Ch. 49 FAAHN (Ch. 9 PPT 2 through 9 AHN) 📖 SG External/Internal Respiration and Exchange, Ch. 49 p. 413 FAAHN (Ch. 9 p. 101 AHN) ▸ Discuss the differences between internal and external respiration. ▸ Discuss the muscles that are employed in the process of respiration. *Class Activity **Take the class to the nursing lab. Using student volunteers, demonstrate how to correctly perform a respiratory assessment.***
Describe the purpose of the respiratory system.	■ Anatomy and physiology of the respiratory system (FAAHN p. 1610, AHN p. 374)	▣ PPT 2 Ch. 49 FAAHN (Ch. 9 PPT 2 AHN) 📖 SG Respiratory Tract, Ch. 49 p. 413 FAAHN (Ch. 9 p. 101 AHN) ▸ Discuss the functions of the respiratory system. ▸ Discuss the impact of impaired respiratory function. *Class Activity **Contact a local chapter of the American Cancer Society or the Heart Association. Ask to borrow the "Smoking Joe" model. This can be used to demonstrate the process of respiration.***

Mosby items and derived items © 2011 by Mosby, Inc., an affiliate of Elsevier Inc.
Some material was previously published.

Adult Health Nursing, 6th ed.
Christensen & Kockrow

OBJECTIVES	CONTENT	TEACHING RESOURCES
List and define the parts of the upper and lower respiratory tracts.	■ Anatomy and physiology of the respiratory system (FAAHN p. 1610, AHN p. 374) ☐ Upper respiratory tract (FAAHN p. 1610, AHN p. 374) – Nose (FAAHN p. 1610, AHN p. 374) – Pharynx (FAAHN p. 1610, AHN p. 374) – Larynx (FAAHN p. 1610, AHN p. 374) – Trachea (FAAHN p. 1610, AHN p. 374) ☐ Lower respiratory tract (FAAHN p. 1613, AHN p. 377) – Bronchial tree (FAAHN p. 1613, AHN p. 377)	⊠▬ PPT 3 Ch. 49 FAAHN (Ch. 9 PPT 3AHN) 🔁 EILR IC Ch. 49 images 1 through 6 FAAHN (Ch. 9 images 1 through 6 AHN) 🔁 EILR TB Ch. 49 question 2 (Ch. 9 question 2 AHN) SG Respiratory Tract, p. 413 FAAHN (Ch. 9 p. 101 AHN) **BOOK RESOURCES** Review Questions for the NCLEX Examination Ch. 49 questions 3, 4 FAAHN (Ch. 9 questions 3, 4 AHN) Fig. 49-1 Structural plan of the respiratory organs (FAAHN p. 1610) (Fig. 9-1 AHN p. 374) Fig. 49-2 Sagittal section through the face and the neck (FAAHN p. 1611) (Fig. 9-2 AHN p. 375) Fig. 49-3 Projections of paranasal sinuses and oral nasal cavities (FAAHN p. 1611) (Fig. 9-3 AHN p. 375) Fig. 49-4 A Sagittal section through the larynx (FAAHN p. 1612) (Fig. 9-4 AHN p. 376) Fig. 49-5 Projection of the lungs and trachea in relation to ribcage and clavicles (FAAHN p. 1612) (Fig. 9-5 AHN p. 376) Fig. 49-6 Alveolus (FAAHN p. 1613) (Fig. 9-6 AHN p. 377) ▶ Discuss the organs in the upper respiratory tract. ▶ Discuss the organs contained in the lower respiratory tract. *Class Activity **Provide an unlabeled diagram of the respiratory system. Give a brief period of time for the students to label the organs in the system.*** *Note: This activity may be performed before the lecture begins to assess student knowledge.*
List the ways in which oxygen and carbon dioxide are transported in the blood.	☐ Mechanics of breathing (FAAHN p. 1613, AHN p. 377) – Thoracic cavity (FAAHN p. 1613, AHN p. 377) – Lungs (FAAHN p. 1613, AHN p. 377) – Respiratory movements and ranges (FAAHN p. 1614, AHN p. 378)	⊠▬ PPT 4 Ch. 49 FAAHN (Ch. 9 PPT 4 AHN) 🔁 EILR IC Ch. 49 image 6 FAAHN (Ch. 9 image 6 AHN) 🔁 EILR TB Ch. 49 question 30 FAAHN (Ch. 9 question 30 AHN) SG Alveolus and Gas Exchange, p. 414 FAAHN (Ch. 9 pp. 102 AHN) **BOOK RESOURCES**

Adult Health Nursing, 6ᵗʰ ed.

Christensen & Kockrow

OBJECTIVES	CONTENT	TEACHING RESOURCES
		Review Questions for the NCLEX Examination Ch. 49 question 5 FAAHN (Ch. 9 question 5 AHN)
		▶ Discuss the steps that take place after oxygen is inhaled into the body.
		▶ Discuss the relationship between the blood's concentration of oxygen and carbon dioxide.
		Class Activity Contact a packing or slaughter house. Obtain the lungs of an animal and place the lungs on a large tray. Attach the bronchi to an ambu-bag. Squeeze the bag to demonstrate the transportation of oxygen.
Discuss the mechanisms that regulate respirations.	☐ Regulation of respiration (FAAHN p. 1614, AHN p. 378) – Nervous control (FAAHN p. 1614, AHN p. 378)	PPT 4 Ch. 49 FAAHN (Ch. 9 PPT 4 AHN) SG Regulators, Ch. 49 p. 415 FAAHN (Ch. 9 p. 103 AHN) **BOOK RESOURCES** Review Questions for the NCLEX Examination Ch. 49 questions 1, 2 FAAHN (Ch. 9 questions 1, 2 AHN) ▶ Discuss the influences of negative pressure in maintaining the lungs' inflation. ▶ Discuss the role of the visceral and parietal pleura in the movement of the lung tissue during respiration. *Class Activity Assess class knowledge and instruct students to write down their perception of how respirations are regulated.*
Identify those signs and symptoms that indicate a patient is experiencing hypoxia.	■ Assessment of the respiratory system (FAAHN p. 1614, AHN p. 378)	EILR TB Ch. 49 question 11 FAAHN (Ch. 9 question 11 AHN) ESLR Review Questions for the NCLEX Examination Ch. 49 question 1 FAAHN (Ch. 9 question 1 AHN) SG Hypoxia and Adventitious Sounds Ch. 49 p. 415 FAAHN (Ch. 9 p. 103 AHN) **BOOK RESOURCES** Table 49-1 Adventitious Breath Sounds (FAAHN p. 1615) (Table 9-1 AHN p. 379) Box 49-1 Signs and Symptoms of Hypoxia (FAAHN p. 1616) (Box 9-1 AHN p. 380) ▶ Discuss the cause of hypoxia. ▶ Discuss the clinical presentation associated with hypoxia.

Adult Health Nursing, 6th ed.

Christensen & Kockrow

OBJECTIVES	CONTENT	TEACHING RESOURCES
		Class Activity **Prepare several hypoxia scenarios (three to five, depending upon the size of the class). Write them on note cards. Group the students to role-play the situations given, relating to the patient presenting with signs and symptoms of hypoxia.**
Differentiate among sonorous wheezes, sibilant wheezes, crackles, and pleural friction rub.	■ Assessment of the respiratory system (FAAHN p. 1614, AHN p. 378)	EILR Open Book Quiz Ch. 49 question 1 FAAHN (Ch. 9 question 1 AHN) SG Hypoxia and Adventitious Sounds Ch. 49 pp. 415-416 FAAHN (Ch. 9 pp. 103-104 AHN) ▸ Discuss the underlying cause of adventitious lung sounds. ▸ Discuss the characteristic sounds associated with the most commonly heard adventitious lung sounds. *Class Activity* **Bring several dual-head stethoscopes to the class. Pair students and have them perform lung assessments on each other.**
Describe the purpose, significance of results, and nursing interventions related to diagnostic examinations of the respiratory system.	■ Laboratory and diagnostic examinations (FAAHN p. 1615, AHN p. 379) □ Chest roentgenogram (FAAHN p. 1615, AHN p. 379) □ Computed tomography (FAAHN p. 1616, AHN p. 380) – Chest CT scan (FAAHN p. 1616, AHN p. 380) □ Pulmonary function testing (PFT) (FAAHN p. 1616, AHN p. 380) □ Mediastinoscopy (FAAHN p. 1616, AHN p. 380) □ Laryngoscopy (FAAHN p. 1617, AHN p. 381) □ Bronchoscopy (FAAHN p. 1617, AHN p. 381) □ Sputum specimen (FAAHN p. 1617, AHN p. 381) □ Cytologic studies (FAAHN p. 1618, AHN p. 382) □ Lung biopsy (FAAHN p. 1618, AHN p. 382)	PPT 5 through 9, Ch. 49 FAAHN (Ch. 9 PPT 5 through 9 AHN) EILR IC Ch. 49 images 7 through 10 FAAHN (Ch. 9 images 7 through 10 AHN) SG Diagnostic Tests, Ch. 49 p. 416 FAAHN (Ch. 9 p. 104 AHN) **BOOK RESOURCES** Review Questions for the NCLEX Examination Ch. 49 questions 9, 10, 26, 35, 37 FAAHN (Ch. 9 questions 9, 10, 26, 35, 37 AHN) Fig. 49-7 Fiberoptic bronchoscope (FAAHN p. 1617) (Fig. 9-7 AHN p. 381) Box 49-2 Guidelines for Sputum Specimen Collection (FAAHN p. 1617) (Box 9-2 AHN p. 381) Box 49-3 Range of Sputum Characteristics (FAAHN p. 1618 (Box 9-3 AHN p. 382) Fig. 49-8 Thoracentesis (FAAHN p. 1618) (Fig. 9-8 AHN p. 382) ▸ Discuss the patient education needs concerning the diagnostic examinations of the respiratory system. ▸ Discuss the consents that must be completed for those tests deemed to be invasive.

ELSEVIER

Mosby items and derived items © 2011 by Mosby, Inc., an affiliate of Elsevier Inc.
Some material was previously published.

Adult Health Nursing, 6th ed.
Christensen & Kockrow

OBJECTIVES	CONTENT	TEACHING RESOURCES
	☐ Thoracentesis (FAAHN p. 1618, AHN p. 382) ☐ Arterial blood gases (ABGs) (FAAHN p. 1618, AHN p. 382) ☐ Pulse oximetry (FAAHN p. 1619, AHN p. 383)	*Class Activity Write three to five scenarios on index cards in which a patient has been scheduled for a diagnostic examination of the respiratory system. Pair the students and distribute the cards. Allow the students a few minutes to role-play the nurse and patient. The nurse is to provide the appropriate patient teaching for the assigned scenario.*
Describe the significance of arterial blood gas values and differentiate between arterial oxygen tension (PaO₂) and arterial oxygen saturation (SaO₂).	☐ Arterial blood gases (ABGs) (FAAHN p. 1618, AHN p. 382)	SG Diagnostic Tests, Ch. 49 p. 416 FAAHN (Ch. 9 p. 104 AHN) **BOOK RESOURCES** Review Questions for the NCLEX Examination Ch. 49 question 29 FAAHN (Ch. 9 question 29 AHN) Box 49-4 Guidelines for Interpreting Arterial Blood Gas Values (FAAHN p. 1619) (Box 9-4 AHN p. 383) Table 49-2 Acid-Base Disturbances and Compensatory Mechanisms (FAAHN p. 1619) (Table 9-2 AHN p. 383) Fig. 49-9 Portable pulse oximeter (FAAHN p. 1620) (Fig. 9-9 AHN p. 384) ▸ Discuss the normal results for an arterial blood gas test. ▸ Discuss the differences between the PaO_2 and the SaO_2 test. *Class Activity Distribute two index cards to each student to develop two NCLEX-style questions relating to arterial blood gas values, arterial oxygen tension, or arterial oxygen saturation. After the questions are completed, collect the cards for a short class review.*

9.1 Homework/Assignments:

9.1 Instructor's Notes/Student Feedback:

LESSON 9.2

CRITICAL THINKING QUESTION

A patient has been recently diagnosed with hypertension. He has been admitted to the hospital to manage his blood pressure. On the first evening of his hospitalization, he calls the nurse's station and reports a nose bleed. What interventions can be performed to stop the bleeding? Later, the patient reports he has had several nose bleeds in recent weeks. What information can be given to the patient regarding these episodes?

Guidelines: A nose bleed or epistaxis results when the nasal membranes become congested. The patient should be assisted into a sitting position, leaning forward. Pinching the nose for a period of 10 to 15 minutes will be helpful. Ice applied over the nose's exterior or allowing the patient to suck on ice will promote venous constriction and reduce or stop the flow of blood. Gauze can be place in the nose, if needed. Epistaxis can be caused by hypertension.

OBJECTIVES	CONTENT	TEACHING RESOURCES
Discuss the etiology and pathophysiology, clinical manifestations, assessment, diagnostic tests, medical management, nursing interventions, and prognosis of the patient with disorders of the upper airway.	☐ Disorders of the upper airway (FAAHN p. 1620, AHN p. 384) ☐ Epistaxis (FAAHN p. 1620, AHN p. 384) – Etiology and pathophysiology (FAAHN p. 1620, AHN p. 384) – Clinical manifestations (FAAHN p. 1620, AHN p. 384) – Assessment (FAAHN p. 1620, AHN p. 384) – Diagnostic tests (FAAHN p. 1620, AHN p. 384) – Medical management (FAAHN p. 1621, AHN p. 385) – Nursing interventions and patient teaching (FAAHN p. 1621, AHN p. 385) – Prognosis (FAAHN p. 1621, AHN p. 385) ☐ Deviated septum and nasal polyps (FAAHN p. 1621, AHN p. 385) – Etiology and pathophysiology (FAAHN p. 1621, AHN p. 385) – Clinical manifestations (FAAHN p. 1621, AHN p. 385)	▦ PPT 10 through 31 Ch. 49 FAAHN (Ch. 9 PPT 10 through 31 AHN) 🔋 EILR TB Ch. 49 questions 4, 19, 23 FAAHN (Ch. 9 questions 4, 19, 23 AHN) 🔋 EILR Open Book Quiz Ch. 49 questions 3 through 7 FAAHN (Ch. 9 questions 3 through 7 AHN) 🔋 ESLR Review Questions for the NCLEX Examination Ch. 49 questions 3, 4 FAAHN (Ch. 9 questions 3, 4 AHN) 📖 Upper Airway Disorders, Ch. 49 pp. 418-419 FAAHN (Ch. 9 pp. 106-107 AHN) **BOOK RESOURCES** Review Questions for the NCLEX Examination Ch. 49 questions 3, 14, 19, 32 FAAHN (Ch. 9 questions 3, 14, 19, 32 AHN) Fig. 49-10 Nasal continuous positive airway pressure (nCPAP) (FAAHN p. 1624) (Fig. 9-10 AHN p. 388) Complementary and Alternative Therapies Respiratory Disorders (FAAHN p. 1627) (AHN p. 391) ▸ Discuss the clinical manifestations associated with an upper airway disorder. ▸ Discuss the populations at an increased risk for the development of an upper airway disorder. *Class Activity **Divide the class into two teams. Each team will develop a list of 25 questions***

OBJECTIVES	CONTENT	TEACHING RESOURCES
	– Assessment (FAAHN p. 1621, AHN p. 385) – Diagnostic tests (FAAHN p. 1621, AHN p. 385) – Medical management (FAAHN p. 1621, AHN p. 385) – Nursing interventions and patient teaching (FAAHN p. 1622, AHN p. 386) – Prognosis (FAAHN p. 1622, AHN p. 386) ☐ Antigen-antibody allergic rhinitis and allergic conjunctivitis (hay fever) (FAAHN p. 1622, AHN p. 386) – Etiology and pathophysiology (FAAHN p. 1622, AHN p. 386) – Clinical manifestations (FAAHN p. 1622, AHN p. 386) – Assessment (FAAHN p. 1622, AHN p. 386) – Diagnostic tests (FAAHN p. 1622, AHN p. 386) – Medical management (FAAHN p. 1622, AHN p. 386) – Nursing interventions and patient teaching (FAAHN p. 1623, AHN p. 387) ☐ Obstructive sleep apnea (FAAHN p. 1623, AHN p. 387) – Etiology and pathophysiology (FAAHN p. 1623, AHN p. 387) – Clinical manifestations/ assessment (FAAHN p. 1623, AHN p. 387) – Diagnostic tests (FAAHN p. 1623, AHN p. 387)	*about upper airway disorders. Select one student from each team to act as the show "host." The host will ask questions of the competing team. Keep score. The team having the most correct answers will win.*

OBJECTIVES	CONTENT	TEACHING RESOURCES
	– Medical management/nursing interventions (FAAHN p. 1624, AHN p. 388)	
	☐ Upper airway obstruction (FAAHN p. 1624, AHN p. 388)	
	– Etiology and pathophysiology (FAAHN p. 1624, AHN p. 388)	
	– Clinical manifestations (FAAHN p. 1624, AHN p. 388)	
	– Assessment (FAAHN p. 1624, AHN p. 388)	
	– Diagnostic tests (FAAHN p. 1624, AHN p. 388)	
	– Medical management (FAAHN p. 1624, AHN p. 388)	
	– Nursing interventions and patient teaching (FAAHN p. 1624, AHN p. 388)	
	– Prognosis (FAAHN p. 1625, AHN p. 389)	
	☐ Respiratory infections (FAAHN p. 1627, AHN p. 391)	
	☐ Acute rhinitis (FAAHN p. 1627, AHN p. 391)	
	– Etiology and pathophysiology (FAAHN p. 1627, AHN p. 391)	
	– Clinical manifestations (FAAHN p. 1627, AHN p. 391)	
	– Assessment (FAAHN p. 1627, AHN p. 391)	
	– Diagnostic tests (FAAHN p. 1627, AHN p. 391)	
	– Medical management (FAAHN p. 1627, AHN p. 391)	
	– Nursing interventions and patient teaching (FAAHN p. 1627, AHN p. 391)	

OBJECTIVES	CONTENT	TEACHING RESOURCES
	– Prognosis (FAAHN p. 1628, AHN p. 392)	
	☐ Acute follicular tonsillitis (FAAHN p. 1628, AHN p. 392)	
	– Etiology and pathophysiology (FAAHN p. 1628, AHN p. 392)	
	– Clinical manifestations (FAAHN p. 1628, AHN p. 392)	
	– Assessment (FAAHN p. 1628, AHN p. 392)	
	– Diagnostic tests (FAAHN p. 1628, AHN p. 392)	
	– Medical management (FAAHN p. 1628, AHN p. 392)	
	– Nursing interventions and patient teaching (FAAHN p. 1628, AHN p. 392)	
	– Prognosis (FAAHN p. 1629, AHN p. 393)	
	☐ Laryngitis (FAAHN p. 1629, AHN p. 393)	
	– Etiology and pathophysiology (FAAHN p. 1629, AHN p. 393)	
	– Clinical manifestations (FAAHN p. 1629, AHN p. 393)	
	– Assessment (FAAHN p. 1629, AHN p. 393)	
	– Diagnostic tests (FAAHN p. 1629, AHN p. 393)	
	– Medical management (FAAHN p. 1629, AHN p. 393)	
	– Nursing interventions and patient teaching (FAAHN p. 1629, AHN p. 393)	
	– Prognosis (FAAHN p. 1629, AHN p. 393)	

Christensen & Kockrow

OBJECTIVES	CONTENT	TEACHING RESOURCES
	☐ Pharyngitis (FAAHN p. 1630, AHN p. 394)	
	– Etiology and pathophysiology (FAAHN p. 1630, AHN p. 394)	
	– Clinical manifestations (FAAHN p. 1630, AHN p. 394)	
	– Assessment (FAAHN p. 1630, AHN p. 394)	
	– Diagnostic tests (FAAHN p. 1630, AHN p. 394)	
	– Medical management (FAAHN p. 1630, AHN p. 394)	
	– Nursing interventions and patient teaching (FAAHN p. 1630, AHN p. 394)	
	– Prognosis (FAAHN p. 1630, AHN p. 394)	
	☐ Sinusitis (FAAHN p. 1630, AHN p. 394)	
	– Etiology and pathophysiology (FAAHN p. 1630, AHN p. 394)	
	– Clinical manifestations (FAAHN p. 1630, AHN p. 394)	
	– Assessment (FAAHN p. 1630, AHN p. 394)	
	– Diagnostic tests (FAAHN p. 1630, AHN p. 394)	
	– Medical management (FAAHN p. 1630, AHN p. 394)	
	– Nursing interventions and patient teaching (FAAHN p. 1631, AHN p. 395)	
	– Prognosis (FAAHN p. 1631, AHN p. 395)	

Christensen & Kockrow

OBJECTIVES	CONTENT	TEACHING RESOURCES
Discuss nursing interventions for the patient with a laryngectomy.	☐ Cancer of the larynx (FAAHN p. 1625, AHN p. 389) – Etiology and pathophysiology (FAAHN p. 1625, AHN p. 389) – Clinical manifestations (FAAHN p. 1625, AHN p. 389) – Assessment (FAAHN p. 1625, AHN p. 389) – Diagnostic tests (FAAHN p. 1625, AHN p. 389) – Medical management (FAAHN p. 1625, AHN p. 389) – Nursing interventions and patient teaching (FAAHN p. 1626, AHN p. 390) – Prognosis (FAAHN p. 1626, AHN p. 390)	⌗ PPT 23, 24 Ch. 49 FAAHN (Ch. 9 PPT 23, 24 AHN) ⊞ EILR TB Ch. 49 questions 3, 9, 20 FAAHN (Ch. 9 questions 3, 9, 20 AHN) ▤ SG Laryngectomy, Ch. 49 p. 419 FAAHN (Ch. 9 p. 107 AHN) ▸ Discuss the priorities of care for the patient who has had a laryngectomy. ▸ Discuss the role of the nurse in providing care to the patient who has had a laryngectomy. *Class Activity Develop four nursing diagnoses for the patient who has had a laryngectomy. Post these diagnoses on the board for student viewing. Ask the students to select a partner. Instruct each pair to develop interventions to accompany the diagnoses. If time allows, encourage students to share their work with the entire class.*

9.2 Homework/Assignments:

9.2 Instructor's Notes/Student Feedback:

Mosby items and derived items © 2011 by Mosby, Inc., an affiliate of Elsevier Inc.
Some material was previously published.

Christensen & Kockrow

LESSON 9.3

CRITICAL THINKING QUESTION

What is the difference between a carcinoma of the lung when it is a primary tumor and when it is a secondary tumor?

Guidelines: A primary tumor of the lung would consist of cells from the respiratory tract and would have had its origin within the lung. A secondary tumor of the lung is a metastasized tumor from another part of the body. The metastasis to the lung is common due to the vascular nature of the lungs.

OBJECTIVES	CONTENT	TEACHING RESOURCES
Discuss the etiology and pathophysiology, clinical manifestations, assessment, diagnostic tests, medical management, nursing interventions, and prognosis of the patient with disorders of the lower airway.	☐ Disorders of the lower airway (FAAHN p. 1631, AHN p. 395) ☐ Acute bronchitis (FAAHN p. 1631, AHN p. 395) – Etiology and pathophysiology (FAAHN p. 1631, AHN p. 395) – Clinical manifestations (FAAHN p. 1631, AHN p. 395) – Assessment (FAAHN p. 1631, AHN p. 395) – Diagnostic tests (FAAHN p. 1631, AHN p. 395) – Medical management (FAAHN p. 1631, AHN p. 395) – Nursing interventions and patient teaching (FAAHN p. 1631, AHN p. 395) – Prognosis (FAAHN p. 1632, AHN p. 396) ☐ Legionnaires' disease (FAAHN p. 1632, AHN p. 396) – Etiology and pathophysiology (FAAHN p. 1632, AHN p. 396) – Clinical manifestations (FAAHN p. 1632, AHN p. 396) – Assessment (FAAHN p. 1632, AHN p. 396) – Diagnostic tests (FAAHN p. 1632, AHN p. 396) – Medical management (FAAHN p. 1632, AHN p. 396) – Nursing interventions and patient teaching (FAAHN p. 1632, AHN p. 396) – Prognosis (FAAHN p. 1633, AHN p. 397)	PPT 35 through 66, Ch. 49 FAAHN (Ch. 9 PPT 35 through 66 AHN) EILR TB Ch. 49 questions 1, 5 through 7, 11 through 13, 21, 24, 31 through 33, 35 FAAHN (Ch. 9 questions 1, 5 through 7, 11 through 13, 21, 24, 31 through 33, 35 AHN) EILR Open Book Quiz Ch. 49 questions 9, 10 FAAHN (Ch. 9 questions 9, 10 AHN) ESLR Review Questions for the NCLEX Examination Ch. 49 question 5, 7, 9 FAAHN (Ch. 9 question 5, 7, 9 AHN) SG Lower Airway Disorders Ch. 49 p. 420 FAAHN (Ch. 9 p. 108 AHN) **BOOK RESOURCES** Review Questions for the NCLEX Examination Ch. 49 question 25 FAAHN (Ch. 9 question 25 AHN) Cultural Considerations: Tuberculosis (FAAHN p. 1635) (AHN p. 399) Health Promotion: Pneumonia (FAAHN p. 1640) (AHN p. 404) Life Span Considerations, Older Adults: Respiratory Disorder (FAAHN p. 1641) (AHN p. 405) Fig. 49-14 Disorders of the airways in patients with chronic bronchitis, asthma, and emphysema (FAAHN p. 1656) (Fig. 9-14 AHN p. 420) Home Care Considerations: Chronic Oxygen Therapy at Home (FAAHN p. 1660) (AHN p.424) ▸ Discuss diagnostic tests used to diagnose disorders of the lower airway.

ELSEVIER

Christensen & Kockrow

OBJECTIVES	CONTENT	TEACHING RESOURCES
	☐ Severe acute respiratory syndrome (FAAHN p. 1633, AHN p. 397)	▸ Discuss the incidence of lower airway disorders in the elderly.
	– Etiology and pathophysiology (FAAHN p. 1633, AHN p. 397)	*Class Activity Invite a speaker to the class to discuss the role of the respiratory therapist in the care of lower airway disorders. If your college/university has a respiratory therapy program, that would be an ideal source for the speaker. If not, contact a local hospital to find an appropriate speaker.*
	– Clinical manifestations (FAAHN p. 1633, AHN p. 397)	
	– Diagnostic tests (FAAHN p. 1633, AHN p. 397)	
	– Medical management (FAAHN p. 1633, AHN p. 397)	
	– Nursing interventions/patient teaching (FAAHN p. 1633, AHN p. 397)	
	– Prognosis (FAAHN p. 1633, AHN p. 397)	
	☐ Anthrax (FAAHN p. 1634, AHN p. 398)	
	– Etiology and pathophysiology (FAAHN p. 1634, AHN p. 398)	
	– Diagnostic tests (FAAHN p. 1634, AHN p. 398)	
	– Medical management (FAAHN p. 1634, AHN p. 398)	
	☐ Pneumonia (FAAHN p. 1639, AHN p. 403)	
	– Etiology and pathophysiology (FAAHN p. 1639, AHN p. 403)	
	– Clinical manifestations (FAAHN p. 1640, AHN p. 404)	
	– Assessment (FAAHN p. 1641, AHN p. 405)	
	– Diagnostic tests (FAAHN p. 1641, AHN p. 405)	
	– Medical management (FAAHN p. 1642, AHN p. 406)	
	– Nursing interventions and patient teaching (FAAHN p. 1642, AHN p. 406)	
	– Prognosis (FAAHN p. 1643, AHN p. 407)	
	☐ Pleurisy (FAAHN p. 1643, AHN p. 407)	

Adult Health Nursing, 6th ed.
Christensen & Kockrow

OBJECTIVES	CONTENT	TEACHING RESOURCES
	– Etiology and pathophysiology (FAAHN p. 1643, AHN p. 407)	
	– Clinical manifestations (FAAHN p. 1643, AHN p. 407)	
	– Assessment (FAAHN p. 1643, AHN p. 407)	
	– Diagnostic tests (FAAHN p. 1643, AHN p. 407)	
	– Medical management (FAAHN p. 1643, AHN p. 407)	
	– Nursing interventions and patient teaching (FAAHN p. 1643, AHN p. 407)	
	– Prognosis (FAAHN p. 1644, AHN p. 408)	
	☐ Atelectasis (FAAHN p. 1646, AHN p. 410)	
	– Etiology and pathophysiology (FAAHN p. 1646, AHN p. 410)	
	– Clinical manifestations (FAAHN p. 1646, AHN p. 410)	
	– Assessment (FAAHN p. 1647, AHN p. 411)	
	– Diagnostic tests (FAAHN p. 1647, AHN p. 411)	
	– Medical management (FAAHN p. 1647, AHN p. 411)	
	– Nursing interventions and patient teaching (FAAHN p. 1647, AHN p. 411)	
	– Prognosis (FAAHN p. 1647, AHN p. 411)	
	☐ Pneumothorax (FAAHN p. 1647, AHN p. 411)	
	– Etiology and pathophysiology (FAAHN p. 1647, AHN p. 411)	
	– Clinical manifestations (FAAHN p. 1648, AHN p. 412)	
	– Assessment (FAAHN p. 1648, AHN p. 412)	
	– Diagnostic tests (FAAHN p. 1648, AHN p. 412)	
	– Medical management (FAAHN p. 1648, AHN p. 412)	

OBJECTIVES	CONTENT	TEACHING RESOURCES
	– Nursing interventions and patient teaching (FAAHN p. 1648, AHN p. 412)	
	– Prognosis (FAAHN p. 1649, AHN p. 413)	
	☐ Lung cancer (FAAHN p. 1649, AHN p. 413)	
	– Etiology and pathophysiology (FAAHN p. 1649, AHN p. 413)	
	– Clinical manifestations (FAAHN p. 1649, AHN p. 413)	
	– Assessment (FAAHN p. 1649, AHN p. 413)	
	– Diagnostic tests (FAAHN p. 1649, AHN p. 413)	
	– Medical management (FAAHN p. 1650, AHN p. 414)	
	– Nursing interventions and patient teaching (FAAHN p. 1650, AHN p. 414)	
	– Prognosis (FAAHN p. 1651, AHN p. 415)	
	☐ Pulmonary edema (FAAHN p. 1651, AHN p. 415)	
	– Etiology and pathophysiology (FAAHN p. 1651, AHN p. 415)	
	– Clinical manifestations (FAAHN p. 1651, AHN p. 415)	
	– Assessment (FAAHN p. 1651, AHN p. 415)	
	– Diagnostic tests (FAAHN p. 1652, AHN p. 416)	
	– Medical management (FAAHN p. 1652, AHN p. 416)	
	– Nursing interventions and patient teaching (FAAHN p. 1652, AHN p. 416)	
	– Prognosis (FAAHN p. 1652, AHN p. 416)	
	☐ Acute respiratory distress syndrome (FAAHN p. 1654, AHN p. 418)	
	– Etiology and pathophysiology (FAAHN p. 1654, AHN p. 418)	

Adult Health Nursing, 6th ed.

Christensen & Kockrow

OBJECTIVES	CONTENT	TEACHING RESOURCES
	– Clinical manifestations (FAAHN p. 1655, AHN p. 419) – Assessment (FAAHN p. 1655, AHN p. 419) – Diagnostic tests (FAAHN p. 1655, AHN p. 419) – Medical management (FAAHN p. 1655, AHN p. 419) – Nursing interventions and patient teaching (FAAHN p. 1655, AHN p. 419) – Prognosis (FAAHN p. 1656, AHN p. 420)	
List five nursing interventions to assist patients with retained pulmonary secretions.	☐ Disorders of the lower airway (FAAHN p. 1631, AHN p. 395)	EILR TB Ch. 49 questions 1 through 4, 8, 21, 24 FAAHN (Ch. 9 questions 1 through 4, 8, 21, 24 AHN) SG Nursing Interventions Ch. 49 p. 422 FAAHN (Ch. 9 p. 110 AHN) **BOOK RESOURCES** Review Questions for the NCLEX Examination Ch. 49 questions 8, 24 FAAHN (Ch. 9 questions 8, 24 AHN) ▸ Discuss documentation that is needed when caring for a patient having retained pulmonary secretions. ▸ Discuss the nursing intervention that can be used to assist patients experiencing retained pulmonary secretions. *Class Activity **Distribute blank nursing care plan forms to the students. Instruct the students to create a short nursing care plan for the patient who has retained pulmonary secretions. After a brief period of time, allow the students to compare notes with a partner.***

Christensen & Kockrow

OBJECTIVES	CONTENT	TEACHING RESOURCES
Differentiate between tuberculosis infection and tuberculosis disease.	☐ Tuberculosis (FAAHN p. 1634, AHN p. 398) – Etiology and pathophysiology (FAAHN p. 1634, AHN p. 398) – Clinical manifestations (FAAHN p. 1635, AHN p. 399) – Assessment (FAAHN p. 1635, AHN p. 399) – Diagnostic tests (FAAHN p. 1636, AHN p. 400) – Medical management (FAAHN p. 1636, AHN p. 400) – Nursing interventions and patient teaching (FAAHN p. 1636, AHN p. 400) – Prognosis (FAAHN p. 1639, AHN p. 403)	▣▤ PPT 43, 44 Ch. 49 FAAHN (Ch. 9 PPT 43, 44 AHN) 🔳 EILR Open Book Quiz Ch. 49 question 8 FAAHN (Ch. 9 question 8 AHN) 🔳 ESLR Review Questions for the NCLEX Examination Ch. 49 question 6 FAAHN (Ch. 9 question 6 AHN) 📖 SG Tuberculosis, Ch. 49 p. 422 FAAHN (Ch. 9 p. 110 AHN) **BOOK RESOURCES** Review Questions for the NCLEX Examination Ch. 49 questions 7, 20 FAAHN (Ch. 9 questions 7, 20 AHN) Box 49-5 High-Risk Groups to Screen for Tuberculosis (FAAHN p. 1635 (Box 9-5 AHN p. 399) ▶ Discuss the mode of transmission for tuberculosis. ▶ Discuss the tests used to diagnose the presence of tuberculosis. *Class Activity Contact the local board of health. Obtain facts and figures concerning the frequency of tuberculosis and the system of reporting within the county. During the class period, assess the students' knowledge of this information.*
List four medications commonly prescribed for the patient with tuberculosis.	– Medical management (FAAHN p. 1636, AHN p. 400) – Nursing interventions and patient teaching (FAAHN p. 1636, AHN p. 400)	▣▤ PPT 44, Ch. 49 FAAHN (Ch. 9 PPT 44 AHN) 📖 SG Tuberculosis Ch. 49 p. 422 FAAHN (Ch. 9 p. 110 AHN) ▶ Discuss the medications used in the management of the patient with tuberculosis. ▶ Discuss the nursing implications in the care of the patient diagnosed with tuberculosis. *Class Activity Place the name of one medication used to treat tuberculosis on each index card and distribute the cards to students who have been paired together. Each pair of students will create a drug card regarding their assigned medication. After completion, the students will present information about the medication to the rest of the class.*

OBJECTIVES	CONTENT	TEACHING RESOURCES
List five nursing assessments or interventions pertaining to the care of the patient with closed-chest drainage.	☐ Pleural effusion/empyema (FAAHN p. 1644, AHN p. 408) – Etiology and pathophysiology (FAAHN p. 1644, AHN p. 408) – Clinical manifestations (FAAHN p. 1644, AHN p. 408) – Assessment (FAAHN p. 1644, AHN p. 408) – Diagnostic tests (FAAHN p. 1644, AHN p. 408) – Medical management (FAAHN p. 1644, AHN p. 408) – Nursing interventions and patient teaching (FAAHN p. 1645, AHN p. 409) – Prognosis (FAAHN p. 1646, AHN p. 410)	🖳 PPT 49, 50, Ch. 49 FAAHN (Ch. 9 PPT 49, 50 AHN) 📧 EILR IC Ch. 49 images 11, 12 FAAHN (Ch. 9 images 11, 12 AHN) 📧 ESLR Review Questions for the NCLEX Examination Ch. 49 question 8 FAAHN (Ch. 9 question 8 AHN) 📓 SG Closed-Chest Drainage, Ch. 49 p. 423 FAAHN (Ch. 9 p. 111 AHN) **BOOK RESOURCES** Review Questions for the NCLEX Examination Ch. 49 questions 11, 30 FAAHN (Ch. 9 questions 11, 30 AHN) Fig. 49-11 A Drainage tube inserted into pleural space (FAAHN p. 1645) (Fig. 9-11 AHN p. 409) Fig. 49-12 Pleur-Evac (FAAHN p. 1645) (Fig. 9-12 AHN p. 409) Box 49-6 Guidelines for Care of Patient with Chest Tubes and Water-Seal Drainage (FAAHN p. 1646) (Box 9-6 AHN p. 410) Fig. 49-13 Pneumothorax (FAAHN p. 1648) (Fig. 9-13 AHN p. 412) ▸ Discuss the clinical conditions that warrant the use of closed-chest drainage apparatus. ▸ Discuss the nursing role in monitoring the patient having closed-chest drainage. *Class Activity Take the class to the nursing lab. Use lab equipment to demonstrate the setup that can be expected with a closed-chest drainage system.*
Discuss three risk factors associated with pulmonary emboli.	☐ Pulmonary embolism (FAAHN p. 1652, AHN p. 416) – Etiology and pathophysiology (FAAHN p. 1652, AHN p. 416) – Clinical manifestations (FAAHN p. 1653, AHN p. 417) – Assessment (FAAHN p. 1653, AHN p. 417) – Diagnostic tests (FAAHN p. 1653, AHN p. 417)	🖳 PPT 61, 62, Ch. 49 FAAHN (Ch. 9 PPT 61, 62 AHN) 📧 EILR TB Ch. 49 question 15 FAAHN (Ch. 9 question 15 AHN) 📧 ESLR Review Questions for the NCLEX Examination Ch. 49 question 2 FAAHN (Ch. 9 question 2 AHN) 📓 SG Pulmonary Emboli, Ch. 49 p. 423 FAAHN (Ch. 9 p. 111 AHN)

Adult Health Nursing, 6th ed.
Christensen & Kockrow

OBJECTIVES	CONTENT	TEACHING RESOURCES
	– Medical management (FAAHN p. 1653, AHN p. 417) – Nursing interventions and patient teaching (FAAHN p. 1654, AHN p. 418) – Prognosis (FAAHN p. 1654, AHN p. 418)	**BOOK RESOURCES** Review Questions for the NCLEX Examination Ch. 49 questions 14, 15, 36 FAAHN (Ch. 9 questions 14, 15, 36 AHN) ▸ Discuss nursing interventions geared toward the prevention of pulmonary emboli. ▸ Discuss the therapies for the patient diagnosed with pulmonary emboli. *Class Activity Divide the students into small groups of four or five students. Ask two of the students to select words relating to pulmonary emboli to use in a game of hangman. During the game, the remaining students will be given clues to solve the puzzle.*

9.3 Homework/Assignments:

9.3 Instructor's Notes/Student Feedback:

LESSON 9.4

CRITICAL THINKING QUESTION

You are assigned to care for a patient who has been hospitalized after having experienced an asthmatic attack. The clinical manifestations of the attack included dyspnea, tachypnea, tachycardia, diaphoresis, and chest tightness. The physician has ordered a series of tests to review the patient's condition. What tests do you anticipate will be performed? What is the significance of each of these tests? What medications might be prescribed?

Guidelines: An asthmatic attack can necessitate hospitalization. Diagnostic testing could include arterial blood gases, pulmonary function tests, a complete blood test, and a sputum culture. The blood gases will be used to determine the arterial values of the body's oxygen, carbon dioxide, bicarbonate, and pH. The severity of the disease can be evaluated with pulmonary function tests. Areas evaluated will include lung volume, ventilation, pulmonary spirometry, and gas exchange. The sputum culture will be used to determine if there is any underlying infection. Pharmacological therapies used to manage asthma include beta-antagonists and inhaled steroids.

OBJECTIVES	CONTENT	TEACHING RESOURCES
Compare and contrast the etiology and pathophysiology, clinical manifestations, assessment, diagnostic tests, medical management, nursing interventions, and prognosis for the patient with chronic obstructive pulmonary disease, including emphysema, chronic bronchitis, asthma, and bronchiectasis.	☐ Chronic obstructive pulmonary disease (FAAHN p. 1656, AHN p. 420) ☐ Emphysema (FAAHN p. 1657, AHN p. 421) – Etiology and pathophysiology (FAAHN p. 1657, AHN p. 421) – Clinical manifestations (FAAHN p. 1657, AHN p. 421) – Assessment (FAAHN p. 1657, AHN p. 421) – Diagnostic tests (FAAHN p. 1658, AHN p. 422) – Medical management (FAAHN p. 1658, AHN p. 422) – Nursing interventions and patient teaching (FAAHN p. 1659, AHN p. 423) – Prognosis (FAAHN p. 1659, AHN p. 423) ☐ Chronic bronchitis (FAAHN p. 1660, AHN p. 424) – Etiology and pathophysiology (FAAHN p. 1660, AHN p. 424) – Clinical manifestations (FAAHN p. 1660, AHN p. 424) – Assessment (FAAHN p. 1660, AHN p. 424)	PPT 70 through 79, Ch. 49 FAAHN (Ch. 9 PPT 70 through 79 AHN) EILR IC Ch. 49 images 14 through 16 FAAHN (Ch. 9 images 14 through 16 AHN) EILR TB Ch. 49 questions 5, 10, 14, 16, 17, 22, 24, 36 FAAHN (Ch. 9 question 5, 10, 14, 16, 17, 22, 24, 36 AHN) ESLR Review Questions for the NCLEX Examination Ch. 49 question 10 FAAHN (Ch. 9 question 10 AHN) SG Chronic Obstructive Pulmonary Disease, Ch. 49 p. 424 FAAHN (Ch. 9 p. 112 AHN) **BOOK RESOURCES** Review Questions for the NCLEX Examination Ch. 49 questions 6, 12, 13, 18, 23, 33 FAAHN (Ch. 9 questions 6, 12, 13, 18, 23, 33 AHN) Home Care Considerations: Chronic Oxygen Therapy at Home (FAAHN p. 1660) (AHN p. 424) Communication (FAAHN p. 1660) (AHN p. 424) Nursing Care Plan 49-1 The Patient with Emphysema (FAAHN p. 1661) (NCP 9-1 AHN p. 425) ▸ Discuss the priorities of care for the patient diagnosed with asthma.

Adult Health Nursing, 6th ed.

Christensen & Kockrow

OBJECTIVES	CONTENT	TEACHING RESOURCES
	– Diagnostic tests (FAAHN p. 1660, AHN p. 424) – Medical management (FAAHN p. 1662, AHN p. 426) – Nursing interventions and patient teaching (FAAHN p. 1662, AHN p. 426) – Prognosis (FAAHN p. 1662, AHN p. 426) ☐ Asthma (FAAHN p. 1662, AHN p. 426) – Etiology and pathophysiology (FAAHN p. 1662, AHN p. 426) – Clinical manifestations (FAAHN p. 1662, AHN p. 426) – Assessment (FAAHN p. 1663, AHN p. 427) – Diagnostic tests (FAAHN p. 1663, AHN p. 427) – Medical management (FAAHN p. 1663, AHN p. 427) – Nursing interventions and patient teaching (FAAHN p. 1664, AHN p. 428) – Prognosis (FAAHN p. 1664, AHN p. 428) ☐ Bronchiectasis (FAAHN p. 1664, AHN p. 428) – Etiology and pathophysiology (FAAHN p. 1664, AHN p. 428) – Clinical manifestations (FAAHN p. 1664, AHN p. 428) – Assessment (FAAHN p. 1664, AHN p. 428) – Diagnostic tests (FAAHN p. 1665, AHN p. 429) – Medical management (FAAHN p. 1665, AHN p. 429) – Nursing interventions and patient teaching (FAAHN p. 1665, AHN p. 429)	▸ Discuss the documentation of respiratory status required by the nurse when caring for the patient diagnosed with chronic obstructive pulmonary disease (COPD), including emphysema, chronic bronchitis, asthma, and bronchiectasis. *Class Activity Develop four role-play scenarios. Divide students into pairs. Assign a scenario to each pair. Instruct each pair to role-play the nurse assigned to provide care to the patient diagnosed with chronic obstructive pulmonary disease (COPD), including emphysema, chronic bronchitis, asthma, and bronchiectasis.*

Christensen & Kockrow

OBJECTIVES	CONTENT	TEACHING RESOURCES
	– Prognosis (FAAHN p. 1665, AHN p. 429)	
Differentiate between medical management of the patient with emphysema and the patient with asthma.	☐ Emphysema (FAAHN p. 1657, AHN p. 421) – Medical management (FAAHN p. 1658, AHN p. 422) ☐ Asthma (FAAHN p. 1662, AHN p. 426) – Medical management (FAAHN p. 1663, AHN p. 427)	🖵■ PPT 67 through 71, Ch. 49 FAAHN (Ch. 9 PPT 67 through 71 AHN) 📖 SG Asthma or Emphysema p. 425 FAAHN (Ch. 9 p. 113 AHN) **BOOK RESOURCES** Review Questions for the NCLEX Examination Ch. 49 questions 16, 17, 21, 22 FAAHN (Ch. 9 questions 16, 17, 21, 22 AHN) Fig. 49-15 Mechanisms of air trapping in emphysema (FAAHN p. 1657) (Fig. 9-15 AHN p. 421) Fig. 49-16 Barrel chest (FAAHN p. 1657) (Fig. 9-16 AHN p. 421) ▸ Discuss the classifications of medications used in the treatment of emphysema and asthma. ▸ Discuss the nursing implications for the medications used in the treatment of emphysema and asthma. *Class Activity **Distribute two index cards to each student. Instruct each student to develop one NCLEX-style question each for asthma and emphysema. Then ask students to gather in groups of four. Allow students the time to quiz their assigned groups using their questions.***
Discuss why low-flow oxygen is required for patients with emphysema.	– Nursing interventions and patient teaching (FAAHN p. 1659, AHN p. 423) – Prognosis (FAAHN p. 1659, AHN p. 423)	🖵■ PPT 71, Ch. 49 FAAHN (Ch. 9 PPT 71 AHN) 🅔 EILR TB Ch. 49 question 22 FAAHN (Ch. 9 question 22 AHN) 📖 SG Asthma or Emphysema, Ch. 49 p. 425 FAAHN (Ch. 9 p. 113 AHN) ▸ Discuss the arterial blood gas readings associated with the patient with emphysema. ▸ Discuss the administration of oxygen for the patient diagnosed with emphysema. *Class Activity **Obtain the delivery systems used to administer oxygen. Bring the items to class. Ask for student volunteers to demonstrate their use.***

OBJECTIVES	CONTENT	TEACHING RESOURCES
State three possible nursing diagnoses for the patient with altered respiratory function.	☐ Nursing process for the patient with a respiratory disorder (FAAHN p. 1665, AHN p. 429) – Assessment (FAAHN p. 1665, AHN p. 429) – Nursing diagnosis (FAAHN p. 1665, AHN p. 429) – Expected outcomes and planning (FAAHN p. 1666, AHN p. 430) – Implementation (FAAHN p. 1666, AHN p. 430) – Evaluation (FAAHN p. 1666, AHN p. 430)	🖩 PPT 79, Ch. 49 FAAHN (Ch. 9 PPT 79 AHN) 📇 EILR TB Ch. 49 question 18 FAAHN (Ch. 9 question 18 AHN) 📓 SG Nursing Diagnoses, Ch. 49 p. 425 FAAHN (Ch. 9 p. 113 AHN) **BOOK RESOURCES** Review Questions for the NCLEX Examination Ch. 49 questions 27, 28, 34 FAAHN (Ch. 9 questions 27, 28, 34 AHN) ▸ Discuss the assessment of the patient diagnosed with altered respiratory function. ▸ Discuss the development of individualized nursing diagnoses applicable to the care of the patient with altered respiratory function. *Class Activity **Distribute blank nursing care plan forms. Divide students into small groups and ask each group to select a respiratory disease Each group will select a different disease. After the disease is selected, instruct the students to determine and prioritize the top three nursing diagnoses for a patient having the selected medical diagnosis.***
Performance Evaluation		📇 EILR TB Ch. 49 questions 1 through 36 FAAHN (Ch. 12 questions 1 through 36 AHN) 📇 EILR Open Book Quiz Ch. 49 questions 1 through 10 FAAHN (Ch. 9 questions 1 through 10 AHN) 📇 ESLR Review Questions for the NCLEX Examination Ch. 49 questions 1 through 10 FAAHN (Ch. 9 questions 1 through 10 AHN) 📓 SG Ch. 49 pp. 413-428 FAAHN (Ch. 9 pp. 101-116 AHN) **BOOK RESOURCES** Nursing Care Plan 49-1 The Patient with Emphysema (FAAHN p. 1661) (NCP 9-1 AHN p. 425)

ELSEVIER

Mosby items and derived items © 2011 by Mosby, Inc., an affiliate of Elsevier Inc.
Some material was previously published.

Adult Health Nursing, 6th ed.
Christensen & Kockrow

OBJECTIVES	CONTENT	TEACHING RESOURCES
		♀ NCP CTQ 1 through 3 (FAAHN p. 1661) (AHN p. 425) Review Questions for the NCLEX Examination Ch. 49 question 1 through 37 FAAHN (Ch. 9 question 1 through 37 AHN)

9.4 Homework/Assignments:

9.4 Instructor's Notes/Student Feedback:

ELSEVIER

Mosby items and derived items © 2011 by Mosby, Inc., an affiliate of Elsevier Inc.
Some material was previously published.

Adult Health Nursing, 6th ed.
Christensen & Kockrow

Slide 1

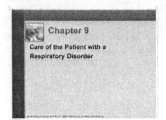

Slide 2

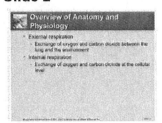

- The respiratory system functions to transport oxygen to the body. This function is vital to the survival of the body's cells and organs.

Slide 3

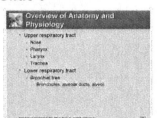

- The respiratory system is divided into two tracts.

- Review the functions of each of the structures of each of the upper and lower respiratory tract.

- How do the functions of the upper and lower respiratory tracts differ?

Slide 4

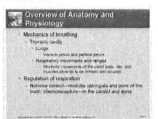

- The best known organs of respiration are the lungs.

- The lungs lie in the chest on either side of the heart.

- The lungs get their blood from the pulmonary artery directly from the heart.

- Describe the concentration of oxygen in the blood.

Slide 5

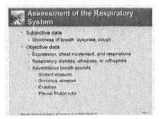

- Impaired functioning of the respiratory system impacts the entire body.

- A reduction in oxygenation prevents the body's cells from carrying out their prescribed functions.

- Every physical examination provides an opportunity to check the functioning of the respiratory system.

- When performing a health assessment, what questions should be asked by the nurse concerning respiratory status?

Christensen & Kockrow

Slide 6

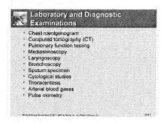

- In the event that complications involving the respiratory system are suspected, diagnostic testing can be ordered.

- Certain types of tests are noninvasive. Others require specific preparation and the completion of consent forms.

- Which of the listed tests are considered invasive? What special preparation is needed prior to performing them?

Slide 7

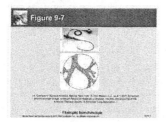

- The bronchoscopy involves the use of an illuminated, flexible scope. The scope is passed through the trachea into the bronchi.

- The physician can perform important assessments when using the bronchoscope. What can be viewed/evaluated using this technology?

- After the test is completed, when can the patient resume eating and drinking?

Slide 8

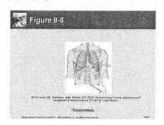

- Thoracentesis involves the perforation of the chest wall and pleural space.

- Discuss indications for performing this test.

- When the test is performed and fluid is removed, a limitation of 1,300 mL is imposed. No more than that can be taken in a 30-minute time period. What dangers exist if more fluid is removed?

Slide 9

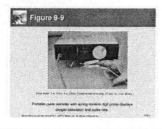

- Pulse oximetry is a noninvasive test used to determine the oxygen saturation level of the blood.

- The test can be performed on the ears, bridge of the nose, fingers, toes, or ear lobes. When attempting to perform the test, what factors might impair the ability of the machine to accurately measure the degree of oxygenation?

- Describe the technology the test uses to evaluate the body's oxygenation level.

Slide 10

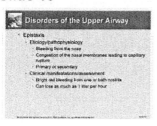

- Nosebleeds are a common occurrence. They can be caused by a variety of events.

- What are potential causes of both primary and secondary epistaxis?

- Corticosteroid use can cause epistaxis. Explain how this results.

- When epistaxis occurs, it can appear to be a large quantity of blood. Fortunately, the episode rarely lasts for a prolonged period.

Adult Health Nursing, 6th ed.

Christensen & Kockrow

Slide 11

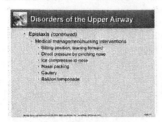

- Identify nursing diagnoses that can be applied to the patient experiencing epistaxis.

Slide 12

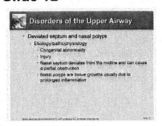

- Obstruction of the nares could occur due to a deviated septum or nasal polyps.

- When performing data collection on the patient suspected of having a nasal obstruction, what subjective data might be reported?

Slide 13

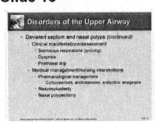

- If the presence of nasal polyps or a deviated septum is suspected, diagnostic testing is indicated.

- What tests can be ordered?

- Treatment might be conservative, using pharmacological therapies. What actions will corticosteroids and antihistamines take to manage polyps?

Slide 14

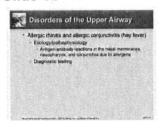

- Allergic rhinitis and allergic conjunctivitis are irritating conditions that plague people of all ages.

- These allergies are often seasonal.

- The reaction involves an antigen-antibody reaction. The ciliary action slows and is accompanied by an increase in mucus secretion. The body mounts a response involving the white blood cells. The increase in capillary permeability and vasodilation act as a catalyst for the characteristic nasal congestion.

- What are potential environmental causes?

Slide 15

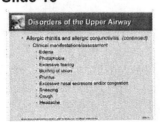

- The clinical manifestations cause distress to the sufferer.

- If not treated, chronic sufferers can develop infections.

- Provide examples of the infections that could result.

Slide 16

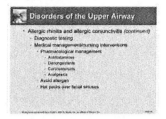

- The clinical picture often presents adequate information to make a diagnosis.

- What diagnostic tests can be used to pinpoint causative agents?

- Discuss the use of patch and scratch testing.

- Compare and contrast the functions of antihistamines, decongestants, and corticosteroids in the medical management of allergic rhinitis and allergic conjunctivitis.

Slide 17

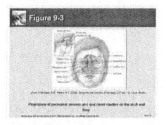

Slide 18

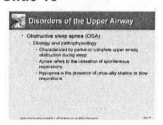

- Sleep apnea is considered a greatly underreported disorder. It is estimated to affect up to 18 million adults in the United States. Many are undiagnosed.

- Discuss the changes that take place during the cycle of apnea.

Slide 19

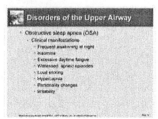

Slide 20

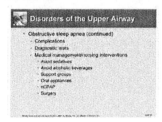

- Describe populations at risk for the development of obstructive sleep apnea. What factors do these individuals have in common?

- Describe polysomnography.

- What impact do sedatives and alcohol use have on sleep apnea?

Slide 21

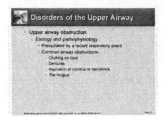

- Upper airway obstruction involves any condition that can produce a reduction in airway expanse.

Slide 22

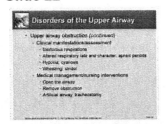

- The presence of an upper airway obstruction is a clinical emergency. There is no need or time for the use of diagnostic testing.

- What will determine the type of management option selected?

- What are the priorities of nursing care for the patient diagnosed with an upper airway obstruction?

Slide 23

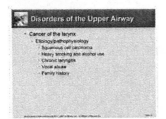

- The number of cases of cancer of the larynx is growing.

- To what can this increase be attributed?

- What populations are most likely to develop cancer of the larynx?

Slide 24

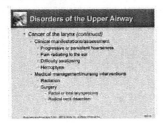

- When a patient presents for medical attention with clinical manifestations consistent with cancer of the larynx, what diagnostic tests might be ordered? What findings will support a diagnosis of cancer?

- When diagnosed, cancer of the larynx is associated with a high rate of metastasis. Why is this cancer associated with rapid spreading?

- What type of prognosis accompanies the diagnosis of cancer of the larynx?

Slide 25

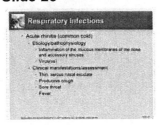

- Most people will become ill with the common cold each year. Although many associate their development only with the winter months, they can occur during any season.

- How is the common cold spread?

ELSEVIER

Mosby items and derived items © 2011, 2007 by Mosby, Inc., an affiliate of Elsevier Inc.
Some material was previously published.

Adult Health Nursing, 6th ed.
Christensen & Kockrow

Slide 26

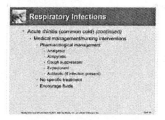

- There is no specific treatment for the common cold. The best action is prevention. What can be done to reduce the transmission of the cold?
- One common misconception involves the need for antibiotics to treat colds. When is the use of an antibiotic indicated? When should it be avoided?

Slide 27

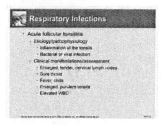

- School-aged children represent the population most commonly affected with tonsillitis.
- What are the usual pathogens involved?

Slide 28

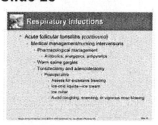

- When a patient presents with the signs and symptoms consistent with tonsillitis, what diagnostic testing may be indicated?
- Identify the special relationship between tonsillitis and group A β-hemolytic streptococci.

Slide 29

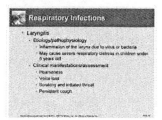

- Laryngitis frequently accompanies or occurs after other respiratory infections.
- It can be acute or chronic.
- The age of the patient impacts the severity. Explain the unique complications associated with laryngitis in children under the age of 5 years.

Slide 30

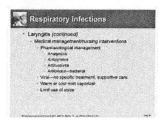

- The care and treatment employed to manage laryngitis are not specific. Individualized comfort measures are utilized.
- Identify two nursing diagnoses relating to the adult patient diagnosed with laryngitis.

Christensen & Kockrow

Slide 31

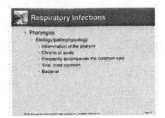

- Pharyngitis is the most common inflammation of the throat. It is normally most contagious 2 to 3 days after the onset of symptoms.

Slide 32

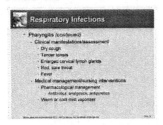

- When performing the data collection on the patient who has presented with the clinical manifestations associated with pharyngitis, describe the health assessment.

Slide 33

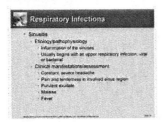

- Sinusitis can be chronic or acute.

- Which sinuses are most commonly affected?

- Discuss the chain of events seen most frequently with sinusitis.

Slide 34

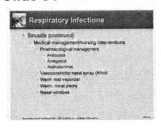

- When the patient presents to the physician with complaints of headaches and congestion, x-rays might be indicated to provide support for the diagnosis. What are typical findings on an x-ray associated with the presence of sinusitis?

- When conservative management of sinusitis is not successful, surgical interventions would be undertaken. Describe potential surgical interventions.

Slide 35

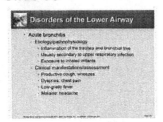

Slide 36

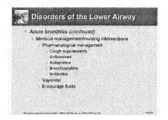

- When providing care to the patient diagnosed with bronchitis, it is important to prevent secondary infections.
- When planning the care of the patient with bronchitis, what are two priority nursing diagnoses for the patient with bronchitis?

Slide 37

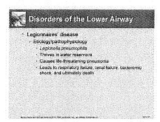

- Legionnaires' disease first became famous in 1976 after participants in a Philadelphia convention became ill.
- Describe the mode of transmission for this disorder.
- Legionnaires' causes a type of pneumonia resulting in lung consolidation and alveolar necrosis.
- Discuss the concepts of lung consolidation and alveolar necrosis.

Slide 38

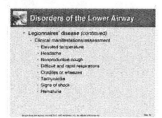

- Prompt diagnosis of Legionnaires' disease is needed to reduce complications.
- What diagnostic tests are performed to confirm the condition?
- What findings support the diagnosis?

Slide 39

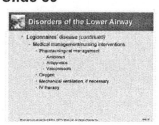

- Management of the patient with Legionnaires' disease might require dialysis in addition to the anticipated respiratory support.
- Why might dialysis be indicated?
- What is the prognosis for Legionnaires' disease?

Slide 40

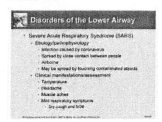

- Discuss which manifestations are early and which will be later developments.

Slide 41

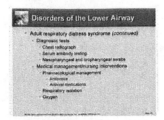

- The focus of SARS is on supportive care and treatment while managing the root cause of the problems.

- Discuss personal protective equipment that may be employed to protect the health care worker.

- Develop two nursing diagnoses for the care and support of the patient or family experiencing a diagnosis of SARS.

Slide 42

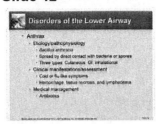

- Anthrax is found in nature. It commonly infects hoofed animals.

- It is transmitted via spores. Describe the action that takes place when the spores are in an acceptable host.

- The disease is not transmitted by contact with an infected person.

- Review the diagnostic tests used to identify an anthrax infection.

- Discuss the use of anthrax as a chemical weapon.

Slide 43

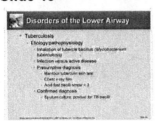

- Tuberculosis (TB) is a chronic pulmonary and extrapulmonary contagious disease.

- Discuss the demographics associated with TB.

- A TB infection differs from the active disease TB. Compare and contrast their differences.

- The number of cases of TB has had several historical fluctuations. Before the 1950s, TB was considered a near epidemic in the Western world. What factors in the 1950s resulted in a reduction in the number of cases?

- The number of TB cases has begun a gradual increase. What factors can help explain the recent increase in the number of cases?

Slide 44

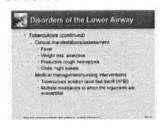

- The treatment/management of TB rely on drug therapies. What drugs are indicated for the treatment of TB?

- What precautions are needed to reduce the spread of disease when the patient with TB is in the hospital environment?

- What education will be needed by the patient and family experiencing a diagnosis of TB?

Mosby items and derived items © 2011, 2007 by Mosby, Inc., an affiliate of Elsevier Inc.
Some material was previously published.

Slide 45

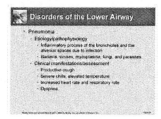

- Pneumonia is most commonly contracted in the winter and early spring months.

- The underlying causes of pneumonia might not only be related to an infection but also to oversedation, inadequate ventilation, or aspiration.

- What populations are at the greatest risk for contracting pneumonia?

Slide 46

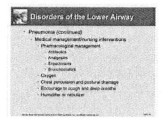

- The clinical manifestations associated with pneumonia will vary between individuals. Most will experience a productive cough. The other signs and symptoms will differ depending upon the causative agent.

- When attempting to pinpoint a diagnosis, what testing will be indicated?

Slide 47

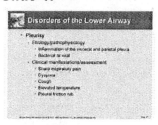

- Pleurisy can occur spontaneously but more often occurs as a complication of other respiratory disorders such as pneumonia, pulmonary infarctions, viral infections, pleural trauma, or early stages of TB or lung tumors.

Slide 48

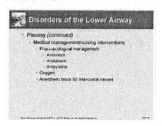

- When providing care for the patient diagnosed with pleurisy, the nurse's responsibilities include both monitoring the patient and providing comfort measures.

- With what frequency should the nursing assessments be performed?

- What is the prognosis for the patient diagnosed with pleurisy?

Slide 49

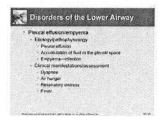

- Pleural effusion rarely results independently. It usually accompanies another disease process. With what diseases is pleural effusion often associated?

Adult Health Nursing, 6th ed.

Christensen & Kockrow

Slide 50

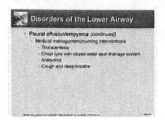

- The focus of nursing care for the patient experiencing pleural effusion involves monitoring, education concerning the disease process, and respiratory care treatments.

Slide 51

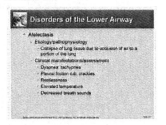

- Atelectasis causes an imbalance in the body between carbon dioxide and oxygen. In this condition, a blockage prevents the normal exchange of gases.

- What are potential causes of atelectasis?

- The location of the occlusion will determine the severity and the clinical manifestations.

Slide 52

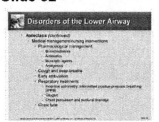

- When caring for the patient diagnosed with atelectasis, what items will need to be included in the nursing assessment?

- What diagnostic tests will be used to confirm the presence of atelectasis?

- What is the prognosis for the patient diagnosed with atelectasis? What factors will aid in determining this?

Slide 53

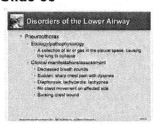

- The disruption in the negative pressure of the pleural space is what impairs the ability of the lung to remain inflated. What events might cause a pneumothorax?

Slide 54

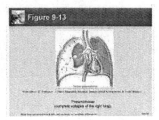

- Ask the students to study the illustration. As they view it, ask them what they anticipate will occur to the initially unaffected side as the pressure forces the lung to remain collapsed and then presses to that side. Ask the students to consider the cardiac implications.

Adult Health Nursing, 6th ed.
Christensen & Kockrow

Slide 55

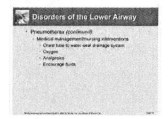

- When providing care to the patient diagnosed with a pneumothorax, what are the priorities for care?
- Identify three nursing diagnoses appropriate for the care of this patient.

Slide 56

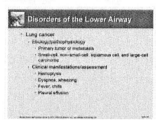

- The number of people in the United States diagnosed with lung cancer has continued to grow over the past several decades.
- To what factors can this increase be attributed?
- List risk factors associated with the development of lung cancer.
- Discuss the concept of "passive smoke."

Slide 57

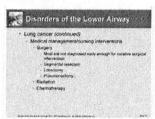

- The plan of treatment is largely determined by the stage of the malignancy when diagnosed.
- Unfortunately, diagnosis is often made late in the disease. This is related to the subtlety and gradual occurrence of clinical manifestations.
- Discuss the areas of the body to which lung cancer is known to metastasize. What types of cancer are associated with spreading to the lungs?
- What is the prognosis for patients with lung cancer?

Slide 58

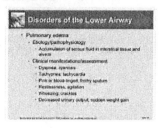

- Pulmonary edema is a serious condition that could result in death unless treated promptly.
- What factors can lead to the occurrence of pulmonary edema?
- Outline the sequence of events that take place during the onset and progression of pulmonary edema.

Slide 59

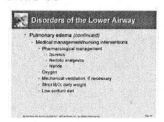

- Prompt diagnosis and treatment of the patient suspected of pulmonary edema is vital for survival. What diagnostic tests are indicated for the disorder? What findings will support the presence of pulmonary edema?
- What information will need to be collected and documented by the nurse?

Christensen & Kockrow

Slide 60

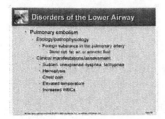

- The most common abnormal occurrence relating to pulmonary perfusion is pulmonary embolus.

- What populations are at highest risk for the development of an embolus? What characteristics place them at this elevated risk?

Slide 61

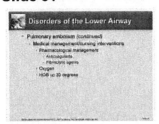

- When events occur that indicate the presence of a pulmonary embolus, what diagnostic tests will be used to support the diagnosis?

- What findings will confirm the presence of the pulmonary embolus?

- The treatment of a pulmonary embolus is long-term and will continue long after the initial hospitalization. What will be included in the long-term care plan of this patient?

Slide 62

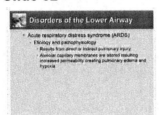

- Causes of ARDS may be viral or bacterial. Identify sources of pulmonary trauma or injury that may also cause the disorder.

Slide 63

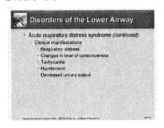

- ARDS manifests 12 to 24 hours after injury.

- Diagnostic testing focuses on pulmonary function testing

Slide 64

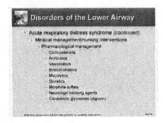

Slide 65

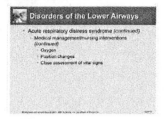

- What is the prognosis for the patient with acute respiratory distress syndrome?

- Identify two nursing diagnoses for the patient with acute respiratory distress syndrome.

Slide 66

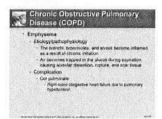

- Emphysema is a chronic obstructive pulmonary disease.

- The initial clinical manifestations often begin between the ages of 50 to 60 years.

- What risk factors are associated with the development of emphysema?

Slide 67

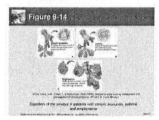

- Compare and contrast the disorders on the chart.

- Which students have cared for patients with any of the diagnoses highlighted during their clinical rotations?

Slide 68

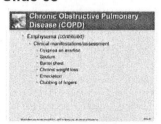

- The physical changes that characteristically accompany emphysema include clubbing of fingers, weight loss resulting in emaciation, and "barrel chesting." What elements in the disease process can explain these changes in appearance?

Slide 69

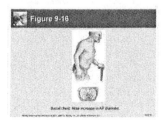

Adult Health Nursing, 6th ed.

Christensen & Kockrow

Slide 70

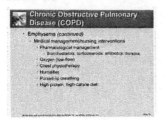

- Emphysema is a disease that has no cure. The treatment plan will be lifelong.
- What are the psychosocial implications associated with the diagnosis of this disease?

Slide 71

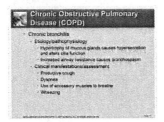

- Criteria needed to achieve a diagnosis of chronic bronchitis involve the presence of a recurrent or chronic, productive cough for at least 3 months a year for a 2-year time period.
- What populations/behaviors are associated with the development of chronic bronchitis?
- Explain in detail the progression of the development of the disease.

Slide 72

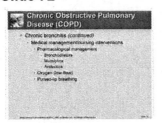

- Initial chest x-rays might not demonstrate abnormalities. Changes might not be evident until the later stages of the disease.
- What laboratory tests could be employed? What findings will support a diagnosis of chronic bronchitis?

Slide 73

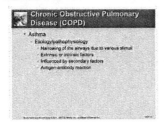

Slide 74

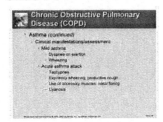

- In addition to mild asthma and acute asthmatic attacks, sufferers can also experience an event known as status asthmaticus. This is a life-endangering episode that does not respond to normal interventions. Explain the process that takes place during status asthmaticus.

Adult Health Nursing, 6th ed.

Mosby items and derived items © 2011, 2007 by Mosby, Inc., an affiliate of Elsevier Inc.
Some material was previously published.

Christensen & Kockrow

Slide 75

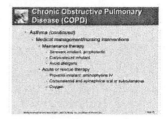

- The medical management of asthma involves maintenance therapy and acute/rescue therapy. Maintenance therapy is geared toward providing medications to allow the patient to live as normally as possible by controlling the symptoms.

- Describe rescue therapy.

Slide 76

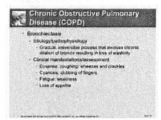

- What conditions might promote the development of bronchiectasis?

- Discuss preventive measures.

Slide 77

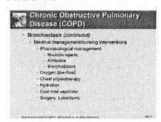

- When suspecting bronchiectasis, what diagnostic testing will be done?

- Outline the prognosis for the patient experiencing bronchiectasis.

Slide 78

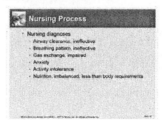

TEACHING FOCUS

In this chapter, the student will be introduced to the care of the patient with a urinary disorder. The student will begin by exploring the structure and function of the urinary system, including urine formation, the components of urine, and the hormones that influence nephron function. Next, the student will have the opportunity to learn about the disorders of the urinary tract, nursing diagnoses related to alterations in urinary function, the changes in body image created by an alteration in urinary function, and the effects of aging and renal disease on the urinary system. The student also will explore teaching methods, community resources, and pharmacotherapeutic and nutritional considerations for the patient with a urinary disorder.

MATERIALS AND RESOURCES

- ☐ Computer/overhead projector (all lessons)
- ☐ White/black board and marker/chalk (all lessons)
- ☐ Copies of diagrams of the kidney, urethra, and bladder for each student (Lesson 10.1)
- ☐ Set of index cards, each labeled with a concern associated with aging and the urinary system (Lesson 10.1)
- ☐ Blank index cards (Lesson 10.1)
- ☐ Blank teaching plans (Lesson 10.3)

LESSON CHECKLIST

Preparations for this lesson include:

- Lecture
- Invite a family social worker to speak with the class about resources available in the community.
- Invite one or two family members of a patient undergoing dialysis to speak with the class.

KEY TERMS

anasarca (FAAHN p. 1703, AHN p. 467)
anuria (FAAHN p. 1707, AHN p. 471)
asthenia (FAAHN p. 1687, AHN p. 451)
azotemia (FAAHN p. 1691, AHN p. 455)
bacteriuria (FAAHN p. 1687, AHN p. 451)
costovertebral angle (FAAHN p. 1691, AHN p. 455)
cytologic evaluation (FAAHN p. 1697, AHN p. 461)
dialysis (FAAHN p. 1710, AHN p. 474)
dysuria (FAAHN p. 1677, AHN p. 441)
hematuria (FAAHN p. 1687, AHN p. 451)

hydronephrosis (FAAHN p. 1693, AHN p. 457)
ileal conduit (FAAHN p. 1714, AHN p. 478)
micturition (FAAHN p. 1693, AHN p. 457)
nephrotoxin (FAAHN p. 1716, AHN p. 480)
nocturia (FAAHN p. 1687, AHN p. 451)
oliguria (FAAHN p. 1703, AHN p. 467)
prostatodynia (FAAHN p. 1690, AHN p. 454)
pyuria (FAAHN p. 1687, AHN p. 451)
residual urine (FAAHN p. 1684, AHN p. 448)
retention (FAAHN p. 1684, AHN p. 448)
urolithiasis (FAAHN p. 1693, AHN p. 457)

ADDITIONAL RESOURCES (AHN)

PPT Ch. 50, 1 through 57 FAAHN (Ch. 10, 1 through 57 AHN)
EILR IC images Ch. 50, 1through 14 FAAHN (Ch. 10, 1 through 14 AHN)
EILR TB questions Ch. 50, 1 through 44 FAAHN (Ch. 10, 1 through 44 AHN)
EILR Open Book Quiz Ch. 50, 1 through 10 FAAHN (Ch. 10, 1 through 10 AHN)
ESLR Review Questions for the NCLEX® Examination Ch. 50, 50-01 through 50-10 FAAHN (Ch. 10, 10-01 through 10-10 AHN)

Legend

PPT
PowerPoint
Slides

EILR
EVOLVE Instructor
Learning Resources:
Image Collection, Test
Bank, Open Book Quizzes

ESLR
EVOLVE Student
Learning Resources:
Review Questions
for the NCLEX
Examination

SG
Study Guide

NCP CTQ
Nursing Care Plan
Critical Thinking
Question

Class Activities are indicated in **bold italic**.

LESSON 10.1

PRETEST

1. The _____ is the functional unit of the kidney.
   a. nephron
   b. renal pelvis
   c. renal pyramid
   d. renal papilla

2. When ketone bodies are located in the urine, it indicates:
   a. potential infection or tumors.
   b. toxicity of the urine related to heavy metal exposure.
   c. the oxidation of fatty acids.
   d. probable kidney disease.

3. When providing care to a patient whose physician has ordered the PSA test, you are questioned about the ordered test. What information will you include in your response?
   a. The PSA is less accurate than the PAP test, but it is the first line of recommended testing at this time.
   b. A PSA result of less than 4 ng/mL is associated with the presence of benign prostatic hypertrophy and prostatitis.
   c. The PSA should be obtained after the physician completes the physical examination.
   d. Elevated PSA results are associated with the presence of prostate cancer.

4. The collection of a creatinine clearance test involves which of the following?
   a. A urine specimen is obtained by using a straight catheter to ensure the specimen is not contaminated.
   b. A blood specimen is collected after the morning meal the day of the test.
   c. The urine will be collected over a 24-hour period.
   d. The collection period begins with the first kept urine specimen.

5. A patient diagnosed with acute renal failure can expect to have which of the following medications prescribed to promote diuresis during the oliguric phase?
   a. Nalidixic Acid
   b. Osmitrol
   c. Triamterene
   d. Furosemide

6. While providing care for a patient who has blood in his urine, which of the following catheters will be most effective?
   a. Malecot
   b. Robinson
   c. Whistle-tip
   d. Suprapubic

7. Reabsorption of water, glucose, and necessary ions back into the blood takes place in the
   _____.
   a. loop of Henle
   b. Bowman's capsule
   c. distal convoluted tubule
   d. glomerulus

8. A patient has been diagnosed with cystitis. Which of the following may have contributed to the development of this condition?
   a. Recent catheterization
   b. The use of steroids
   c. Immobility
   d. Hypertension

9. A patient who has been experiencing urinary difficulty has been diagnosed with benign prostatic hypertrophy. Which of the following statements by the patient indicates the need for further teaching?
   a. "The physician may prescribe medications to manage my condition."
   b. "The insertion of a Foley catheter can help relieve my discomfort."
   c. "I may need radiation to manage this condition."
   d. "Surgery may be indicated to manage this condition."

10. When providing care for the patient diagnosed with nephritis, which of the following dietary changes is indicated?
    a. Increase protein to promote healing
    b. Increase calories to increase energy
    c. Increase sodium to replenish blood levels
    d. Reduce calcium to assist the kidney's filtration responsibilities

Answers:

1. a	2. c	3. d	4. c	5. b
6. c	7. a	8. a	9. c	10. b

BACKGROUND ASSESSMENT

Question: You are assigned to provide care to a 71-year-old woman. She has been hospitalized for complications of diabetes and has been incontinent. To reduce the risk of skin breakdown, her physician has ordered an indwelling Foley catheter. What care is needed for the catheter? What documentation will be required?

Answer: An indwelling Foley catheter must have appropriate care to prevent infection or other complications. Once anchored, catheter care is needed at least twice daily. Mild soap and water should be used. The catheter bag must be kept below the level of the bladder to prevent reflux of urine. The bag will need to be emptied as indicated at least once per shift. It is the responsibility of the nurse to ensure there is adequate urine drainage. Documentation must include placement of the catheter and information concerning the characteristics of the urine drained. The amount of urine must be recorded at the end of each shift.

Question: A 23-year-old woman has been diagnosed with, and treatment has been prescribed for, a urinary tract infection. As you are giving her the prescriptions written by her physician, she states, "I don't know why this keeps happening to me. This is the third time I have been diagnosed with this problem." What information should she be given? What populations have a higher incidence of urinary tract infections?

Answer: Urinary tract infections result when pathogens enter the system. They are more common in women because of the shorter length of their urethras. Other groups at higher risk include the elderly, immobile patients, and those experiencing multiorgan impairments. Preventive care information should be provided. Prevention includes voiding after sex, increased fluid intake, and good personal hygiene habits. She should be advised to take the entire prescribed course of medication.

CRITICAL THINKING QUESTION

You are assigned to care for a patient who has been prescribed a spironolactone (Aldactone). The patient has questions concerning the medication. He reports he has family members who take diuretics. He is concerned about the need to increase the amount of potassium in his diet and the need for potassium supplements. Based upon your knowledge about this medication, what information will be needed by the patient?

Guidelines: Spironolactone (Aldactone) is a diuretic. It is considered a potassium-sparing diuretic. This means it does not deplete the amount of potassium. Potassium supplements and increased potassium-containing foods will not be needed in relation to these medications. There are diuretic medications that do deplete potassium. Fortunately, the medication prescribed to the patient is not one of them.

OBJECTIVES	CONTENT	TEACHING RESOURCES
Describe the structures of the urinary system, including functions.	■ Anatomy and physiology of the urinary system (FAAHN p. 1670, AHN p. 434) □ Kidneys (FAAHN p. 1670, AHN p. 434) – Gross anatomical structure (FAAHN p. 1671, AHN p. 435) – Microscopic structure (FAAHN p. 1671, AHN p. 435)	PPT 2 through 6, Ch. 50 FAAHN (Ch. 10 PPT 2 through 6 AHN) EILR IC Ch. 50 images 1, 2, 5 FAAHN (Ch. 10 images 1, 2, 5 AHN) EILR TB Ch. 50 question 3 FAAHN (Ch. 10 question 3 AHN) EILR Open Book Quiz Ch. 50 question 1 FAAHN (Ch. 10 question 1 AHN) ESLR Review Questions for the NCLEX Examination Ch. 50 question 1 FAAHN (Ch. 10 question 1 AHN) SG Ch. 50 Structures, p. 429; Renal Tubules, p. 431 FAAHN (Ch. 10 pp. 117, 119 AHN) **BOOK RESOURCES** Fig. 50-1 Locations of the urinary system organs (FAAHN p. 1671) (Fig. 10-1 AHN p. 435) Fig. 50-2 Coronal section through right kidney (FAAHN p. 1671) (Fig. 10-2 AHN p. 435) Fig. 50-3 The nephron unit (FAAHN p. 1672) (Fig. 10-3 AHN p. 436) Fig. 50-4 Cross-section from the four segments of the renal tubule (FAAHN p. 1673) (Fig. 10-4 AHN p. 437) Fig. 50-5 the male urinary bladder, cut to show the interior (FAAHN p. 1674) (Fig. 10-5 AHN p. 438) Review Questions for the NCLEX Examination Ch. 50 questions 1, 9 FAAHN (Ch. 10 questions 1, 9 AHN)

OBJECTIVES	CONTENT	TEACHING RESOURCES
		▸ Discuss the anatomy and physiology of the urinary system. *Class Activity Distribute diagrams of the kidney, urethra, and bladder. Instruct the students to label the major parts of each. Allow only a brief period of time for this task. After the answers are reviewed, reward any student with all answers correct. This reward can consist of a piece of fruit or pencils.*
List the three processes involved in urine formation.	– Microscopic structure (FAAHN p. 1671, AHN p. 435)	▰ EILR IC Ch. 50 images 3, 4 FAAHN (Ch. 10 images 3, 4 AHN) ▰ EILR Open Book Quiz Ch. 50 question 12 FAAHN (Ch. 10 question 12 AHN) ▰ SG Urine Ch. 50 p. 430 FAAHN (Ch. 10 p. 118 AHN) **BOOK RESOURCES** Fig. 50-4 Cross-section from the four segments of the renal tubule (FAAHN p. 1673) (Fig. 10-4 AHN p. 437) Table 50-1 Functions of Parts of the Nephron in Urine Formation (FAAHN p. 1673) (Table 10-1 AHN p. 437) Box 50-1 Major Functions of the Kidneys (FAAHN p. 1674) (Box 10-1 AHN p. 438) ▸ Discuss the three processes involved in the formation of urine. ▸ Discuss the impact on the patient if any one of the processes is not functioning. *Class Activity Ask each student to take out a sheet of paper. Instruct each student to illustrate the manner in which urine is formed.*
Name three hormones and their influence on nephron function.	– Microscopic structure (FAAHN p. 1671, AHN p. 435)	▰ SG Hormones, Ch. 50 p. 430 FAAHN (Ch. 10 p. 118 AHN) ▸ Discuss the hormones involved in the urinary system. ▸ Discuss the implications of hormonal imbalances on the urinary system. *Class Activity Instruct each student to develop two or three NCLEX-style questions concerning the hormonal influence on the nephrons. After the questions are completed,*

Adult Health Nursing, 6th ed.
Christensen & Kockrow

OBJECTIVES	CONTENT	TEACHING RESOURCES
		ask each student to spend a few minutes with a peer to quiz each other verbally using the questions. After time has passed, call for a switch and ask the students to meet with another classmate. This drill can be continued as long as time permits.
Compare the normal components of urine with the abnormal components.	☐ Urine composition and characteristics (FAAHN p. 1674, AHN p. 438) ☐ Urine abnormalities (FAAHN p. 1674, AHN p. 438) ■ Laboratory and diagnostic examinations (FAAHN p. 1675, AHN p. 439) ☐ Urinalysis (FAAHN p. 1675, AHN p. 439) ☐ Specific gravity (FAAHN p. 1676, AHN p. 440) ☐ Blood (serum) urea nitrogen (FAAHN p. 1676, AHN p. 440) ☐ Blood (serum) creatinine (FAAHN p. 1676, AHN p. 440) ☐ Creatinine clearance (FAAHN p. 1676, AHN p. 440) ☐ Prostate-specific antigen (FAAHN p. 1676, AHN p. 440) ☐ Osmolality (FAAHN p. 1677, AHN p. 441) ☐ Kidney-ureter-bladder radiography (FAAHN p. 1677, AHN p. 441) ☐ Intravenous pyelogram (IVP)/ intravenous urography (FAAHN p. 1677, AHN p. 441) ☐ Retrograde pyelography (FAAHN p. 1677, AHN p. 441) ☐ Voiding cystourethrography (FAAHN p. 1677, AHN p. 441) ☐ Endoscopic procedures (FAAHN p. 1677, AHN p. 441) ☐ Renal angiography (FAAHN p. 1678, AHN p. 442) ☐ Renal venogram (FAAHN p. 1678, AHN p. 442)	⊠▤ PPT 7, 8 Ch. 50 FAAHN (Ch. 10 PPT 7, 8 AHN) ▰ ESLR Review Questions for the NCLEX Examination Ch. 50 questions 3, 4 FAAHN (Ch. 10 questions 3, 4 AHN) ▱sg SG Urine, Ch. 50 p. 430 FAAHN (Ch. 10 p. 118 AHN) **BOOK RESOURCES** Cultural Considerations: Urinary Disorder Ch. 50 p. 1675 FAAHN (Ch. 10 p. 439 AHN) Table 50-2 Urinalysis (FAAHN p. 1676) (Table 10-2 AHN p. 440) Review Questions for the NCLEX Examination Ch. 50 questions 12, 35 FAAHN (Ch. 10 questions 12, 35 AHN) ▸ Discuss the normal components of urine. ▸ Discuss testing performed on urine to determine composition. *Class Activity Obtain a laboratory reporting sheet. Make copies and distribute to the class. Instruct the students to view the normal and abnormal results. Ask the students to work together and make suggestions concerning the implications of each abnormality.*

Christensen & Kockrow

OBJECTIVES	CONTENT	TEACHING RESOURCES
	☐ Computed tomography (FAAHN p. 1678, AHN p. 442)	
	☐ Magnetic resonance imaging (MRI) (FAAHN p. 1678, AHN p. 442)	
	☐ Renal scan (FAAHN p. 1678, AHN p. 442)	
	☐ Ultrasonography (FAAHN p. 1678, AHN p. 442)	
	☐ Transrectal ultrasound (FAAHN p. 1678, AHN p. 442)	
	☐ Renal biopsy (FAAHN p. 1678, AHN p. 442)	
	☐ Urodynamic studies (FAAHN p. 1678, AHN p. 442)	
Identify the effects of aging on urinary system function.	☐ Normal aging of the urinary system (FAAHN p. 1675, AHN p. 439)	*e* EILR TB Ch. 50 question 40 FAAHN (Ch. 10 question 40 AHN) *e* ESLR Review Questions for the NCLEX Examination Ch. 50 question 2 FAAHN (Ch. 10 question 2 AHN) SG Aging, Ch. 50 p. 436 FAAHN (Ch. 10 p. 124 AHN) **BOOK RESOURCES** Life Span Considerations, Older Adult: Urinary Disorder (FAAHN p. 1675) (AHN p. 439) ▸ Discuss the changes anticipated in the urinary system with aging. ▸ Discuss the preventive care an individual can incorporate into daily life to maintain function of the urinary system. *Class Activity Prepare index cards for distribution. On each card record a concern associated with aging and the urinary system. Distribute cards to half of the class. Next, randomly pair the students. The students with the index cards will role-play the patient. The students without cards will act as the nurse. The role of the nurse is to collect information regarding the problems associated with aging and the urinary system. After a brief time period, instruct the students to identify two individualized nursing diagnoses for their assigned disorder.*

OBJECTIVES	CONTENT	TEACHING RESOURCES
Appraise the changes in body image created when the patient experiences an alteration in urinary function.	☐ Normal aging of the urinary system (FAAHN p. 1675, AHN p. 439)	⎚ EILR TB Ch. 50 question 30 FAAHN (Ch. 10 question 30 AHN) ⎚ ESLR Review Questions for the NCLEX Examination Ch. 50 question 5 FAAHN (Ch. 10 question 5 AHN) ⎚ SG Body Image, Ch. 50 p. 435 FAAHN (Ch. 10 p. 123 AHN) **BOOK RESOURCES** ▸ Discuss the psychosocial implications associated with urinary dysfunction. ▸ Discuss the assessment of coping mechanisms. *Class Activity **Prepare a scenario that has the patient seeking care for a urinary dysfunction. Divide the students into pairs and assign each student the role of patient or nurse. After the experience, ask the groups to discuss as a class the difficulty experienced in discussing such personal matters.***

Incorporate pharmaco-therapeutic and nutritional considerations into the nursing care plan of the patient with a urinary disorder.	■ Medication considerations (FAAHN p. 1679, AHN p. 443)
	
	☐ Diuretics to enhance urinary output (FAAHN p. 1679, AHN p. 443)
	
	  – Thiazide diuretics (FAAHN p. 1679, AHN p. 443)
	
	  – Loop (or high ceiling) diuretics (FAAHN p. 1679, AHN p. 443)
	
	  – Potassium-sparing diuretics (FAAHN p. 1680, AHN p. 444)
	
	  – Osmotic diuretics (FAAHN p. 1680, AHN p. 444
	
	  – Carbonic anhydrase inhibitor diuretics (FAAHN p. 1680, AHN p. 444)
	
	  – Nursing interventions (FAAHN p. 1680, AHN p. 444)
	
	☐ Medications for urinary tract infections (FAAHN p. 1680, AHN p. 444)
	
	  – Nursing interventions (FAAHN p. 1681, AHN p. 445)
		▦ PPT 9 Ch. 50 FAAHN (Ch. 10 PPT 9 AHN)
		
		⎚ EILR TB Ch. 50 questions 7, 19, 21, 22, 25, 26, 29, 32, 33, 39, 41 FAAHN (Ch. 10 questions 7, 19, 21, 22, 25, 26, 29, 32, 33, 39, 41 AHN)
		
		⎚ EILR Open Book Quiz Ch. 50 questions 4, 5 FAAHN (Ch. 10 questions 4, 5 AHN)
		
		⎚ SG Drugs and Nutrition, Ch. 50 p. 436 FAAHN (Ch. 10 p. 124 AHN)
		
		BOOK RESOURCES
		
		Table 50-3 Medications that Affect the Urinary System Table (FAAHN p. 1679) (Table 10-3 AHN p. 443)
		
		Box 50-2 Acid-Ash and Alkaline-Ash Foods (FAAHN p. 1681) (Box 10-2 AHN p. 445)
		
		Review Questions for the NCLEX Examination Ch. 50 questions 8 through 10, 12, 27, 32 through 34 FAAHN (Ch. 10 questions 8 through 10, 12, 27, 32 through 34 AHN)
		
		▸ Discuss the nursing implications when planning to administer medications to treat/manage a urinary dysfunction.
		
		▸ Discuss the patient teaching needed for the patient prescribed medications to manage a urinary dysfunction.

ELSEVIER

OBJECTIVES	CONTENT	TEACHING RESOURCES
	■ Nutritional considerations (FAAHN p. 1681, AHN p. 445)	*Class Activity Pass index cards to students and ask them to develop two NCLEX-style questions relating to nutritional or pharmacotherapeutic topics. Use these questions in a class review of content.*
Prioritize the special needs of the patient with urinary dysfunction.	■ Maintaining adequate urinary drainage (FAAHN p. 1681, AHN p. 445) ☐ Types of catheters (FAAHN p. 1681, AHN p. 445) ☐ Nursing interventions and patient teaching (FAAHN p. 1682, AHN p. 446) – Self-catheterization (FAAHN p. 1683, AHN p. 447) – Bladder training (FAAHN p. 1683, AHN p. 447) ☐ Prognosis (FAAHN p. 1684, AHN p. 448)	PPT 10, 11 Ch. 50 FAAHN (Ch. 10 PPT 10, 11 AHN) EILR IC Ch. 50 image 6 FAAHN (Ch. 10 image 6 AHN) EILR TB Ch. 50 questions 4, 9 through 13, 35, 42, 43 FAAHN (Ch. 10 questions 4, 9 through 13, 35, 42, 43 AHN) EILR Open Book Quiz Ch. 50 question 8 FAAHN (Ch. 10 question 8 AHN) SG Special Needs, Ch. 50 p. 434 FAAHN (Ch. 10 p. 122 AHN) SG Kock Pouch, Ch. 50 p. 446 FAAHN (Ch. 10 p. 124 AHN) **BOOK RESOURCES** Fig. 50-6 Commonly used catheters (FAAHN p. 1682) (Fig. 10-6 AHN p. 446) Review Questions for the NCLEX Examination Ch. 50 questions 3, 4, 7, 11, 13 through 18, 22 FAAHN (Ch. 10 questions 3, 4, 7, 11, 13 through 18, 22 AHN) ▶ Discuss the assessment of patient needs when faced with health concerns involving a urinary function disorder. ▶ Discuss the development of patient-focused goals for the patient diagnosed with a urinary disorder. *Class Activity Instruct each student to develop two nursing diagnoses associated with care of a urinary disorder. After the diagnoses are completed, instruct students to share their work with a partner.*

Christensen & Kockrow

10.1 Homework/Assignments:

10.1 Instructor's Notes/Student Feedback:

LESSON 10.2

CRITICAL THINKING QUESTION

While you are working in an emergency room, a patient presents with complaints of severe flank pain, nausea, and vomiting. There is no temperature. A urine specimen reveals hematuria. Based upon your knowledge, what do you anticipate the medical diagnosis will be? What diagnostic tests will be ordered to confirm this diagnosis? What treatment will be employed to manage this patient's condition?

Guidelines: The clinical manifestations listed above are consistent with urolithiasis (kidney stones). These stones result from mineral formation in the urinary tract. When these stones become large enough to become lodged or move in the tract, pain will result. Potential diagnostic tests may include KUP, IVP, ultrasound, cystoscopy and urinalysis. This condition could be conservatively managed. The patient will be given analgesics, antibiotics, and emotional support. Fluid intake will be encouraged to allow the stone to migrate downward and, it is hoped, be voided. The nurses caring for the patient will be required to strain all urine. Intake and output will be monitored. Patients not able to pass the stone might undergo more invasive techniques.

OBJECTIVES	CONTENT	TEACHING RESOURCES
Describe the alterations in renal function associated with disorders of the urinary tract.	■ Disorders of the urinary system (FAAHN p. 1684, AHN p. 448) □ Alterations in voiding patterns (FAAHN p. 1684, AHN p. 448) □ Urinary retention (FAAHN p. 1684, AHN p. 448) – Etiology and pathophysiology (FAAHN p. 1684, AHN p. 448) – Clinical manifestations (FAAHN p. 1684, AHN p. 448) – Assessment (FAAHN p. 1684, AHN p. 448) – Medical management (FAAHN p. 1684, AHN p. 448) – Nursing interventions (FAAHN p. 1684, AHN p. 448) □ Urinary incontinence (FAAHN p. 1684, AHN p. 448) – Etiology and pathophysiology (FAAHN p. 1685, AHN p. 449) – Clinical manifestations (FAAHN p. 1685, AHN p. 449) – Assessment (FAAHN p. 1685, AHN p. 449) – Medical management (FAAHN p. 1685, AHN p. 449)	PPT 12 through 52 Ch. 50 FAAHN (Ch. 10 PPT 12 through 52 AHN) EILR IC Ch. 50 images 7, 8 FAAHN (Ch. 10 images 7, 8 AHN) EILR TB Ch. 50 questions 8, 14 through 18, 20, 23, 27, 28, 31, 34, 36 through 38, 44 FAAHN (Ch. 10 questions 8, 14 through 18, 20, 23, 27, 28, 31, 34, 36 through 38, 44 AHN) EILR Open Book Quiz Ch. 50 questions 2, 3, 6, 7, 9, 10 FAAHN (Ch. 10 questions 2, 3, 6, 7, 9, 10 AHN) ESLR Review Questions for the NCLEX Examination Ch. 50 questions 6 through 10, FAAHN (Ch. 10 questions 6 through 10 AHN) SG Alterations Ch. 50 p. 432 FAAHN (Ch. 10 p. 120 AHN) **BOOK RESOURCES** Complementary and Alternative Therapies: Urinary Disorders (FAAHN p. 1688) (AHN p. 452) Safety Alert! Cystitis (FAAHN p. 1689) (AHN p. 453) Fig. 50-7 Location and methods of removing renal calculi from upper urinary tract (FAAHN p. 1694) (Fig. 10-7 AHN p. 458) Box 50-3 Four Prostatecomy Techniques (FAAHN p. 1699) (Box 10-3 AHN p. 463)

OBJECTIVES	CONTENT	TEACHING RESOURCES
	– Nursing interventions (FAAHN p. 1686, AHN p. 450)	Fig. 50-8 Four types of prostatectomies (FAAHN p. 1699) (Fig. 10-8 AHN p. 463)
	☐ Neurogenic bladder (FAAHN p. 1686, AHN p. 450)	Health Promotion: The Patient with Nephritis (FAAHN p. 1705) (AHN p. 469)
	– Etiology and pathophysiology (FAAHN p. 1686, AHN p. 450)	Nursing Care Plan 50-1 The Patient with End-Stage Renal Disease (FAAHN p. 1709) (NCP 10-1 AHN p. 473)
	– Clinical manifestations (FAAHN p. 1686, AHN p. 450)	◌ NCP CTQ 1 through 3 (FAAHN p. 1710) (AHN p. 474)
	– Assessment (FAAHN p. 1686, AHN p. 450)	Box 50-4 Nursing Intervention Guidelines for the Patient Undergoing Hemodialysis (FAAHN p. 1711) (Box 10-4 AHN p. 475)
	– Diagnostic tests (FAAHN p. 1686, AHN p. 450)	Fig. 50-9 External arteriovenous shunt (FAAHN p. 1711) (Fig. 10-9 AHN p. 475)
	– Medical management (FAAHN p. 1686, AHN p. 450)	Fig. 50-10 Internal arteriovenous fistula (FAAHN p. 1711) (Fig. 10-10 AHN p. 475)
	– Nursing interventions and patient teaching (FAAHN p. 1687, AHN p. 451)	Communication: Psychosocial Aspects of Care for Patients Receiving Dialysis (FAAHN p. 1712) (AHN p. 476)
	■ Inflammatory and infectious disorders of the urinary system (FAAHN p. 1687, AHN p. 451)	Fig. 50-11 Peritoneal dialysis (FAAHN p. 1712) (Fig. 10-11 AHN p. 476)
	☐ Urinary tract infections (FAAHN p. 1687, AHN p. 451)	Box 50-5 Nursing Intervention Guidelines for the Patient Undergoing Peritoneal Dialysis (FAAHN p. 1713) (Box 10-5 AHN p. 477)
	– Etiology and pathophysiology (FAAHN p. 1687, AHN p. 451)	Table 50-4 Surgical Procedures for Urinary Dysfunction (FAAHN p. 1713) (Table 10-4 AHN p. 477)
	– Clinical manifestations (FAAHN p. 1687, AHN p. 451)	Fig. 50-12 Kidney transplantation (FAAHN p. 1714) (Fig. 10-12 AHN p. 478)
	– Assessment (FAAHN p. 1687, AHN p. 451)	Fig. 50-13 Ileal conduit or ileal loop (FAAHN p. 1715) (Fig. 10-13 AHN p. 479)
	– Diagnostic tests (FAAHN p. 1687, AHN p. 451)	Fig. 50-14 Kock pouch (FAAHN p. 1715) (Fig. 10-14 AHN p. 479)
	– Medical management (FAAHN p. 1688, AHN p. 452)	Review Questions for the NCLEX Examination Ch. 50 questions 5, 6, 21, 23 through 26, 28, 29, 31 FAAHN (Ch. 10 questions 4, 5, 21, 23 through 26, 28, 29, 31 AHN)
	– Nursing interventions (FAAHN p. 1688, AHN p. 452)	
	☐ Urethritis (FAAHN p. 1688, AHN p. 452)	▶ Discuss populations at risk for the development of urinary tract infections.
	– Etiology and pathophysiology (FAAHN p. 1688, AHN p. 452)	▶ Discuss preventive health measures that can be taken to reduce the risk of developing urinary tract infections.
	– Clinical manifestations (FAAHN p. 1688, AHN p. 452)	

Adult Health Nursing, 6th ed.

Christensen & Kockrow

OBJECTIVES	CONTENT	TEACHING RESOURCES
	– Assessment (FAAHN p. 1688, AHN p. 452)	*Class Activity Assign each student to a small group of three or four students. Instruct each group to develop three NCLEX-style questions for its assigned urinary disorder. The disorders to be assigned should include cystitis, interstitial cystitis, pyelonephritis, and urethritis. After the questions are completed, collect the finished copies and use them in a class review of the content.*
	– Diagnostic tests (FAAHN p. 1688, AHN p. 452)	
	– Medical management (FAAHN p. 1688, AHN p. 452)	
	– Nursing interventions (FAAHN p. 1689, AHN p. 453)	
	☐ Cystitis (FAAHN p. 1689, AHN p. 453)	
	– Etiology and pathophysiology (FAAHN p. 1689, AHN p. 453)	
	– Clinical manifestations (FAAHN p. 1689, AHN p. 453)	
	– Assessment (FAAHN p. 1689, AHN p. 453)	
	– Diagnostic tests (FAAHN p. 1689, AHN p. 453)	
	– Medical management (FAAHN p. 1689, AHN p. 453)	
	– Nursing interventions and patient teaching (FAAHN p. 1689, AHN p. 453)	
	– Prognosis (FAAHN p. 1689, AHN p. 453)	
	☐ Interstitial cystitis (FAAHN p. 1689, AHN p. 453)	
	– Etiology and pathophysiology (FAAHN p. 1689, AHN p. 453)	
	– Clinical manifestations (FAAHN p. 1690, AHN p. 454)	
	– Assessment (FAAHN p. 1690, AHN p. 454)	
	– Medical management (FAAHN p. 1690, AHN p. 454)	
	– Nursing interventions and patient teaching (FAAHN p. 1690, AHN p. 454)	
	– Prognosis (FAAHN p. 1690, AHN p. 454)	

Adult Health Nursing, 6th ed.
Christensen & Kockrow

OBJECTIVES	CONTENT	TEACHING RESOURCES
	☐ Prostatitis (FAAHN p. 1690, AHN p. 454)	
	– Etiology and pathophysiology (FAAHN p. 1690, AHN p. 454)	
	– Clinical manifestations (FAAHN p. 1690, AHN p. 454)	
	– Diagnostic tests (FAAHN p. 1690, AHN p. 454)	
	– Assessment (FAAHN p. 1691, AHN p. 455)	
	– Medical management (FAAHN p. 1691, AHN p. 455)	
	– Nursing interventions and patient teaching (FAAHN p. 1691, AHN p. 455)	
	– Prognosis (FAAHN p. 1691, AHN p. 455)	
	☐ Pyelonephritis (FAAHN p. 1691, AHN p. 455)	
	– Etiology and pathophysiology (FAAHN p. 1691, AHN p. 455)	
	– Clinical manifestations (FAAHN p. 1691, AHN p. 455)	
	– Assessment (FAAHN p. 1691, AHN p. 455)	
	– Diagnostic tests (FAAHN p. 1691, AHN p. 455)	
	– Medical management (FAAHN p. 1691, AHN p. 455)	
	– Nursing interventions and patient teaching (FAAHN p. 1692, AHN p. 456)	
	– Prognosis (FAAHN p. 1692, AHN p. 456)	
	■ Obstructive disorders of the urinary tract (FAAHN p. 1692, AHN p. 456)	
	☐ Urinary obstruction (FAAHN p. 1692, AHN p. 456)	
	– Etiology and pathophysiology (FAAHN p. 1692, AHN p. 456)	
	– Clinical manifestations (FAAHN p. 1692, AHN p. 456)	
	– Assessment (FAAHN p. 1692, AHN p. 456)	

OBJECTIVES	CONTENT	TEACHING RESOURCES
	– Diagnostic tests (FAAHN p. 1692, AHN p. 456) – Medical management (FAAHN p. 1692, AHN p. 456) – Nursing interventions (FAAHN p. 1693, AHN p. 457) – Prognosis (FAAHN p. 1693, AHN p. 457) ☐ Hydronephrosis (FAAHN p. 1693, AHN p. 457) – Etiology and pathophysiology (FAAHN p. 1693, AHN p. 457) – Clinical manifestations (FAAHN p. 1693, AHN p. 457) – Assessment (FAAHN p. 1693, AHN p. 457) – Diagnostic tests (FAAHN p. 1693, AHN p. 457) – Medical management (FAAHN p. 1693, AHN p. 457) – Nursing interventions and patient teaching (FAAHN p. 1693, AHN p. 457) – Prognosis (FAAHN p. 1693, AHN p. 457) ☐ Urolithiasis (FAAHN p. 1693, AHN p. 457) – Etiology and pathophysiology (FAAHN p. 1693, AHN p. 457) – Clinical manifestations (FAAHN p. 1694, AHN p. 458) – Assessment (FAAHN p. 1694, AHN p. 458) – Diagnostic tests (FAAHN p. 1694, AHN p. 458) – Medical management (FAAHN p. 1694, AHN p. 458) – Nursing interventions and patient teaching (FAAHN p. 1694, AHN p. 458) – Prognosis (FAAHN p. 1695, AHN p. 459) ■ Tumors of the urinary system (FAAHN p. 1695, AHN p. 459)	

Christensen & Kockrow

OBJECTIVES	CONTENT	TEACHING RESOURCES

	☐ Renal tumors (FAAHN p. 1695, AHN p. 459)
	
	  – Etiology and pathophysiology (FAAHN p. 1695, AHN p. 459)
	
	  – Clinical manifestations (FAAHN p. 1695, AHN p. 459)
	
	  – Assessment (FAAHN p. 1695, AHN p. 459)
	
	  – Diagnostic tests (FAAHN p. 1695, AHN p. 459)
	
	  – Medical management (FAAHN p. 1696, AHN p. 460)
	
	  – Nursing interventions and patient teaching (FAAHN p. 1696, AHN p. 460)
	
	  – Prognosis (FAAHN p. 1696, AHN p. 460)
	
	☐ Renal cysts (FAAHN p. 1696, AHN p. 460)
	
	  – Etiology and pathophysiology (FAAHN p. 1696, AHN p. 460)
	
	  – Clinical manifestations (FAAHN p. 1696, AHN p. 460)
	
	  – Assessment (FAAHN p. 1697, AHN p. 461)
	
	  – Diagnostic tests (FAAHN p. 1697, AHN p. 461)
	
	  – Medical management (FAAHN p. 1697, AHN p. 461)
	
	  – Nursing interventions (FAAHN p. 1697, AHN p. 461)
	
	  – Prognosis (FAAHN p. 1697, AHN p. 461)
	
	☐ Tumors of the urinary bladder (FAAHN p. 1697, AHN p. 461)
	
	  – Etiology and pathophysiology (FAAHN p. 1697, AHN p. 461)
	
	  – Clinical manifestations (FAAHN p. 1697, AHN p. 461)
	
	  – Assessment (FAAHN p. 1697, AHN p. 461)	

OBJECTIVES	CONTENT	TEACHING RESOURCES
	− Diagnostic tests (FAAHN p. 1697, AHN p. 461)	
	− Medical management (FAAHN p. 1697, AHN p. 461)	
	− Nursing interventions and patient teaching (FAAHN p. 1697, AHN p. 461)	
	− Prognosis (FAAHN p. 1698, AHN p. 462)	
	■ Conditions affecting the prostate gland (FAAHN p. 1698, AHN p. 462)	
	☐ Benign prostatic hypertrophy (FAAHN p. 1698, AHN p. 462)	
	− Etiology and pathophysiology (FAAHN p. 1698, AHN p. 462)	
	− Clinical manifestations (FAAHN p. 1698, AHN p. 462)	
	− Assessment (FAAHN p. 1698, AHN p. 462)	
	− Diagnostic tests (FAAHN p. 1698, AHN p. 462)	
	− Medical management (FAAHN p. 1698, AHN p. 462)	
	− Nursing interventions (FAAHN p. 1699, AHN p. 463)	
	− Prognosis (FAAHN p. 1700, AHN p. 464)	
	☐ Cancer of the prostate (FAAHN p. 1700, AHN p. 464)	
	− Etiology and pathophysiology (FAAHN p. 1700, AHN p. 464)	
	− Clinical manifestations (FAAHN p. 1700, AHN p. 464)	
	− Assessment (FAAHN p. 1700, AHN p. 464)	
	− Diagnostic tests (FAAHN p. 1700, AHN p. 464)	
	− Medical management (FAAHN p. 1701, AHN p. 465)	
	− Nursing interventions and patient teaching (FAAHN p. 1702, AHN p. 466)	
	− Prognosis (FAAHN p. 1702, AHN p. 466)	

OBJECTIVES	CONTENT	TEACHING RESOURCES
	☐ Urethral strictures (FAAHN p. 1702, AHN p. 466)	
	– Etiology and pathophysiology (FAAHN p. 1702, AHN p. 466)	
	– Clinical manifestations (FAAHN p. 1702, AHN p. 466)	
	– Assessment (FAAHN p. 1702, AHN p. 466)	
	– Diagnostic tests (FAAHN p. 1702, AHN p. 466)	
	– Medical management (FAAHN p. 1702, AHN p. 466)	
	– Nursing interventions (FAAHN p. 1703 AHN p. 467)	
	– Prognosis (FAAHN p. 1703, AHN p. 467)	
	☐ Urinary tract trauma (FAAHN p. 1703, AHN p. 467)	
	– Etiology and pathophysiology (FAAHN p. 1703, AHN p. 467)	
	– Clinical manifestations (FAAHN p. 1703, AHN p. 467)	
	– Assessment (FAAHN p. 1703, AHN p. 467)	
	– Diagnostic tests (FAAHN p. 1703, AHN p. 467)	
	– Medical management (FAAHN p. 1703, AHN p. 467)	
	– Nursing interventions (FAAHN p. 1703, AHN p. 467)	
	– Prognosis (FAAHN p. 1703, AHN p. 467)	
	■ Immunological disorders of the kidney (FAAHN p. 1703, AHN p. 467)	
	☐ Nephrotic syndrome (FAAHN p. 1703, AHN p. 467)	
	– Etiology and pathophysiology (FAAHN p. 1703, AHN p. 467)	
	– Clinical manifestations (FAAHN p. 1703, AHN p. 467)	

OBJECTIVES	CONTENT	TEACHING RESOURCES
	– Assessment (FAAHN p. 1703, AHN p. 467)	
	– Diagnostic tests (FAAHN p. 1704, AHN p. 468)	
	– Medical management (FAAHN p. 1704, AHN p. 468)	
	– Nursing interventions and patient teaching (FAAHN p. 1704, AHN p. 468)	
	– Prognosis (FAAHN p. 1704, AHN p. 468)	
	☐ Nephritis (FAAHN p. 1704, AHN p. 468)	
	– Acute glomerulonephritis (FAAHN p. 1704, AHN p. 468)	
	– Chronic glomerulonephritis (FAAHN p. 1705, AHN p. 469)	
	☐ Renal failure (FAAHN p. 1706, AHN p. 470)	
	☐ Acute renal failure (FAAHN p. 1706, AHN p. 470)	
	– Etiology and pathophysiology (FAAHN p. 1706, AHN p. 470)	
	– Clinical manifestations (FAAHN p. 1706, AHN p. 470)	
	– Assessment (FAAHN p. 1706, AHN p. 470)	
	– Diagnostic tests (FAAHN p. 1706, AHN p. 470)	
	– Medical management (FAAHN p. 1707, AHN p. 471)	
	– Nursing interventions and patient teaching (FAAHN p. 1707, AHN p. 471)	
	– Prognosis (FAAHN p. 1707, AHN p. 471)	
	☐ Chronic renal failure (end-stage renal disease) (FAAHN p. 1707, AHN p. 471)	
	– Etiology and pathophysiology (FAAHN p. 1707, AHN p. 471)	

Christensen & Kockrow

OBJECTIVES	CONTENT	TEACHING RESOURCES
	– Clinical manifestations (FAAHN p. 1707, AHN p. 471)	
	– Assessment (FAAHN p. 1707, AHN p. 471)	
	– Diagnostic tests (FAAHN p. 1708, AHN p. 472)	
	– Medical management (FAAHN p. 1708, AHN p. 472)	
	– Nursing interventions and patient teaching (FAAHN p. 1708, AHN p. 472)	
	■ Care of the patient requiring dialysis (FAAHN p. 1710, AHN p. 474)	
	□ Hemodialysis (FAAHN p. 1710, AHN p. 474)	
	– Medical management (FAAHN p. 1710, AHN p. 474)	
	– Nursing interventions (FAAHN p. 1711, AHN p. 475)	
	□ Peritoneal dialysis (FAAHN p. 1711, AHN p. 475)	
	– Nursing interventions (FAAHN p. 1711, AHN p. 475)	
	– Prognosis (FAAHN p. 1713, AHN p. 477)	
	■ Surgical procedures for urinary dysfunction (FAAHN p. 1713, AHN p. 477)	
	□ Nephrectomy (FAAHN p. 1713, AHN p. 477)	
	– Patient teaching (FAAHN p. 1713, AHN p. 477)	
	– Prognosis (FAAHN p. 1713, AHN p. 477)	
	□ Nephrostomy (FAAHN p. 1713, AHN p. 477)	
	□ Kidney transplantation (FAAHN p. 1714, AHN p. 478)	
	– Patient teaching (FAAHN p. 1714, AHN p. 478)	

OBJECTIVES	CONTENT	TEACHING RESOURCES
	– Prognosis (FAAHN p. 1714, AHN p. 478)	
	☐ Urinary diversion (FAAHN p. 1714, AHN p. 478)	
	– Patient teaching (FAAHN p. 1715, AHN p. 479)	
	– Prognosis (FAAHN p. 1715, AHN p. 479)	

10.2 Homework/Assignments:

10.2 Instructor's Notes/Student Feedback:

Adult Health Nursing, 6th ed.
Christensen & Kockrow

LESSON 10.3

CRITICAL THINKING QUESTION

A 30-year-old female has recently had surgery performed for a urinary diversion. The first day after the surgery, the patient appears extremely interested in her care and the care of the device. She is concerned about the odor of the urine, asking, "What can we do about that smell?" What information can be given to her concerning the inquiry?

Guidelines: The urinary diversion device will be a challenge to care for. The smell can be a clue to underlying conditions and concerns. Dietary intake can impact the odor. The avoidance of odor-producing foods, such as onions, beans, and cabbage, high fiber wheat, and simple sugars, will be helpful. There are drops and tablets available that can be placed in the bag to reduce/prevent odors. An excessive odor could signal an infection. The patient should also be advised that regular drainage of the bag will also be helpful.

OBJECTIVES	CONTENT	TEACHING RESOURCES
Discuss the effects of renal disease on family function.	☐ Hemodialysis (FAAHN p. 1710, AHN p. 474) – Medical management (FAAHN p. 1710, AHN p. 474) – Nursing interventions (FAAHN p. 1711, AHN p. 475) ☐ Kidney transplantation (FAAHN p. 1714, AHN p. 478) – Patient teaching (FAAHN p. 1714, AHN p. 478) ☐ Urinary diversion (FAAHN p. 1714, AHN p. 478) – Patient teaching (FAAHN p. 1715, AHN p. 479)	▰ EILR TB Ch. 50 question 5 FAAHN (Ch. 10 question 5 AHN) ▰ SG Patient/Family Support Ch. 50 p. 437 FAAHN (Ch. 10 p. 125 AHN) **BOOK RESOURCES** Health Promotion: The Patient with Renal Failure (FAAHN p. 1708) (AHN p. 472) Nursing Care Plan 50-1 The Patient with End-Stage Renal Disease FAAHN p. 1709 (NCP 10-1 AHN p. 473) Box 50-4 Nursing Intervention Guidelines for the Patient Undergoing Hemodialysis FAAHN p. 1711 (Box 10-4 AHN p. 475) Communication: Psychosocial Aspects of Care for Patients Receiving Dialysis (FAAHN p. 1712) (AHN p. 476) Home Care Considerations: Urinary Diversion Warning Signs (FAAHN p. 1716) (AHN p. 480) ▸ Discuss the assessment of patient coping mechanisms. ▸ Discuss both adaptive and maladaptive coping mechanisms. *Class Activity Invite one or two family members of a patient undergoing dialysis to visit with the class. Ask them to speak about the stresses experienced by the patient and family.* *Note: The local hospital unit might be able to provide a listing of speakers on this topic.*

Adult Health Nursing, 6th ed.
Christensen & Kockrow

Address patient concerns in teaching about altered sexuality secondary to urinary disorders and treatments.	– Medical management (FAAHN p. 1701, AHN p. 465) – Nursing interventions and patient teaching (FAAHN p. 1702, AHN p. 466)	SG Patient/Family Support Ch. 50 p. 437 FAAHN (Ch. 10 p. 125 AHN) ▶ Discuss therapies used in the management of prostate cancer that may result in a loss of sexual function. ▶ Discuss the emotional support needs of a patient receiving treatments that may result in a loss of sexual function *Class Activity Ask members of the class to work in pairs to develop two nursing diagnoses.*
Investigate community resources for support for the patient and significant others as they face lifestyle changes from chronic urinary disorders and treatment.	☐ Kidney transplantation (FAAHN p. 1714, AHN p. 478) – Patient teaching (FAAHN p. 1714, AHN p. 478) – Prognosis (FAAHN p. 1714, AHN p. 478) ☐ Urinary diversion (FAAHN p. 1714, AHN p. 478) – Patient teaching (FAAHN p. 1715, AHN p. 479) – Prognosis (FAAHN p. 1715, AHN p. 479)	PPT 55 through 57 Ch. 50 FAAHN (Ch. 10 PPT 55 through 57 AHN) EILR TB Ch. 50 question 6 FAAHN (Ch. 10 question 6 AHN) SG Patient/Family Support Ch. 50 p. 437 FAAHN (Ch. 10 p. 125 AHN) ▶ Discuss the emotional needs of the patient and family experiencing treatment for a chronic urinary disorder. ▶ Discuss community resources to consider when developing a long-range plan of care for the patient facing a chronic urinary disorder. *Class Activity Invite a family social worker to the class to discuss resources available in the community.*
Select nursing diagnoses related to alterations in urinary function.	☐ Nursing process for patients with a urinary disorder (FAAHN p. 1716, AHN p. 480) – Assessment (FAAHN p. 1716, AHN p. 480) – Nursing diagnoses (FAAHN p. 1716, AHN p. 480) – Expected outcomes and planning (FAAHN p. 1716, AHN p. 480) – Implementation (FAAHN p. 1716, AHN p. 480) – Evaluation (FAAHN p. 1716, AHN p. 481)	PPT 58, Ch. 50 FAAHN (Ch. 10 PPT 58 AHN) EILR TB Ch. 50 question 24 FAAHN (Ch. 10 question 24 AHN) SG Nursing Diagnoses, Ch. 50 p. 433 FAAHN (Ch. 10 p. 121 AHN) ▶ Discuss the priorities of care for the patient experiencing a urinary disorder. ▶ Discuss the development of a care plan for the patient diagnosed with a urinary disorder. *Class Activity Assign the students to groups of three or four. Randomly assign each group a urinary disorder. Instruct each group to develop two nursing interventions and patient-centered goals for the assigned disorder.*

Design culturally sensitive care of the patient with a urinary disorder.	☐ Nursing process for patients with a urinary disorder (FAAHN p. 1716, AHN p. 480)	SG Patient/Family Support Ch. 50 p. 437 FAAHN (Ch. 10 p. 125 AHN) ▸ Discuss the role of a cultural assessment in the care of the patient experiencing a urinary disorder. *Class Activity Ask each student to write down three impacts that culture will have on the needs of the patient being treated for a urinary disorder. Allow only a few minutes for this activity. Next, allow the students to share their thoughts and perspectives.*
	– Assessment (FAAHN p. 1716, AHN p. 480)	
	– Nursing diagnoses (FAAHN p. 1716, AHN p. 480)	
	– Expected outcomes and planning (FAAHN p. 1716, AHN p. 480)	
	– Implementation (FAAHN p. 1716, AHN p. 480)	
	– Evaluation (FAAHN p. 1716, AHN p. 481)	
Performance Evaluation		**E** EILR TB Ch. 50 questions 1 through 44 FAAHN (Ch. 10 questions 1 through 44 AHN) **E** EILR Open Book Quiz Ch. 50 question 1 through 10 FAAHN (Ch. 10 questions 1 through 10 AHN) **SG** SG Ch. 50 pp. 429 through 440 FAAHN (Ch. 10 pp. 117 through 128 AHN) **BOOK RESOURCES** Nursing Care Plan 50-1 The Patient with End-Stage Renal Disease (FAAHN p. 1709) (NCP 10-1 AHN p. 473) 💡 NCP CTQ 1 through 3 (FAAHN p. 1709) (AHN p. 473) Review Questions for the NCLEX Examination Ch. 50 questions 1 through 35 FAAHN (Ch. 10 questions 1 through 35 AHN)

10.3 Homework/Assignments:

10.3 Instructor's Notes/Student Feedback:

Adult Health Nursing, 6th ed.
Christensen & Kockrow

Slide 1

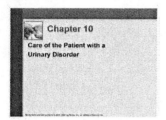

Slide 2

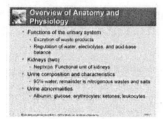

- As the body takes in nutrients to meet the body's requirements to sustain life, the breakdown of these elements results in waste products. The management of these waste products is handled by the urinary system.

- How is the body impacted by the different substances ingested by the body?

Slide 3

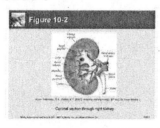

- The kidneys are dark red, bean-shaped organs. They are located, one on each side, toward the back of the body, just below the diaphragm.

- Describe the parts of the kidney.

Slide 4

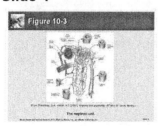

Slide 5

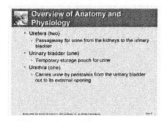

- The urinary system is comprised of two ureters, the bladder, and one urethra.

- What is the function of each of the parts listed?

Christensen & Kockrow

Slide 6

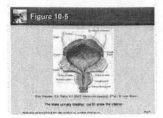

Slide 7

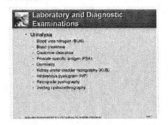

- When attempting to diagnose a disorder of the urinary system, the first line of testing involves the urine. The urine provides clues into many disorders.

- Collection of the specimen will vary by test.

- What is each of the listed tests used to evaluate? What education should the nurse provide to the patient regarding each of the listed tests?

Slide 8

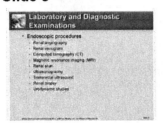

- In addition to analyzing the urine, detecting disorders of the urinary system can also include scanning or biopsy procedures.

- Review each of the tests listed and discuss the nursing implications for each.

Slide 9

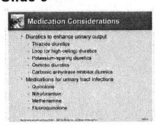

- Diuretics' method of action is accomplished by increasing the kidney's filtration of elements.

- In what disorders are the use of diuretics prescribed?

- There are different types of diuretics. What are examples of each type of diuretic? How do the types differ?

- In the event of an infection of the urinary system, antimicrobial medications can be prescribed. What nursing implications are indicated with each of the medications listed?

Slide 10

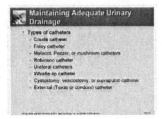

- Catheters are indicated when a patient's condition does not allow successful elimination of urine. In what cases is each of the catheter types indicated?

ELSEVIER

Mosby items and derived items © 2011, 2007 by Mosby, Inc., an affiliate of Elsevier Inc.
Some material was previously published.

Adult Health Nursing, 6th ed.
Christensen & Kockrow

Slide 11

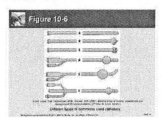

- Pictured are the types of catheters.

- Discuss the types and the times when their use is indicated.

- What are the nursing responsibilities associated with the care of a patient having an indwelling urinary catheter?

Slide 12

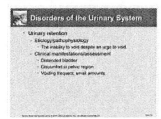

- When urinary retention results, what potential hazards exist?

- What nursing assessments are indicated to determine the presence of urinary retention?

Slide 13

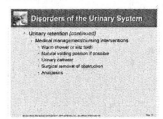

- Numerous interventions can be attempted to manage urinary retention. What are the goals of management?

- Ask students what interventions they have used or have observed being used in the clinical environment to manage urinary retention.

Slide 14

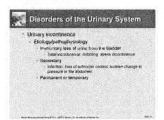

- Urinary incontinence is a common problem experienced by women.

- What subjective data should be assessed? What questions might assist the nurse in obtaining the needed information?

- What are potential causes of incontinence?

- Postmenopausal women have a greater risk for the development of urinary incontinence. What is the relationship between this stage in the lifespan of a woman and incontinence?

Slide 15

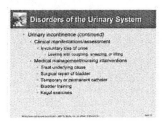

- The goals of management are the treatment of the underlying causes of incontinence.

- Urinary incontinence is an embarrassing problem. What role does the nurse have in assisting the patient at this difficult time?

ELSEVIER

Mosby items and derived items © 2011, 2007 by Mosby, Inc., an affiliate of Elsevier Inc.
Some material was previously published.

Adult Health Nursing, 6th ed.
Christensen & Kockrow

Slide 16

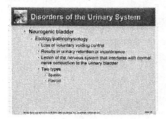

- A neurogenic bladder can be caused by a variety of factors. What are examples of potential causes?

Slide 17

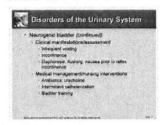

- When performing an assessment of a neurogenic bladder, the primary focus is locating the underlying cause and preventing complications.

- In addition to the observation of clinical manifestations, what diagnostic tests might be indicated?

- Medication therapies can be instituted in the management of a neurogenic bladder. What is the rationale for the use of these medications?

Slide 18

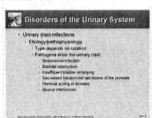

- Urinary tract infections result when pathogens enter the urinary tract. There are populations at risk for their development. Why are these people/groups at an increased risk?

- Compare and contrast urethritis, cystitis, interstitial cystitis, prostatitis, and pyelonephritis.

Slide 19

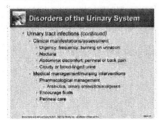

- Urinary tract infections can lead to increasingly complicated medical problems. Prevention of urinary tract infections is possible in many cases. What interventions can be instituted to reduce their incidence?

- Complementary and alternative therapies can be used to manage/prevent urinary tract infections.

Slide 20

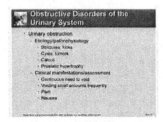

- An obstruction at any location within the urinary tract can adversely affect functioning. The onset of the obstruction can be sudden or result over a long period of time. What are potential causes for each of the categories listed above?

ELSEVIER

Mosby items and derived items © 2011, 2007 by Mosby, Inc., an affiliate of Elsevier Inc. Some material was previously published.

Adult Health Nursing, 6th ed.
Christensen & Kockrow

Slide 21

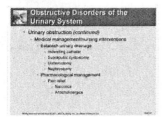

- When an obstruction is suspected, diagnostic tests will be performed to detect the location and cause. What tests can be anticipated for this purpose?
- What factors will determine the prognosis for a patient experiencing a urinary obstruction?

Slide 22

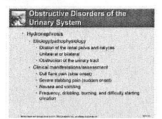

- When urine cannot adequately pass through the renal pelvis, potential damage can result. This is the pathophysiology of hydronephrosis.
- Not all patients experiencing hydronephrosis experience visible symptoms.
- The onset of hydronephrosis can be rapid or result after a long-term assault on the urinary system.
- Differentiate between the signs and symptoms that present both rapidly and slowly.
- What objective data will be collected from the patient demonstrating the clinical manifestations associated with hydronephrosis?

Slide 23

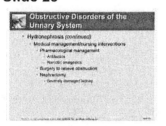

- In addition to the clinical picture presented, a series of diagnostic tests will be ordered to confirm the diagnosis and determine the degree of damage.
- What tests can be anticipated?
- Management options will vary, depending on the severity of the disease and the patient's response to treatment.
- What are the responsibilities of the nurse when providing care to this patient?
- What complications can occur as a result of hydronephrosis?

Slide 24

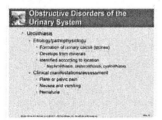

- Kidney stones are a painful event. Although there is no exact cause for their occurrence, there are predisposed populations and risk factors associated with their development.
- What populations experience kidney stones most frequently?
- What lifestyle changes can be implemented to reduce the risk in identified populations?

ELSEVIER

Adult Health Nursing, 6th ed.

Christensen & Kockrow

Slide 25

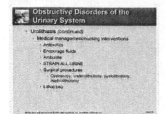

- When a patient presents with clinical manifestations associated with developing kidney stones, diagnostic tests will be performed to support the diagnosis.

- What tests can be anticipated? What findings will support the presence of kidney stones?

Slide 26

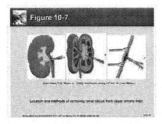

Slide 27

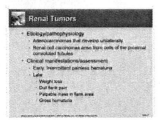

- Men are affected more commonly by renal tumors than women.

- Unfortunately, finding a renal tumor occurs late, when the tumor is quite large.

- What risk factors support the development of renal tumors? Which of these risk factors are modifiable?

Slide 28

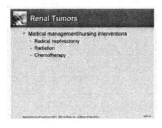

- Discuss the role of the nurse in the care of the patient diagnosed with renal tumors.

- What is the anticipated prognosis of the patient who has renal tumors?

Slide 29

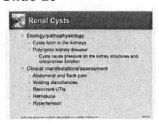

- Single cysts might never be detected because they might not hinder kidney functioning.

- Polycystic kidney disease is a genetic condition in which numerous cysts form in the kidney.

- What impact does the presence of cysts have on the kidney's ability to function?

Christensen & Kockrow

Slide 30

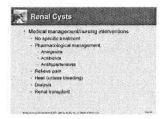

- When preparing to confirm a diagnosis of polycystic kidney disease, laboratory tests can be ordered. In addition, the physician could order screening tests to view the kidney. How will the kidney appear if the condition is present?

Slide 31

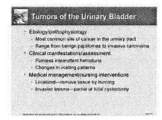

- Tumors of the urinary system are more common in men than women. Other than gender, what are some other risk factors for the development of these tumors?

- Often, the diagnosis of tumors of the bladder does not take place until the disease is advanced and the tumors are quite large. To what can this delay in diagnosis be attributed?

- What diagnostic tests might be ordered when evaluating tumors of the urinary system?

Slide 32

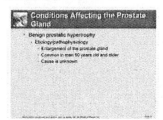

- The man's urethra is surrounded by the prostate gland. What is the function of the prostate gland?

- As men age, the gland might increase in size, causing problems. Although the cause is not known for certain, what theories could explain this occurrence?

Slide 33

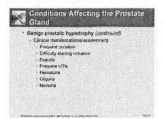

Slide 34

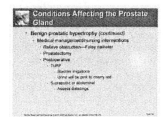

- When a patient presents with complaints involving the prostate gland, what diagnostic tests can be anticipated?

- Review the technique needed to examine the prostate gland.

- What findings will support a prostate disorder?

- When an enlarged prostate is diagnosed, what will determine the course of treatment?

Christensen & Kockrow

Slide 35

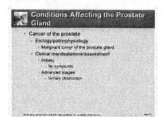

- Unfortunately, when cancer of the prostate gland is present, metastasis can result. What body structures are most prone to becoming sites of metastasis?
- Why is this type of cancer at a high risk for spreading?

Slide 36

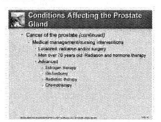

- What prognosis is associated with cancer of the prostate?

Slide 37

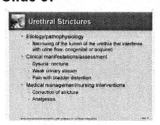

- Urethral stricture can be a painful condition. Identify potential causes of acquired urethral strictures.
- Discuss the assessment of a patient presenting with suspected urethral strictures.
- What questions should be asked during the data collection phase and the physical examination?

Slide 38

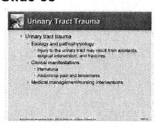

- Urinary tract trauma may result from lacerations and contusions to urinary tract structures.
- What diagnostic tests may be ordered to assess for the presence of urinary tract trauma?

Slide 39

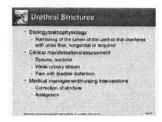

- Nephrotic syndrome is a grouping of interrelated clinical manifestations in which the permeability of the glomerulus is altered, resulting in changes in the composition of both blood and urine.
- Provide a detailed discussion of the resulting changes in the blood and urine.
- How might the urine of the patient experiencing nephrotic syndrome appear?

Slide 40

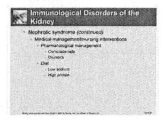

- The goal of treatment is geared at locating and treating the underlying causes. What are potential causes of nephrotic syndrome?

- What is the prognosis for the patient diagnosed with nephrotic syndrome? What impact does this condition have on the body's immune response?

Slide 41

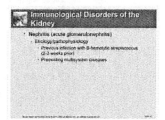

- Nephritis results from an inflammation of the kidney. Multiple disorders belong to this classification.

- Acute glomerulonephritis results after an immune response is triggered by an illness in the body. Explain the pathophysiological mechanism of the condition.

Slide 42

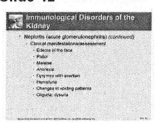

- Discuss the objective and subjective data that should be collected for the patient suspected of having acute glomerulonephritis.

Slide 43

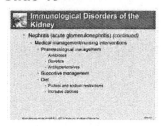

- The physician will order a series of tests to confirm a diagnosis. These tests will include BUN, serum creatinine, potassium levels, erythrocyte sedimentation rate, antistreptolysin-O titer, and urinalysis. What test findings will support the diagnosis?

- The treatment is aimed at caring for the presenting symptoms. What are the nursing responsibilities relating to patient education?

Slide 44

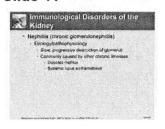

- Glomerulonephritis may be acute or chronic. How do the two types differ?

- Does the patient diagnosed with acute glomerulonephritis have the risk of developing chronic glomerulonephritis? If so, how?

ELSEVIER

Mosby items and derived items © 2011, 2007 by Mosby, Inc., an affiliate of Elsevier Inc.
Some material was previously published.

Adult Health Nursing, 6th ed.

Christensen & Kockrow

Slide 45

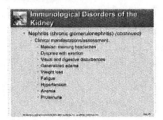

- Patients suffering from chronic glomerulonephritis could exhibit alterations in mental functioning/abilities. What is the underlying cause of these changes on cognition? What questions/assessment tools can be used in the assessment process?

Slide 46

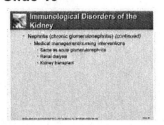

- Management of chronic glomerulonephritis involves treating the side effects of the disorder. Dialysis could be indicated. What will dialysis accomplish?

- What is the role of the nurse in providing care of this patient?

- Identify the prognosis for the patient with chronic glomerulonephritis.

Slide 47

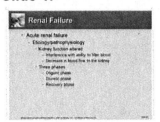

- Renal failure is a serious medical problem. The onset could be the result of chronic urinary dysfunction or an unexpected rapidly progressing disease process.

- There are predisposing factors associated with the onset of renal failure. Identify some of the more common factors.

- What role can be played by nurses in preventing the onset of renal failure?

Slide 48

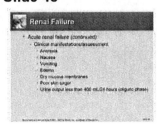

- The progression of renal failure is typically described in phases. During each phase, there are a series of characteristic events. What occurs during each phase?

- Discuss the role of the nurse regarding the assessment and education in each phase.

Slide 49

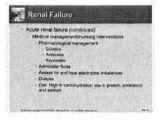

- The clinical findings associated with renal failure will be combined with laboratory testing to confirm a diagnosis. What tests can be anticipated? What results will confirm the onset of renal failure?

- What are the goals of medical management for acute renal failure?

- Recovery from acute renal failure can occur. What factors will affect the body's ability to regain renal function?

ELSEVIER

Adult Health Nursing, 6th ed.

Christensen & Kockrow

Slide 50

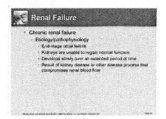

- In some cases, it might be impossible for the body's kidneys to resume functioning. This total loss of function results in end-stage renal failure.

- What populations are at highest risk for this to happen?

Slide 51

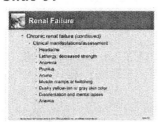

- The presenting symptoms of chronic renal failure are very individualized. The patient's overall health status will have a large impact on the clinical presentation.

Slide 52

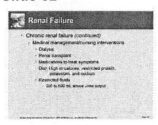

- The goals of medical management are to safeguard renal function as long as possible.

- Dialysis, dietary modification, and drug therapy could be instituted.

- The patient in renal failure will face numerous challenges concerning the prescribed diet. What elements are restricted in the diet? What is the underlying rationale for the dietary restrictions?

- Review the actual foods limited in the care of a patient in chronic renal failure.

Slide 53

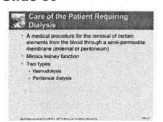

- When the kidneys fail to adequately remove toxins from the body, dialysis is instituted.

- The physician could order either peritoneal dialysis or hemodialysis. How do these procedures differ? Which patients are most suited for each type?

- What emotional stressors are associated with dialysis?

Slide 54

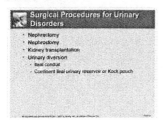

- Surgical intervention might be needed if less invasive measures of treatment are not successful in managing urinary disorders.

- Review the procedure of each of the listed surgeries. When is each of them performed?

- What is the role of the nurse in the preoperative and postoperative phases of care for the patient undergoing surgical management of a urinary disorder?

Christensen & Kockrow

Slide 55

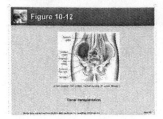

Slide 56

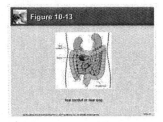

Slide 57

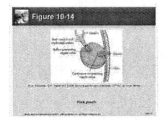

Slide 58

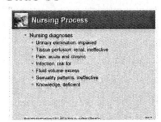

ELSEVIER

Mosby items and derived items © 2011, 2007 by Mosby, Inc., an affiliate of Elsevier Inc.
Some material was previously published.

Adult Health Nursing, 6th ed.
Christensen & Kockrow

11 Care of the Patient with an Endocrine Disorder

TEACHING FOCUS

In this chapter, the student will be introduced to the care of the patient with an endocrine disorder. The student will begin by exploring the structure and function of the endocrine system, including the endocrine glands, their hormones, the action of their hormones, the negative feedback system, and the role of the hypothalamus. The student then will have the opportunity to learn the etiology and pathophysiology, clinical manifestations, assessment, diagnostic tests, medical management, nursing interventions, patient teaching, and prognosis for disorders of the endocrine system.

MATERIALS AND RESOURCES

- ☐ Computer/overhead projector (all lessons)
- ☐ White/black board and marker/chalk (all lessons)
- ☐ Pencils, fruit, or other items to use as small prizes (Lesson 11.1)
- ☐ Sheets of unlined paper (Lesson 11.1)
- ☐ Small note cards (Lesson 11.1)
- ☐ Ball or other soft object than can be passed around the room (Lesson 11.4)
- ☐ Several scenarios involving diabetic patients (Lesson 11.4)
- ☐ Supplies used to administer insulin and a manikin. If a manikin is unavailable, an orange may be used in demonstrating administration of insulin (Lesson 11.4).
- ☐ Blank drug cards (Lesson 11.4)
- ☐ Telephone books (Lesson 11.4)

LESSON CHECKLIST

Preparations for this lesson include:
- Lecture
- Invite a nurse employed in an endocrine disorder treatment facility or in family practice to speak with the class about the treatment of endocrine gland disorders.
- Secure use of the nursing lab
- Invite a clinical dietitian to speak with the class about dietary management for the diabetic patient.

KEY TERMS

Chvostek's sign (FAAHN p. 1734, AHN p. 498)

dysphagia (FAAHN p. 1733, AHN p. 497)

endocrinologist (FAAHN p. 1727, AHN p. 491)

glycosuria (FAAHN p. 1747, AHN p. 511)

hirsutism (FAAHN p. 1741, AHN p. 505)

hyperglycemia (FAAHN p. 1747, AHN p. 511)

hypocalcemia (FAAHN p. 1739, AHN p. 503)

hypoglycemia (FAAHN p. 1754, AHN p. 518)

hypokalemia (FAAHN p. 1740, AHN p. 504)

idiopathic hyperplasia (FAAHN p. 1725, AHN p. 489)

ketoacidosis (FAAHN p. 1747, AHN p. 511)

ketone bodies (FAAHN p. 1746, AHN p. 510)

lipodystrophy (FAAHN p. 1753, AHN p. 517)

neuropathy (FAAHN p. 1758, AHN p. 522)

polydipsia (FAAHN p. 1747, AHN p. 511)

polyphagia (FAAHN p. 1747, AHN p. 511)

polyuria (FAAHN p. 1747, AHN p. 511)

Trousseau's sign (FAAHN p. 1734, AHN p. 498)

turgor (FAAHN p. 1729, AHN p. 493)

type 1 diabetes mellitus (FAAHN p. 1745, AHN p. 509)

type 2 diabetes mellitus (FAAHN p. 1746, AHN p. 510)

ADDITIONAL RESOURCES (AHN)

PPT Ch. 51, 1 through 60 FAAHN (Ch. 11, 1 through 60 AHN)

EILR IC images Ch 51, 1 through 18 FAAHN (Ch. 11, 1 through 18 AHN)

EILR TB questions Ch. 51, 1 through 42 FAAHN (Ch. 11, 1 through 42 AHN)

EILR Open Book Quiz Ch. 51, 1 through 10 FAAHN (Ch. 11, 1 through 10 AHN)

ESLR Review Questions for the NCLEX® Examination Ch. 51, 51-01 through 51-10 FAAHN (Ch. 11, 11-01 through 11-10 AHN)

Legend

PPT
PowerPoint
Slides

EILR
EVOLVE Instructor
Learning Resources:
Image Collection, Test
Bank, Open Book Quizzes

ESLR
EVOLVE Student
Learning Resources:
Review Questions
for the NCLEX
Examination

SG
Study Guide

NCP CTQ
Nursing Care Plan
Critical Thinking
Question

Class Activities are indicated in **bold italic**.

LESSON 11.1

PRETEST

1. The _____ is known as the "master gland."
   a. thyroid gland
   b. pituitary gland
   c. parathyroid gland
   d. adrenal gland

2. When a patient experiences a reduction in blood glucose levels, which of the following hormones is secreted in response?
   a. Insulin
   b. Carbohydrates
   c. Glucagon
   d. Progesterone

3. The body's response to stressors is known as "fight or flight." What part of the body is responsible for this phenomenon?
   a. Adrenal medulla
   b. Anterior pituitary gland
   c. Posterior pituitary gland
   d. Cerebellum

4. When interpreting the results of the serum thyroxine test, which of the following results is within a normal range?
   a. 1 to 3.5 ng/dL
   b. 5 to 12 mcg/dL
   c. 65 to 195 ng/dL
   d. 0.3 to 5.4 mcg/mL

5. When providing teaching for the parents of a child diagnosed with dwarfism, which of the following points should be included in the information presented?
   a. The child will appear older than his peers as a result of the condition.
   b. A dental consultation will be indicated to assist with the difficulties anticipated as the "baby" teeth erupt.
   c. Sexual development will be delayed.
   d. The child will most likely experience sterility.

6. You are assigned to plan the care for a patient diagnosed with acromegaly. What considerations should be incorporated into the plan?
   a. To compensate for the increase in body size, the caloric count of the patient should be closely monitored.
   b. Narcotic analgesics are indicated for the pain experienced.
   c. Bed rest will be indicated during acute episodes.
   d. The diet should be soft and easy to chew.

Adult Health Nursing, 6th ed.
Christensen & Kockrow

7. The evaluation of urine and serum test results are indicated in the care of a patient suspected of diabetes insipidus. Which of the following results is associated with this condition?
   a. Urine specific gravity 1.003 to 1.008
   b. Serum sodium 139 mEq/L
   c. Serum osmolality 280 mOsm/kg
   d. Urine specific gravity 1.001 to 1.005

8. Which of the following medications can be associated with the onset of inappropriate secretion of an antidiuretic hormone?
   a. Opiates
   b. NSAIDs
   c. Antibiotics
   d. Oral contraceptives

9. Medical management of hyperthyroidism can include:
   a. methimazole.
   b. calcium.
   c. thyroglobulin.
   d. vitamin D.

10. An insulin with a rapid onset is prescribed. Which of the following listed below will meet the criteria?
    a. NPH
    b. Lente
    c. Lantus
    d. Humalog

Answers:

1. b	2. c	3. a	4. b	5. c
6. d	7. d	8. a	9. a	10. d

BACKGROUND ASSESSMENT

Question: Nutrition plays a vital role in the successful control of diabetes. When planning a diet appropriate for a diabetic patient, what are the primary requirements? What factors will determine the caloric intake? How is the diet composed?

Answer: The diet is a very personalized part of a diabetic's plan of care. A balanced diet is needed to keep the blood glucose levels below the desired 126 mg/dL. The diet is normally divided into three balanced meals with two snacks per day. The number of daily calories or food exchanges used will be determined by several interrelated factors. The age of the patient and activity level will be the largest determinants. The diet will reflect a reduced sugar and fat content. It is recommended that 45% to 50% of the total calories come from carbohydrates and 10% to 20% from proteins, and the fat content should not exceed 30%. It is important to remember that not all carbohydrate and protein foods will have the same effect on the body's blood glucose levels.

Question: A patient presents to the clinic with complaints of fatigue, weight gain, anorexia, and constipation. During the interview, you note that her voice is hoarse and difficult to hear at times. She appears to be exhausted after the assessment. Based upon your knowledge, with what endocrine disorder do you anticipate she will be diagnosed? What diagnostic testing will be used to confirm the diagnosis? How will the condition be managed?

Answer: The assessment findings point to a diagnosis of hypothyroidism. This disorder is due to the thyroid gland's inability to secrete adequate hormones for the body. A diagnosis will be confirmed by the clinical picture and the results of diagnostic testing. These tests will include a TSH, T3, T4, and free T4 levels. Management will entail the replacement of the thyroid hormone by medications. The dosages will start low and gradually increase until the desired levels are obtained. The patient will have serum monitoring of hormone levels every 6 to 8 weeks until a therapeutic level is achieved. After this level is reached, the patient will be evaluated annually. The treatment will involve lifelong medications.

Mosby items and derived items © 2011 by Mosby, Inc., an affiliate of Elsevier Inc.
Some material was previously published.

Adult Health Nursing, 6th ed.

Christensen & Kockrow

CRITICAL THINKING QUESTION

A patient has been hospitalized due to complications of his hypoparathyroidism. During the admission assessment, the patient reported he had been experiencing headaches, nausea, and abdominal discomfort. As you collect the data, you note he is also jittery and nervous. After the admission paperwork has been completed, the physician has ordered that the patient be placed on a high-calcium diet and that intravenous calcium supplementation be administered. After the second treatment, the patient contacts the nurse's station and reports that he is feeling weak and dizzy. What actions should the nurse take? What do you suspect has occurred?

Guidelines: The patient could be experiencing complications associated with intravenous calcium administration. The vital signs will need to be taken, and the infusion will need to be stopped. A complete assessment of the patient will be needed. Specific findings associated with this condition include vomiting, disorientation, anorexia, abdominal pain, and weakness. Additional areas for observation include the vital signs. The physician will need to be notified of the episode and the findings of the assessment.

OBJECTIVES	CONTENT	TEACHING RESOURCES
List and describe the endocrine glands and their hormones.	■ Anatomy and physiology of the endocrine system (FAAHN p. 1721, AHN p. 485) □ Endocrine glands and hormones (FAAHN p. 1721, AHN p. 485) – Pituitary gland (FAAHN p. 1721, AHN p. 485) – Thyroid gland (FAAHN p. 1721, AHN p. 485) – Parathyroid glands (FAAHN p. 1722, AHN p. 486) – Adrenal glands (FAAHN p. 1722, AHN p. 486) – Adrenal cortex (FAAHN p. 1722, AHN p. 486) – Adrenal medulla (FAAHN p. 1722, AHN p. 486) – Pancreas (FAAHN p. 1723, AHN p. 487) – Female sex glands (FAAHN p. 1724, AHN p. 488) – Male sex glands (FAAHN p. 1724, AHN p. 488) – Thymus gland (FAAHN p. 1724, AHN p. 488) – Pineal gland (FAAHN p. 1724, AHN p. 488)	PPT 2 through 6, Ch. 51 FAAHN (Ch. 11 PPT 2 through 6 AHN) EILR IC Ch. 51 images 1, 4, 5 FAAHN (Ch. 11 images 1, 4, 5 AHN) EILR TB Ch. 51 questions 31, 42 FAAHN (Ch. 11 questions 31, 42 AHN) EILR Open Book Quiz Ch. 51 question 1 FAAHN (Ch. 11 question 1 AHN) SG Glands and Hormones, Ch. 51 p. 441 FAAHN (Ch. 11 p. 129 AHN) Structure of the Adrenal Glands Ch. 51 p. 446 FAAHN (Ch. 11 p. 134 AHN) **BOOK RESOURCES** Fig. 51-1 Location of the endocrine glands in the female and male bodies (FAAHN p. 1721) (Fig. 11-1 AHN p. 485) Fig. 51-4 Thyroid and parathyroid glands (FAAHN p. 1723) (Fig. 11-4 AHN p. 487) Fig. 51-5 Structure of the adrenal gland (FAAHN p. 1724) (Fig. 11-5 AHN p. 488) Review Questions for the NCLEX Examination Ch. 51 questions 1, 2 FAAHN (Ch. 11 question 1, 2 AHN) □ Discuss the categories/classifications of glands. □ Discuss endocrine glands and the hormones they secrete. *Class Activity* **Divide the students into small groups. Instruct each group to draw a stick figure and label the location of the endocrine**

OBJECTIVES	CONTENT	TEACHING RESOURCES
		glands in the body. The group who finishes the task first wins a small prize (fruit or pencils). **Note: Use this task before the lecture to assess existing knowledge of the students.**
Define the negative feedback system.	■ Anatomy and physiology of the endocrine system (FAAHN p. 1721, AHN p. 485) ☐ Endocrine glands and hormones (FAAHN p. 1721, AHN p. 485)	🔲 EILR TB Ch. 51 question 1 FAAHN (Ch. 11 question 1 AHN) 🔲 ESLR Review Questions for the NCLEX Examination Ch. 51 question 1 FAAHN (Ch. 11 question 1 AHN) 📖 SG Hormonal Imbalance Ch. 51 p. 443 FAAHN (Ch. 11 p. 131 AHN) ▸ Discuss the rate of hormonal release based upon the negative feedback system. ▸ Discuss the pituitary gland and why it is known as the "master gland." *Class Activity Provide sheets of unlined paper to students. Ask them to sketch their impression of the steps that occur when the negative feedback system is functioning appropriately. Post the sketches on the board. Allow the students to look them over.*
Explain the action of the hormones on their target organs.	☐ Endocrine glands and hormones (FAAHN p. 1721, AHN p. 485) – Pituitary gland (FAAHN p. 1721, AHN p. 485) – Thyroid gland (FAAHN p. 1721, AHN p. 485) – Parathyroid glands (FAAHN p. 1722, AHN p. 486) – Adrenal glands (FAAHN p. 1722, AHN p. 486) – Adrenal cortex (FAAHN p. 1722, AHN p. 486) – Adrenal medulla (FAAHN p. 1722, AHN p. 486) – Pancreas (FAAHN p. 1723, AHN p. 487) – Female sex glands (FAAHN p. 1724, AHN p. 488)	🔲 PPT 2 through 4 Ch. 51 FAAHN (Ch. 11 PPT 2 through 4 AHN) 🔲 EILR IC Ch. 51 image 2 FAAHN (Ch. 11 image 2 AHN) 🔲 ESLR Review Questions for the NCLEX Examination Ch. 51 question 2 FAAHN (Ch. 11 question 2 AHN) 📖 SG Glands and Hormones, Ch. 51 p. 441 FAAHN (Ch. 11 p. 129 AHN) **BOOK RESOURCES** Fig. 51-2 Pituitary hormones (FAAHN p. 1722) (Fig. 11-2 AHN p. 486) Review Questions for the NCLEX Examination Ch. 51 questions 3, 4 FAAHN (Ch. 11 question 3, 4 AHN) ▸ Discuss which hormone is secreted by each of the endocrine glands. ▸ Discuss the function of each of the endocrine gland hormones.

OBJECTIVES	CONTENT	TEACHING RESOURCES
	– Male sex glands (FAAHN p. 1724, AHN p. 488) – Thymus gland (FAAHN p. 1724, AHN p. 488) – Pineal gland (FAAHN p. 1724, AHN p. 488)	*Class Activity Play a quick game of "round robin." Ask students questions about the endocrine glands and their hormones. The questions should be kept short with brief answers. This will provide a quick review for the students.*
Describe how the hypothalamus controls the anterior and posterior pituitary glands.	– Pituitary gland (FAAHN p. 1721, AHN p. 485)	SG Hormonal Imbalance Ch. 51 pp. 443-446 FAAHN (Ch. 11 pp. 131-134 AHN) **BOOK RESOURCES** Fig. 51-3 Names and functions of anterior pituitary hormones (FAAHN p. 1723) (Fig. 11-3 AHN p. 487) ▶ Discuss the anatomic relationship between the hypothalamus and the pituitary gland. ▶ Discuss the mechanism that promotes hormone release by the pituitary glands. *Class Activity Write the names of each of the anterior and posterior pituitary glands, and the hormones secreted by the glands, on small note cards. Ask each student to select one card from the bag. After the selection has been taken, instruct the students to link with the students having cards that correspond to their hormone or gland. Once the groups have been formed, instruct them to review the manner in which hormones or glands are controlled by the hypothalamus.*

11.1 Homework/Assignments:

11.1 Instructor's Notes/Student Feedback:

LESSON 11.2

CRITICAL THINKING QUESTION

What are the symptoms of hypoglycemia that must be taught to the patient who has just been diagnosed with diabetes mellitus?

Guidelines: The person who has just been diagnosed with diabetes mellitus must be able to tell the difference between hyperglycemia and hypoglycemia. The signs of hypoglycemia usually have a slow onset with shakiness, palpitations, vertigo, diaphoresis, hunger, pallor, fatigue, confusion, irritable behavior, and visual disturbances. If the patient is not given glucose, the patient could become comatose. The condition can be a medical emergency if the person is not given glucose while still alert.

OBJECTIVES	CONTENT	TEACHING RESOURCES
Discuss the etiology/ pathophysiology, clinical manifestations, assessment, diagnostic tests, medical management, nursing interventions, patient teaching, and prognosis for patients with acromegaly, gigantism, dwarfism, diabetes insipidus, syndrome of inappropriate antidiuretic hormone (SIADH), hyperthyroidism, hypothyroidism, goiter, thyroid cancer, hyperparathyroidism, hypoparathyroidism, Cushing syndrome, and Addison's disease.	■ Disorders of the pituitary gland (hypophysis) (FAAHN p. 1725, AHN p. 489) □ Acromegaly (FAAHN p. 1725, AHN p. 489) – Etiology and pathophysiology (FAAHN p. 1725, AHN p. 489) – Clinical manifestations (FAAHN p. 1725, AHN p. 489) – Assessment (FAAHN p. 1725, AHN p. 489) – Diagnostic tests (FAAHN p. 1725, AHN p. 489) – Medical management (FAAHN p. 1725, AHN p. 489) – Nursing interventions and patient teaching (FAAHN p. 1725, AHN p. 489) – Prognosis (FAAHN p. 1727, AHN p. 491) □ Gigantism (FAAHN p. 1727, AHN p. 491) – Etiology and pathophysiology (FAAHN p. 1727, AHN p. 491) – Clinical manifestations (FAAHN p. 1727, AHN p. 491) – Assessment (FAAHN p. 1727, AHN p. 491) – Diagnostic tests (FAAHN p. 1727, AHN p. 491) – Medical management (FAAHN p. 1727, AHN p. 491)	▣ PPT 7 through 45, Ch. 51 FAAHN (Ch. 11 PPT 7 through 45 AHN) 🖪 EILR IC Ch. 51 images 6 through 11 FAAHN (Ch. 11 images 6 through 11 AHN) 🖪 EILR TB Ch. 51 questions 2 through 4, 6, 8 through 12, 15, 19, 24, 27, 28, 30, 32, 33, 34, 41 FAAHN (Ch. 11 questions 2 through 4, 6, 8 through 10, 11, 12, 15, 19, 24, 27, 28, 30, 32, 33, 34, 41 AHN) 🖪 EILR Open Book Quiz Ch. 51 question 2 through 5, 7, 8 FAAHN (Ch. 11 question 2 through 5, 7, 8, AHN) 🖪 ESLR NCLEX-Style Review Questions Ch. 51 questions 3, 6 through 8 FAAHN (Ch. 11 questions 3, 6 through 8 AHN) 📖 SG Hormonal Imbalance Ch. 51 pp. 443-446 FAAHN (Ch. 11 pp. 131-134 AHN) **BOOK RESOURCES** Fig. 51-6 Common facial features associated with pituitary tumor (FAAHN p. 1725) (Fig. 11-6 AHN p. 489) Table 51-1 Medications for Endocrine Disorders (FAAHN p. 1726) (Table 11-1 AHN p. 490) Fig. 51-7 Exophthalmos of Graves' disease (FAAHN p. 1731) (Fig. 11-7 AHN p. 495) Table 51-2 Medications Commonly Used to Treat Hyperthyroidism and Hypothyroidism (FAAHN p. 1733) (Table 11-2 AHN p. 497)

OBJECTIVES	CONTENT	TEACHING RESOURCES
	– Nursing interventions and patient teaching (FAAHN p. 1727, AHN p. 491)	Fig. 51-8 Person with myxedema (FAAHN p. 1735) (Fig. 11-8 AHN p. 499)
	– Prognosis (FAAHN p. 1727, AHN p. 491)	Fig. 51-9 Adult cretin (FAAHN p. 1735) (Fig. 11-9 AHN p. 499)
	☐ Dwarfism (FAAHN p. 1728, AHN p. 492)	Fig. 51-10 Simple goiter (FAAHN p. 1737) (Fig. 11-10 AHN p. 501)
	– Etiology and pathophysiology (FAAHN p. 1728, AHN p. 492)	Review Questions for the NCLEX Examination Ch. 51 questions 5, 7, 8, 13, 24 through 28, 32 through 34 FAAHN (Ch. 11 question 5, 7, 8, 13, 24 through 28, 32 through 34 AHN)
	– Clinical manifestations (FAAHN p. 1728, AHN p. 492)	
	– Assessment (FAAHN p. 1728, AHN p. 492)	▶ Discuss the clinical manifestations associated with a disorder of the pituitary gland.
	– Diagnostic tests (FAAHN p. 1728, AHN p. 492)	▶ Discuss the use of diagnostic scanning tests to confirm a diagnosis for disorders of the pituitary gland.
	– Medical management (FAAHN p. 1728, AHN p. 492)	
	– Nursing interventions and patient teaching (FAAHN p. 1728, AHN p. 492)	*Class Activity **Invite a guest speaker to the class. Ask the speaker to discuss the care and treatment of endocrine gland disorders. Note: Nurses employed in family practice or endocrine disorder treatment facilities would be beneficial. If none of these options are available in your community, you can invite a patient who personally has experienced a pituitary disorder to speak to the class.***
	– Prognosis (FAAHN p. 1728, AHN p. 492)	
	☐ Diabetes insipidus (FAAHN p. 1728, AHN p. 492)	
	– Etiology and pathophysiology (FAAHN p. 1728, AHN p. 492)	*Class Activity **Demonstrate physiological changes caused by acromegaly. Start at the hairline and move down the body.***
	– Clinical manifestations (FAAHN p. 1728, AHN p. 492)	
	– Assessment (FAAHN p. 1728, AHN p. 492)	
	– Diagnostic tests (FAAHN p. 1729, AHN p. 493)	
	– Medical management (FAAHN p. 1729, AHN p. 493)	
	– Nursing interventions and patient teaching (FAAHN p. 1729, AHN p. 493)	
	– Prognosis (FAAHN p. 1729, AHN p. 493)	
	☐ Syndrome of inappropriate antidiuretic hormone (FAAHN p. 1729, AHN p. 493)	

ELSEVIER

OBJECTIVES	CONTENT	TEACHING RESOURCES
	– Etiology and pathophysiology (FAAHN p. 1729, AHN p. 493)	
	– Clinical manifestations (FAAHN p. 1730, AHN p. 494)	
	– Assessment (FAAHN p. 1730, AHN p. 494)	
	– Diagnostic tests (FAAHN p. 1730, AHN p. 494)	
	– Medical management (FAAHN p. 1730, AHN p. 494)	
	– Nursing interventions and patient teaching (FAAHN p. 1730, AHN p. 494)	
	– Prognosis (FAAHN p. 1731, AHN p. 495)	
	■ Disorders of the thyroid and parathyroid glands (FAAHN p. 1731, AHN p. 495)	
	☐ Hyperthyroidism (FAAHN p. 1731, AHN p. 495)	
	– Etiology and pathophysiology (FAAHN p. 1731, AHN p. 495)	
	– Clinical manifestations (FAAHN p. 1731, AHN p. 495)	
	– Assessment (FAAHN p. 1732, AHN p. 496)	
	– Diagnostic tests (FAAHN p. 1732, AHN p. 496)	
	– Medical management (FAAHN p. 1732, AHN p. 496)	
	– Nursing interventions and patient teaching (FAAHN p. 1733, AHN p. 497)	
	– Prognosis (FAAHN p. 1734, AHN p. 498)	
	☐ Hypothyroidism (FAAHN p. 1734, AHN p. 498)	
	– Etiology and pathophysiology (FAAHN p. 1734, AHN p. 498)	
	– Clinical manifestations (FAAHN p. 1735, AHN p. 499)	

Christensen & Kockrow

OBJECTIVES	CONTENT	TEACHING RESOURCES
	– Assessment (FAAHN p. 1735, AHN p. 499)	
	– Diagnostic tests (FAAHN p. 1735, AHN p. 499)	
	– Medical management (FAAHN p. 1736, AHN p. 500)	
	– Nursing interventions and patient teaching (FAAHN p. 1736, AHN p. 500)	
	– Prognosis (FAAHN p. 1736, AHN p. 500)	
	☐ Simple (colloid) goiter (FAAHN p. 1736, AHN p. 500)	
	– Etiology and pathophysiology (FAAHN p. 1736, AHN p. 500)	
	– Clinical manifestations (FAAHN p. 1736, AHN p. 500)	
	– Assessment (FAAHN p. 1736, AHN p. 500)	
	– Medical management (FAAHN p. 1737, AHN p. 501)	
	– Nursing interventions and patient teaching (FAAHN p. 1737, AHN p. 501)	
	– Prognosis (FAAHN p. 1737, AHN p. 501)	
	☐ Cancer of the thyroid (FAAHN p. 1737, AHN p. 501)	
	– Etiology and pathophysiology (FAAHN p. 1737, AHN p. 501)	
	– Clinical manifestations (FAAHN p. 1737, AHN p. 501)	
	– Assessment (FAAHN p. 1737, AHN p. 501)	
	– Diagnostic tests (FAAHN p. 1737, AHN p. 501)	
	– Medical management (FAAHN p. 1738, AHN p. 502)	
	– Nursing interventions and patient teaching (FAAHN p. 1738, AHN p. 502)	

OBJECTIVES	CONTENT	TEACHING RESOURCES
	– Prognosis (FAAHN p. 1738 AHN p. 502)	
	☐ Hyperparathyroidism (FAAHN p. 1738, AHN p. 502)	
	– Etiology and pathophysiology (FAAHN p. 1738, AHN p. 502)	
	– Clinical manifestations (FAAHN p. 1738, AHN p. 502)	
	– Assessment (FAAHN p. 1738, AHN p. 502)	
	– Diagnostic tests (FAAHN p. 1738, AHN p. 502)	
	– Medical management (FAAHN p. 1738, AHN p. 502)	
	– Nursing interventions and patient teaching (FAAHN p. 1739, AHN p. 503)	
	– Prognosis (FAAHN p. 1739, AHN p. 503)	
	☐ Hypoparathyroidism (FAAHN p. 1739, AHN p. 503)	
	– Etiology and pathophysiology (FAAHN p. 1739, AHN p. 503)	
	– Clinical manifestations (FAAHN p. 1739, AHN p. 503)	
	– Assessment (FAAHN p. 1739, AHN p. 503)	
	– Diagnostic tests (FAAHN p. 1740, AHN p. 504)	
	– Medical management (FAAHN p. 1740, AHN p. 504)	
	– Nursing interventions and patient teaching (FAAHN p. 1740, AHN p. 504)	
	– Prognosis (FAAHN p. 1740, AHN p. 504)	
	■ Disorders of the adrenal glands (FAAHN p. 1740, AHN p. 504)	
	☐ Adrenal hyperfunction (Cushing syndrome) (FAAHN p. 1740, AHN p. 504)	

Christensen & Kockrow

OBJECTIVES	CONTENT	TEACHING RESOURCES
	– Etiology and pathophysiology (FAAHN p. 1740, AHN p. 504)	
	– Clinical manifestations (FAAHN p. 1740, AHN p. 504)	
	– Assessment (FAAHN p. 1741, AHN p. 505)	
	– Diagnostic tests (FAAHN p. 1741, AHN p. 505)	
	– Medical management (FAAHN p. 1741, AHN p. 505)	
	– Nursing interventions and patient teaching (FAAHN p. 1741, AHN p. 505)	
	– Prognosis (FAAHN p. 1742, AHN p. 506)	
	☐ Adrenal hypofunction (Addison's disease) (FAAHN p. 1742, AHN p. 506)	
	– Etiology and pathophysiology (FAAHN p. 1742, AHN p. 506)	
	– Clinical manifestations (FAAHN p. 1742, AHN p. 506)	
	– Assessment (FAAHN p. 1742, AHN p. 506)	
	– Diagnostic tests (FAAHN p. 1743, AHN p. 507)	
	– Medical management (FAAHN p. 1743, AHN p. 507)	
	– Nursing interventions and patient teaching (FAAHN p. 1743, AHN p. 507)	
	– Prognosis (FAAHN p. 1744, AHN p. 508)	
	☐ Pheochromocytoma (FAAHN p. 1744, AHN p. 508)	
	– Etiology and pathophysiology (FAAHN p. 1744, AHN p. 508)	
	– Clinical manifestations (FAAHN p. 1744, AHN p. 508)	
	– Assessment (FAAHN p. 1744, AHN p. 508)	

OBJECTIVES	CONTENT	TEACHING RESOURCES
	– Diagnostic tests (FAAHN p. 1744, AHN p. 508)	
	– Medical management (FAAHN p. 1744, AHN p. 508)	
	– Nursing interventions and patient teaching (FAAHN p. 1744, AHN p. 508)	
	– Prognosis (FAAHN p. 1745, AHN p. 509)	

11.2 Homework/Assignments:

11.2 Instructor's Notes/Student Feedback:

LESSON 11.3

CRITICAL THINKING QUESTION

After experiencing an unsuccessful attempt to manage hyperthyroidism with medication therapy, a patient has just had surgery for removal of the thyroid gland. After receiving the patient from the postoperative recovery unit, an assessment is completed. The patient is restless and hoarse. An assessment of the vital signs reveals a temperature of 98.1, pulse 108, respirations 25, and blood pressure 95/70. The dressing is clean, dry, and intact. Are these findings normal? Is there need for concern or further action at this time?

Guidelines: The assessment reveals voice hoarseness. A slight hoarseness is normal initially. The patient will need to be reminded to rest his voice. The potentially problematic areas in the assessment involve the patient's presentation of restlessness and the vital signs. Both of these can signal bleeding. Bleeding is a serious potential complication after a thyroidectomy. In addition to the dressing, the back and sides of the neck will need to be assessed. The patient's comfort level will need to be evaluated. Pain can increase the pulse and respiratory rate. The patient's previously recorded vital signs should be reviewed to determine if this is normal for him. The physician will need to be apprised of the findings and actions taken.

OBJECTIVES	CONTENT	TEACHING RESOURCES
List four tests used in the diagnosis of hyperthyroidism.	☐ Hyperthyroidism (FAAHN p. 1731, AHN p. 495) – Etiology and pathophysiology (FAAHN p. 1731, AHN p. 495) – Clinical manifestations (FAAHN p. 1731, AHN p. 495) – Assessment (FAAHN p. 1732, AHN p. 496) – Diagnostic tests (FAAHN p. 1732, AHN p. 496) – Medical management (FAAHN p. 1732, AHN p. 496) – Nursing interventions and patient teaching (FAAHN p. 1733, AHN p. 497) – Prognosis (FAAHN p. 1734, AHN p. 498)	▣ PPT 18 through 22, Ch. 51 FAAHN (Ch. 11 PPT 18 through 22 AHN) ▣ SG Thyroid Disorders, Ch. 51 p. 447 FAAHN (Ch. 11 p. 135 AHN) **BOOK RESOURCES** Box 51-1 Diagnostic Tests for Hyperthyroidism (FAAHN p. 1732) (Box 11-1 AHN p. 496) ▸ Discuss the findings that will confirm a diagnosis of hyperthyroidism. ▸ Discuss the education that is indicated for the patient scheduled to undergo diagnostic testing for hyperthyroidism. *Class Activity Instruct each student to develop two NCLEX-style questions relating to the diagnostic tests used to assess hyperthyroidism. Collect the written questions and use them in a brief oral review of the content or as a test review.*
Explain how to test for Chvostek's sign, Trousseau's sign, and carpopedal spasms.	☐ Hyperthyroidism (FAAHN p. 1731, AHN p. 495) – Etiology and pathophysiology (FAAHN p. 1731, AHN p. 495) – Clinical manifestations (FAAHN p. 1731, AHN p. 495) – Assessment (FAAHN p. 1732, AHN p. 496)	▣ PPT 22, Ch. 51 FAAHN (Ch. 11 PPT 22 AHN) 🅔 EILR TB Ch. 51 question 18 FAAHN (Ch. 11 question 18 AHN) 🅔 EILR Open Book Quiz Ch. 51 question 6 FAAHN (Ch. 11 question 6 AHN)

OBJECTIVES	CONTENT	TEACHING RESOURCES
	− Diagnostic tests (FAAHN p. 1732, AHN p. 496) − Medical management (FAAHN p. 1732, AHN p. 496) − Nursing interventions and patient teaching (FAAHN p. 1733, AHN p. 497) − Prognosis (FAAHN p. 1734, AHN p. 498)	SG Thyroid Disorders Ch. 51 p. 447 FAAHN (Ch. 11 p. 135 AHN) **BOOK RESOURCES** Review Questions for the NCLEX Examination Ch. 51 question 30 FAAHN (Ch. 11 question 30 AHN) ▶ Discuss the underlying cause associated with the manifestation of Chvostek's and Trousseau's signs. ▶ Discuss the medical management that will be indicated in the event Chvostek's and Trousseau's signs are assessed. *Class Activity **Demonstrate the assessment of Chvostek's and Trousseau's signs.***
List two significant complications that may occur after thyroidectomy.	☐ Hyperthyroidism (FAAHN p. 1731, AHN p. 495) − Etiology and pathophysiology (FAAHN p. 1731, AHN p. 495) − Clinical manifestations (FAAHN p. 1731, AHN p. 495) − Assessment (FAAHN p. 1732, AHN p. 496) − Diagnostic tests (FAAHN p. 1732, AHN p. 496) − Medical management (FAAHN p. 1732, AHN p. 496) − Nursing interventions and patient teaching (FAAHN p. 1733, AHN p. 497) − Prognosis (FAAHN p. 1734, AHN p. 498)	PPT 22 Ch. 51 FAAHN (Ch. 11 PPT 22 AHN) EILR TB Ch. 51 questions 7, 13, 14, 40 FAAHN (Ch. 11 questions 7, 13, 14, 40 AHN) ESLR Review Questions for the NCLEX Examination Ch. 43 question 4 FAAHN (Ch. 3 question 4 AHN) SG Thyroid Disorders Ch. 51 p. 447 FAAHN (Ch. 11 p. 135 AHN) **BOOK RESOURCES** Review Questions for the NCLEX Examination Ch. 51 questions 6, 9 FAAHN (Ch. 11 question 6, 9 AHN) ▶ Discuss the conditions that warrant a thyroidectomy. ▶ Discuss the nursing assessments required of a patient during the postoperative period after undergoing a thyroidectomy. *Class Activity **Utilize the nursing lab for this activity. Ask for a student volunteer. Ask the volunteer to lie on the bed. Demonstrate the appropriate positioning and movement of a patient who has had a thyroidectomy during the immediate postoperative period.***

Christensen & Kockrow

Discuss the medications commonly used to treat hyperthyroidism and hypothyroidism.	☐ Hyperthyroidism (FAAHN p. 1731, AHN p. 495) – Etiology and pathophysiology (FAAHN p. 1731, AHN p. 495) – Clinical manifestations (FAAHN p. 1731, AHN p. 495) – Assessment (FAAHN p. 1732, AHN p. 496) – Diagnostic tests (FAAHN p. 1732, AHN p. 496) – Medical management (FAAHN p. 1732, AHN p. 496) – Nursing interventions and patient teaching (FAAHN p. 1733, AHN p. 497) – Prognosis (FAAHN p. 1734, AHN p. 498) ☐ Hypothyroidism (FAAHN p. 1734, AHN p. 498) – Etiology and pathophysiology (FAAHN p. 1734, AHN p. 498) – Clinical manifestations (FAAHN p. 1735, AHN p. 499) – Assessment (FAAHN p. 1735, AHN p. 499) – Diagnostic tests (FAAHN p. 1735, AHN p. 499) – Medical management (FAAHN p. 1736, AHN p. 500) – Nursing interventions and patient teaching (FAAHN p. 1736, AHN p. 500) – Prognosis (FAAHN p. 1736, AHN p. 500)	PPT 21, 26 Ch. 51 FAAHN (Ch. 11 PPT 21, 26 AHN) EILR TB Ch. 51 question 35 FAAHN (Ch. 11 question 35 AHN) ESLR Review Questions for the NCLEX Examination Ch. 51 question 5 FAAHN (Ch. 11 question 5AHN) SG Thyroid Disorders, Ch. 51 p. 447 FAAHN (Ch. 11 p. 135 AHN) **BOOK RESOURCES** Table 51-1 Medications for Endocrine Disorders (FAAHN p. 1726) (Table 11-1 AHN p. 490) ▸ Discuss the nursing implications associated with administration of medications used to treat both hyperthyroidism and hypothyroidism. ▸ Discuss the common side effects associated with the medications used to treat both hyperthyroidism and hypothyroidism. *Class Activity Instruct each student to prepare a drug card for a medication used to treat hyperthyroidism and hypothyroidism as assigned by the instructor. After the cards are completed, divide the class into small groups. Each group should not have more than one or two students with the same drug. Allow the students a brief period of time to present their drug card information to the small group.*

| Differentiate between the clinical manifestations of Cushing syndrome and those of Addison's disease. | ■ Disorders of the adrenal glands (FAAHN p. 1740, AHN p. 504)

☐ Adrenal hyperfunction (Cushing syndrome) (FAAHN p. 1740, AHN p. 504)

– Etiology and pathophysiology (FAAHN p. 1740, AHN p. 504)

– Clinical manifestations (FAAHN p. 1740, AHN p. 504)

– Assessment (FAAHN p. 1741, AHN p. 505)

– Diagnostic tests (FAAHN p. 1741, AHN p. 505)

– Medical management (FAAHN p. 1741, AHN p. 505)

– Nursing interventions and patient teaching (FAAHN p. 1741, AHN p. 505)

– Prognosis (FAAHN p. 1742, AHN p. 506)

☐ Adrenal hypofunction (Addison's disease) (FAAHN p. 1742, AHN p. 506)

– Etiology and pathophysiology (FAAHN p. 1742, AHN p. 506)

– Clinical manifestations (FAAHN p. 1742, AHN p. 506)

– Assessment (FAAHN p. 1742, AHN p. 506)

– Diagnostic tests (FAAHN p. 1743, AHN p. 507)

– Medical management (FAAHN p. 1743, AHN p. 507)

– Nursing interventions and patient teaching (FAAHN p. 1743, AHN p. 507)

– Prognosis (FAAHN p. 1744, AHN p. 508) | PPT 37 through 44, Ch. 51 FAAHN (Ch. 11 PPT 37 through 44 AHN)

SG Adrenal Disorders, Ch. 51 p. 448 FAAHN (Ch. 11 p. 136 AHN)

BOOK RESOURCES

Table 51-2 Medications Commonly Used to Treat Hyperthyroidism and Hypothyroidism (FAAHN p. 1733) (Table 11-2 AHN p. 497)

▸ Discuss the etiology of Cushing syndrome.

▸ Discuss the etiology of Addison's disease.

Class Activity Separate the students into three teams. Each team will be assigned one of the steroidal hormones produced by the adrenal glands. Instruct each team to develop a short presentation, no longer than 3 minutes, concerning the functions of its assigned hormone and the physiological impacts of a deficiency and an oversecretion of the hormone. |
| Describe the etiology/ pathophysiology, clinical manifestations, assessment, diagnostic tests, medical management, | ■ Disorders of the pancreas (FAAHN p. 1745, AHN p. 509)

☐ Diabetes mellitus (FAAHN p. 1745, AHN p. 509)

– Etiology (FAAHN p. 1745, AHN p. 509) | PPT 46 through 59, Ch. 51 FAAHN (Ch. 11 PPT 46 through 59 AHN)

EILR IC Ch. 51 images 12 through 18 FAAHN (Ch. 11 images 12 through 18 AHN)

EILR TB Ch. 51 questions 20, 22, 25 FAAHN (Ch. 1 questions 20, 22, 25 AHN) |

Christensen & Kockrow

| nursing interventions, patient teaching, and prognosis for the patient with diabetes mellitus. | – Types of diabetes mellitus (FAAHN p. 1745, AHN p. 509)
– Pathophysiology (FAAHN p. 1746, AHN p. 510)
– Clinical manifestations (FAAHN p. 1747, AHN p. 511)
– Assessment (FAAHN p. 1747, AHN p. 511)
– Diagnostic tests (FAAHN p. 1747, AHN p. 511)
– Medical management (FAAHN p. 1748, AHN p. 512)
– Nursing interventions and patient teaching (FAAHN p. 1757, AHN p. 521)
– Prognosis (FAAHN p. 1764, AHN p. 528) | ■SG SG Diabetes Mellitus, Ch. 51 p. 448 FAAHN (Ch. 11 p. 136 AHN)

BOOK RESOURCES

Table 51-3 Nursing Assessment of Patients with Cushing's Syndrome or Addison's Disease (FAAHN p. 1743) (Table 11-3 AHN p. 507)

Box 51-2 Diagnostic Tests for Diabetes Mellitus (FAAHN p. 1748) (Box 11-2 AHN p. 512)

Complementary and Alternative Therapies: Endocrine Disorders (FAAHN p. 1757) (ANH p. 521)

Review Questions for the NCLEX Examination Ch. 51 questions 7, 10 through 12, 15, 35 FAAHN (Ch. 11 questions 7, 10 through 12, 15, 35 AHN)

▸ Discuss the diagnostic tests used to confirm a diagnosis of diabetes mellitus.

▸ Discuss the teaching that will be needed for the patient undergoing testing for suspected diabetes mellitus.

Class Activity Divide the students into three groups. The groups will be as follows: pathophysiology/etiology, clinical manifestations, and medical management. Within each group, further divide into two subgroups. Divide the subgroups into type 1 diabetes and the other into type 2 diabetes. Instruct the groups to determine the appropriate information for their topic and subgroup. When completed, each of the larger groups will share their information. |

11.3 Homework/Assignments:

11.3 Instructor's Notes/Student Feedback:

Mosby items and derived items © 2011 by Mosby, Inc., an affiliate of Elsevier Inc.
Some material was previously published.

Adult Health Nursing, 6th ed.
Christensen & Kockrow

LESSON 11.4

CRITICAL THINKING QUESTION

A 20-year-old patient hospitalized for management of recently diagnosed diabetes mellitus type 1 is assigned to your care for the evening shift. While you are completing the routine shift assessment, she vents her frustration concerning her condition. She states, "This diagnosis is a drag." When questioned, she reports she had been feeling tired, thirsty, and hungry for the past few months. The disorder was diagnosed during a routine physical examination. She reports being squeamish about giving herself injections. She asks when she will be "well enough" to switch to pills to control her blood sugar. What information concerning her desired mode of medication administration should be given to her? In addition to the prescribed medications, what can she do to control her blood sugar and reduce the amount of insulin needed?

Guidelines: Patients diagnosed with type 1 diabetes mellitus depend on insulin to control their blood glucose. Oral hypoglycemic medications cannot be used for this population. She will be able to control her blood glucose level by closely following the prescribed diet and participating in a regular exercise program.

OBJECTIVES	CONTENT	TEACHING RESOURCES
Differentiate between the signs and symptoms of hyperglycemia and hypoglycemia.	– Pathophysiology (FAAHN p. 1746, AHN p. 510) – Medical management (FAAHN p. 1748, AHN p. 512)	PPT 47 through 49, Ch. 51 FAAHN (Ch. 11 PPT 47 through 49 AHN) EILR TB Ch. 51 questions 37, 38 FAAHN (Ch. 11 questions 37, 38 AHN) ESLR Review Questions for the NCLEX Examination Ch. 51 question 9 FAAHN (Ch. 11 question 9 AHN) SG Signs of Problems, Ch. 51 p. 452 FAAHN (Ch. 11 p. 140 AHN) ▸ Discuss the serum glucose results associated with the clinical manifestations of hypoglycemia and hyperglycemia. ▸ Discuss the events that can cause hyperglycemia and hypoglycemia. *Class Activity Instruct the students to stand. Pass a small object around the room. As each student is passed the object, he/she must state a fact about hyperglycemia or hypoglycemia. After he/she states the information, the student can sit down. Continue until each person is seated.*

| Differentiate among the signs and symptoms of diabetic ketoacidosis, hyperglycemic hyperosmolar nonketotic coma, and hypoglycemic reaction. | – Pathophysiology (FAAHN p. 1746, AHN p. 510)

– Medical management (FAAHN p. 1748, AHN p. 512) | PPT 57 through 58, Ch. 51 FAAHN (Ch. 11 PPT 57 through 58 AHN)

EILR TB Ch. 51 question 23 FAAHN (Ch. 11 question 23 AHN)

SG Signs of Problems, Ch. 51 p. 452 FAAHN (Ch. 11 p. 140 AHN)

BOOK RESOURCES

Table 51-5 Types of Insulin (FAAHN pp. 1751-1752) (Table 11-5 AHN pp. 515-516)

Safety Alert! Emergency Care for Hypoglycemic Reaction (FAAHN p. 1760) (AHN p. 524)

Safety Alert! Emergency Care for Hyperglycemic Reaction (Diabetic Ketoacidosis) (FAAHN p. 1761) (AHN p. 525)

Review Questions for the NCLEX Examination Ch. 51 questions 16, 31 FAAHN (Ch. 11 questions 16, 31 AHN)

▶ Discuss the signs and symptoms associated with diabetic ketoacidosis, hyperosmolar nonketotic coma, and hypoglycemic reaction.

▶ Discuss the emergency care for managing the patient experiencing a hypoglycemic reaction.

Class Activity Instruct each student to develop two quiz questions relating to the signs and symptoms of diabetic ketoacidosis, hyperosmolar nonketotic coma, and hypoglycemic coma. After the students have completed their questions, ask them to share the questions with at least two other students. |

Christensen & Kockrow

| Explain the roles of nutrition, exercise, and medication in the control of diabetes mellitus. | – Medical management (FAAHN p. 1748, AHN p. 512)

 – Nursing interventions and patient teaching (FAAHN p. 1757, AHN p. 521)

 – Prognosis (FAAHN p. 1764, AHN p. 528) | ⊠▤ PPT 51 through 57, Ch. 51 FAAHN (Ch. 11 PPT 51 through 57 AHN)

 🔲 EILR IC Ch. 51 images 12 through 17 FAAHN (Ch. 11 images 12 through 17 AHN)

 🔲 EILR TB Ch. 51questions 5, 17 FAAHN (Ch. 11 questions 5, 17 AHN)

 📙 SG Diabetes Management Ch. 51 p. 451 FAAHN (Ch. 11 p. 139 AHN)

 BOOK RESOURCES

 Review Questions for the NCLEX Examination Ch. 51 questions 18, 29 FAAHN (Ch. 11 questions 18, 29 AHN)

 ▸ Discuss the education needed concerning dietary compliance for the management of diabetes.

 ▸ Discuss the impact of exercise on the blood's glucose level.

 *Class Activity **Invite a guest speaker to the class. The topic will include dietary management for the diabetic patient.***

 Note: A clinical dietitian will provide a good presentation and can be located at a local health care facility. |
| Discuss how oral agents work to improve the mechanisms by which insulin and glucose are produced and used by the body. | – Medical management (FAAHN p. 1748, AHN p. 512) | ⊠▤ PPT 56 Ch. 51 FAAHN (Ch. 11 PPT 56 AHN)

 📙 SG Insulin Ch. 51 pp. 449-451 FAAHN (Ch. 11 pp. 137-139 AHN)

 BOOK RESOURCES

 Table 51-5 Types of Insulin (FAAHN p. 1751) (Table 11-5 AHN p. 515)

 Table 51-6 Five Classes of Oral Hypoglycemics (FAAHN p. 1756) (Table 11-6 AHN p. 520)

 Review Questions for the NCLEX Examination Ch. 51 question 21 FAAHN (Ch. 11 question 21 AHN)

 ▸ Discuss the action of oral agents in the treatment of diabetes. |

Christensen & Kockrow

		▸ Discuss the differences between the classifications of oral hypoglycemic agents. *Class Activity Role play. Ask for three student volunteers. Assign one student to play the role of the nurse and the other two students to be the patient and support person. In the scenario, the patient has just been prescribed oral agents to manage type 2 diabetes mellitus. The nurse will be providing information concerning the use of these medications. After the skit, allow time to review and offer suggestions concerning information that should be included.*
Discuss the two new subcutaneous insulin-enhancing drugs exenatide (Byetta) and pramlintide (Symlin) and their mechanisms of action.	– Medications (p. 1750 FAAHN) (p. 514 AHN)	**SG** SG Insulin, Ch. 51 pp. 449-451 FAAHN (Ch. 11 pp. 137-139 AHN) ▸ Discuss the use of exenatide (Byetta) and pramlintide (Symlin). *Class Activity Assign the students to work in small groups of three or four. Assign each group either exenatide (Byetta) or pramlintide (Symlin). Working in small groups, develop drug cards for the nurse planning to administer one of the medications. After the cards are completed, allow class time to review the cards. Use this time to distinguish differences between the two medications.*
Discuss the various insulin types and their characteristics.	– Medical management (FAAHN p. 1748, AHN p. 512) – Nursing interventions and patient teaching (FAAHN p. 1757, AHN p. 521) –Prognosis (FAAHN p. 1764, AHN p. 528)	PPT 54, Ch. 51 FAAHN (Ch. 11 PPT 54 AHN) EILR IC Ch. 51 images 14, 15, 17 FAAHN (Ch. 11 images 14, 15, 17 Ch. 11 AHN) EILR TB Ch. 51 questions 16, 36, 39 FAAHN (Ch. 11 questions 16, 36, 39 AHN) **SG** SG Insulin, pp. 449-451 FAAHN (Ch. 11 pp. 137-139 AHN) **BOOK RESOURCES** Fig. 51-11 Common characteristics of Cushing syndrome (FAAHN p. 1741) (Fig. 11-11 AHN p. 505) Table 51-4 Comparison of Type 1 and Type 2 Diabetes Mellitus (FAAHN p. 1746) (Table 11-4 AHN p. 510)

		Fig. 51-12 Glucose sensor for self-monitoring of blood glucose (FAAHN p. 1748) (Fig. 11-12 AHN p. 512)
		Review Questions for the NCLEX Examination Ch. 51 questions 14, 17, 22, 23 FAAHN (Ch. 11 question 14, 17, 22, 23 AHN)
		▶ Discuss the timing of insulin administration in relation to dietary intake.
		▶ Discuss the onset and peak of action for the commonly prescribed types of insulin.
		Class Activity Develop a set of scenarios. Assign the scenarios to each group. Allow the groups to determine nursing interventions related to each type of insulin and list appropriate insulin reactions.
Discuss the proper way to draw up and administer insulin.	– Medical management (FAAHN p. 1748, AHN p. 512)	PPT 55, Ch. 51 FAAHN (Ch. 11 PPT 55 AHN)
		EILR IC Ch. 51 image 16 FAAHN (Ch. 11 image 16 AHN)
		EILR TB Ch. 51 question 29 FAAHN (Ch. 11 question 29 AHN)
		SG Insulin, Ch. 51 pp. 449-451 FAAHN (Ch. 11 pp. 137-139 AHN)
		BOOK RESOURCES
		Fig. 51-13 U/100 Insulin and disposable U/100 insulin syringe (FAAHN p. 1750) (Fig 11-13 AHN p. 514)
		Fig. 51-14 Commercially available insulin preparations (FAAHN p. 1753) (Fig. 11-14 AHN p. 517)
		Fig. 51-15 A NovoPen insulin pen (FAAHN p. 1753) (Fig. 11-15 AHN p. 517)
		Fig. 51-16 Rotation of sites for insulin injections (FAAHN p. 1755) (Fig. 11-16 AHN p. 519)
		Box 51-4 Technique for Insulin Injection (FAAHN p. 1755) (Box 11-4 AHN p. 519)
		Fig. 51-17 Medtronic MiniMed Insulin pump (FAAHN p. 1755) (Fig. 11-17 AHN p. 519)
		▶ Discuss the sites for the administration of insulin.
		▶ Discuss common concerns associated with insulin administration.

Adult Health Nursing, 6th ed.

Christensen & Kockrow

		Class Activity Bring to class the supplies needed to administer insulin. Demonstrate the correct administration technique for the class. *Note: If manikins are not available to demonstrate administration, an orange can be used.*
Discuss the various classes of oral hypoglycemic medications to treat type 2 diabetes mellitus.	– Medical management (FAAHN p. 1748, AHN p. 512)	PPT 56, Ch. 51 FAAHN (Ch. 11 PPT 56 AHN) EILR TB Ch. 51 question 26 FAAHN (Ch. 11 question 26 AHN) EILR Open Book Quiz Ch. 51 question 10 FAAHN (Ch. 11 question 10 AHN) SG Insulin, Ch. 51 pp. 449-451 FAAHN (Ch. 11 pp. 137-139 AHN) **BOOK RESOURCES** Table 51-5 Types of Insulin (FAAHN p. 1751) (Table 11-5 AHN p. 515) Complementary and Alternative Therapies: Endocrine Disorders (FAAHN p. 1757) (AHN p. 521) ▸ Discuss patients who are candidates for the use of oral hypoglycemic agents. ▸ Discuss contraindications for the use of oral hypoglycemic agents. *Class Activity Using audiovisual aids, post blank drug cards. As a class, develop the drug cards for each of the classifications of oral hypoglycemic medications. After completion, these cards can be copied and distributed to the students for use as a study aid.*
Discuss the acute and long-term complications of diabetes mellitus.	– Nursing interventions and patient teaching (FAAHN p. 1757, AHN p. 521) –Prognosis (FAAHN p. 1764, AHN p. 528)	PPT 57, 58, Ch. 51 FAAHN (Ch. 11 PPT 57, 58 AHN) EILR IC Ch. 51 image 18 FAAHN (Ch. 11 image 18 AHN) ESLR Review Questions for the NCLEX Examination Ch. 43 question 10 FAAHN (Ch. 3 question 10 AHN) SG Complications of Diabetes Ch. 51 p. 453 FAAHN (Ch. 11 p. 141 AHN)

		BOOK RESOURCES
		Fig. 51-18 Long-term complications of diabetes mellitus (p. 1762 FAAHN) (Fig 11-18 AHN p. 526)
		▸ Discuss the signs and symptoms that should be taught to the patient about diabetes complications.
		▸ Discuss preventive measures that can be taken by the diabetic to reduce complications.
		Class Activity Assign each student a body system. Group the students by body system. Instruct each group to gather information and identify the impact of diabetes on its assigned body system.
List five nursing interventions that foster self-care in the activities of daily living of the patient with diabetes mellitus.	– Nursing interventions and patient teaching (FAAHN p. 1757, AHN p. 521) ☐ Nursing process for patients with an endocrine disorder (FAAHN p. 1764, AHN p. 528) – Assessment (FAAHN p. 1764, AHN p. 528) – Nursing diagnoses (FAAHN p. 1764, AHN p. 528) – Expected outcomes and planning (FAAHN p. 1764, AHN p. 528) – Implementation (FAAHN p. 1765, AHN p. 529) – Evaluation (FAAHN p. 1765, AHN p. 529)	PPT 51 through 57, Ch. 51 FAAHN (Ch. 11 PPT 51 through 57 AHN) SG Diabetes Management, Ch. 51 p. 451 FAAHN (Ch. 11 p. 139 AHN) **BOOK RESOURCES** Evidence-Based Practice: Changes in Diabetes Self-Care Behaviors (FAAHN p. 1749) (AHN p. 513) Health Promotion: Foot Care for the Patient with Diabetes Mellitus (FAAHN p. 1758) (AHN p. 522) Life Span Considerations, Older Adults: Endocrine Disorder (FAAHN p. 1759) (AHN p. 523) Nursing Care Plan 51-1 The Patient with Diabetes Mellitus (FAAHN p. 1759) (NCP 11-1 p. 523 AHN) NCP CTQ 1 through 3 (FAAHN p. 1760) (AHN p. 524) Communication : Importance of Proper Foot Care for Patients with Diabetes (FAAHN p. 1763) (AHN p. 527) Home Care Considerations: Diabetes Mellitus (FAAHN p. 1764) (AHN p. 528) Cultural Considerations: Chronic Conditions (FAAHN p. 1764) (AHN p. 528) Review Questions for the NCLEX Examination Ch. 51 questions 19, 20, 36 FAAHN (Ch. 11 questions 19, 20, 36 AHN)

Adult Health Nursing, 6th ed.
Christensen & Kockrow

		▸ Discuss the responsibilities of the nurse in promoting self-care activities for the patient living with a diagnosis of diabetes mellitus.
		Class Activity Divide the class into groups of three. Instruct each group to write down the areas that it anticipates would be of concern to the diabetic patient. Then each group will be asked to brainstorm to develop a listing of community-based resources available to assist the patient and family in meeting these concerns.
		Note: This will be useful to stimulate dialogue and critical thinking. Providing telephone books can help the students.
Performance Evaluation		▰ EILR TB Ch. 51 questions 1 through 42 FAAHN (Ch. 11 questions 1 through 42 AHN)
		▰ EILR Open Book Quiz Ch. 51 questions 1 through 10 FAAHN (Ch. 11 questions 1 through 10 AHN)
		SG Ch. 51 pp. 441-456 FAAHN (Ch. 11 pp. 129-144 AHN)
		BOOK RESOURCES
		Nursing Care Plan 51-1 The Patient with Diabetes Mellitus (FAAHN p. 1759) (NCP 11-1 p. 523 AHN)
		♀ NCP CTQ 1-3 (FAAHN p. 1760) (AHN p. 524)
		Review Questions for the NCLEX Examination Ch. 51 questions 1 through 37 FAAHN (Ch. 11 questions 1 through 37 AHN)

11.4 Homework/Assignments:

11.4 Instructor's Notes/Student Feedback:

Adult Health Nursing, 6th ed.
Christensen & Kockrow

Slide 1

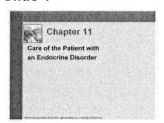

Slide 2

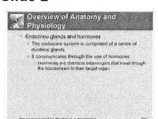

- The body's glands are divided into two categories: endocrine and exocrine. Review how these two types differ.

Slide 3

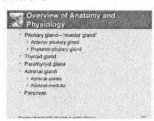

- The pituitary gland is known as the "master gland." Why has this moniker been applied?

Slide 4

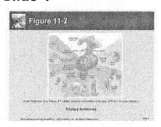

- The pituitary gland is responsible for the secretion of eight different hormones. Hormones play a vital function in the human body.

- What is the definition of hormones and the roles they play?

Slide 5

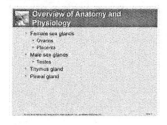

- The endocrine glands are responsible for the regulation of numerous physiological processes in the body, including reproductive functions. The ovaries, located in the lower abdomen, secrete estrogen, which is responsible for the development of secondary sexual characteristics.

- The placenta is a unique organ. It is present in the woman only during pregnancy. What are the functions of the placenta? What hormones are secreted by the placenta?

- What hormone is secreted by the testes? What bodily changes result from this substance?

Christensen & Kockrow

Slide 6

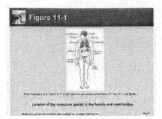

Slide 7

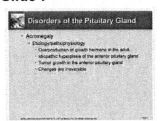

- Acromegaly is a relatively rare disorder. Onset of the disorder is usually in the third or fourth decade of life.

Slide 8

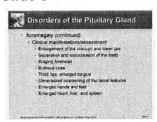

- The characteristic clinical manifestations of acromegaly occur throughout the body. When collecting information from patients, what subjective data should be obtained?

- What questions should be asked of this patient?

Slide 9

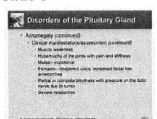

- The significant changes in appearance associated with acromegaly have the potential to have psychosocial implications. What nursing diagnoses may be applicable to the psychosocial needs of the patient diagnosed with acromegaly?

Slide 10

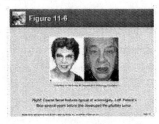

- The photograph on the left represents the individual prior to the diagnosis of acromegaly. The physiological impact of the disease is apparent in the photograph on the right side.

ELSEVIER

Mosby items and derived items © 2011, 2007 by Mosby, Inc., an affiliate of Elsevier Inc.
Some material was previously published.

Adult Health Nursing, 6th ed.
Christensen & Kockrow

Slide 11

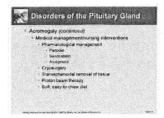

- The patient experiencing acromegaly will often experience 7 to 9 years between the diagnosis of the disorder and the onset of clinical manifestations. What factors could be associated with this delay in a definitive diagnosis?

- When acromegaly is suspected, the diagnosis will be made based upon the patient's health history, clinical manifestations, and the results of screening tests. What tests can be anticipated? What findings will support a positive diagnosis?

- Why are analgesics prescribed for the patient with acromegaly?

- After diagnosis and treatment, what prognosis can the acromegalic patient anticipate?

Slide 12

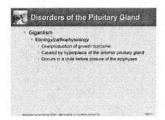

- The secretion of growth hormone is responsible for the growth and development of the body's tissues. When growth hormone is produced in excess, gigantism can result.

- Review the epiphyses. What are they, and why is gigantism impacted by their development?

Slide 13

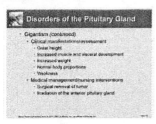

- Clinical manifestations associated with gigantism resemble an "overgrowth." Despite their large size, the affected patients experience weakness.

- What causes this weakness?

- What nursing care will be needed for the patient diagnosed with gigantism?

Slide 14

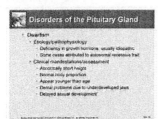

- A deficiency in growth hormone can result in dwarfism. Dwarfism is associated with the expected short stature. What other body systems will be affected?

Slide 15

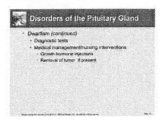

- When a deficiency of growth hormone occurs, what diagnostic workup can be anticipated?

- What psychosocial implications are associated with a diagnosis of dwarfism?

- When diagnosed and treated, what is the long-term prognosis?

ELSEVIER

Slide 16

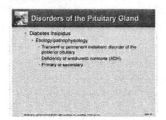

- Diabetes insipidus results when antidiuretic hormone secretion or function goes awry. What physiological function does antidiuretic hormone have in the body?

- What factors can cause this dysfunction?

Slide 17

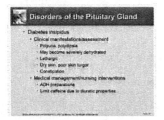

- Patients experiencing diabetes insipidus might feel the need to consume several liters of fluid and then void thousands of milliliters daily.

- Review the physiological significance caused by this massive fluid output. Which electrolytes are most compromised with the condition?

- If the patient wishes to drink so much fluid, what are the dangers of being allowed to do so?

Slide 18

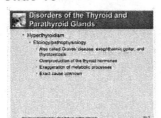

- Hyperthyroidism occurs more commonly in women than men.

- It results when there is an elevation in thyroid hormone secretion.

- Although there is no exact known cure, there are supported theories in existence. Discuss these circulating theories.

Slide 19

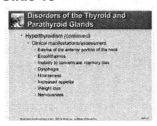

- When collecting data, what subjective data should be solicited? Provide examples of questions to include in the patient interview.

Slide 20

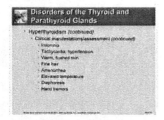

Slide 21

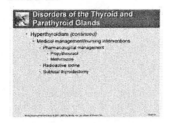

- When hyperthyroidism is suspected, a full diagnostic workup is warranted. What tests can be anticipated? What findings will support a positive diagnosis for the condition?

- The condition can be managed with the use of medications as well as surgical intervention. When medications are prescribed, what is their mode of action?

Slide 22

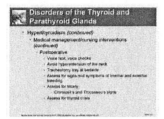

- Surgical intervention is indicated for those cases for which drug therapy is not appropriate.

- When surgery is planned, what are the preoperative goals for the patient?

- During the postoperative period the patient's environment is monitored. What characteristics are desired for the patient's care environment? Why?

- Outline the critical elements in the postoperative assessment.

- Demonstrate the assessment for Chvostek's and Trousseau's signs.

Slide 23

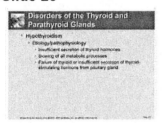

- Hypothyroidism is a common disorder. What populations are affected most?

- What conditions can cause hypothyroidism?

Slide 24

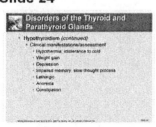

- Hypothyroidism can affect both newborns and adults. What medical terminology is used to refer to the condition in newborns? In adults?

Slide 25

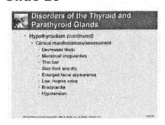

- The reduction of thyroid hormone will result in a generalized slowing of metabolic processes. All systems are implicated in the condition.

- In addition to determining the physical signs and symptoms, what psychosocial factors should be assessed?

- What nursing care will be indicated to meet both the physical and psychological needs of the patient?

ELSEVIER

Adult Health Nursing, 6th ed.

Christensen & Kockrow

Slide 26

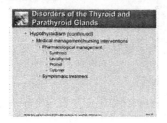

- When hypothyroidism is suspected, a series of tests will be performed to make a diagnosis. What tests can be anticipated? What results will support a diagnosis of hypothyroidism?

- When medications are prescribed to treat the disorder, what patient teaching is indicated?

Slide 27

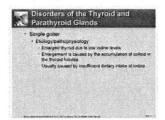

- A simple goiter is also known as a colloid goiter. What does the term colloid mean?

- Explain the interrelationship between the T3 levels and TSH secretion.

Slide 28

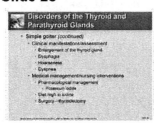

- The diagnosis is usually made based upon the clinical presentation of the patient.

- What are potential topics for patient education concerning the diagnosis?

- When considering a diet high in iodine, what should be encouraged in the patient's intake?

- What is the prognosis for a simple goiter?

Slide 29

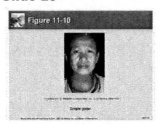

Slide 30

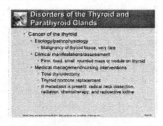

- While there are few cases of thyroid cancer in the United States, there is an anticipated increase on the horizon. To what factors is this expected increase attributed?

- There are populations in which thyroid cancer occurs more frequently: females and whites.

- When thyroid cancer is suspected, diagnostic tests are used to make a positive diagnosis. What results will confirm a diagnosis?

- Review the prognosis associated with a diagnosis of thyroid cancer.

ELSEVIER

Adult Health Nursing, 6th ed.
Christensen & Kockrow

Slide 31

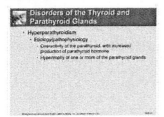

- Hyperparathyroidism results when the parathyroid gland produces the parathyroid hormone in excess. This disorder affects women between the ages of 30 and 70 years of age.

- What underlying conditions can cause this to occur?

Slide 32

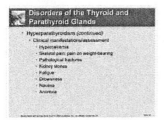

- Hypercalcemia is the primary manifestation. What series of events will accompany hypercalcemia?

- Why is there pain associated with this disease?

- The cardiovascular system may be impacted by hyperparathyroidism. What will occur if this system becomes involved?

Slide 33

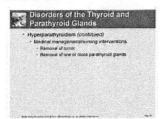

- When hyperparathyroidism is suspected, a series of diagnostic tests will be performed. A radiographic examination of the skeleton might be ordered. What results would be anticipated to support a positive diagnosis?

- Additional tests will include serum alkaline phosphate and calcium levels.

Slide 34

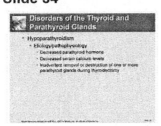

- A reduction of parathyroid hormones will result in hypoparathyroidism.

- What will cause this disorder to occur?

Slide 35

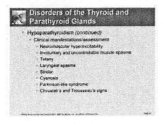

- The signs and symptoms of this disorder occur when the serum levels of calcium become compromised.

- In addition to the objective manifestations, what subjective signs might be present?

Slide 36

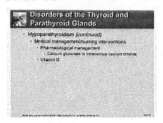

- The management of hypoparathyroidism involves the administration of calcium gluconate or calcium chloride. What nursing implications accompany these medications?
- When developing a plan of care for this patient, what dietary recommendations should be made?

Slide 37

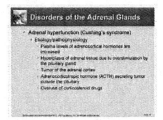

- The adrenal cortex consists of three layers. A specific hormone is secreted by each layer.
- The hormones secreted by the adrenal cortex are steroids.
- Identify the hormones produced by the adrenal cortex.

Slide 38

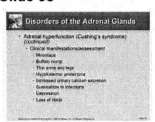

- The changes exhibited by an oversecretion of adrenal hormones often cause a drastic change in appearance.
- In addition to the outward manifestations exhibited, there are blood imbalances. The blood glucose is elevated. What causes this to occur?
- Discuss the changes in electrolyte balance.

Slide 39

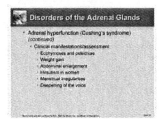

Slide 40

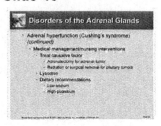

- The diagnosis of Cushing's syndrome is made by combining the patient's physical symptoms with diagnostic tests for confirmation.
- The diagnostic tests that might be performed include serum levels and scanning tests. What tests can be anticipated to confirm a diagnosis?
- What are the goals of nursing care for the Cushing's syndrome patient in the initial period after diagnosis?

ELSEVIER

Adult Health Nursing, 6th ed.
Christensen & Kockrow

Slide 41

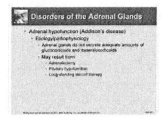

- What populations have the greatest incidence of Addison's disease?

Slide 42

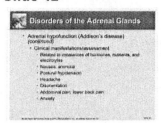

- Patients experiencing hypofunction of the adrenal glands present with a broad range of symptoms.

- What electrolytes are imbalanced? What manifestations will be noted with these imbalances?

- Anxiety is a chief concern for these patients. What should the nurse assess to determine the coping abilities of the patient?

Slide 43

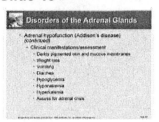

- The patient suspected of Addison's disease can present with integumentary changes. Hyperpigmentation often results. What causes this to occur? When assessing the patient for these changes, where should the nurse focus the observations?

- Assessment of vital signs is also important as the patient could experience alterations in body temperature.

- Review the physiological changes that cause an adrenal crisis to occur.

Slide 44

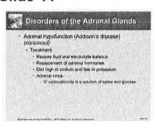

- After diagnosis, the patient with Addison's disease will require close nursing assessments. Identify the primary patient-centered goals.

Slide 45

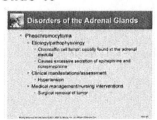

- Pheochromocytoma is a rare occurrence.

- The tumor may be benign or malignant. Most are benign.

- What complications may result from this condition?

Christensen & Kockrow

Slide 46

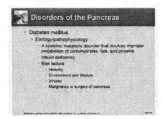

- Diabetes is a chronic metabolic disorder.
- The exact cause of diabetes is unknown, although there are several factors that are associated with its development.

Slide 47

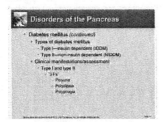

- There are several types of diabetes mellitus. Although each type is different, the common theme involves the body's inability to adequately metabolize glucose.
- The two most common types of DM are type I diabetes mellitus (IDDM) and type II (noninsulin dependent) diabetes mellitus.
- How do these types differ in presentation?

Slide 48

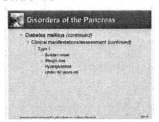

- Typically Type I diabetes mellitus demonstrates a rapid onset. It is characterized by a progressive destruction of beta-cell function. What theories explain potential causes of this type of DM?
- This type of DM is significantly less common than type II.

Slide 49

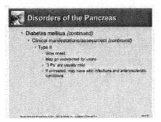

- What populations are most affected by type II diabetes?

Slide 50

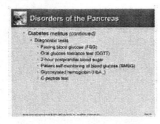

- When making a diagnosis for diabetes mellitus, both the patient's clinical manifestations and the diagnostic screening test results will be utilized.
- What glucose screening results signify a probable diagnosis of diabetes?
- When tests are scheduled, what patient education is required to ensure preoperative compliance and dependable results?

Adult Health Nursing, 6th ed.

Slide 51

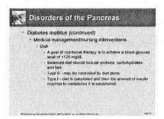

- One of the largest components of diabetic management involves the diet. The diet will need to be individualized.

- What factors should be assessed concerning individual dietary preferences? What role will culture play?

Slide 52

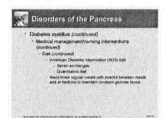

- The exchange system is a common means of developing a diet for patients. What are the underlying principles to this type of diet?

Slide 53

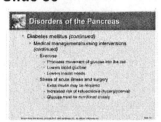

- Successful diabetes management involves control of a series of interrelated factors. In addition to diet, exercise, illness, and stress play a role in the body's glucose levels.

- What advice should be given to patients regarding the incorporation of exercise into their plan of care?

Slide 54

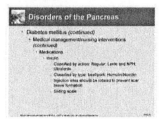

- Insulin administration is needed to sustain the lives of type I diabetes mellitus patients. The type of insulin prescribed will be based upon the individual needs of the patients.

- Review the types of insulin.

Slide 55

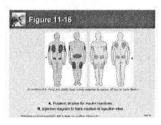

- Insulin is administered via subcutaneous injection. The selection of the site for administration is vital for a diabetic. Where in the body can insulin be injected? How do these sites differ?

- Discuss the means to rotate injection sites.

Slide 56

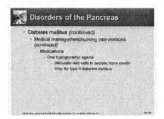

- Oral hypoglycemic medications are used by those diagnosed with type II diabetes mellitus. How do these medications work?

- In what patient populations are they contraindicated?

Slide 57

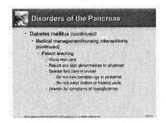

- Successful management of diabetes requires patient teaching. The patient must be assessed for readiness to learn. Education is best completed with an emphasis on repetition. What behaviors signal a readiness to learn?

- How can learning be evaluated?

Slide 58

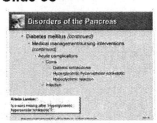

- When diabetes is not successfully managed, life-threatening complications can result. What are the signs and symptoms of each complication?

Slide 59

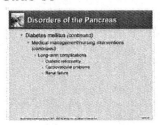

- The longer an individual lives with diabetes, the greater the risk of complications. Discuss the ways a patient can reduce long-term complications.

Slide 60

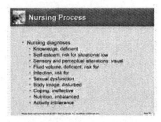

Christensen & Kockrow

12 Lesson Plan
Care of the Patient with a Reproductive Disorder

TEACHING FOCUS

In this chapter, the student will be introduced to the care of the patient with a reproductive disorder. The student will begin by exploring the structure and function of the reproductive system, including the organs of the male and female reproductive tracts, menstruation, and the hormones of the menstrual cycle. The student will then have the opportunity to learn the etiology and pathophysiology, clinical manifestations, assessment, diagnostic tests, medical management, nursing interventions, patient teaching, and prognosis for a variety of male and female reproductive disorders.

MATERIALS AND RESOURCES

- ☐ Computer/overhead projector (all lessons)
- ☐ White/black board and marker/chalk (all lessons)
- ☐ Unlabeled diagrams of the male and female pelvis (Lesson 12.1)
- ☐ Free pamphlets or reminders cards from a local breast-screening clinic to distribute to students (Lesson 12.1)
- ☐ Ball or other soft object that can be tossed around the classroom (Lesson 12.2)
- ☐ Educational materials concerning cancers of the female reproductive system from a local cancer treatment facility (Lesson 12.2)
- ☐ Breast assessment teaching guides from the American Cancer Society (Lesson 12.3)
- ☐ Blank paper (Lesson 12.3)
- ☐ A testicular model to be used to demonstrate the detection of testicular cancer (12.4)

LESSON CHECKLIST

Preparations for this lesson include:
- Lecture
- Invite a survivor of breast cancer to speak with the class.
- Invite a representative of a family planning center or Planned Parenthood to discuss available services.

KEY TERM

amenorrhea (FAAHN p. 1782, AHN p. 546)
candidiasis (FAAHN p. 1827, AHN p. 591)
carcinoma in situ (FAAHN p. 1801, AHN p. 565)
chancre (FAAHN p. 1825, AHN p. 589)
Chlamydia trachomatis (FAAHN p. 1827, AHN p. 591)
circumcision (FAAHN p. 1820, AHN p. 584)
climacteric (FAAHN p. 1787, AHN p. 551)
colporrhaphy (FAAHN p. 1798, AHN p. 562)
colposcopy (FAAHN p. 1778, AHN p. 542)
cryptorchidism (FAAHN p. 1821, AHN p. 585)
culdoscopy (FAAHN p. 1778, AHN p. 542)
curettage (FAAHN p. 1780, AHN p. 544)
dysmenorrhea (FAAHN p. 1782, AHN p. 546)
endometriosis (FAAHN p. 1796, AHN p. 560)
epididymitis (FAAHN p. 1820, AHN p. 584)

fistula (FAAHN p. 1797, AHN p. 561)
introitus (FAAHN p. 1798, AHN p. 562)
laparoscopy (FAAHN p. 1778, AHN p. 542)
mammography (FAAHN p. 1780, AHN p. 544)
menorrhagia (FAAHN p. 1782, AHN p. 546)
metrorrhagia (FAAHN p. 1783, AHN p. 547)
panhysterosalpingo-oophorectomy (FAAHN p. 1805, AHN p. 569)
Papanicolaou (Pap) test (smear) (FAAHN p. 1778, AHN p. 542)
phimosis (FAAHN p. 1820, AHN p. 584)
procidentia (FAAHN p. 1798, AHN p. 562)
sentinel lymph node mapping (FAAHN p. 1810, AHN p. 574)
trichomoniasis (FAAHN p. 1826, AHN p. 590)

ADDITIONAL RESOURCES (AHN)

PPT Ch. 52, 1 through 87 FAAHN (Ch. 12, 1 through 87 AHN)
EILR IC images Ch. 52, 1 through 21 FAAHN (Ch. 12, 1 through 21 AHN)
EILR TB questions Ch. 52, 1 through 39 FAAHN (Ch. 12, 1 through 39 AHN)
EILR Open Book Quiz Ch. 52, 1 through 10 FAAHN (Ch. 12, 1 through 10 AHN)
ESLR Review Questions for the NCLEX® Examination Ch. 52, 52-01 through 52-10 FAAHN (Ch. 12, 12-01 through 12-10 AHN)

Christensen & Kockrow

Legend

PPT
PowerPoint
Slides

EILR
EVOLVE Instructor
Learning Resources:
Image Collection, Test
Bank, Open Book Quizzes

ESLR
EVOLVE Student
Learning Resources:
Review Questions
for the NCLEX
Examination

SG
Study Guide

NCP CTQ
Nursing Care Plan
Critical Thinking
Question

Class Activities are indicated in **bold italic**.

LESSON 12.1

PRETEST

1. The American Cancer Society makes which of the following recommendations concerning the use of mammography for women who do not have any remarkable risk factors?
   a. Mammograms should be done annually beginning at age 35 for all patients.
   b. Patients should begin to have annual mammograms beginning at age 40.
   c. Mammography baseline examinations should begin at age 30.
   d. Mammograms should be performed every 2 years after age 45.

2. The use of lotions and deodorants has what influence on a mammogram?
   a. Lotions and deodorants do not impact the accuracy of a mammogram.
   b. Lotions and deodorants can cause false positive responses on the mammogram's interpretation.
   c. Whereas lotion doesn't influence mammogram readings, deodorant can cause a false negative interpretation.
   d. Lotions and deodorants can cause false negative responses on the interpretation of a mammogram.

3. A 35-year-old patient has been diagnosed with a vaginal yeast infection. Based upon your knowledge, what medication might be ordered for treatment?
   a. Acyclovir
   b. Danazol
   c. Premarin
   d. Metronidazole

4. While reviewing the medical records of a 36-year-old patient, you notice she has been seen at the clinic with complaints of dyspareunia. You recognize this medical terminology refers to:
   a. painful intercourse.
   b. painful menstrual cramps.
   c. an estrogen imbalance.
   d. the presence of vaginal dryness.

5. A 42-year-old woman presents with complaints of vaginal irritations and dyspareunia. Her physician diagnoses her with atrophic vaginitis. She asks how she contracted this disorder. What information should be included in the patient education?
   a. Reduced estrogen levels have caused vaginal changes resulting in the symptoms being experienced.
   b. Excessive douching is associated with the development of this disorder.
   c. An increase in the normal pH of the vaginal vault has caused the changes being experienced.
   d. This disorder is associated with sexual contact with an infected partner.

6. A 22-year-old female is hospitalized with complaints of a sore throat, headache, nausea, vomiting, and fever. During data collection, you note she has a red macular palmar rash on her hands and feet. What diagnosis do you anticipate for this patient?
   a. Pelvic inflammatory disease
   b. Endometriosis
   c. Systemic bacterial vaginosis
   d. Toxic shock syndrome

ELSEVIER

Mosby items and derived items © 2011 by Mosby, Inc., an affiliate of Elsevier Inc.
Some material was previously published.

Adult Health Nursing, 6th ed.
Christensen & Kockrow

7. During a routine visit to her physician, a 23-year-old patient asks how often she should have a breast examination. What information will you provide to the patient?
   a. "You need to perform a self breast exam monthly, and your breasts need to be examined annually by the physician."
   b. "You will need to perform a self breast exam each month, and your physician will examine them every 2 years."
   c. "As long as you are examining your breasts at home monthly, there is no need to begin annual examinations until you begin to experience menopausal signs and symptoms."
   d. "Perform a self breast exam monthly, and then follow up for a breast exam with your physician every 3 years."

8. A 32-year-old man has been diagnosed with a primary episode of genital herpes. What medication do you anticipate will be prescribed?
   a. Tetracycline
   b. Penicillin
   c. Zovirax
   d. Rocephin

9. A patient reports to the clinic with complaints of dysuria, pruritus, and a frothy green discharge. These clinical manifestations are associated with:
   a. trichomoniasis
   b. herpes simplex
   c. gonorrhea
   d. syphilis

10. _____ refers to the number of births a woman has experienced.
   a. Gravidity
   b. Parity
   c. Metorrhagia
   d. Dysmenorrhea

Answers:

1. b	2. b	3. d	4. a	5. a
6. d	7. d	8. c	9. a	10. b

BACKGROUND ASSESSMENT

Question: A 34-year-old woman reports to the physician's office. She has concerns about not yet having become pregnant. She states she and her husband have been trying to conceive for the past 5 months. She asks "to be tested." She states, "Obviously there is something wrong with me." She is tearful and asks for your input. What information should she be given?

Answer: The patient should be advised that there might not be anything wrong with her. Her concerns are being voiced prematurely. A couple is not considered infertile until being unable to conceive after 1 year of sexual intercourse without using birth control. It is still too early for testing to begin. The nurse should assess the patient's knowledge of the appropriate timing of intercourse in relation to her menstrual cycle. Emotional support is also indicated.

Question: During a routine physical examination, a patient reports she has been experiencing frequent yeast infections. During the discussion, she reports she does not understand why she keeps getting the infection since she douches at least every other day. What information should be given to the patient regarding her concerns?

Answer: Frequent yeast infections should be reported to the physician for investigation. Repeated outbreaks can signal an underlying disorder. The patient's hygiene behaviors, that is, frequent douching, increase the likelihood of developing yeast infections. Douching disturbs the normal pH of the vagina.

CRITICAL THINKING QUESTION

A 25-year-old woman reports to the clinic with concerns about changes in her menstrual cycle. She has not had a period for nearly 3 months, and she states she does not think she is pregnant. She asks what can be done for her. What medical term is used for this condition? What assessment information

ELSEVIER

Adult Health Nursing, 6th ed.

Christensen & Kockrow

should be obtained? What diagnostic tests can be anticipated? What are some potential causes that can be associated with her complaints?

Guidelines: The patient is experiencing amenorrhea. Potential causes of amenorrhea include pregnancy, frequent vigorous exercise, an emotional disorder, an eating disorder, and hormonal imbalances. Assessment information gathered or reviewed would include a complete personal and family medical history, the presence of factors that can impact the menstrual cycle, the history of amenorrhea, and recent drug intake. Diagnostic testing could include a pregnancy test; pelvic examination; blood, urine, and hormonal analysis; and a Pap test. Management will be determined by the cause of the condition.

OBJECTIVES	CONTENT	TEACHING RESOURCES
List and describe the functions of the organs of the male and female reproductive tracts.	■ Anatomy and physiology of the reproductive system (FAAHN p. 1770, AHN p. 534) □ Male reproductive system (FAAHN p. 1770, AHN p. 534) – Testes (testicles) (FAAHN p. 1770, AHN p. 534) – Ductal system (FAAHN p. 1770, AHN p. 534) – Accessory glands (FAAHN p. 1770, AHN p. 534) – Urethra and penis (FAAHN p. 1771, AHN p. 535) – Sperm (FAAHN p. 1771, AHN p. 535) □ Female reproductive system (FAAHN p. 1771, AHN p. 535) – Ovaries (FAAHN p. 1772, AHN p. 536) – Fallopian tubes (oviducts) (FAAHN p. 1772, AHN p. 536) – Uterus (FAAHN p. 1772, AHN p. 536) – Vagina (FAAHN p. 1773, AHN p. 537) – External genitalia (FAAHN p. 1773, AHN p. 537) – Accessory glands (FAAHN p. 1773, AHN p. 537) – Perineum (FAAHN p. 1773, AHN p. 537) – Mammary glands (breasts) (FAAHN p. 1773, AHN p. 537) – Menstrual cycle (FAAHN p. 1774, AHN p. 538)	▨ PPT 2 through 10, Ch. 52 FAAHN (Ch. 12 PPT 2 through 10 AHN) 🔗 EILR IC Ch. 52 images 1 through 7, 14 FAAHN (Ch. 12 images 1 through 7, 14 AHN) 🔗 EILR TB Ch. 52 question 39 FAAHN (Ch. 12 question 39 AHN) 🔗 ESLR Review Questions for the NCLEX Examination Ch. 52 question 1 FAAHN (Ch. 12 question 1 AHN) 📖 SG Functions, Ch. 52 p. 457 FAAHN (Ch. 12 p. 145 AHN) 📖 SG Sectional View of the Uterus, Ch. 52 p. 461 FAAHN (Ch. 12 p. 149 AHN) **BOOK RESOURCES** Fig. 52-1 Longitudinal section of the male pelvis showing the location of the male reproductive organs (FAAHN p. 1770) (Fig. 12-1 AHN p. 534) Fig. 52-2 Male sex cell (spermatozoon) greatly enlarged (*left*) (FAAHN p. 1771) (Fig. 12-2 AHN p. 535) Fig. 52-3 Longitudinal section of the female pelvis showing the location of the female reproductive organs (FAAHN p. 1772) (Fig. 12-3 AHN p. 536) Fig. 52-4 Sectioned view of the uterus showing relationship to the ovaries and the vagina (FAAHN p. 1772) (Fig. 12-4 AHN p. 536) Fig. 52-5 External female genitalia (vulva) (FAAHN p. 1773) (Fig. 12-5 AHN p. 537) Fig. 52-6 Lateral view of the breast (sagittal section) (FAAHN p. 1774) (Fig. 12-6 AHN p. 538)

Christensen & Kockrow

OBJECTIVES	CONTENT	TEACHING RESOURCES
		Fig. 52-7 Mammalian ovary showing successive stages of ovarian (graafian) follicle and ovum development. Begin with the first stage (egg nest) and follow around clockwise to the final stage (corpus albicans). (FAAHN p. 1775) (Fig. 12-7 AHN p. 539) ▸ Discuss the functions of the male reproductive system. ▸ Discuss the functions of the female reproductive system. ***Class Activity Provide unlabeled diagrams of the male and female pelvis. Allow 3 to 5 minutes for students to label the primary anatomical organs for each picture.*** ***Note: It would be helpful do this prior to lecture. This will allow an assessment of student knowledge.***
Discuss menstruation and the hormones necessary for a complete menstrual cycle.	– Menstrual cycle (FAAHN p. 1774, AHN p. 538)	SG Menstrual Disturbances, Ch. 52 p. 459 FAAHN (Ch. 12 p. 147 AHN) ▸ Discuss the role of the hormones to maintain healthful functioning of the menstrual cycle. ▸ Discuss the impact on the woman's health if the hormone levels become imbalanced. ***Class Activity Review the roles of each of the hormones on the woman's cycle and have students list each of them on the board.***
Discuss the impact of illness on the patient's sexuality.	☐ Effects of normal aging on the reproductive systems (FAAHN p. 1774, AHN p. 538) ■ Human sexuality (FAAHN p. 1774, AHN p. 538) ☐ Sexual identity (FAAHN p. 1775, AHN p. 539) ☐ Taking a sexual history (FAAHN p. 1776) (AHN p. 540) ☐ Illness and sexuality (FAAHN p. 1777, AHN p. 541)	PPT 11, Ch. 52 FAAHN (Ch. 12 PPT 11 AHN) EILR TB Ch. 52 question 31 FAAHN (Ch. 12 question 31 AHN) ESLR Review Questions for the NCLEX Examination Ch. 52 question 2 FAAHN (Ch. 12 question 2 AHN) SG Sexuality, Ch.52 p. 458 FAAHN (Ch. 12 p. 146 AHN)

Christensen & Kockrow

OBJECTIVES	CONTENT	TEACHING RESOURCES
		BOOK RESOURCES
		Life Span Considerations, Older Adults: Reproductive Disorders (FAAHN p. 1775) (AHN p. 539)
		Health Promotion: Factors that Can Interfere with the Promotion of Sexual Health (FAAHN p. 1776) (AHN p. 540)
		Box 52-1 Requirements for Taking a Sexual History (FAAHN p. 1776) (Box 12-1 AHN p. 540)
		Health Promotion: Self-Help Organizations that Publish Sexuality Pamphlets (FAAHN p. 1777) (AHN p. 541)
		Box 52-2 Brief Sexual History (FAAHN p. 1777) (Box 12-2 AHN p. 541)
		▸ Discuss the differences between sex and sexuality.
		▸ Discuss the psychological concerns associated with the onset of problems in the reproductive system.
		Class Activity Separate students into pairs. Assign the groups to role-play. Assign one student the role of patient and the other the clinic-employed nurse. The patient is to report concerns associated with impaired functioning of the reproductive system. The other student will act as the nurse gathering data. This exercise will demonstrate the difficulty encountered by the patient reporting this type of physical concern.
		Note: It would be most beneficial to have the students paired with students they are less familiar with. This will highlight the difficulty encountered when discussing sexual concerns with strangers.
Discuss nursing interventions for the patient undergoing diagnostic studies related to the reproductive system.	■ Laboratory and diagnostic examinations (FAAHN p. 1777, AHN p. 541) □ Diagnostic tests for the female (FAAHN p. 1777, AHN p. 541) – Colposcopy (FAAHN p. 1778, AHN p. 542)	🖳 PPT 12, 13, Ch. 52 FAAHN (Ch. 12 PPT 12, 13 AHN) ▨ EILR TB Ch. 52 questions 30, 32, 33, 34, 35 FAAHN (Ch. 12 questions 30, 32, 33, 34, 35 AHN) ▨ EILR Open Book Quiz Ch. 52 question 2 FAAHN (Ch. 12 question 2 AHN)

Mosby items and derived items © 2011 by Mosby, Inc., an affiliate of Elsevier Inc. Some material was previously published.

Adult Health Nursing, 6th ed.

Christensen & Kockrow

OBJECTIVES	CONTENT	TEACHING RESOURCES
	– Culdoscopy (FAAHN p. 1778, AHN p. 542) – Laparoscopy (FAAHN p. 1778, AHN p. 542) – Papanicolaou (Pap) test (smear) (FAAHN p. 1778, AHN p. 542) – Biopsy (FAAHN p. 1779, AHN p. 543) – Other diagnostic studies (FAAHN p. 1780, AHN p. 544) ☐ Diagnostic tests for men (FAAHN p. 1781, AHN p. 545) – Testicular biopsy (FAAHN p. 1781, AHN p. 545) – Semen analysis (FAAHN p. 1781, AHN p. 545) – Prostatic smears (FAAHN p. 1781, AHN p. 545) – Cystoscopy (FAAHN p. 1781, AHN p. 545) – Other diagnostic studies (FAAHN p. 1781, AHN p. 545)	▄ ESLR Review Questions for the NCLEX Examination Ch. 52 question 3 FAAHN (Ch. 12 question 3 AHN) ▄ SG Diagnostic Studies, Ch. 52 p. 461 FAAHN (Ch. 12 p. 149 AHN) **BOOK RESOURCES** Review Questions for the NCLEX Examination Ch. 52 question 13 FAAHN (Ch.12 question 13 AHN) Box 52-3 Endoscopic Procedures for Visualization of Pelvic Organs (FAAHN p. 1778) (Box 12-3 AHN p. 542) Box 52-4 Nursing Interventions for the Patient Undergoing Diagnostic Studies (FAAHN p. 1782) (Box 12-4 AHN p. 546) ▸ Discuss the education needed for the patient undergoing diagnostic study related to the reproductive system. ▸ Discuss the nurse's responsibilities caring for the patient undergoing diagnostic testing for concerns about the reproductive system. *Class Activity **Divide the students into groups of four. Instruct each group to prepare a teaching care plan for two of the female diagnostic tests. To conserve time, instruct each group to present findings to only one other group. This will ensure that each student becomes more familiar with at least four diagnostic examinations.***
Discuss the importance of the Papanicolaou smear test in early detection of cervical cancer and mammography as a screening procedure for breast cancer.	– Papanicolaou (Pap) test (smear) (FAAHN p. 1778, AHN p. 542)	▄ EILR TB Ch. 52 question 13 FAAHN (Ch. 12 question 13 AHN) ▄ SG Pap Smear, Ch. 52 p. 473 FAAHN (Ch. 12 p. 151 AHN) **BOOK RESOURCES** Review Questions for the NCLEX Examination Ch. 52 question 21 FAAHN (Ch.12 question 21 AHN)

Adult Health Nursing, 6th ed.

Christensen & Kockrow

OBJECTIVES	CONTENT	TEACHING RESOURCES
		Table 52-1 Pap Test Interpretation Classifications and Action (FAAHN p. 1779) (Box 12-1 AHN p. 543)
		▸ Discuss the recommended frequency for the Papanicolaou smear test and the mammography screening procedure.
		▸ Discuss the nursing care of the patient undergoing the Papanicolaou smear and the mammography screening procedure.
		Class Activity Contact a local breast screening clinic. Ask for free pamphlets or reminder cards to distribute to the class for their personal use. Provide a brief discussion of the materials as they are distributed.
List nursing interventions for patients with menstrual disturbances.	■ The reproductive cycle (FAAHN p. 1782, AHN p. 546) □ Menarche (FAAHN p. 1782, AHN p. 546) □ Disturbances of menstruation (FAAHN p. 1782, AHN p. 546) □ Amenorrhea (FAAHN p. 1783, AHN p. 547) – Etiology and pathophysiology (FAAHN p. 1783, AHN p. 547) – Assessment (FAAHN p. 1783, AHN p. 547) – Diagnostic tests (FAAHN p. 1783, AHN p. 547) – Medical management (FAAHN p. 1783, AHN p. 547) – Nursing interventions and patient teaching (FAAHN p. 1783, AHN p. 547) □ Dysmenorrhea (FAAHN p. 1783, AHN p. 547) – Etiology and pathophysiology (FAAHN p. 1783, AHN p. 547) – Assessment (FAAHN p. 1783, AHN p. 547) – Diagnostic tests (FAAHN p. 1784, AHN p. 548) – Medical management (FAAHN p. 1784, AHN p. 548)	⊠ PPT 14 through 23, Ch. 52 FAAHN (Ch. 12 PPT 14 through 23 AHN) 🔲 EILR Open Book Quiz Ch. 52 question 1 FAAHN (Ch. 12 question 1 AHN) 🔲 ESLR Review Questions for the NCLEX Examination Ch. 52 questions 4 through 6 FAAHN (Ch. 12 question 4 through 6 AHN) 📖 SG Menstrual Disturbances, Ch. 52 p. 459 FAAHN (Ch. 12 p. 147 AHN) **BOOK RESOURCES** Review Questions for the NCLEX Examination Ch. 52 question 24 FAAHN (Ch.12 question 24 AHN) Health Promotion: Health Teaching for Menstruation (FAAHN p. 1782) (AHN p. 546) Table 52-1 Medications for Reproductive Disorders (FAAHN p. 1784) (Table 12-1 AHN p. 548) Fig. 52-9 Common sites of endometriosis (FAAHN p. 1796) (Fig. 12-9 AHN p. 560) Complementary & Alternative Therapies: Male and Female Reproductive Disorders (p. 1833 FAAHN) (p. 597 AHN)

ELSEVIER

Christensen & Kockrow

OBJECTIVES	CONTENT	TEACHING RESOURCES
	– Nursing interventions and patient teaching (FAAHN p. 1784, AHN p. 548)	▶ Discuss the terminology used to describe menstrual abnormalities.
	☐ Abnormal uterine bleeding (menorrhagia and metorrhagia) (FAAHN p. 1784, AHN p. 548)	▶ Discuss the normal menstrual cycle.
	☐ Premenstrual syndrome (FAAHN p. 1786, AHN p. 550)	*Class Activity Have students relate what they know or have heard from relatives about menopausal symptoms and how these symptoms are being managed (food, teas, OTC medications, hormone replacement therapy).*
	– Etiology and pathophysiology (FAAHN p. 1786, AHN p. 550)	
	– Clinical manifestations (FAAHN p. 1786, AHN p. 550)	*Class Activity Ask students to express their feelings about TV/radio ads for impotence drugs.*
	– Assessment (FAAHN p. 1787, AHN p. 551)	
	– Diagnostic tests (FAAHN p. 1787, AHN p. 551)	*Class Activity Without identifying anyone, ask students if they have direct knowledge of someone using current reproductive technology to conceive.*
	– Medical management (FAHN p. 1787, AHN p. 551)	
	– Nursing interventions and patient teaching (FAAHN p. 1787, AHN p. 551)	
	☐ Menopause (FAAHN p. 1787, AHN p. 551)	
	– Etiology and pathophysiology (FAAHN p. 1787, AHN p. 551)	
	– Clinical manifestations (FAAHN p. 1788, AHN p. 552)	
	– Assessment (FAAHN p. 1788, AHN p. 552)	
	– Diagnostic tests (FAAHN p. 1788, AHN p. 552)	
	– Medical management (FAAHN p. 1788, AHN p. 552)	
	– Nursing interventions and patient teaching (FAAHN p. 1789, AHN p. 553)	
	☐ Male climacteric (FAAHN p. 1789, AHN p. 553)	
	– Etiology and pathophysiology (FAAHN p. 1789, AHN p. 553)	
	– Clinical manifestations (FAAHN p. 1790, AHN p. 554)	
	– Assessment (FAAHN p. 1790, AHN p. 554)	

Mosby items and derived items © 2011 by Mosby, Inc., an affiliate of Elsevier Inc.
Some material was previously published.

Christensen & Kockrow

OBJECTIVES	CONTENT	TEACHING RESOURCES
	– Diagnostic tests (FAAHN p. 1790, AHN p. 554)	
	– Nursing interventions and patient teaching (FAAHN p. 1790, AHN p. 554)	
	☐ Erectile dysfunction (FAAHN p. 1790, AHN p. 554)	
	– Medical management (FAAHN p. 1790, AHN p. 554)	
	– Nursing interventions and patient teaching (FAAHN p. 1791, AHN p. 555)	
	☐ Infertility (FAAHN p. 1791, AHN p. 555)	
	– Etiology and pathophysiology (FAAHN p. 1791, AHN p. 555)	
	– Assessment (FAAHN p. 1791, AHN p. 555)	
	– Diagnostic tests (FAAHN p. 1791, AHN p. 555)	
	– Medical management (FAAHN p. 1792, AHN p. 556)	
	– Nursing interventions (FAAHN p. 1792, AHN p. 556)	
	– Prognosis (FAAHN p. 1792, AHN p. 556)	

12.1 Homework/Assignments:

Instruct each student to interview a patient who has had a surgical procedure not related to the reproductive system. This interview must take place prior to the class discussion relating to reproductive surgeries. After the lecture, compare and contrast the types of concerns and limitations for the differing types of surgical patients. See Teaching Resources in next lesson.

12.1 Instructor's Notes/Student Feedback:

ELSEVIER

Adult Health Nursing, 6th ed.
Christensen & Kockrow

LESSON 12.2

CRITICAL THINKING QUESTION

An 18-year-old female reports to the clinic with complaints of "blisters" on her genitals. In addition to open lesions on her labia, the pelvic examination also reveals leukorrhea and swollen lymph nodes. When questioned further, she states she feels "achy and tired." After the examination, the physician diagnoses her with genital herpes. Upon receiving the diagnosis, she becomes tearful. She asks how this could have happened. After regaining her composure, she asks how this illness will be cured. What information will need to be provided to this patient?

Guidelines: She should be advised that genital herpes is a viral infection. It is spread by contact with infected individuals. Her misconception that herpes can be "cured" must be corrected. Herpes cannot be permanently cured. After the initial outbreak, herpes can reoccur. Herpes can be managed with lifestyle changes and medication. Medication therapies involve the use of antiviral drugs such as Zovirax and Valtrex. During outbreaks the goals are to increase comfort and to prevent infection and transmission to others. Patient teaching must include a discussion of safe sexual practices.

OBJECTIVES	CONTENT	TEACHING RESOURCES
Discuss the etiology/ pathophysiology, clinical manifestations, assessment, diagnostic tests, medical management, nursing interventions, patient teaching, and prognosis for infections of the female reproductive tract.	■ Inflammatory and infections of the female reproductive tract (FAAHN p. 1792, AHN p. 556) □ Simple vaginitis (FAAHN p. 1793, AHN p. 557) – Etiology and pathophysiology (FAAHN p. 1793, AHN p. 557) – Clinical manifestations (FAAHN p. 1793, AHN p. 557) – Assessment (FAAHN p. 1793, AHN p. 557) – Diagnostic tests (FAAHN p. 1793, AHN p. 557) – Medical management (FAAHN p. 1793, AHN p. 557) – Nursing interventions and patient teaching (FAAHN p. 1793, AHN p. 557) – Prognosis (FAAHN p. 1793, AHN p. 557) □ Senile vaginitis or atrophic vaginitis (FAAHN p. 1793, AHN p. 557) □ Cervicitis (FAAHN p. 1794, AHN p. 558) □ Pelvic inflammatory disease (FAAHN p. 1794, AHN p. 558)	⊠ PPT 26 through 49, Ch. 52 FAAHN (Ch. 12 PPT 26 through 49 AHN) 🖰 EILR IC Ch. 52 images 11 through 13 FAAHN (Ch. 12 images 11 through 13 AHN) 🖰 EILR TB Ch. 52 questions 7, 15, 36 FAAHN (Ch. 12 question 7, 15, 36 AHN) 🖰 EILR Open Book Quiz Ch. 52 questions 3, 5, 6 FAAHN (Ch. 12 questions 3, 5, 6 AHN) 🖰 ESLR Review Questions for the NCLEX Examination Ch. 52 questions 7, 8 FAAHN (Ch.12 questions 7, 8 AHN) 🖾 SG Infections of the Female Reproductive Tract, Ch. 52 p. 463 FAAHN (Ch. 12 p. 151 AHN) **BOOK RESOURCES** Review Questions for the NCLEX Examination Ch. 52 questions 8, 26 FAAHN (Ch.12 questions 8, 26 AHN) Table 52-2 Medications for Reproductive Disorders (p. 1785 FAAHN) (p. 549 AHN) Figure 52-11 Uterine prolapse (FAAHN p. 1798) (Fig. 12-11 p. 562) Figure 52-13 **A**, Cystocele. **B**, Rectocele (FAAHN p. 1799) (Fig. 12-13 p. 563)

OBJECTIVES	CONTENT	TEACHING RESOURCES
	– Etiology and pathophysiology (FAAHN p. 1794, AHN p. 558) – Clinical manifestations (FAAHN p. 1794, AHN p. 558) – Assessment (FAAHN p. 1794, AHN p. 558) – Diagnostic tests (FAAHN p. 1794, AHN p. 558) – Medical management (FAAHN p. 1794, AHN p. 558) – Nursing interventions and patient teaching (FAAHN p. 1794, AHN p. 558) – Prognosis (FAAHN p. 1795, AHN p. 559) ☐ Toxic shock syndrome (FAAHN p. 1795, AHN p. 559) – Etiology and pathophysiology (FAAHN p. 1795, AHN p. 559) – Clinical manifestations (FAAHN p. 1795, AHN p. 559) – Assessment (FAAHN p. 1795, AHN p. 559) – Diagnostic tests (FAAHN p. 1795, AHN p. 559) – Medical management (FAAHN p. 1795, AHN p. 559) – Nursing interventions and patient teaching (FAAHN p. 1795, AHN p. 559) – Prognosis (FAAHN p. 1796, AHN p. 560)	▸ Discuss the high-risk behaviors associated with contracting infections of the female reproductive tract. ▸ Discuss the signs and symptoms of the infections of the female reproductive tract. *Class Activity Toss a ball around the class. As the ball is caught by each student, that student will be asked to make a true statement concerning infections of the female reproductive tract.*
Discuss four important points to be addressed in discharge planning for the patient with pelvic inflammatory disease (PID).	☐ Pelvic inflammatory disease (FAAHN p. 1794, AHN p. 558) – Etiology and pathophysiology (FAAHN p. 1794, AHN p. 558) – Clinical manifestations (FAAHN p. 1794, AHN p. 558) – Assessment (FAAHN p. 1794, AHN p. 558)	▦ PPT 30, 31 Ch. 52 FAAHN (Ch.12 PPT 31, 32 AHN) ▰ EILR TB Ch. 52 question 17 FAAHN (Ch. 17 question 12 AHN) ▨ SG Pelvic Inflammatory Disease, Ch. 52 p. 464 FAAHN (Ch. 12 p. 152 AHN)

Christensen & Kockrow

OBJECTIVES	CONTENT	TEACHING RESOURCES
	– Diagnostic tests (FAAHN p. 1794, AHN p. 558) – Medical management (FAAHN p. 1794, AHN p. 558) – Nursing interventions and patient teaching (FAAHN p. 1794, AHN p. 558) – Prognosis (FAAHN p. 1795, AHN p. 559)	**BOOK RESOURCES** Review Questions for the NCLEX Examination Ch. 52 question 25 FAAHN (Ch.12 question 25 AHN) ▸ Discuss the populations at highest risk for the development of pelvic inflammatory disease (PID). ▸ Discuss the implications of a diagnosis of pelvic inflammatory disease on a woman's reproductive health. *Class Activity **Have the class modify a nursing care plan for the patient diagnosed with pelvic inflammatory disease.***
List four nursing diagnoses pertinent to the patient with endometriosis.	■ Disorders of the female reproductive system (FAAHN p. 1796, AHN p. 560) ☐ Endometriosis (FAAHN p. 1796, AHN p. 560) – Etiology and pathophysiology (FAAHN p. 1796, AHN p. 560) – Clinical manifestations (FAAHN p. 1796, AHN p. 560) – Assessment (FAAHN p. 1796, AHN p. 560) – Diagnostic tests (FAAHN p. 1796, AHN p. 560) – Medical management (FAAHN p. 1796, AHN p. 560) – Nursing interventions and patient teaching (FAAHN p. 1797, AHN p. 561) – Prognosis (FAAHN p. 1797, AHN p. 561) ☐ Relaxed pelvic muscles (FAAHN p. 1798, AHN p. 562) – Displaced uterus (FAAHN p. 1798, AHN p. 562) – Uterine prolapse (FAAHN p. 1798, AHN p. 562) ☐ Leiomyomas of the uterus (FAAHN p. 1799, AHN p. 563)	PPT 34, 35, Ch. 52 FAAHN (Ch.12 PPT 34, 35 AHN) EILR IC Ch. 52 image 9 FAAHN (Ch. 12 image 9 AHN) SG Endometriosis, Ch. 52 p. 464 FAAHN (Ch. 12 p. 152 AHN) **BOOK RESOURCES** Review Questions for the NCLEX Examination Ch. 52 question 23 FAAHN (Ch.12 question 23 AHN) Box 52-1 Requirements for Taking a Sexual History (p. 1776 FAAHN) (p. 540 AHN) Fig. 52-9 Common sites of endometriosis (FAAHN p. 1796) (Fig. 12-9 AHN p. 560) ▸ Discuss clinical manifestations associated with a diagnosis of endometriosis. ▸ Discuss risk factors associated with a diagnosis of endometriosis. *Class Activity **Divide students into groups of four. Assign each group the task of investigating an aspect of endometriosis. Topics to be reviewed include: pathophysiology, clinical manifestations, management, and prognosis. Allow each student group 3 minutes to present their group's findings.***

Christensen & Kockrow

OBJECTIVES	CONTENT	TEACHING RESOURCES
	– Etiology and pathophysiology (FAAHN p. 1799, AHN p. 563)	
	– Clinical manifestations (FAAHN p. 1799, AHN p. 563)	
	– Assessment (FAAHN p. 1800, AHN p. 564)	
	– Diagnostic tests (FAAHN p. 1800, AHN p. 564)	
	– Medical management (FAAHN p. 1800, AHN p. 564)	
	– Nursing interventions and patient teaching (FAAHN p. 1800, AHN p. 564)	
	– Prognosis (FAAHN p. 1800, AHN p. 564)	
	☐ Ovarian cysts (FAAHN p. 1800, AHN p. 564)	
	– Etiology and pathophysiology (FAAHN p. 1800, AHN p. 564)	
	– Clinical manifestations (FAAHN p. 1800, AHN p. 564)	
	– Medical management (FAAHN p. 1800, AHN p. 564)	
	– Nursing interventions (FAAHN p. 1800, AHN p. 564)	
	– Prognosis (FAAHN p. 1800, AHN p. 564)	
Identify the clinical manifestations of a vaginal fistula.	☐ Vaginal fistula (FAAHN p. 1797, AHN p. 561) – Etiology and pathophysiology (FAAHN p. 1797, AHN p. 561) – Clinical manifestations (FAAHN p. 1797, AHN p. 561) – Assessment (FAAHN p. 1797, AHN p. 561) – Diagnostic tests (FAAHN p. 1797, AHN p. 561) – Medical management (FAAHN p. 1797, AHN p. 561)	PPT 36, 37, Ch. 52 FAAHN (Ch. 12 PPT 36, 37 AHN) EILR IC Ch. 52 image 10 FAAHN (Ch. 12 image 10 AHN) EILR TB Ch. 52 question 37 FAAHN (Ch. 12 question 37 AHN) SG Fistula, Ch. 52 p. 465 FAAHN (Ch. 12 p. 153 AHN) **BOOK RESOURCES** Review Questions for the NCLEX Examination Ch. 52 question 12 FAAHN (Ch.12 question 12 AHN)

OBJECTIVES	CONTENT	TEACHING RESOURCES
	– Nursing interventions (FAAHN p. 1797, AHN p. 561) – Prognosis (FAAHN p. 1798, AHN p. 562)	Fig. 52-10 Types of fistulas that may develop in the vagina and the uterus (FAAHN p. 1797) (Fig. 12-10 AHN p. 561) ▸ Discuss the causes of fistula development. ▸ Discuss populations at risk for fistula development. *Class Activity Ask the students to list on the board the implications of a fistula for the overall health status of a patient.*
Describe the common problems with cystocele and rectocele, and the related medical management and nursing interventions.	☐ Relaxed pelvic muscles (FAAHN p. 1798, AHN p. 562) – Displaced uterus (FAAHN p. 1798, AHN p. 562) – Uterine prolapse (FAAHN p. 1798, AHN p. 562) – Cystocele and rectocele (FAAHN p. 1798, AHN p. 562)	PPT 43 through 45, Ch. 52 FAAHN (Ch. 12 PPT 43 through 45 AHN) EILR TB Ch. 52 question 19 FAAHN (Ch. 12 question 19 AHN) SG Cystocele and Rectocele, Ch. 52 p. 466 FAAHN (Ch. 12 p. 154 AHN) **BOOK RESOURCES** Review Questions for the NCLEX Examination Ch. 52 question 20 FAAHN (Ch.12 question 20 AHN) Health Promotion: Kegel Exercises (p. 1789 FAAHN) (p. 553 AHN) Fig. 52-11 Uterine prolapse (FAAHN p. 1798) (Fig. 12-11 AHN p. 562) Fig. 52-12 **A,** Cystocele. **B,** Rectocele (FAAHN p. 1799) (Fig. 12-12 AHN p. 563) ▸ Discuss factors contributing to the development of cystoceles and rectoceles. *Class Activity Have the students call out the symptoms and treatment options for cystoceles and rectoceles.*
Discuss the etiology, pathophysiology, clinical manifestations, assessment, diagnostic tests, medical management, nursing	■ Cancer of the female reproductive tract (FAAHN p. 1800, AHN p. 564) ☐ Cancer of the cervix (FAAHN p. 1801, AHN p. 565) – Etiology and pathophysiology (FAAHN p. 1801, AHN p. 565) – Clinical manifestations (FAAHN p. 1801, AHN p. 565)	PPT 49 through 55, Ch. 52 FAAHN (Ch. 12 PPT 49 through 55 AHN) EILR TB Ch. 52 questions 3, 11 FAAHN (Ch. 12 questions 3, 11 AHN) EILR Open Book Quiz Ch. 52 question 7 FAAHN (Ch. 12 question 7 AHN)

Christensen & Kockrow

OBJECTIVES	CONTENT	TEACHING RESOURCES
interventions, patient teaching, and prognosis for cancers of the female reproductive system.	– Assessment (FAAHN p. 1801, AHN p. 565) – Diagnostic tests (FAAHN p. 1801, AHN p. 565) – Medical management (FAAHN p. 1802, AHN p. 566) – Nursing interventions and patient teaching (FAAHN p. 1802, AHN p. 566) – Prognosis (FAAHN p. 1802, AHN p. 566) ☐ Cancer of the endometrium (FAAHN p. 1803, AHN p. 567) – Etiology and pathophysiology (FAAHN p. 1803, AHN p. 567) – Clinical manifestations (FAAHN p. 1803, AHN p. 567) – Assessment (FAAHN p. 1803, AHN p. 567) – Diagnostic tests (FAAHN p. 1803, AHN p. 567) – Medical management (FAAHN p. 1803, AHN p. 567) – Nursing interventions and patient teaching (FAAHN p. 1803, AHN p. 567) – Prognosis (FAAHN p. 1803, AHN p. 567) ☐ Cancer of the ovary (FAAHN p. 1803, AHN p. 567) – Etiology and pathophysiology (FAAHN p. 1803, AHN p. 567) – Clinical manifestations (FAAHN p. 1804, AHN p. 568) – Assessment (FAAHN p. 1804, AHN p. 568) – Diagnostic tests (FAAHN p. 1804, AHN p. 568) – Medical management (FAAHN p. 1804, AHN p. 568)	▨ SG Cancer of the Reproductive System, Ch. 52 p. 467 FAAHN (Ch. 12 p. 155 AHN) **BOOK RESOURCES** Review Questions for the NCLEX Examination Ch. 52 questions 1, 29 FAAHN (Ch.12 questions 1, 29 AHN) Cultural Considerations: Cancer of Female Reproductive System (FAAHN p. 1801) (AHN p. 565) ▸ Discuss the incidence of cancers of the reproductive system. ▸ Discuss the clinical manifestations associated with cancers of the reproductive system. *Class Activity Contact a local cancer treatment facility. Ask for educational materials concerning cancers of the female reproductive system. Use these materials in a class discussion.*

Christensen & Kockrow

OBJECTIVES	CONTENT	TEACHING RESOURCES
	– Nursing interventions (FAAHN p. 1804, AHN p. 568) – Prognosis (FAAHN p. 1805, AHN p. 569) ☐ Hysterectomy (FAAHN p. 1805, AHN p. 569) ☐ Vaginal hysterectomy (FAAHN p. 1805, AHN p. 569) ☐ Abdominal hysterectomy (FAAHN p. 1805, AHN p. 569) – Nursing interventions (FAAHN p. 1805, AHN p. 569) – Patient teaching (FAAHN p. 1806, AHN p. 570)	
Identify four nursing diagnoses pertinent to ovarian cancer.	☐ Cancer of the ovary (FAAHN p. 1803, AHN p. 567) – Etiology and pathophysiology (FAAHN p. 1803, AHN p. 567) – Clinical manifestations (FAAHN p. 1804, AHN p. 568) – Assessment (FAAHN p. 1804, AHN p. 568) – Diagnostic tests (FAAHN p. 1804, AHN p. 568) – Medical management (FAAHN p. 1804, AHN p. 568) – Nursing interventions (FAAHN p. 1804, AHN p. 568) – Prognosis (FAAHN p. 1805, AHN p. 569)	🖼 PPT 53 through 55, Ch. 52 FAAHN (Ch. 12 PPT 53 through 55 AHN) 📙 SG Cancer of the Reproductive System, Ch. 43 p. 467 FAAHN (Ch. 3 p. 155 AHN) ▶ Discuss potential concerns associated with a diagnosis of ovarian cancer. ▶ Discuss setting priorities for the nursing care of the patient diagnosed with ovarian cancer. *Class Activity Ask the students to cluster in small groups of three or four. Assign the task of modifying a nursing care plan for the patient with ovarian cancer. The care plan should include two or three priority nursing diagnoses and at least three interventions with rationales for each diagnosis.*
Describe the preoperative and postoperative nursing interventions for the patient requiring major surgery of the female reproductive system.	■ Cancer of the female reproductive tract (FAAHN p. 1800, AHN p. 564) ☐ Cancer of the cervix (FAAHN p. 1801, AHN p. 565) – Etiology and pathophysiology (FAAHN p. 1801, AHN p. 565) – Clinical manifestations (FAAHN p. 1801, AHN p. 565)	🖼 PPT 56, Ch. 52 FAAHN (Ch. 12 PPT 56 AHN) 📧 EILR IC Ch. 52 image 20 FAAHN (Ch. 12 image 20 AHN) 📧 EILR TB Ch. 52 questions 1, 21, 22, 24 FAAHN (Ch. 12 question 1, 21, 22, 24 AHN)

ELSEVIER

OBJECTIVES	CONTENT	TEACHING RESOURCES
	– Assessment (FAAHN p. 1801, AHN p. 565)	EILR Open Book Quiz Ch. 52 question 8 FAAHN (Ch. 12 question 8 AHN)
	– Diagnostic tests (FAAHN p. 1801, AHN p. 565)	
	– Medical management (FAAHN p. 1802, AHN p. 566)	ESLR Review Questions for the NCLEX Examination Ch. 52 question 9 FAAHN (Ch. 12 question 9 AHN)
	– Nursing interventions and patient teaching (FAAHN p. 1802, AHN p. 566)	SG Surgery Ch. 52 p. 465 FAAHN (Ch. 12 p. 153 AHN)
	– Prognosis (FAAHN p. 1802, AHN p. 566)	**BOOK RESOURCES**
	☐ Cancer of the endometrium (FAAHN p. 1803, AHN p. 567)	Review Questions for the NCLEX Examination Ch. 52 questions 6, 7, 18, 19 FAAHN (Ch.12 question 6, 7, 18, 19 AHN)
	– Etiology and pathophysiology (FAAHN p. 1803, AHN p. 567)	▸ Discuss the surgical implications of the female reproductive system.
	– Clinical manifestations (FAAHN p. 1803, AHN p. 567)	▸ Discuss the postoperative considerations for the patient who has had surgery for a reproductive concern.
	– Assessment (FAAHN p. 1803, AHN p. 567)	*Class Activity Instruct each student to interview a patient who has had a surgical procedure not related to the reproductive system. This interview must take place prior to the class discussion relating to reproductive surgeries. After the lecture, compare and contrast the types of concerns and limitations for the differing types of surgical patients.*
	– Diagnostic tests (FAAHN p. 1803, AHN p. 567)	
	– Medical management (FAAHN p. 1803, AHN p. 567)	
	– Nursing interventions and patient teaching (FAAHN p. 1803, AHN p. 567)	
	– Prognosis (FAAHN p. 1803, AHN p. 567)	
	☐ Cancer of the ovary (FAAHN p. 1803, AHN p. 567)	
	– Etiology and pathophysiology (FAAHN p. 1803, AHN p. 567)	
	– Clinical manifestations (FAAHN p. 1804, AHN p. 568)	
	– Assessment (FAAHN p. 1804, AHN p. 568)	
	– Diagnostic tests (FAAHN p. 1804, AHN p. 568)	
	– Medical management (FAAHN p. 1804, AHN p. 568)	

Mosby items and derived items © 2011 by Mosby, Inc., an affiliate of Elsevier Inc. Some material was previously published.

OBJECTIVES	CONTENT	TEACHING RESOURCES

	– Nursing interventions (FAAHN p. 1804, AHN p. 568)
	
	  – Prognosis (FAAHN p. 1805, AHN p. 569)
	
	☐ Hysterectomy (FAAHN p. 1805, AHN p. 569)
	
	☐ Vaginal hysterectomy (FAAHN p. 1805, AHN p. 569)
	
	☐ Abdominal hysterectomy (FAAHN p. 1805, AHN p. 569)
	
	  – Nursing interventions (FAAHN p. 1805, AHN p. 569)
	
	  – Patient teaching (FAAHN p. 1806, AHN p. 570)	

12.2 Homework/Assignments:

12.2 Instructor's Notes/Student Feedback:

ELSEVIER

Mosby items and derived items © 2011 by Mosby, Inc., an affiliate of Elsevier Inc.
Some material was previously published.

Adult Health Nursing, 6th ed.

Christensen & Kockrow

LESSON 12.3

CRITICAL THINKING QUESTION

You are assigned to care for a patient who had a simple mastectomy on her right breast a few days earlier. The physician has written for her discharge the following morning. As you are caring for her, she states she is nervous about going home. She voices concerns about when she will look "more normal." She states she and her doctor decided to wait until after the chemotherapy is completed before undergoing reconstruction. What should be included in her patient teaching with regard to her home care and her verbalized concerns?

Guidelines: The patient's demeanor indicates a readiness to learn. Wound care must be taught. She must understand the importance of protecting her surgical site. The right arm must be safeguarded. Things to be avoided for the right side include infection, reduced circulation, burns, and dragging or pulling the affected side. She must understand the signs and symptoms to report to her physician, including redness, swelling, and pain. Exercise of the affected side is also necessary. This exercise will aid in the prevention of muscle contractures and promote circulation. She has also verbalized an interest in her physical appearance. Since the reconstruction will be "on hold," she should seek the advice and approval of her physician concerning the use of breast prosthesis.

OBJECTIVES	CONTENT	TEACHING RESOURCES
Describe six important points to emphasize in the teaching of breast self-examination.	■ Disorders of the female breast (FAAHN p. 1806, AHN p. 570) ☐ Fibrocystic breast condition (FAAHN p. 1806, AHN p. 570) – Etiology and pathophysiology (FAAHN p. 1806, AHN p. 570) – Clinical manifestations (FAAHN p. 1807, AHN p. 571) – Diagnostic tests (FAAHN p. 1807, AHN p. 571) – Medical management (FAAHN p. 1807, AHN p. 571) – Nursing interventions and patient teaching (FAAHN p. 1807, AHN p. 571) ☐ Acute mastitis (FAAHN p. 1807, AHN p. 571) ☐ Chronic mastitis (FAAHN p. 1807, AHN p. 571) ☐ Breast cancer (FAAHN p. 1807, AHN p. 571) – Etiology and pathophysiology (FAAHN p. 1807, AHN p. 571) – Clinical manifestations (FAAHN p. 1808, AHN p. 572)	PPT 57 through 61, Ch. 52 FAAHN (Ch.12 PPT 57 through 61 AHN) EILR IC Ch. 52 image 15 FAAHN (Ch. 12 image 15 AHN) EILR TB Ch. 52 questions 14, 20, 23, 26, 27 FAAHN (Ch. 12 questions 14, 20, 23, 26, 27 AHN) SG Breast Self-Examination, Ch. 43 p. 468 FAAHN (Ch. 3 p. 156 AHN) **BOOK RESOURCES** Review Questions for the NCLEX Examination Ch. 52 question 2, 13 through 15 FAAHN (Ch.12 question 2, 13 through 15 AHN) Box 52-5 Predisposing Factors for Women at High Risk for Breast Cancer (FAAHN p. 1807) (Box 12-5 AHN p. 571) Fig. 52-14 **A,** Lymph nodes of the axilla. **B,** Lymphatic drainage of the breast (FAAHN p. 1808) (Fig. 12-14 AHN p. 572) Fig. 52-15 Methods for palpation (FAAHN p. 1808) (Fig. 12-15 AHN p. 572) Patient Teaching: Breast Self-Examination (FAAHN p. 1809) (AHN p. 573)

OBJECTIVES	CONTENT	TEACHING RESOURCES
	– Diagnostic tests (FAAHN p. 1808, AHN p. 572) – Medical management (FAAHN p. 1810, AHN p. 574) – Nursing interventions (FAAHN p. 1813, AHN p. 577) – Patient teaching (FAAHN p. 1815, AHN p. 579) – Breast reconstruction (FAAHN p. 1817, AHN p. 581) – Prognosis (FAAHN p. 1819, AHN p. 583)	Box 52-6 TNM System for Staging Breast Cancer (FAAHN p. 1811) (Box 12-6 AHN p. 575) ▸ Discuss the frequency of breast exams recommended by the American Cancer Society. ▸ Discuss the procedure to perform the self breast examination. *Class Activity Contact the local chapter of the American Cancer Society. Request breast assessment teaching guides. Demonstrate and discuss their use in the classroom. Encourage the students to take the guides home to their friends and families.*
Compare four surgical approaches for cancer of the breast.	☐ Breast cancer (FAAHN p. 1807, AHN p. 571) – Etiology and pathophysiology (FAAHN p. 1807, AHN p. 571) – Clinical manifestations (FAAHN p. 1808, AHN p. 572) – Diagnostic tests (FAAHN p. 1808, AHN p. 572) – Medical management (FAAHN p. 1810, AHN p. 574) – Nursing interventions (FAAHN p. 1813, AHN p. 577) – Patient teaching (FAAHN p. 1815, AHN p. 579) – Breast reconstruction (FAAHN p. 1817, AHN p. 581) – Prognosis (FAAHN p. 1819, AHN p. 583)	▦ PPT 59, 60 Ch. 52 FAAHN (Ch. 12 PPT 59, 60 AHN) ▱ EILR IC Ch. 52 image 17 FAAHN (Ch. 12 image 17 AHN) ▤ SG Treating Breast Cancer, Ch. 52 p. 468 FAAHN (Ch. 12 p.156 AHN) **BOOK RESOURCES** Review Questions for the NCLEX Examination Ch. 52 question 3, 16 FAAHN (Ch.12 question 3, 16 AHN) Nursing Care Plan 52-1 The Patient Undergoing Modified Radical Mastectomy (FAAHN p. 1813) (NCP 12-1 AHN p. 577) ⚲ NCP CTQ 1 through 3 (FAAHN p. 1814) (AHN p. 578) Fig. 52-17 Transverse rectus abdominis musculocutaneous (TRAM) flap (FAAHN p. 1818) (Fig. 12-17 AHN p. 582) Table 52-3 Prognosis and Nodal Involvement in Breast Cancer (FAAHN p. 1819) (Table 12-3 AHN p. 583) ▸ Discuss the factors used to determine the surgical procedure to manage cancer of the breast. ▸ Discuss the psychosocial considerations for the patient planning to be treated surgically for breast cancer.

OBJECTIVES	CONTENT	TEACHING RESOURCES
		Class Activity Invite a breast cancer survivor to speak to the class. Topics to be addressed include care and concerns after discharge from the health care facility. *NOTE: Have this speaker address the Objective below as well.*
Discuss adjuvant therapies for breast cancer.	– Medical management (FAAHN p. 1810, AHN p. 574)	PPT 61, Ch. 52 FAAHN (Ch. 12 PPT 61 AHN) SG Treating Breast Cancer, Ch. 52 p. 468 FAAHN (Ch. 12 p. 156 AHN) ▸ Discuss the mode of action for each of the adjuvant therapies for breast cancer. ▸ Discuss the psychosocial needs of the patient undergoing adjuvant therapies for the treatment of breast cancer.
Discuss nursing interventions for the patient who has had a modified radical mastectomy.	– Nursing interventions (FAAHN p. 1813, AHN p. 577) – Patient teaching (FAAHN p. 1815, AHN p. 579) – Breast reconstruction (FAAHN p. 1817, AHN p. 581) – Prognosis (FAAHN p. 1819, AHN p. 583)	PPT 61, Ch. 52 FAAHN (Ch. 12 PPT x through x AHN) EILR TB Ch. 52 questions 5, 21, 38 FAAHN (Ch. 12 questions 5, 21, 38 AHN) ESLR Review Questions for the NCLEX Examination Ch. 52 question 10 FAAHN (Ch. 12 question 10 AHN) SG Postoperative Care, Ch. 52 p. 470 FAAHN (Ch. 12 p. 158 AHN) **BOOK RESOURCES** Review Questions for the NCLEX Examination Ch. 52 questions 9, 17 FAAHN (Ch.12 questions 9, 17 AHN) Box 52-7 Hand and Arm Care after Breast Surgery (p. 1816 FAAHN) (Box 12-7 p. 580 AHN) ▸ Discuss the nursing assessment required for the patient who has had a modified radical mastectomy. *Class Activity Have the class list on the board the dos and don'ts in the postoperative period for the patient who has had a modified radical mastectomy.*

ELSEVIER

Adult Health Nursing, 6th ed.
Christensen & Kockrow

List several discharge planning instructions for the patient who has undergone a modified radical mastectomy.	– Patient teaching (FAAHN p. 1815, AHN p. 579)	PPT 61 Ch. 52 FAAHN (Ch. 12 PPT 61 AHN) EILR IC image Ch. 52 image 16 FAAHN (Ch. 12 image 16 AHN) EILR TB Ch. 52 questions 6, 12 FAAHN (Ch. 12 questions 6, 12 AHN) SG Postoperative Care, Ch. 43 p. 470 FAAHN (Ch. 3 p. 158 AHN) **BOOK RESOURCES** Box 52-7 Hand and Arm Care after Breast Surgery (p. 1816 FAAHN) (Box 12-7 p. 580 AHN) Fig. 52-16 Exercises after mastectomy (FAAHN p. 1816) (Fig. 12-16 AHN p. 580) Box 52-8 Postmastectomy Arm Exercises (FAAHN p. 1817) (Box 12-8 AHN p. 581) Home Care Considerations: Cancer of the Breast (p. 1819 FAAHN, p. 583 AHN) ▸ Discuss the assessment of readiness in the patient preparing for discharge after undergoing a modified radical mastectomy. *Class Activity Pass a paper around the room and ask each student to add a discharge instruction for the patient who has had a modified radical mastectomy.*

12.3 Homework/Assignments:

Have each student locate an article on the Internet concerning an inflammatory disorder of the male reproductive system. The day of the lecture, group students by the disorder selected. Allow each group to meet for 5 minutes and share their findings with each other. See next lesson.

12.3 Instructor's Notes/Student Feedback:

LESSON 12.4

CRITICAL THINKING QUESTION

While at her routine annual physical, a woman reports she has a 16-year-old son. She states that she recently read an article about testicular cancer. She has several questions about this disease. What should she be told?

Guidelines: Testicular cancer is a malignancy that most often occurs in young men ages 15 to 35. It is relatively rare. Factors associated with the development of this cancer include a failure of the testes to descend, testicular atrophy, and scrotal trauma. Clinical manifestations include enlarged scrotum, a dull ache, pain in the testicles, and a scrotal mass. Males should be taught to begin monthly self-testicular exams beginning at age 16. The mother should be encouraged to speak with her son or make an appointment for him to speak with the physician privately.

OBJECTIVES	CONTENT	TEACHING RESOURCES
Discuss the etiology, pathophysiology, clinical manifestations, assessment, diagnostic tests, medical management, nursing interventions, patient teaching, and prognosis for inflammatory disorders of the male reproductive system.	■ Inflammatory disorders of the male reproductive system (FAAHN p. 1819, AHN p. 583) □ Prostatitis (FAAHN p. 1819, AHN p. 583) – Etiology and pathophysiology (FAAHN p. 1819, AHN p. 583) – Clinical manifestations (FAAHN p. 1819, AHN p. 583) – Diagnostic tests (FAAHN p. 1819, AHN p. 583) – Medical management (FAAHN p. 1819, AHN p. 583) – Nursing interventions (FAAHN p. 1819, AHN p. 583) – Prognosis (FAAHN p. 1820, AHN p. 584) □ Epididymitis (FAAHN p. 1820, AHN p. 584) – Etiology and pathophysiology (FAAHN p. 1820, AHN p. 584) – Clinical manifestations (FAAHN p. 1820, AHN p. 584) – Diagnostic tests (FAAHN p. 1820, AHN p. 584) – Medical management (FAAHN p. 1820, AHN p. 584) – Nursing interventions (FAAHN p. 1820, AHN p. 584)	PPT 62 through 66, Ch. 52 FAAHN (Ch. 12 PPT 62 through 66 AHN) EILR IC Ch. 52 images 8, 21 FAAHN (Ch. 12 images 8, 21 AHN) EILR TB Ch. 52 questions 10, 26 FAAHN (Ch. 12 questions 10, 26 AHN) EILR Open Book Quiz Ch. 52 questions 4, 9, 10 FAAHN (Ch.12 questions 4, 9, 10 AHN) ▶ Discuss the similarities and differences between the inflammatory disorders of the male reproductive system. ▶ Discuss the psychosocial implications of the diagnosis and screening for inflammatory disorders of the male reproductive system. *Class Activity In the class session prior to this lecture, have each student locate an article on the Internet concerning an inflammatory disorder of the male reproductive system. The day of the lecture, group students by the disorder selected. Allow each group to meet for 5 minutes and share their findings with each other.*

ELSEVIER

Mosby items and derived items © 2011 by Mosby, Inc., an affiliate of Elsevier Inc.
Some material was previously published.

Adult Health Nursing, 6th ed.
Christensen & Kockrow

OBJECTIVES	CONTENT	TEACHING RESOURCES
	– Prognosis (FAAHN p. 1820, AHN p. 584) ■ Disorders of the male genital organs (FAAHN p. 1820, AHN p. 584) ☐ Phimosis and paraphimosis – Etiology (FAAHN p. 1820, AHN p. 584) – Medical management (FAAHN p. 1820, AHN p. 584) – Nursing interventions (FAAHN p. 1820, AHN p. 584)	
Distinguish between hydrocele and varicocele.	■ Disorders of the male genital organs (FAAHN p. 1820, AHN p. 584) ☐ Hydrocele (FAAHN p. 1821, AHN p. 585) – Etiology and pathophysiology (FAAHN p. 1821, AHN p. 585) – Medical management (FAAHN p. 1821, AHN p. 585) – Nursing interventions (FAAHN p. 1821, AHN p. 585) – Prognosis (FAAHN p. 1821, AHN p. 585) ☐ Varicocele (FAAHN p. 1821, AHN p. 585)	PPT 67, 68 Ch. 52 FAAHN (Ch.12 PPT 67, 68 AHN) EILR TB Ch. 52 question 25 FAAHN (Ch. 12 question 25 AHN) SG Hydrocele and Varicocele, Ch. 52 p. 471 FAAHN (Ch. 12 p. 159 AHN) ▸ Discuss the clinical manifestations associated with hydrocele and varicocele. *Class Activity **Have the students list on the board the nursing implications of a hydrocele and varicocele on male reproductive health.***
Discuss the importance of monthly testicular self-examination beginning at 15 years of age.	■ Cancer of the male reproductive tract (FAAHN p. 1821, AHN p. 585) ☐ Cancer of the testis (testicular cancer (FAAHN p. 1821, AHN p. 585) – Etiology and pathophysiology (FAAHN p. 1821, AHN p. 585) – Clinical manifestations (FAAHN p. 1821, AHN p. 585) – Diagnostic tests (FAAHN p. 1821, AHN p. 585) – Medical management (FAAHN p. 1821, AHN p. 585)	PPT 69, 70 Ch. 52 FAAHN (Ch.12 PPT 69, 70 AHN) EILR IC Ch. 52 image 18 FAAHN (Ch. 12 image 18 AHN) EILR TB Ch. 52 questions 8, 9 FAAHN (Ch. 12 questions 8, 9 AHN) SG Testicular Self-Examination, Ch. 52 p. 472 FAAHN (Ch. 12 p. 160 AHN) **BOOK RESOURCES** Patient Teaching: Testicular Self-Examination (FAAHN p. 1822) (AHN p. 586) Fig. 52-18 Testicular self-examination (FAAHN p. 1822) (Fig. 12-18 AHN p. 586)

Christensen & Kockrow

OBJECTIVES	CONTENT	TEACHING RESOURCES
	– Nursing interventions and patient teaching (FAAHN p. 1821, AHN p. 585)	▸ Discuss the clinical manifestations of testicular cancer.
	– Prognosis (FAAHN p. 1822, AHN p. 586)	▸ Discuss the recommended screening for testicular cancer.
	□ Cancer of the penis (FAAHN p. 1822, AHN p. 586)	*Class Activity Bring a testicular model to class to demonstrate the assessment and examination used to detect testicular cancer.*
	– Etiology and pathophysiology (FAAHN p. 1822, AHN p. 586)	
	– Clinical manifestations (FAAHN p. 1822, AHN p. 586)	
	– Diagnostic tests (FAAHN p. 1822, AHN p. 586)	
	– Medical management (FAAHN p. 1822, AHN p. 586)	
	– Nursing interventions (FAAHN p. 1822, AHN p. 586)	
Discuss patient education related to prevention of sexually transmitted diseases.	■ Sexually transmitted infections (FAAHN p. 1822, AHN p. 586)	PPT 71 through 86 Ch. 52 FAAHN (Ch.12 PPT 71 through 86 AHN)
	□ Genital herpes (FAAHN p. 1823, AHN p. 587)	EILR IC Ch. 52 image 19 FAAHN (Ch. 52 image 19 AHN)
	– Etiology and pathophysiology (FAAHN p. 1823, AHN p. 587)	EILR TB Ch. 52 questions 16, 18, 28, 29 FAAHN (Ch. 12 questions 16, 18, 28, 29 AHN)
	– Clinical manifestations (FAAHN p. 1823, AHN p. 587)	SG Sexually Transmitted Infections, Ch. 52 p. 472 FAAHN (Ch. 12 p. 160 AHN)
	– Diagnostic tests (FAAHN p. 1824, AHN p. 588)	**BOOK RESOURCES**
	– Medical management (FAAHN p. 1824, AHN p. 588)	Review Questions for the NCLEX Examination Ch. 52 questions 4, 8, 10, 11, 27, 30 FAAHN (Ch.12 question 4, 8, 10, 11, 27, 30 AHN)
	– Nursing interventions and patient teaching (FAAHN p. 1824, AHN p. 588)	Safety Alert! Sexually Transmitted Infections (FAAHN p. 1823) (AHN p. 587)
	– Prognosis (FAAHN p. 1824, AHN p. 588)	Fig. 52-19 Herpes simplex virus type 2 in a male and female patient. Vesicular lesions on **A,** penis, and **B,** perineum (FAAHN p. 1824) (Fig. 12-19 AHN p. 588)
	□ Syphilis (FAAHN p. 1824, AHN p. 588)	
	– Etiology and pathophysiology (FAAHN p. 1824, AHN p. 588)	
	– Clinical manifestations (FAAHN p. 1825, AHN p. 589)	Box 52-9 Prevention of Sexually Transmitted Infections (FAAHN p. 1828) (Box 12-9 AHN p. 592)

OBJECTIVES	CONTENT	TEACHING RESOURCES
	– Diagnostic tests (FAAHN p. 1825, AHN p. 589)	Fig. 52-20 Tubal ligation (FAAHN p. 1829) (Fig. 12-20 AHN p. 593)
	– Medical management (FAAHN p. 1825, AHN p. 589)	Fig. 52-21 Vasectomy (FAAHN p. 1829) (Fig. 12-21 AHN p. 593)
	– Nursing interventions (FAAHN p. 1825, AHN p. 589)	▸ Discuss the signs and symptoms of each of the sexually transmitted diseases.
	– Prognosis (FAAHN p. 1825, AHN p. 589)	▸ Discuss the care and medical management for each of the sexually transmitted diseases.
	☐ Gonorrhea (FAAHN p. 1825, AHN p. 589)	*Class Activity Invite a representative of a local family planning center or Planned Parenthood to visit the class and discuss available services.*
	– Etiology and pathophysiology (FAAHN p. 1825, AHN p. 589)	
	– Clinical manifestations (FAAHN p. 1825, AHN p. 589)	
	– Diagnostic tests (FAAHN p. 1826, AHN p. 590)	
	– Medical management (FAAHN p. 1826, AHN p. 590)	
	– Nursing interventions and patient teaching (FAAHN p. 1826, AHN p. 590)	
	– Prognosis (FAAHN p. 1826, AHN p. 590)	
	☐ Trichomoniasis (FAAHN p. 1826, AHN p. 590)	
	– Etiology and pathophysiology (FAAHN p. 1826, AHN p. 590)	
	– Clinical manifestations (FAAHN p. 1826, AHN p. 590)	
	– Diagnostic tests (FAAHN p. 1827, AHN p. 591)	
	– Medical management (FAAHN p. 1827, AHN p. 591)	
	– Nursing interventions and patient teaching (FAAHN p. 1827, AHN p. 591)	
	– Prognosis (FAAHN p. 1827, AHN p. 591)	
	☐ Candidiasis (FAAHN p. 1827, AHN p. 591)	

OBJECTIVES	CONTENT	TEACHING RESOURCES
	– Etiology and pathophysiology (FAAHN p. 1827, AHN p. 591)	
	– Clinical manifestations (FAAHN p. 1827, AHN p. 591)	
	– Diagnostic tests (FAAHN p. 1827, AHN p. 591)	
	– Medical management (FAAHN p. 1827, AHN p. 591)	
	– Nursing interventions and patient teaching (FAAHN p. 1827, AHN p. 591)	
	– Prognosis (FAAHN p. 1827, AHN p. 591)	
	☐ Chlamydia (FAAHN p. 1827, AHN p. 591)	
	– Etiology and pathophysiology (FAAHN p. 1827, AHN p. 591)	
	– Clinical manifestations (FAAHN p. 1828, AHN p. 592)	
	– Diagnostic tests (FAAHN p. 1828, AHN p. 592)	
	– Medical management (FAAHN p. 1828, AHN p. 592)	
	– Nursing interventions and patient teaching (FAAHN p. 1828, AHN p. 592)	
	– Prognosis (FAAHN p. 1828, AHN p. 592)	
	☐ Acquired immunodeficiency syndrome (FAAHN p. 1828, AHN p. 592)	
	■ Family planning (FAAHN p. 1828, AHN p. 592)	
	☐ Nursing process for patients with reproductive disorders (FAAHN p. 1829, AHN p. 596)	
	– Data collection for females (FAAHN p. 1829, AHN p. 596)	
	– Data collection for males (FAAHN p. 1829, AHN p. 596)	

Christensen & Kockrow

OBJECTIVES	CONTENT	TEACHING RESOURCES
	– Nursing diagnosis (FAAHN p. 1829, AHN p. 596)	
	– Expected outcomes and planning (FAAHN p. 1829, AHN p. 596)	
	– Implementation (FAAHN p. 1829, AHN p. 596)	
	– Evaluation (FAAHN p. 1829, AHN p. 596)	
Performance Evaluation		![] EILR TB Ch. 52 questions 1 through 39 FAAHN (Ch. 12 questions 1 through 39 AHN)
		![] EILR Open Book Quiz Ch. 43 questions 1 through 10 FAAHN (Ch. 12 questions 1 through 10 AHN)
		![] ESLR Review Questions for the NCLEX Examination Ch. 43 questions 1 through 10 FAAHN (Ch. 12 questions 1 through 10 AHN)
		![] SG Ch. 52 pp. 457 through 476 FAAHN (Ch. 12 pp. 145 through 164 AHN)
		BOOK RESOURCES
		Nursing Care Plan 52-1 The Patient Undergoing Modified Radical Mastectomy (FAAHN p. 1813) (NCP 12-1 AHN p. 577)
		⚲ NCP CTQ 1 through 3 (FAAHN p. 1814) (AHN p. 578)
		Review Questions for the NCLEX Examination Ch. 52 question 1 through 30 FAAHN (Ch. 12 question 1 through 30 AHN)

12.4 Homework/Assignments:

12.4 Instructor's Notes/Student Feedback:

Slide 1

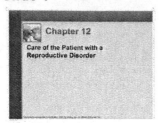

Slide 2

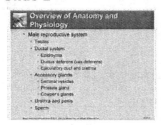

- The organs of the male reproductive system include the testes, the ductal system, the accessory glands, and the penis. What are the three functions of the male reproductive system?

Slide 3

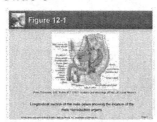

- Outline the role played by the primary structures of the male reproductive system. **NOTE:** Point to the structures as they are discussed. This will aid the student in visualizing the structure during the discussion of the function.

Slide 4

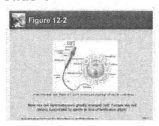

Slide 5

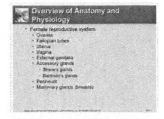

- The organs of the female reproductive system include the ovaries, uterus, fallopian tubes, and vagina.

Christensen & Kockrow

Slide 6

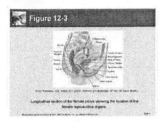

- What roles are played by the organs of the female reproductive system? **NOTE:** Point to the structures as they are discussed.

Slide 7

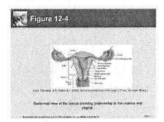

- The sectioned view of the uterus illustrates the relationship between the uterus, ovaries and vagina.

- The ovum mature in the ovaries. Once mature, they are released in response to hormonal levels. What is the term for this process? *Ovulation.*

- After leaving the ovaries, the ovum travels through the fallopian tubes toward the uterus. It is at this time sperm have the opportunity to unite with the egg cell. What is the term for this process? *Fertilization.*

Slide 8

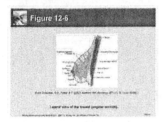

- This is a lateral view of the breast. Breasts function to provide nutrition to the baby.

- The size of the breast is determined by the quantity of adipose tissue.

- What hormone is responsible for the production of milk?

- What hormone is responsible for the release of milk?

Slide 9

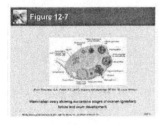

- Note the stages of ovarian follicle development. Hormones control the process of egg maturation. What hormones play a role in this process?

- After the egg's release from the ovary, if fertilized, the resulting union is the beginning of a pregnancy.

- If fertilization does not occur, the hormone levels are reduced. At that time, what physiological process begins?

Slide 10

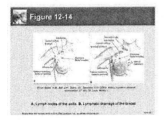

Slide 11

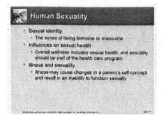

- Sexuality and sex differ. Sexuality refers to the sense of being a man or woman. The term "sex" refers to the biologic aspects of sexual activity.

- Sexual and reproductive health can impact overall emotional and physical well-being.

- The aging process plays a significant role in sexual health.

- What are some of the changes associated with aging that impact the health of the reproductive system?

- Biologic identity begins at conception. Influences on this identity include hormones, environment, and culture.

- What occurs when there is a conflict between the sexual orientation and the physiological identity?

Slide 12

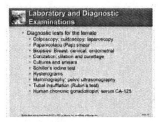

- The diagnostic tests for the female reproductive system can be divided into two groups. One group includes those tests that are recommended by physicians to be completed on a scheduled basis for screening purposes. The second group of tests is ordered when there is a specific disorder or concern within the system.

- Which of the examinations is ordered on a scheduled basis? *The pap smear and the mammogram.*

- What are the recommended parameters for pap smears by the American Cancer Society? What events/situations may warrant an increase in testing frequency?

- Mammography is a radiologic examination of the breast's soft tissue. Baseline screening should begin for women between the ages of 35 to 39 years. After age 40, the examinations should be done annually.

- Provide an explanation of the remaining tests.

Slide 13

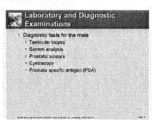

- The testicular biopsy is performed to detect abnormal cells and the presence of sperm. A small incision is initiated to perform the examination. What will the postprocedure nursing care focus be?

- Semen analysis is employed to evaluate the presence of or quantity of the sperm. The sperm specimen can be collected by manual stimulation or with a condom.

- Prostatic smears can be used to locate and identify microorganisms and cancer cells in the prostate.

- Cystoscopy is used to examine the prostate and bladder by using a lighted scope through the urethra to the bladder.

- The PSA test is performed to assess levels of the prostate-specific antigen in the bloodstream. Elevated levels are associated with cancer.

Adult Health Nursing, 6th ed.
Christensen & Kockrow

Slide 14

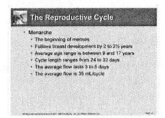

- What factors will impact the age of onset of menstruation?

Slide 15

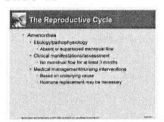

- Amenorrhea refers to the absence of menstrual flow. What are some potential causes of amenorrhea? How do primary and secondary amenorrhea differ?

- Identify two nursing diagnoses for the patient experiencing amenorrhea.

Slide 16

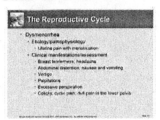

- Painful menstruation is known as dysmenorrhea. The causes of dysmenorrhea can relate to an endocrine imbalance, an increase in prostaglandin secretions, or chronic illness, fatigue, and anemia.

- Compare and contrast primary and secondary dysmenorrhea.

Slide 17

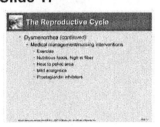

- The treatment options available for dysmenorrhea are individualized according to the specific cause and the individual needs of the patient. Review the rationale for the treatment options listed. How do they increase the patient's comfort?

- What diagnostic tests can be utilized to evaluate dysmenorrhea?

Slide 18

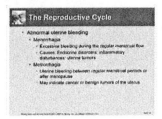

- Abnormal uterine bleeding can signal an underlying disease process. What nursing assessments are indicated when caring for the patient experiencing menorrhagia and metrorrhagia?

- Attributing causes of menorrhagia differ for younger and older women. What difference are these differences?

ELSEVIER

Christensen & Kockrow

Slide 19

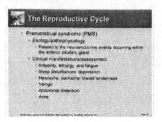

- An estimated 30% to 50% of women experience PMS.

- PMS is not a disease but a grouping of symptoms.

- What are some supported theories for the cause of PMS?

- The clinical manifestations of PMS can vary greatly between patients. The symptoms typically occur 7 to 10 days before the menstrual period and resolve within the first 3 days after the onset of bleeding.

- What are common myths and rumors associated with PMS?

Slide 20

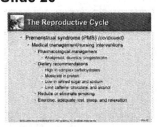

- When caring for the patient experiencing PMS, what should be included in the nursing interventions?

- What nursing diagnoses apply to the patient with PMS?

Slide 21

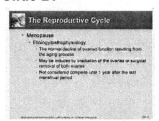

- Menopause begins in most women between the ages of 35 to 60 years. It is characterized by infrequent ovulation, decreased menstrual function, and finally the cessation of menstrual flow.

- Discuss some of the misinformation associated with menopause.

Slide 22

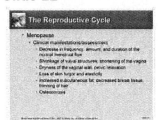

- The clinical manifestations associated with menopause occur from the loss of estrogen. Women experiencing menopause face numerous physical changes. What impact do these changes have on a woman's life?

Slide 23

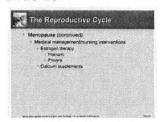

- Medical management of menopause can include hormone replacement therapy. What are some of the implications and concerns associated with the administration of estrogen therapy?

- What nonpharmacologic remedies can be used to manage the symptoms of menopause?

Mosby items and derived items © 2011, 2007 by Mosby, Inc., an affiliate of Elsevier Inc.
Some material was previously published.

Christensen & Kockrow

Slide 24

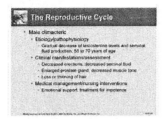

- The climacteric is less evident in men than women.

- The experienced impact on men is often psychological in nature.

- Ask the class what information they may have heard about the male climacteric. How many students have heard of this phenomenon?

Slide 25

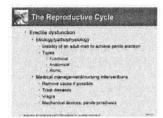

- Impotence has several forms and is a serious concern for men.

- Review the differing types of impotence.

- What concerns can impotence cause in men?

- What teaching should be given to the man who is prescribed medications to manage erectile dysfunction?

Slide 26

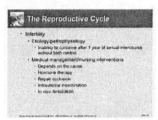

- Infertility is defined as inability to conceive after 1 year of sexual intercourse without birth control. Age and fertility in women are closely related. Females are most fertile between 20 and 29 years of age. Male fertility does not significantly drop with aging.

- Review diagnostic tests used to evaluate fertility.

- What are some potential causes of infertility? How can infertility impact a couple's relationship?

Slide 27

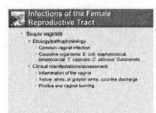

- Vaginitis is a common vaginal infection.

- When evaluating a patient for complaints associated with a vaginal infection, what should be included in the nursing assessment?

Slide 28

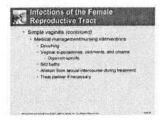

- In addition to collecting the patient's report of vaginal irritation, the physician will perform a diagnostic examination. There is typically a vaginal examination and cultures of the organisms to determine the appropriate treatment. An examination is performed to check for inflammation of the vagina and surrounding tissues.

Christensen & Kockrow

Slide 29

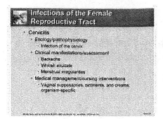

Slide 30

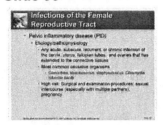

Slide 31

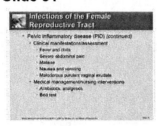

- Pelvic inflammatory disease is an infection of the pelvic cavity and reproductive organs. PID can be mild or severe.

- The impact of PID could be significant. It can be associated with the development of scar tissue in the reproductive cavity and infertility.

- What diagnostic tests are used to evaluate the patient who presents with complaints associated with PID?

- Outline the patient education that should accompany a diagnosis of PID.

Slide 32

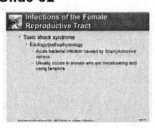

- Although toxic shock syndrome can be diagnosed in men, women, and children, it is most commonly seen in women of childbearing age.

Slide 33

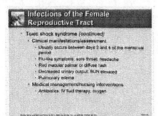

- The onset of clinical manifestations is sudden.

- There are no diagnostic tests for this disease. Diagnosis is made based upon the clinical presentation.

- Because the disease is often seen in menstruating women, what preventative patient teaching should be provided?

ELSEVIER

Mosby items and derived items © 2011, 2007 by Mosby, Inc., an affiliate of Elsevier Inc.
Some material was previously published.

Adult Health Nursing, 6th ed.
Christensen & Kockrow

Slide 34

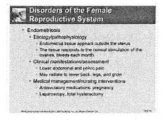

- Endometriosis is the presence of endometrial tissue outside the endometrial cavity.

- What populations experience a higher incidence of endometriosis?

- What nursing care should accompany a diagnosis of endometriosis?

- Discuss the impact of endometriosis on a woman's reproductive health.

Slide 35

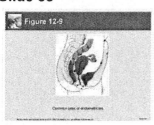

- This figure illustrates the common locations for endometriosis. What theories support how this tissue appears outside of the uterine cavity?

Slide 36

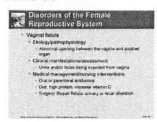

- A fistula is an opening between two normally separated passages. Fistulas are named for the area of the body involved.

- Identify potential causes of fistulas.

Slide 37

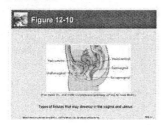

Slide 38

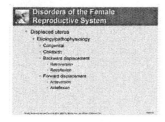

- The uterus may be in an abnormal position due to a number of factors. The causes of this displacement can be congenital or due to muscular changes, causing a shift from the normal position. What events could precipitate muscular changes and cause a displacement of the uterus?

Adult Health Nursing, 6th ed.

Christensen & Kockrow

Slide 39

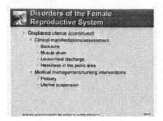

Slide 40

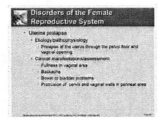

Slide 41

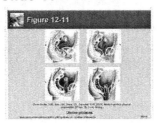

- The degree of prolapse directly influences the type and severity of symptoms experienced by the patient.

- What are the clinical manifestations associated with the differing degrees of uterine prolapse?

Slide 42

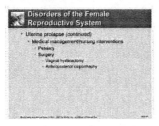

- The management of uterine prolapse can involve the use of a positioning device or surgical interventions. What factors will be used to determine which medical management options will be employed?

- The pessary is a device used to provide uterine support. How does the device work? What education should be provided about its use?

- In the event surgical intervention is selected, what procedure will be performed? How does this procedure manage the problem?

Slide 43

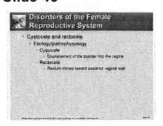

- The weakness in supporting muscle, tissues, and ligaments can cause a displacement of the bladder, vagina, or rectum.

- What events could be associated with the weakening of supportive structures?

Adult Health Nursing, 6th ed.
Christensen & Kockrow

Slide 44

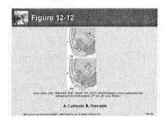

Slide 45

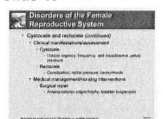

- Describe the nursing care that accompanies the surgical repair for cystoceles and rectoceles.

Slide 46

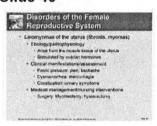

- Leiomyomas are the most common benign tumor of the female reproductive tract.

- What populations have a higher incidence of leiomyoma development?

Slide 47

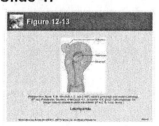

- Note the potential locations for leiomyomas. What implications do they have regarding infertility?

Slide 48

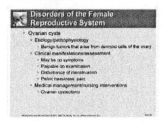

ELSEVIER

Mosby items and derived items © 2011, 2007 by Mosby, Inc., an affiliate of Elsevier Inc.
Some material was previously published.

Adult Health Nursing, 6th ed.
Christensen & Kockrow

Slide 49

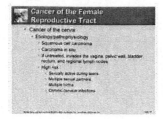

- Cancer is the second leading cause of death in women.

- Cervical cancer is a disease that impacts women in their childbearing years.

- The Pap smear is a screening tool to identify problematic cervical cell changes.

- What are medical recommendations concerning the screening for cervical cancer?

Slide 50

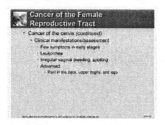

Slide 51

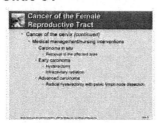

- With consideration to the age and population most affected with cervical cancer, what are the implications on the woman's reproductive health?

- The incidence of cervical cancer is greater among Hispanic, African American, and American Indian women than among white women. The mortality rate for minorities is more than twice that of white women. What might explain these figures?

Slide 52

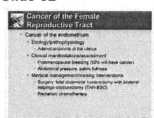

- Cancer of the endometrium occurs more frequently in postmenopausal women. What factors could aid in explaining this phenomenon?

- To assist with early detection of this cancer, patient teaching is vital. What should be included in the teaching plan for women concerning prevention and early detection?

Slide 53

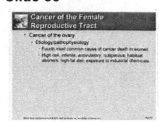

Mosby items and derived items © 2011, 2007 by Mosby, Inc., an affiliate of Elsevier Inc.
Some material was previously published.

Christensen & Kockrow

Slide 54

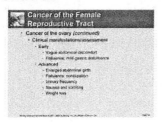

- Ovarian cancer is often overlooked due to the vague symptoms reported.

- What diagnostic tests will be employed to identify ovarian cancer?

Slide 55

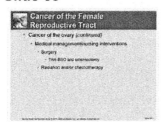

- Conditions involving hormonal issues, disease process, and other disorders can necessitate surgical intervention. The removal of the uterus is known as a hysterectomy.

- There are differing types of hysterectomies. The medical terminology used to refer to the surgical procedure is based upon the type of surgical incision and the organs affected.

- Which of the procedures listed will induce menopause?

Slide 56

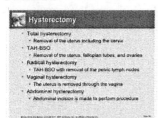

- A variety of procedures can be performed under the heading of a hysterectomy. Review how each of them differ.

- Explain differences in postoperative care between the procedures.

- Identify factors that may determine which procedure is performed on a patient.

Slide 57

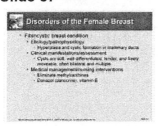

- Fibrocystic breast disease refers to development of benign tumors of the breast. These tumors rarely ever become cancerous and are almost never seen in most menopausal women.

- What factors associated with menopause can explain why it does not normally occur after menopause?

Slide 58

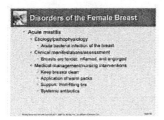

ELSEVIER

Adult Health Nursing, 6th ed.
Christensen & Kockrow

Slide 59

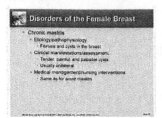

- Compare and contrast acute and chronic mastitis.

Slide 60

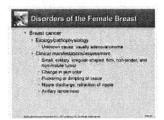

- Breast cancer is the most common cancer in women.
- Only lung cancer outranks breast cancer in the number of deaths per year.
- What populations are at highest risk for the development of breast cancer?
- Outline steps that women can take to reduce their risk for the development of breast cancer.

Slide 61

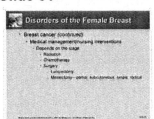

- Once a diagnosis of breast cancer is made, the patient and her physician must determine the best course of treatment. What factors are used to determine the best management plan?
- Explain the concept of cancer staging.
- What are the responsibilities of the nurse when caring for a women diagnosed with breast cancer?

Slide 62

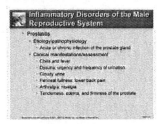

- Prostatitis is an infection of the prostate gland. It most commonly occurs because of a bacterial infection in the bloodstream or from an infection that has descended from the kidneys.
- What diagnostic tests are used to confirm prostatitis?

Slide 63

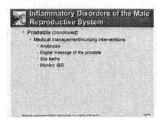

- Identify the role of the nurse in the care of the patient diagnosed with prostatitis.
- What is the prognosis for prostatitis, and what impact does it have on male reproductive health?

Christensen & Kockrow

Slide 64

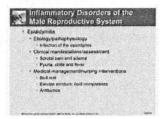

- Epididymitis is a commonly occurring infection of the male reproductive tract. Common causative organisms include *Escherichia coli*, Streptococcus, and *Neisseria gonorrhoeae*.

- What events are associated with the development of epididymitis?

Slide 65

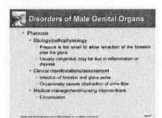

- Phimosis results when the foreskin over the glans penis is too small and cannot be retracted.

- It can cause a localized infection. How does this disorder promote this manifestation?

Slide 66

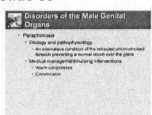

- Discuss conditions that may contribute to the development of paraphimosis.

Slide 67

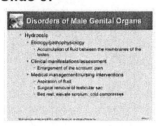

- What are potential causes of hydrocele?

- What will determine the course of treatment for the patient diagnosed with hydrocele?

Slide 68

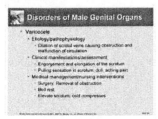

- Identify two nursing diagnoses for the patient with varicocele.

Adult Health Nursing, 6th ed.

Christensen & Kockrow

Slide 69

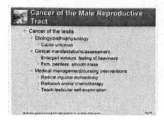

- Testicular cancer is the most common malignancy in men ages 15 to 35 years.

- What populations are at highest risk for the development of testicular cancer?

- What are the recommendations concerning the use of self-testicular examinations?

Slide 70

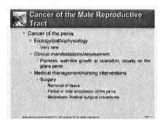

- Cancer of the penis is not frequently seen.

- It is associated with a few select groups of men. Who are they?

Slide 71

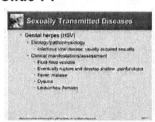

- Genital herpes is a common sexually transmitted disease.

- Being viral in nature, it is a disease characterized by periods of remissions and outbreaks. The frequency and severity of the outbreaks will vary between individuals.

- What is the relationship between herpes simplex type I and herpes simplex type II?

Slide 72

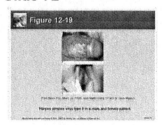

Slide 73

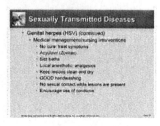

- Although there is no cure for herpes simplex, the disease can be managed with the use of antiviral medications such as acyclovir (Zovirax). What is the desired mode of action by the antiviral medication?

- Herpes simplex is a lifelong disease. What impact will the diagnosis have on the psychological well-being of the patient?

ELSEVIER

Adult Health Nursing, 6th ed.

Christensen & Kockrow

Slide 74

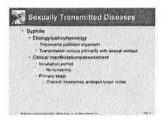

- Syphilis is the third most frequently reported communicable disease in the United States.
- It continues to be more common in young, heterosexual, minority groups.
- Why would these populations be at an increased risk for the disease?

Slide 75

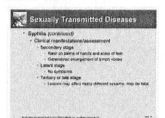

- The development of syphilis is classified by stages. Each of the stages has a unique set of clinical manifestations.

Slide 76

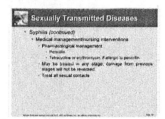

- The goal of treatment for syphilis focuses on the complete annihilation of all traces of the disease.
- In the late stage of development, the damage already present cannot be reversed.
- Review the implications associated with the treatment of syphilis in pregnancy.

Slide 77

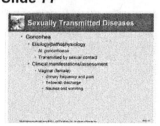

- Gonorrhea is the most commonly reported communicable disease in the United States.
- It is most often seen in young adults.
- Gonorrhea is not limited to only the genital organs. The mouth and throat can also be affected.
- Discuss the "Ping-Pong" effect.

Slide 78

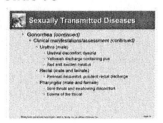

- What diagnostic tests can be used to confirm the presence of gonorrhea?

ELSEVIER

Adult Health Nursing, 6th ed.
Christensen & Kockrow

Slide 79

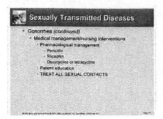

- When treating a patient for gonorrhea, what follow-up care is needed?
- Once a diagnosis has been made, what are the responsibilities for reporting the disease to the proper authorities? Is this a requirement?

Slide 80

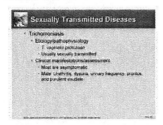

- Trichomoniasis is known as "Trich."
- It is most often transmitted sexually. There are other means of transmission including dirty douche nozzles, douche containers, and washcloths. A baby can also become infected from his mother.
- Since many carriers are asymptomatic, what problems does this create?

Slide 81

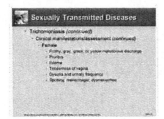

Slide 82

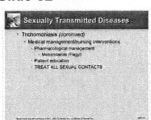

- Treatment of all sexual contacts is needed to prevent the spread of infection. What information, if any, is the patient required to provide to the health authorities?

Slide 83

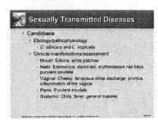

- Candidiasis is a fungal infection. It may be known as "yeast" or "thrush."
- It is common infection.
- What populations are at highest risk for the development of candidiasis?

Adult Health Nursing, 6th ed.
Christensen & Kockrow

Slide 84

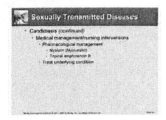

- In addition to antifungal medications, what other nonpharmacologic interventions can be helpful in the management of candidiasis?

Slide 85

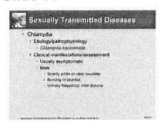

- It is estimated that chlamydia may be the most common sexually transmitted disease.

Slide 86

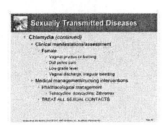

- Chlamydia is often asymptomatic. The lack of reportable symptoms results in untreated infections and continued transmission of the disease.

- Chlamydia has a serious impact on the reproductive health of men and women. Discuss the implications of an untreated chlamydia infection.

Slide 87

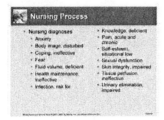

Christensen & Kockrow

TEACHING FOCUS

In this chapter, the student will be introduced to the care of the patient with a visual or auditory disorder. The student will begin by exploring the structure and function of the major sense organs. The student then will have the opportunity to learn the diagnostic studies and age-related changes of the visual and auditory systems. Next, the student will be introduced to a variety of visual and auditory conditions, including their etiology and pathophysiology, clinical manifestations, assessment, diagnostic tests, medical management, nursing interventions, patient teaching, and prognosis. Finally, the student will have the opportunity to learn various nursing care procedures and considerations for people with eye and ear disorders, surgery, or impairments.

MATERIALS AND RESOURCES

- ☐ Computer/overhead projector (all lessons)
- ☐ White/black board and marker/chalk (all lessons)
- ☐ Small finger-food items in each of the four taste sensations (Lesson 13.1)
- ☐ Unlabeled diagram of the eye for each student (Lesson 13.1)
- ☐ Pencils, markers, fruit, or other small items that can be used as prizes (Lesson 13.1)
- ☐ Otoscope (Lesson 13.1)
- ☐ Snellen eye charts and Amsler's grids (Lesson 13.1)
- ☐ Tuning fork (Lesson 13.2)
- ☐ Petroleum jelly and several pairs of sunglasses (Lesson 13.2)
- ☐ Scenario describing a patient who had recent ear surgery (Lesson 13.3)
- ☐ List of surgical procedures for the eye and ear (Lesson 13.3)

LESSON CHECKLIST

Preparations for this lesson include:

- Lecture
- Invite an audiologist to class to demonstrate the care of hearing aids.

KEY TERM

astigmatism (FAAHN p. 1847, AHN p. 611)
audiometry (FAAHN p. 1868, AHN p. 632)
cataract (FAAHN p. 1853, AHN p. 617)
conjunctivitis (FAAHN p. 1850, AHN p. 614)
cryotherapy (FAAHN p. 1856, AHN p. 620)
diabetic retinopathy (FAAHN p. 1854, AHN p. 618)
enucleation (FAAHN p. 1865, AHN p. 629)
exophthalmos (FAAHN p. 1843, AHN p. 607)
glaucoma (FAAHN p. 1859, AHN p. 623)
hyperopia (FAAHN p. 1847, AHN p. 611)
keratitis (FAAHN p. 1851, AHN p. 615)
keratoplasty (FAAHN p. 1865, AHN p. 629)
labyrinthitis (FAAHN p. 1875, AHN p. 639)
mastoiditis (FAAHN p. 1872, AHN p. 636)

miotic (FAAHN p. 1860, AHN p. 624)
mydriatic (FAAHN p. 1844, AHN p. 608)
myopia (FAAHN p. 1847, AHN p. 611)
myringotomy (FAAHN p. 1881, AHN p. 645)
radial keratotomy (FAAHN p. 1848, AHN p. 612)
retinal detachment (FAAHN p. 1858, AHN p. 622)
Sjögren's syndrome (FAAHN p. 1851, AHN p. 615)
Snellen's test (FAAHN p. 1844, AHN p. 608)
stapedectomy (FAAHN p. 1880, AHN p. 644)
strabismus (FAAHN p. 1847, AHN p. 611)
tinnitus (FAAHN p. 1872, AHN p. 636)
tympanoplasty (FAAHN p. 1880, AHN p. 644)
vertigo (FAAHN p. 1875, AHN p. 639)

ADDITIONAL RESOURCES (AHN)

PPT Ch. 53, 1 through 55 FAAHN (Ch. 13, 1 through 55 AHN)
EILR IC images Ch. 53, 1 through 15 FAAHN (Ch. 13, 1 through 15 AHN)
EILR TB questions Ch. 53, 1 through 39 FAAHN (Ch. 3, 1 through 39 AHN)
EILR Open Book Quiz Ch. 53, 1 through 10 FAAHN (Ch. 13, 1 through 10 AHN)
ESLR Review Questions for the NCLEX® Examination Ch. 53, 53-01 through 53-10 FAAHN (Ch. 13, 13-01 through 13-10 AHN)

Christensen & Kockrow

Legend

PPT
PowerPoint
Slides

EILR
EVOLVE Instructor
Learning Resources:
Image Collection, Test
Bank, Open Book Quizzes

ESLR
EVOLVE Student
Learning Resources:
Review Questions
for the NCLEX
Examination

SG
Study Guide

NCP CTQ
Nursing Care Plan
Critical Thinking
Question

Class Activities are indicated in **bold italic**.

LESSON 13.1

PRETEST

1. When explaining the physiology of vision, it is important to understand that convergence involves:
   a. the bending of light rays as they pass through the structures of the eye.
   b. the medial movement of both eyes allowing light rays from the object to hit the same point on both retinas.
   c. the ability of the eyes to focus on objects at differing distances.
   d. the inability of the aging eye to focus on objects at increasing distances.

2. A young man diagnosed as colorblind has which of the following impairments?
   a. A dietary deficiency of vitamin A
   b. The absence of cones
   c. The absence of rods
   d. A reduction in aqueous humor

3. The area of the tongue responsible for the sensation of bitter flavors is:
   a. the posterior portion.
   b. the right side.
   c. the tip of the tongue.
   d. the left side.

4. When caring for a patient having a history of glaucoma, which of the pre-procedural medications will be contraindicated?
   a. Mydriatic drops
   b. Miotic drops
   c. Cycloplegic drops
   d. Antibiotic ointment

5. A patient has just finished seeing the physician concerning an eye disorder. After seeing the physician, the patient states he has been diagnosed with myopia. Based upon your understanding, which of the following statements is correct?
   a. There is an inability of the eyes to focus in the same direction.
   b. The rays of light entering the eye are focusing behind the retina.
   c. There is an elongation of the eyeball, causing light rays to focus in front of the retina.
   d. One eye turns inward in the direction of the nose.

6. When assessing a patient who has developed cataracts associated with drug/medication use, which of the following medications will be implicated?
   a. Chemotherapeutic medications
   b. Nonsteroidal anti-inflammatory medications
   c. Marijuana
   d. Corticosteroids

ELSEVIER

Mosby items and derived items © 2011 by Mosby, Inc., an affiliate of Elsevier Inc.
Some material was previously published.

Adult Health Nursing, 6th ed.
Christensen & Kockrow

7. A patient presents to the physician with complaints of an increasing lack of coordination with voluntary movements. Which of the following diagnostic tests can be anticipated?
   a. Past-point test
   b. Romberg test
   c. Rinne test
   d. Weber's test

8. When planning the care of a patient diagnosed with Ménière's disease, which of the following dietary recommendations will be incorporated?
   a. Sodium restriction
   b. Protein restrictions
   c. Push fluid intake during daytime hours
   d. Potassium restriction

9. After having surgery to treat a hearing loss, the patient asks when she can resume her normal activities. What information will be included in the patient education?
   a. "You may wash your hair 48 hours after surgery."
   b. "You may return to work in 4 to 6 weeks."
   c. "You can take trips in the car only after 3 to 4 weeks."
   d. "Physical activity will be limited for the first week postoperatively."

10. When caring for a patient who underwent a stapedectomy, the patient voices concern because he is unable to note any improvement in hearing since the procedure. What information is the best response by the nurse?
    a. "I will need to contact your physician to communicate this setback."
    b. "Improvements in hearing will not be noted until after the swelling subsides."
    c. "The physician will see you tomorrow."
    d. "Don't worry, your hearing will begin to improve tomorrow."

Answers:

1. b	2. b	3. a	4. a	5. c
6. d	7. a	8. a	9. d	10. b

BACKGROUND ASSESSMENT

Question: A patient reports to the physician's office with complaints of reddened, bloodshot eyes. The patient states, "I do not drink. I always get enough sleep and feel rested." He voices concerns and questions about why he has these symptoms even though he does not have behaviors associated with them. How should you respond to his queries?

Answer: Red eyes are caused by a dilation of the blood vessels of the conjunctiva. They could become dilated due to irritation or congestion. There are causes for "bloodshot eyes" other than alcohol use and a lack of sleep. Other causes for the condition include environmental irritants and illness. A comprehensive investigation should be made into the potential causes of the condition. His physician might determine the need to schedule additional testing.

Question: A deaf male patient has been hospitalized for the management of diabetes. What are the most important factors to be included in the plan of care? What behaviors should be avoided?

Answer: When caring for a deaf patient, it is important to determine his preferred manner of communication. If he reads lips, you must be sure to turn and face him during the interaction. When speaking with the patient, do not cover your mouth, eat, or chew gum. These actions could hinder the patient's abilities to read lips. Be observant of nonverbal behaviors demonstrated both by the patient and yourself. If the patient exhibits fatigue or inattention, it may not be an optimal time for interaction. Avoid appearances of annoyance. Do not rush the conversation. Extra time might be required. Provide written or photo guides to accompany patient education to reinforce content.

CRITICAL THINKING QUESTION

During a routine health physical, a patient reports changes in his vision. He states these changes have become increasingly prevalent during the past 2 to 3 years. The patient is currently 78 years old. He asks questions about what other changes can be anticipated in his visual abilities relating to aging. What information should be provided the patient? What recommendations concerning preventive behaviors can be made to the patient at this time?

Guidelines: The sense of vision experiences changes associated with aging as does the rest of the body. Changes in vision include reduced color perception and discrimination, decreased abilities to adapt to changes in light, reduced tear production, and changes in depth perception. As an individual ages, an increase in cataracts, retinal detachment, macular degeneration, and glaucoma results. To combat and reduce complications, patients are encouraged to have regular screening examinations with their health care provider. Patients should also receive education concerning the dangers of UV exposure, dietary influences, and medication interactions.

OBJECTIVES	CONTENT	TEACHING RESOURCES
List the major sense organs and discuss their anatomic position.	■ Anatomy and physiology of the sensory system (FAAHN p. 1838, AHN p. 602) □ Anatomy of the eye (FAAHN p. 1838, AHN p. 602) □ Accessory structures of the eye (FAAHN p. 1838, AHN p. 602) □ Structure of the eyeball (FAAHN p. 1838, AHN p. 602) □ Chambers of the eye (FAAHN p. 1839, AHN p. 603) □ Physiology of vision (FAAHN p. 1840, AHN p. 604) □ Anatomy and physiology of the ear (FAAHN p. 1840, AHN p. 604) □ External ear (FAAHN p. 1840, AHN p. 604) □ Middle ear (FAAHN p. 1840, AHN p. 604) □ Internal ear (FAAHN p. 1841, AHN p. 605) □ Other special senses (FAAHN p. 1842, AHN p. 606) □ Taste and smell (FAAHN p. 1842, AHN p. 606) □ Touch (FAAHN p. 1842, AHN p. 606) □ Position and movement (FAAHN p. 1842, AHN p. 606)	PPT 2 through 11, Ch. 53 FAAHN (Ch. 13 PPT 2 through 11 AHN) EILR TB Ch. 53 question 39 FAAHN (Ch. 13 question 39 AHN) ESLR Review Questions for the NCLEX Examination Ch. 53 question 1 FAAHN (Ch. 13 question 1 AHN) SG Sensory Organs, Ch. 53 p. 477 FAAHN (Ch. 13 p. 165 AHN) SG Lacrimal Apparatus, Ch. 53 p. 481 FAAHN (Ch. 13 p. 169 AHN) ▶ Discuss the physical structure of both the eye and ear. ▶ Discuss the senses of taste and smell. *Class Activity Note: This activity can be used as a quick fill-in or an icebreaker. Provide small finger food items in each of the four taste sensations. Pair students. Blindfold one student in each team. Ask the blindfolded students to taste items with the assistance of the "sighted" partner. Remember to ask the students to place the foods in the correct areas of the tongue to reinforce which of the tongue locations are associated with which sensation.*

Mosby items and derived items © 2011 by Mosby, Inc., an affiliate of Elsevier Inc. Some material was previously published.

Christensen & Kockrow

OBJECTIVES	CONTENT	TEACHING RESOURCES
List the parts of the eye and define the function of each part.	☐ Anatomy of the eye (FAAHN p. 1842, AHN p. 602) ☐ Accessory structures of the eye (FAAHN p. 1842, AHN p. 602) ☐ Structure of the eyeball (FAAHN p. 1842, AHN p. 602) ☐ Chambers of the eye (FAAHN p. 1843, AHN p. 603) ☐ Physiology of vision (FAAHN p. 1844, AHN p. 604)	▦ PPT 2 through 6, Ch. 53 FAAHN (Ch. 13 PPT 2 through 6 AHN) 🗲 EILR IC Ch. 53 images 1 through 3 FAAHN (Ch. 13 images 1 through 3 AHN) 🗲 EILR TB Ch. 53 question 22 FAAHN (Ch. 13 question 22 AHN) 🗲 ESLR Review Questions for the NCLEX Examination Ch. 53 question 2 FAAHN (Ch. 13 question 2 AHN) 📖 SG Sensory Organs, Ch. 53 p. 477 FAAHN (Ch. 13 p. 165 AHN) **BOOK RESOURCES** Review Questions for the NCLEX Examination Ch. 53 question 32 FAAHN (Ch. 13 question 32 AHN) Fig. 53-1 Lacrimal apparatus (FAAHN p. 1842) (Fig. 13-1 AHN p. 602) Fig. 53-2 Horizontal section through the left eyeball (FAAHN p. 1843) (Fig. 13-2 AHN p.603) ▸ Discuss the physiology of vision. Include a review of each of the four basic processes needed to formulate an image. ▸ Discuss the functions of the eye's accessory organs. *Class Activity Provide students with an unlabeled diagram of the eye. Allow students 3 to 5 minutes to label the structures of the eye. The student who has the most correct answers in the time allowed wins a small prize. Ideas for prizes can include pencils, markers, or fruit.*
List the three divisions of the ear and discuss the function of each.	☐ Anatomy and physiology of the ear (FAAHN p. 1840, AHN p. 604) ☐ External ear (FAAHN p. 1840, AHN p. 604) ☐ Middle ear (FAAHN p. 1840, AHN p. 604) ☐ Internal ear (FAAHN p. 1841, AHN p. 605)	▦ PPT 7 through 10, Ch. 53 FAAHN (Ch. 13 PPT 7 through 10 AHN) 🗲 EILR IC Ch. 53 images 3, 4 FAAHN (Ch. 13 images 3, 4 AHN) 🗲 EILR TB Ch. 53 question 24 FAAHN (Ch. 13 question 24 AHN) 📖 SG Sensory Organs, Ch. 53 p. 477 FAAHN (Ch. 13 p. 165 AHN)

Adult Health Nursing, 6th ed.

Christensen & Kockrow

OBJECTIVES	CONTENT	TEACHING RESOURCES
	□ Other special senses (FAAHN p. 1842, AHN p. 606) □ Taste and smell (FAAHN p. 1842, AHN p. 606) □ Touch (FAAHN p. 1842, AHN p. 606) □ Position and movement (FAAHN p. 1842, AHN p. 606)	**BOOK RESOURCES** Fig. 53-3 External, middle, and inner ear (FAAHN p. 1840) (Fig. 13-3 AHN p. 604) Fig. 53-4 (FAAHN p. 1841) (Fig. 13-4 AHN p.605) ▸ Discuss the divisions and functions of the ear. *Class Activity **Demonstrate an examination of the ear using an otoscope. After the demonstration is complete, allow students to use the otoscope.***
Describe two changes in the sensory system that occur as a result of the normal aging process.	▪ Normal aging of the sensory system (FAAHN p. 1842, AHN p. 606)	*E* EILR TB Ch. 53 question 32 FAAHN (Ch. 13 question 32 AHN) *E* EILR Open Book Quiz Ch. 53 question 1 FAAHN (Ch. 13 question 1 AHN) *E* ESLR Review Questions for the NCLEX Examination Ch. 53 question 3 FAAHN (Ch. 13 question 3 AHN) *SG* SG Aging, Ch. 53 p. 479 FAAHN (Ch. 13 p. 167 AHN) **BOOK RESOURCES** Life Span Considerations, Older Adults: Disorders of the Sensory System (FAAHN p. 1843) (AHN p. 607) ▸ Discuss the physiological changes in the human eye associated with aging. Include a discussion of how these changes impact visual ability. ▸ Discuss preventive health behaviors that could be instituted to preserve functioning of the sensory organs. *Class Activity **Instruct each student to interview two older adults. The students are to ask the adults to describe their current visual and auditory abilities. The adults will also be asked to explain how their vision has changed over the past 10 years. In the next class session, allow students to share their findings. See Homework box below.***

Adult Health Nursing, 6th ed.

Christensen & Kockrow

OBJECTIVES	CONTENT	TEACHING RESOURCES
Describe age-related changes in the visual and auditory systems and differences in assessment findings.	■ Normal aging of the sensory system (FAAHN p. 1842, AHN p. 606) ■ Nursing considerations for care of the patient with an eye disorder (FAAHN p. 1842, AHN p. 606)	SG Aging, Ch. 53 p. 479 FAAHN (Ch. 13 p. 167 AHN) **BOOK RESOURCES** Table 53-1 Normal Findings of the Adult Eye (FAAHN p. 1843) (Table 13-1 AHN p. 607) ▶ Discuss the recommended frequency for medical examinations of the eyes and ears for older adults. ▶ Discuss the psychosocial implications associated with aging of the sensory organs. *Class Activity **Divide the class into small groups (no larger than four students per group). Mix younger students with older students. Instruct each group to investigate the presence of any sensory impairment experienced by the group's members. Do these impairments involve age-related changes? Are there differences noted between the younger and older group members?***
Describe the purpose, significance of results, and nursing responsibilities related to diagnostic studies of the visual and auditory systems.	■ Laboratory and diagnostic examinations (FAAHN p. 1842, AHN p. 606)	PPT 12, Ch. 53 FAAHN (Ch. 13 PPT 53 AHN) EILR IC Ch. 53 images 12 through 14 FAAHN (Ch. 13 images 12 through 14 AHN) EILR TB Ch. 53 questions 1, 34 FAAHN (Ch. 13 questions 1, 34 AHN) EILR Open Book Quiz Ch. 53 question 2 FAAHN (Ch. 13 question 2 AHN) SG Diagnostic Studies, Ch. 53 p. 480 FAAHN (Ch. 13 p. 168 AHN) **BOOK RESOURCES** Review Questions for the NCLEX Examination Ch. 53 questions 6, 25 FAAHN (Ch. 13 question 6, 25 AHN) Table 53-2 Major Diagnostic Eye Tests (FAAHN p. 1844) (Table 13-2 AHN p. 608) Cultural Considerations: Phacoemulsification of a cataractous lens through a self-sealing, scleral-tunnel incision. Note the circular opening in the anterior lens capsule (FAAHN p. 1854) (AHN p. 618)

Christensen & Kockrow

OBJECTIVES	CONTENT	TEACHING RESOURCES
		Fig. 53-10 **A,** In the normal eye, the optic cup is pink with little cupping. **B,** In the glaucomatous eye, the optic disk is bleached and optic cupping is present. (FAAHN p. 1860) (Fig. 13-10 AHN p. 624) Fig. 53-11 Measurement of intraocular pressure with the Schiøtz tonometer (FAAHN p. 1861) (Fig. 13- 11AHN p. 625) Fig. 53-12 Applanation tonometry (FAAHN p. 1861) (Fig. 13-12 AHN p. 625) Fig. 53-13 Weber's tuning fork test (FAAHN p. 1868) (Fig 13-13 AHN p. 632) Fig. 53-14 Rinne tuning fork test (FAAHN p. 1868) (Fig. 13-14 AHN p. 632) ▸ Discuss the recommendations of eye care professionals for screening examinations. ▸ Discuss the role of the nurse when preparing a patient for diagnostic examinations of the eyes and ears. *Class Activity Obtain or develop Snellen eye exam charts and Amsler's grids. Place students in areas of the room where the temporary eye exam stations are located. Allow students to complete examinations on a partner.*

13.1 Homework/Assignments:

Instruct each student to interview two older adults. The students are to ask the subjects to describe their current visual and auditory abilities. The subjects will also be asked to explain how their vision has changed over the past 10 years. In the next class session, allow students to share their findings.

13.1 Instructor's Notes/Student Feedback:

Adult Health Nursing, 6th ed.
Christensen & Kockrow

LESSON 13.2

CRITICAL THINKING QUESTION

You are assigned to care for a patient who has been recently diagnosed with type 2 diabetes mellitus. The patient is experiencing the "normal" anxiety expected with this type of diagnosis. During patient education, she states, "I have heard so much about diabetics having problems with their vision and later going blind." What information should be provided the patient?

Guidelines: Diabetics do have a higher incidence of eye-related complications. These complications occur more frequently in diabetic patients whose blood glucose levels are poorly controlled. The incidence of occurrence of eye complications increases the longer an individual has diabetes. The most common disorder affecting the eyes of diabetics is diabetic retinopathy. It is characterized by microaneurysms, hemorrhage, exudates, and the formation of new vessels and connective tissue. An estimated 80% of patients having diabetes will be affected with an eye disorder. There are interventions that can reduce the likelihood of developing eye complications. These steps include close compliance with the prescribed diet, exercise, and medication schedule. A diabetic should also have regularly scheduled eye examinations and report any visual changes or disturbances to the physician.

OBJECTIVES	CONTENT	TEACHING RESOURCES
Discuss the refractory errors of astigmatism, strabismus, myopia, and hyperopia, including etiology, pathophysiology, clinical manifestations, assessment, diagnostic tests, medical management, nursing interventions, and patient teaching.	■ Disorders of the eye (FAAHN p. 1843, AHN p. 607) ☐ Blindness and near blindness (FAAHN p. 1843, AHN p. 607) – Etiology and pathophysiology (FAAHN p. 1843, AHN p. 607) – Clinical manifestations (FAAHN p. 1845, AHN p. 609) – Assessment (FAAHN p. 1845, AHN p. 609) – Medical management (FAAHN p. 1845, AHN p. 609) – Nursing interventions and patient teaching (FAAHN p. 1846, AHN p. 610) – Prognosis (FAAHN p. 1846, AHN p. 610) ☐ Refractory errors (FAAHN p. 1846, AHN p. 610) – Astigmatism, strabismus, myopia, and hyperopia (FAAHN p. 1847, AHN p. 611)	PPT 13 through 17, Ch. 53 FAAHN (Ch. 13 PPT 13 through 17 AHN) EILR TB Ch. 53 questions 5, 11, 16, 35 FAAHN (Ch. 13 questions 5, 11, 16, 35 AHN) EILR Open Book Quiz Ch. 53 questions 3 through 5 FAAHN (Ch. 13 questions 3 through 5 AHN) ESLR Review Questions for the NCLEX Examination Ch. 53 question 4 FAAHN (Ch. 13 question 4 AHN) SG Refractory Eyes Disorders, Ch. 53 p. 481 FAAHN (Ch. 13 p. 169 AHN) **BOOK RESOURCES** Box 53-1 Guidelines for Communicating with Blind People (FAAHN p. 1846) (Box 13-1 AHN p. 610) Fig. 53-5 Sighted-guide technique (FAAHN p. 1846) (Figure 13-5 AHN p. 610) Table 53-3 Common Refractory Errors (FAAHN p. 1847) (Table 13-3 AHN p. 611) Health Promotion: Contact Lens Care (FAAHN p. 1849) (AHN p. 613) ▶ Discuss the differences in the types of refractory disorders. ▶ Discuss surgical treatment options for the patient with a refractory disorder.

Christensen & Kockrow

OBJECTIVES	CONTENT	TEACHING RESOURCES
Describe inflammatory conditions of the eye including etiology, pathophysiology, clinical manifestations, assessment, diagnostic tests, medical management, nursing interventions, patient teaching, and prognosis.	■ Disorders of the eye (FAAHN p. 1843, AHN p. 607) ☐ Inflammatory and infectious disorders of the eye (FAAHN p. 1849, AHN p. 613) – Hordeolum, chalazion, and blepharitis (FAAHN p. 1849, AHN p. 613) – Inflammation of the conjunctiva (FAAHN p. 1850, AHN p. 614) ☐ Inflammation of the cornea (FAAHN p. 1851, AHN p. 615) – Etiology and pathophysiology (FAAHN p. 1851, AHN p. 615) – Clinical manifestations (FAAHN p. 1851, AHN p. 615) – Assessment (FAAHN p. 1851, AHN p. 615) – Diagnostic tests (FAAHN p. 1851, AHN p. 615) – Medical management (FAAHN p. 1851, AHN p. 615) – Nursing interventions and patient teaching (FAAHN p. 1851, AHN p. 615) – Prognosis (FAAHN p. 1851, AHN p. 615)	PPT 18 through 23, Ch. 53 FAAHN (Ch. 13 PPT 18 through 23 AHN) EILR TB Ch. 53 questions 12, 20 FAAHN (Ch. 13 questions 12, 20 AHN) SG Noninfectious Eye Disorders Ch. 53 p. 483 FAAHN (Ch. 13 p. 171 AHN) SG Inflammatory Eye Disorders, p. 482 FAAHN (Ch. 13 p. 170 AHN) **BOOK RESOURCES** Review Questions for the NCLEX Examination Ch. 53 question 24 FAAHN (Ch. 13 question 24 AHN) Health Promotion: Contact Lens Care (FAAHN p. 1849) (AHN p. 613) Table 53-4 Common Infections and Inflammatory Disorders of the Lid (FAAHN p. 1849) (Table 13-4 AHN p. 613) Table 53-1 Medications for Eye Disorders (FAAHN p. 1861) (Table 13-1 AHN p. 625) ▶ Discuss behaviors that increase the risk for the development of an inflammatory eye condition. ▶ Discuss the clinical manifestations associated with the development of inflammatory eye disorders. *Class Activity Take a class survey. Ask each student to take out a piece of paper. Question the students concerning their personal eye hygiene behaviors. Allow volunteers to share their perception of their level of risk for the development of an inflammatory eye condition.*
Discuss Sjögren syndrome, ectropion and entropion, including etiology, pathophysiology, clinical manifestations, diagnostic tests, medical management, nursing interventions, and prognosis.	■ Disorders of the eye (FAAHN p. 1843, AHN p. 607) ☐ Noninfectious disorders of the eye (FAAHN p. 1851, AHN p. 615) – Dry eye disorders (FAAHN p. 1851, AHN p. 615) ☐ Ectropion and entropion (FAAHN p. 1852, AHN p. 616) – Etiology and pathophysiology (FAAHN p. 1852, AHN p. 616)	PPT 24, Ch. 53 FAAHN (Ch. 13 PPT 24 AHN) EILR TB Ch. 53 question 6 FAAHN (Ch. 13 question 6 AHN) SG Non Infectious Eye Disorders, Ch. 53 p. 483 FAAHN (Ch. 13 p. 171 AHN) **BOOK RESOURCES** Table 53-5 Medications for Eye Disorders (FAAHN p. 1861) (Table 13-5 AHN p. 625)

ELSEVIER

OBJECTIVES	CONTENT	TEACHING RESOURCES
	– Clinical manifestations (FAAHN p. 1852, AHN p. 616) – Assessment (FAAHN p. 1852, AHN p. 616) – Diagnostic tests (FAAHN p. 1852, AHN p. 616) – Medical management (FAAHN p. 1852, AHN p. 616) – Nursing interventions (FAAHN p. 1852, AHN p. 616) – Prognosis (FAAHN p. 1853, AHN p. 617)	▶ Discuss potential causes of ectropion. ▶ Discuss nursing education for the patient with dry eye disorders.
Compare the nature of cataracts, diabetic retinopathy, macular degeneration, retinal detachment and glaucoma, including the etiology, pathophysiology, clinical manifestations, assessment, diagnostic tests, medical management, nursing interventions, patient teaching, and prognosis.	☐ Disorders of the lens (FAAHN p. 1853, AHN p. 617) – Cataracts (FAAHN p. 1853, AHN p. 617) ☐ Disorders of the retina (FAAHN p. 1854, AHN p. 618) – Diabetic retinopathy (FAAHN p. 1854, AHN p. 618) – Age-related macular degeneration (FAAHN p. 1857, AHN p. 621) – Retinal detachment (FAAHN p. 1858, AHN p. 622) ☐ Glaucoma (FAAHN p. 1859, AHN p. 623) – Etiology and pathophysiology (FAAHN p. 1859, AHN p. 623) – Clinical manifestations (FAAHN p. 1860, AHN p. 624) – Assessment (FAAHN p. 1860, AHN p. 624) – Diagnostic tests (FAAHN p. 1860, AHN p. 624)	▣ PPT 25 through 35, Ch. 53 FAAHN (Ch. 13 PPT 25 through 35 AHN) 🖝 EILR IC Ch. 53 images 6 through 11 FAAHN (Ch. 13 images 6 through 11 AHN) 🖝 EILR TB Ch. 53 questions 13, 15, 19, 27 FAAHN (Ch. 13 questions 13, 15, 19, 27 AHN) 🖝 EILR Open Book Quiz Ch. 53 questions 6 through 8 FAAHN (Ch. 13 question 6 through 8 AHN) 🖝 ESLR Review Questions for the NCLEX Examination Ch. 53 question 5 through 7 FAAHN (Ch. 13 question 5 through 7 AHN) 📓 SG Non Infectious Eye Disorders, Ch. 53 p. 483 FAAHN (Ch. 13 p. 171 AHN) **BOOK RESOURCES** Review Questions for the NCLEX Examination Ch. 53 questions 1, 7, 22, 27, 33 FAAHN (Ch. 13 questions 1, 7, 22, 27, 33 AHN) Fig. 53-8 Retinal break with detachment: surgical repair by scleral buckling technique (FAAHN p. 1846) (Fig. 13-5 AHN p. 610) Fig. 53-6 Cataract, visible in the left eye as white opacity of the lens, is seen through the pupil (FAAHN p. 1853) (Fig. 13-6 AHN p. 617) Fig. 53-7 Phacoemulsification of a cataractous lens through a self-sealing, scleral-tunnel incision. Note the circular opening in the

OBJECTIVES	CONTENT	TEACHING RESOURCES
	– Medical management (FAAHN p. 1861, AHN p. 625) – Nursing interventions and patient teaching (FAAHN p. 1863, AHN p. 627) – Prognosis (FAAHN p. 1863, AHN p. 627)	anterior lens capsule (FAAHN p. 1854) (Fig. 13-7 AHN p. 618) Cultural Considerations: Hearing and Visual Problems (FAAHN p. 1854) (AHN p. 618) Nursing Care Plan 53-1 The Patient with Cataracts (FAAHN p. 1855) (NCP 13-1 AHN p. 619) 💡 NCP CTQ 1 through 3 (FAAHN p. 1855) (AHN p. 619) Patient Teaching: After Eye Surgery (FAAHN p. 1856) (AHN p. 620) Patient Teaching: Retinal Detachment (FAAHN p. 1859) (AHN p. 623) Fig. 53-9 **A,** Primary open-angle glaucoma (POAG). Congestion in the trabecular mesh-work reduces the outfl ow of aqueous humor. **B,** Acute angle-closure glaucoma (AACG) (FAAHN p. 1860) (Fig. 13-9 AHN p. 624) Fig. 53-10 **A,** In the normal eye, the optic cup is pink with little cupping. **B,** In the glaucomatous eye, the optic disk is bleached and optic cupping is present (FAAHN p. 1860) (Fig. 13-10 AHN p. 624) Table 53-5 Medications for Eye Disorders (FAAHN p. 1861) (Table 13-5 AHN p. 625) Fig. 53-11 Measurement of intraocular pressure with the Schiøtz tonometer (FAAHN p. 1861) (Fig. 13-11 AHN p. 625) Fig. 53-12 Applanation tonometry (FAAHN p. 1861) (Fig. 13-12 AHN p. 625) ▶ Discuss the populations who experience higher incidence of developing glaucoma, cataracts, macular degeneration, and retinal detachment. ▶ Discuss the prognosis associated with glaucoma, cataracts, macular degeneration, and retinal detachment. *Class Activity **Develop a patient education care plan focusing on the information that will be provided to a patient scheduled for surgical treatment of cataracts.***

Mosby items and derived items © 2011 by Mosby, Inc., an affiliate of Elsevier Inc.
Some material was previously published.

Discuss corneal injuries including etiology/ pathophysiology, clinical manifestations, assessment, diagnostic tests, medical management, nursing interventions, patient teaching, and prognosis.	☐ Corneal injuries (FAAHN p. 1863, AHN p. 627) – Etiology and pathophysiology (FAAHN p. 1863, AHN p. 627) – Clinical manifestations (FAAHN p. 1864, AHN p. 628) – Assessment (FAAHN p. 1864, AHN p. 628) – Diagnostic tests (FAAHN p. 1864, AHN p. 628) – Medical management (FAAHN p. 1864, AHN p. 628) – Nursing interventions and patient teaching (FAAHN p. 1864, AHN p. 628) – Prognosis (FAAHN p. 1865, AHN p. 629)	▦ PPT 36, 37 Ch. 53 FAAHN (Ch. 13 PPT 36, 37 AHN) 🅔 EILR Open Book Quiz Ch. 53 question s 4, 8 FAAHN (Ch. 13 questions 4, 8 AHN) 🅔 ESLR Review Questions for the NCLEX Examination Ch. 53 question 8 FAAHN (Ch. 13 question 8 AHN) 📕 SG Corneal Injuries, Ch. 53 p. 485 FAAHN (Ch. 13 p. 173 AHN) **BOOK RESOURCES** Review Questions for the NCLEX Examination Ch. 53 questions 9, 15 FAAHN (Ch. 13 questions 9, 15 AHN) Safety Alert! Eye Safety Measures (FAAHN p. 1865) (AHN p. 629) ▸ Discuss behaviors associated with corneal injuries. ▸ Discuss the treatment options available for the patient who has been diagnosed with corneal injuries. ***Class Activity Divide the students into groups of four. Instruct the students to develop three to five NCLEX-style questions concerning corneal injuries. After the questions are completed, allow the groups to exchange questions. This will facilitate review and class interaction.***
Describe the various surgeries of the eye, including the nursing interventions and prognosis.	☐ Surgeries of the eye (FAAHN p. 1865, AHN p. 629) ☐ Enucleation (FAAHN p. 1865, AHN p. 629) – Nursing interventions (FAAHN p. 1865, AHN p. 629) – Prognosis (FAAHN p. 1865, AHN p. 629) ☐ Keratoplasty (corneal transplant) (FAAHN p. 1865, AHN p. 629) – Nursing interventions (FAAHN p. 1866, AHN p. 630)	▦ PPT 38 Ch. 53 FAAHN (Ch. 13 PPT 38 AHN) 🅔 EILR IC image Ch. 53 image 15 FAAHN (Ch. 13 image 15 AHN) 🅔 ESLR Review Questions for the NCLEX Examination Ch. 53 question 8 FAAHN (Ch. 13 question 8 AHN) 📕 SG Treatment of the Eye and Ear, Ch. 53 p. 487 FAAHN (Ch. 13 p. 175 AHN) **BOOK RESOURCES** Review Questions for the NCLEX Examination Ch. 53 questions 10, 11, 19, 28, 29 FAAHN (Ch. 13 questions 10, 11, 19, 28, 29 AHN) Communication: Nursing-Patient Dialogue

Mosby items and derived items © 2011 by Mosby, Inc., an affiliate of Elsevier Inc.
Some material was previously published.

Christensen & Kockrow

	– Prognosis (FAAHN p. 1866, AHN p. 630) ☐ Photocoagulation (FAAHN p. 1866, AHN p. 630) – Nursing interventions (FAAHN p. 1866, AHN p. 630) – Prognosis (FAAHN p. 1866, AHN p. 630) ☐ Vitrectomy (FAAHN p. 1866, AHN p. 630) – Nursing interventions and patient teaching (FAAHN p. 1867, AHN p. 631) – Prognosis (FAAHN p. 1867, AHN p. 631)	Regarding Postoperative Eye Surgery (FAAHN p. 1856) (AHN p. 620) Patient Teaching: After Eye Surgery (FAAHN p. 1856) (AHN p. 620)
Differentiate between conductive and sensorineural hearing loss.	■ Nursing considerations for care of the patient with an ear disorder (FAAHN p. 1867, AHN p. 631) ■ Laboratory and diagnostic examinations (FAAHN p. 1867, AHN p. 631) ☐ Otoscopy (FAAHN p. 1867, AHN p. 631) ☐ Tuning fork tests (FAAHN p. 1867, AHN p. 631) – Audiometric testing (FAAHN p. 1868, AHN p. 632) – Vestibular testing (FAAHN p. 1868, AHN p. 632) ■ Disorders of the ear (FAAHN p. 1869, AHN p. 633) ☐ Loss of hearing (deafness) (FAAHN p. 1869, AHN p. 633) – Types of hearing loss (FAAHN p. 1869, AHN p. 633) – Clinical manifestations (FAAHN p. 1870, AHN p. 634) – Assessment (FAAHN p. 1870, AHN p. 634)	PPT 39 through 43, Ch. 53 FAAHN (Ch. 13 PPT 39 through 43, AHN) EILR TB Ch. 53 question 36 FAAHN (Ch. 13 question 36 AHN) ESLR Review Questions for the NCLEX Examination Ch. 53 question 9, 10 FAAHN (Ch. 13 question 9, 10 AHN) SG Hearing Loss, Ch. 53 p. 487 FAAHN (Ch. 13 p. 175 AHN) **BOOK RESOURCES** Review Questions for the NCLEX Examination Ch. 53 questions 2, 13 FAAHN (Ch. 13 questions 2, 13 AHN) Box 53-2 Behavioral Clues Indicating Hearing Loss (FAAHN p. 1867) (Box 13-2 AHN p. 631) Fig. 53-13 Weber's tuning fork test (FAAHN p. 1868) (Fig. 13-13 AHN p. 632) Fig. 53-14 Rinne tuning fork test (FAAHN p. 1868) (Fig. 13-14 AHN p. 632) Health Promotion: Facilitating Communication for People with Impaired Hearing (FAAHN p. 1869) (AHN p. 633) ▸ Discuss the recommendations concerning the schedule of auditory screenings.

ELSEVIER

	– Diagnostic tests (FAAHN p. 1870, AHN p. 634) – Medical management (FAAHN p. 1870, AHN p. 634) – Nursing interventions (FAAHN p. 1870, AHN p. 634) – Patient teaching (FAAHN p. 1870, AHN p. 634) – Prognosis (FAAHN p. 1871, AHN p. 635)	▶ Discuss the type of hearing loss that is identified by each of the diagnostic tests. *Class Activity **Obtain a tuning fork. Demonstrate the use of the tool to perform Weber's and Rinne testing. Have the students demonstrate as well.***
Describe the appropriate care of the hearing aid.	– Nursing interventions (FAAHN p. 1870, AHN p. 634)	⊠▬ PPT 44, Ch. 53 FAAHN (Ch. 13 PPT 44 AHN) SG Care of the Hearing Aid, Ch. 53 p. 486 FAAHN (Ch. 13 p. 174 AHN) **BOOK RESOURCES** Box 53-3 Care of the Hearing Aid (FAAHN p. 1870) (Box 13-3 AHN p. 634) ▶ Discuss the types of hearing losses that may benefit from the use of a hearing aid. ▶ Discuss the psychological impact of wearing a hearing aid. *Class Activity **Invite an audiologist to class to demonstrate the care of hearing aids.***
List tips for communicating with hearing- and sight-impaired people.	■ Blindness and near blindness (FAAHN p. 1843, AHN p. 607) ☐ Nursing interventions and patient teaching (FAAHN p. 1846, AHN p. 610) ■ Disorders of the ear (FAAHN p. 1869, AHN p. 633) ☐ Loss of hearing (deafness) (FAAHN p. 1869, AHN p. 633)	🖥 EILR IC image Ch. 53 image 5 FAAHN (Ch. 13 image 5 AHN) 🖥 EILR TB Ch. 53 questions 14, 18, 26, 38 FAAHN (Ch. 13 questions 14, 18, 26, 38 AHN) SG Caring for Patients with Sensory Impairments, Ch. 53 p. 489 FAAHN (Ch. 13 p. 177 AHN) **BOOK RESOURCES** Box 53-1 Guidelines for Communicating with Blind People (FAAHN p. 1846) (Box 13-1 AHN p. 610) Fig. 53-5 Sighted-guide technique (FAAHN p. 1846) (Fig. 13-5 AHN p. 610)

Christensen & Kockrow

		▶ Discuss the correct manner of providing patient education to a hearing-impaired patient.
		▶ Discuss the behavioral cues that accompany impairments in vision and hearing.
		Class Activity Bring sunglasses and petroleum jelly to class. Smear the glasses with the jelly. This will obstruct the visual field. Assign each student a "buddy." Instruct one student in each pair to wear the glasses. The other student will have the responsibility for assisting the visually impaired student. Allow the pairs 10 minutes to navigate around the room.
Identify communication resources for people with visual and/ or hearing impairment.	■ Blindness and near blindness (FAAHN p. 1843, AHN p. 607) □ Nursing interventions and patient teaching (FAAHN p. 1846, AHN p. 610) ■ Disorders of the ear (FAAHN p. 1869, AHN p. 633) □ Loss of hearing (deafness) (FAAHN p. 1869, AHN p. 633)	PPT 15, Ch. 53 FAAHN (Ch. 13 PPT 15 AHN) SG Caring for Patients with Sensory Impairments, Ch. 53 p. 489 FAAHN (Ch. 13 p. 177 AHN) ▶ Discuss the degrees of visual impairment. ▶ Discuss referrals that could be indicated for the visually or hearing impaired patient. *Class Activity Divide the students into two groups. Assign one group visual impairments and the other group hearing impairments. Instruct each student to investigate community and Internet resources. Ask the students to develop a list of at least three resource agencies for their assigned population. Allow 3 to 5 minutes for sharing resources located by each group.*

13.2 Homework/Assignments:

13.2 Instructor's Notes/Student Feedback:

LESSON 13.3

CRITICAL THINKING QUESTION

While you are working at an ambulatory clinic, you are performing an assessment on an 18-year-old patient who has come in with complaints of severe, throbbing pain in the ear. The patient's vital signs reflect an elevated temperature of 101.1 and a pulse of 96. Further questioning of the patient reveals he recently had an upper respiratory infection. What do you anticipate will be the medical diagnosis? What treatment will most likely be prescribed?

Guidelines: The patient has acute otitis media. This is an infection or inflammation of the middle ear. To aid in confirming the diagnosis, the patient should be asked about the onset of symptoms and the incidence of any recent respiratory infection. Diagnosis will be made based upon the clinical presentation. The ear canal will be assessed for redness, swelling, and discharge. If purulent drainage is present, it can be cultured to identify causative organisms. Management will involve treating the pathogens with antibiotics. Interventions will also focus on reducing the discomfort using compresses or analgesics. Antipyretics can also be used to reduce the fever.

OBJECTIVES	CONTENT	TEACHING RESOURCES
Describe major ear inflammatory and infectious disorders including etiology/pathophysiology, clinical manifestations, assessment, diagnostic tests, medical management, nursing interventions, patient teaching and prognosis.	☐ Inflammatory and infectious disorders of the ear (FAAHN p. 1871, AHN p. 635) – External otitis (FAAHN p. 1871, AHN p. 635) – Acute otitis media (FAAHN p. 1872, AHN p. 636) – Labyrinthitis (FAAHN p. 1875, AHN p. 639) – Obstructions of the ear (FAAHN p. 1875, AHN p. 639)	PPT 45 through 49, Ch. 53 FAAHN (Ch. 13 PPT 45 through 49 AHN) EILR TB Ch. 53 questions 25, 28, 30, 31, 37 FAAHN (Ch. 13 questions 25, 28, 30, 31, 37 AHN) SG Inflammatory /Infectious Ear Disorders, Ch. 53 p. 487 FAAHN (Ch. 13 p. 175 AHN) **BOOK RESOURCES** Patient Teaching: Ear Infection (FAAHN p. 1875) (AHN p. 639) Patient Teaching: Vertigo (FAAHN p. 1876) (AHN p. 640) ▶ Discuss the populations associated with the development of inflammatory and infectious ear disorders. ▶ Discuss preventive teaching that is needed for patients diagnosed with inflammatory or infectious ear disorders that will reduce reinfection. *Class Activity Group students into four small working groups. Assign each group an infectious/inflammatory disorder of the ear. Instruct each group to develop a short presentation for the disorder. This presentation is not to exceed 5 minutes.*

Christensen & Kockrow

Discuss noninfectious disorders of the ear, including etiology, pathophysiology, clinical manifestations, assessment, diagnostic tests, medical management, nursing interventions, and patient teaching.	☐ Noninfectious disorders of the ear (FAAHN p. 1876, AHN p. 640)
	
	  – Otosclerosis (FAAHN p. 1876, AHN p. 640)
	
	  – Ménière's disease (FAAHN p. 1877, AHN p. 641)
		⊠ PPT 50 through 54, Ch. 53 FAAHN (Ch. 13 PPT 50 through 54 AHN)
		
		⊞ EILR TB Ch. 53 questions 9, 17, 21, 29 FAAHN (Ch. 13 questions 9, 17, 21, 29 AHN)
		
		⊞ SG Noninfectious Ear Disorders, Ch. 53 p. 488 FAAHN (Ch. 13 p. 176 AHN)
		
		BOOK RESOURCES
		
		Table 53-5 (FAAHN p. 937) (Table 13-5 AHN p. 625)
		
		Nursing Care Plan 53-2 (FAAHN p. 1879) (NCP 13-2 AHN p. 643)
		
		💡 NCP CTQ 1 through 3 (FAAHN p. 1879) (AHN p. 643)
		
		▶ Discuss the safety implications associated with providing care to a patient diagnosed with Ménière's disease.
		
		▶ Discuss the psychosocial implications associated with a disorder in which hearing is impaired.
		
		***Class Activity** Divide the class into pairs. Instruct each pair to develop three NCLEX-style questions relating to noninfectious disorders of the ear. After the questions are completed, redistribute them to other pairs. Review.*

Describe the various surgeries of the ear, including the nursing interventions, patient teaching, and prognosis.	☐ Surgeries of the ear (FAAHN p. 1880, AHN p. 644)
	
	☐ Stapedectomy (FAAHN p. 1880, AHN p. 644)
	
	  – Nursing interventions (FAAHN p. 1880, AHN p. 644)
	
	  – Prognosis (FAAHN p. 1880, AHN p. 644)
	
	☐ Tympanoplasty (FAAHN p. 1880, AHN p. 644)
	
	  – Nursing interventions (FAAHN p. 1880, AHN p. 644)
	
	  – Prognosis (FAAHN p. 1881, AHN p. 645)
		⊠ PPT 53, Ch. 53 FAAHN (Ch. 13 PPT 53 AHN)
		
		⊞ EILR TB Ch. 53 questions 7, 23 FAAHN (Ch. 13 questions 7, 23 AHN)
		
		⊞ EILR Open Book Quiz Ch. 53 question 10 FAAHN (Ch. 13 question 10 AHN)
		
		⊞ SG Treatment of the Eye and Ear, Ch. 53 p. 487 FAAHN (Ch. 13 p. 175 AHN)
		
		BOOK RESOURCES
		
		Table 53-5 Medications for Eye Disorders (FAAHN p. 1861) (Table 13-5 AHN p. 625)

	☐ Myringotomy (FAAHN p. 1881, AHN p. 645)
	
	   – Nursing interventions and patient teaching (FAAHN p. 1881, AHN p. 645)
	
	   – Prognosis (FAAHN p. 1881, AHN p. 645)
	
	☐ Cochlear implant (FAAHN p. 1881, AHN p. 645)
		Patient Teaching: After Ear Surgery (FAAHN p. 1880) (AHN p. 644)
		
		Fig. 53-15 Cochlear implant (FAAHN p. 1881) (Fig. 13-15 AHN p. 645)
		
		▸ Discuss the physical limitations imposed on a patient after undergoing ear surgery.
		
		▸ Discuss the postoperative positioning for the patient who has had ear surgery.
		
		Class Activity Provide a scenario to the class concerning a patient who has had recent ear surgery. Instruct each student to document priorities of care for the patient. Allow a few minutes for sharing results with the entire class.

Describe home health considerations for people with eye or ear disorders, surgery, or visual and hearing impairments.	☐ Nursing process for the patient with a visual or auditory disorder (FAAHN p. 1881, AHN p. 645)
	
	   – Assessment (FAAHN p. 1882, AHN p. 646)
	
	   – Nursing diagnosis (FAAHN p. 1882, AHN p. 646)
	
	   – Expected outcomes and planning (FAAHN p. 1882, AHN p. 646)
	
	   – Implementation (FAAHN p. 1882, AHN p. 646)
	
	   – Evaluation (FAAHN p. 1882, AHN p. 646)
		▱ EILR IC image Ch. 53 image 5 FAAHN (Ch. 13 image 5 AHN)
		
		▱ EILR TB Ch. 53 questions 2, 3 FAAHN (Ch. 13 questions 2, 3 AHN)
		
		▱ EILR Open Book Quiz Ch. 53 question 9 FAAHN (Ch. 13 question 9 AHN)
		
		▱ SG Caring for Patients with Sensory Impairments, Ch. 53 p. 489 FAAHN (Ch. 13 p. 177 AHN)
		
		BOOK RESOURCES
		
		Health Promotion: Contact Lens Care (FAAHN p. 1849) (AHN p. 613)
		
		Cultural Considerations: Hearing and Visual Problems (FAAHN p. 1854) (AHN p. 618)
		
		▸ Discuss the safety concerns associated with the home environment of a patient having a visual or auditory impairment.
		
		▸ Discuss the use of devices that can be used to enhance the quality and safety of the home environment for the patient experiencing a visual or auditory impairment.
		
		Class Activity Using audiovisual aids, display a nursing care plan form. Employing class participation, modify a nursing care plan for the care of a hearing-impaired patient in the home environment.

Adult Health Nursing, 6th ed.

Christensen & Kockrow

Provide patient instructions regarding care of the eye and ear in accordance with written protocol.	☐ Nursing process for the patient with a visual or auditory disorder (FAAHN p. 1881, AHN p. 645) – Assessment (FAAHN p. 1882, AHN p. 646) – Nursing diagnosis (FAAHN p. 1882, AHN p. 646) – Expected outcomes and planning (FAAHN p. 1882, AHN p. 646) – Implementation (FAAHN p. 1882, AHN p. 646) – Evaluation (FAAHN p. 1882, AHN p. 646)	PPT 55, Ch. 53 FAAHN (Ch. 13 PPT 55 AHN) EILR TB Ch. 53 question 10 FAAHN (Ch. 13 question 10 AHN) SG Patient Teaching, Ch. 53 p. 490 FAAHN (Ch. 13 p. 178 AHN) ▸ Discuss the home care of a patient during the postoperative period after having surgery performed on the eye or ear. ▸ Discuss the support system that should be included in the discharge plans of a patient after a surgical procedure on the eye or ear. ***Class Activity Divide the class into small groups. Assign each group a surgical procedure for the eye or ear. Allow the groups to meet for 5 minutes. During this time the students will be instructed to discuss the assessments that must be provided during the immediate postoperative period.***
Performance Evaluation		EILR TB Ch. 53 questions 1 through 39 FAAHN (Ch. 13 questions 1 through 39 AHN) EILR Open Book Quiz Ch. 53 questions 1 through 10 FAAHN (Ch. 13 questions 1 through 10 AHN) ESLR Review Questions for the NCLEX Examination Ch. 43 questions 1 through 10 FAAHN (Ch. 13 questions 1 through 10 AHN) SG Ch. 53 pp. 477 through 492 FAAHN (Ch. 13 pp. 165 through 180 AHN) **BOOK RESOURCES** Nursing Care Plan 53-1 The Patient with Cataracts (FAAHN p. 1855) (NCP 13-1 AHN p. 619) NCP CTQ 1 through 3 (FAAHN p. 1855) (AHN p. 619) Nursing Care Plan 53-2 (FAAHN p. 1879) (NCP 13-2 AHN p. 643)

Adult Health Nursing, 6th ed.
Christensen & Kockrow

		☿ NCP CTQ 1 through 3 (FAAHN p. 1879) (AHN p. 643) Review Questions for the NCLEX Examination Ch. 53 questions 1 through 34 FAAHN (Ch. 13 questions 1 through 34 AHN)

13.3 Homework/Assignments:

13.3 Instructor's Notes/Student Feedback:

Slide 1

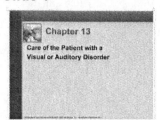

Slide 2

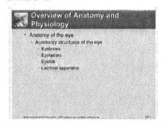

- Only a small portion of the eye is visible to the outside. The sophisticated interrelated system is housed mostly unseen in the cranium.

- Many of the eye's accessory organs are more visible to the outside world.

- What are the functions of the accessory organs?

Slide 3

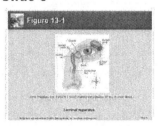

Slide 4

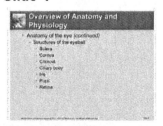

- The anatomy of the eye is divided into three layers or tunics.

- In which layer does each of the eye structures reside?

- How do the characteristics of each of the tunics differ?

Slide 5

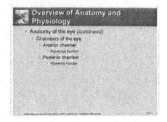

- There are two chambers within the eye. These chambers are defined by the separating lens.

- The anterior chamber contains aqueous humor. This fluid can be likened to the blood plasma. What functions does the aqueous humor have?

- The posterior chamber contains the vitreous humor. It is a gel-like substance.

- How do these two substances differ?

Slide 6

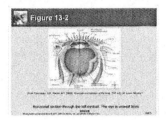

Slide 7

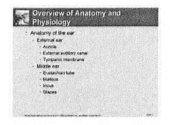

- The process of hearing is complicated. The ear must take in sounds, interpret the sounds, and maintain the body's balance.

- There are three divisions of the ear.

- What is the function of the external ear?

- What role is played by the middle ear?

Slide 8

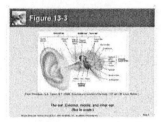

- Point out the distinct separations between the ear's sections.

Slide 9

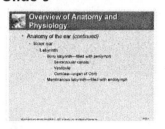

- The inner ear contains the most sensitive portions of the body's auditory system.

- It is the inner ear that has the responsibility for maintaining equilibrium and housing the hair cells that receive the sound messages and transmit them to the brain for interpretation.

Slide 10

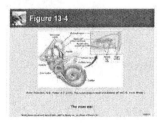

- Trace the path taken by sound waves as they travel through the inner ear. What is the impact if there are impairments within this portion of the ear?

Slide 11

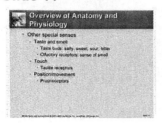

- In addition to hearing and sight, the body has four other senses.

- Taste is a sensation of both necessity and pleasure.

- Specific areas of the tongue have unique and specialized tasting abilities. Which areas are able to taste the four primary "flavors"?

- The sense of smell is conducted by olfactory receptors. These receptors are found in the roof of the nasal canal. Trace the route and mode of the interpretation for odors encountered by the body.

Slide 12

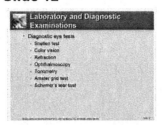

- The management of eye care is handled by a series of professionals. These professions include the optometrist, optician, and ophthalmologist. How do the roles and responsibilities for each of these eye care professionals differ?

- Review each of the diagnostic eye tests.

Slide 13

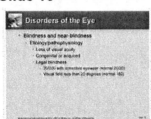

- An estimated 1 million people in the United States are legally blind. How do the terms "legally blind" and "totally blind" differ? What functional differences do the two populations have?

Slide 14

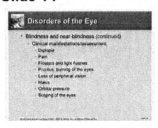

- The clinical manifestations associated with blindness and near-blindness differ depending upon the severity and type of disease process or disorder.

- The patient's abilities to deal with blindness are individualized. What emotional responses can be seen with this population?

Slide 15

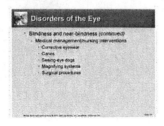

- Regardless of the underlying cause of blindness or the degree of sight loss experienced, visually impaired patients might require nursing interventions. These interventions could be supportive, educational, or geared to assistance with care interventions.

- Outline guidelines for interacting with blind people.

Christensen & Kockrow

Slide 16

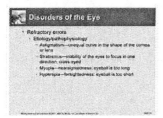

- Refraction refers to the bending of light rays as they pass through the eyes. It is this bending that allows light to focus on the retina.

- In each of the disorders of refraction, where do the images "fall" once they enter the eyes?

Slide 17

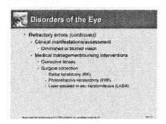

- When patients present with suspected refractory errors, what diagnostic tests can be anticipated?

- What patient education is needed to accompany each of the examinations?

- Refractory errors can be treated with special lenses or surgical intervention. What criteria are used to determine the appropriate management option?

- Review the process of each of the surgical corrective procedures.

Slide 18

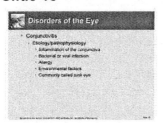

- Conjunctivitis is a common inflammatory eye disorder. Discuss the different ways the disorder is transmitted.

- In the event the source of the inflammation is bacterial, what are some of the more common bacteria? What viruses are most often implicated?

- Identify populations in which conjunctivitis is seen most commonly. Why are these groups at an increased risk?

Slide 19

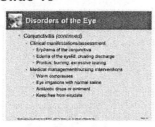

- Conjunctivitis presents with a unique set of clinical manifestations. Diagnosis is based upon the patient's clinical presentation, or the exudates can be cultured to determine the causative organism.

- Once conjunctivitis is diagnosed, what is the role of the nurse?

Slide 20

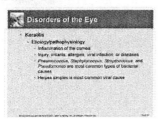

- Keratitis can be superficial or involve the layers of the epithelial tissues.

- What populations are at greatest risk for the development of the condition? Why?

Christensen & Kockrow

Slide 21

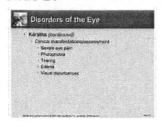

- The presentation of keratitis is most closely associated with pain. When the patient seeks treatment, what information will need to be solicited by the nurse?

- What should be included in the documentation of the presenting problem?

Slide 22

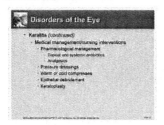

- The treatment of keratitis will include antibiotic therapy. These antibiotics can be topical or systemic depending on the degree of the inflammation.

- What classification of medication will be contraindicated in the management of keratitis? Why?

- What is the rationale for the use of pressure dressings and compresses?

Slide 23

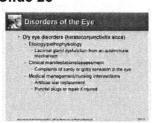

- Dry eye disorders include several ocular disturbances characterized by a reduced tear secretion or increased evaporation of tearing. The treatment is focused on managing the underlying cause.

- It is common for artificial tears to be prescribed for the management of dry eye disorders. When prescribed, these artificial lubricants need to be used with caution. Elaborate on the dangers/difficulties that can accompany excessive use of artificial tears.

- What is the implication if the "dry eyes" are also accompanied by a dry mouth?

Slide 24

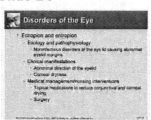

- How do ectropion and entropion differ?

- Discuss the nursing assessment for the patient presenting with ectropion or entropion.

- What is the prognosis for the patient diagnosed with ectropion and entropion?

Slide 25

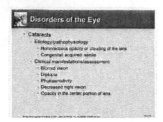

- Cataracts are common disorders of the lens. They are often associated with aging as the lens will lose clarity as time passes.

- Cataracts can be linked to other events. What exposures are tied to the development of cataracts? What is the root cause of congenital cataracts?

Adult Health Nursing, 6th ed.

Christensen & Kockrow

Slide 26

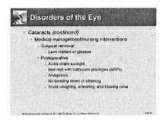

- The only way to permanently manage cataracts is surgery. The decision to have the cataract operatively treated must be agreed upon by both the patient and family.

- There are different surgical procedures that may be performed to manage cataracts. How do they differ?

- What activities are contraindicated during the postoperative phase? Why?

Slide 27

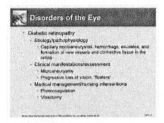

- Diabetic retinopathy is a disorder of the retina. The vast majority of diabetics encounter problems with retinopathy within 15 years of the onset of diabetes. Why does diabetes place patients at an increased risk?

- What can diabetics do to reduce the likelihood of developing retinopathy?

Slide 28

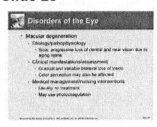

- Macular degeneration is the most common disorder resulting in the loss of sight for Americans 50 years and older.

- Macular degeneration can be classified as "wet" or "dry." How do these types differ? With the loss of central and near vision, what types of complaints can the nurse expect the patient to verbalize?

- When attempting to diagnose macular degeneration, ophthalmoscopy and Amsler's grid can be used. What findings will confirm a diagnosis?

Slide 29

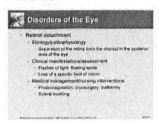

- When retinal detachment occurs, the retina separates from the choroid and vitreous humor begins to leak. The changes that result in retinal detachment can be slow and progressive or acute and due to trauma.

- Diagnostics involve an assessment of visual acuity, ophthalmoscopy, slit lamp exam, or ultrasound examinations. What findings will support the diagnosis?

- What can cause retinal detachment?

Slide 30

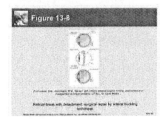

Christensen & Kockrow

Slide 31

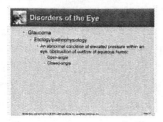

- An estimated 12% to 15% of blindness in America is associated with glaucoma.

- Glaucoma is a group of disorders characterized by three factors: increased or elevated ocular pressure, optic nerve atrophy, and the loss of peripheral vision.

- What populations might experience an increased incidence of this disease?

- Compare and contrast open- and closed-angle glaucoma.

Slide 32

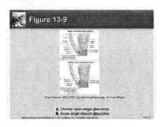

- Acute angle and chronic angle differ in their underlying cause. How does open angle differ from closed angle?

Slide 33

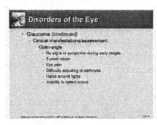

- In addition to reviewing clinical manifestations reported by the patient, what types of objective data should be obtained?

Slide 34

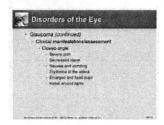

Slide 35

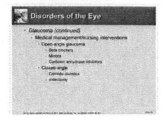

- The management of glaucoma might include both medications and surgical intervention.

- When prescription medications are utilized to manage the condition, what is their method of action?

- Patients with glaucoma require specialized nursing instruction. What should be included in their teaching care plan?

ELSEVIER

Mosby items and derived items © 2011, 2007 by Mosby, Inc., an affiliate of Elsevier Inc.
Some material was previously published.

Adult Health Nursing, 6th ed.
Christensen & Kockrow

Slide 36

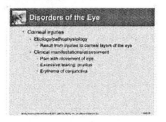

- The cornea is the outermost layer of the eye.

- When the cornea is injured, bleeding will not occur. Why?

- What types of events or situations can precipitate corneal injuries?

- Pain might or might not result with a corneal injury. What factors will aid in determining the presence or degree of pain?

Slide 37

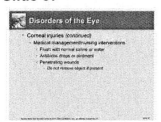

- The degree of corneal injury will determine the means of treatment. What should be included in the nursing assessment and documentation?

Slide 38

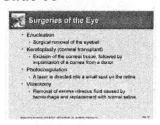

- Disorders of the eye may be managed by surgical intervention. Examples of surgical procedures on the eyes include enucleation, keratoplasty, photocoagulation, and vitrectomy.

- What should the nurse include in the preoperative plan of care?

- When caring for the patient who has had eye surgery, what clinical manifestations indicate potential problems and should be reported to the surgeon?

Slide 39

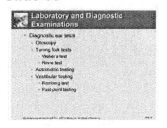

- Auditory testing can be conducted for routine screening purposes or to evaluate reported problems.

- What behavioral cues could indicate a hearing loss?

- What input should be solicited from the family concerning the patient that may point to an auditory impairment?

Slide 40

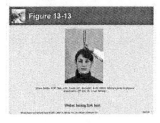

- Weber's test is used to determine auditory acuity and if an impairment is a conductive hearing loss or a sensorineural hearing loss. How do these types of hearing impairments differ?

Christensen & Kockrow

Slide 41

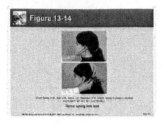

- The Rinne test is employed to distinguish between conductive and sensorineural hearing loss. Describe the differences between the two types of hearing loss.

- What are the nursing responsibilities when assisting with the Rinne test?

Slide 42

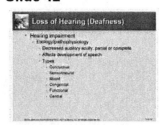

- Hearing impairments are a common disability in the United States.

- They are often a chronic condition that can have a significant impact on one's life.

- Compare and contrast the different types of hearing impairments.

Slide 43

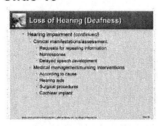

- Treatments prescribed for a hearing impairment will be determined by the underlying cause of the loss.

- Cochlear implants are used in patients having profound bilateral sensorineural hearing loss. How do these implants work?

Slide 44

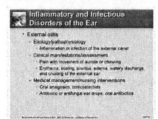

- Also known as "swimmer's ear," external otitis involves an infection or inflammation of the external ear canal. The condition can be chronic or acute.

- To what factors can external otitis be attributed?

Slide 45

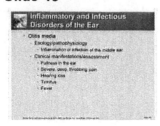

- The most common disorder of the middle ear is otitis media.

- Identify the potential causes of this disorder.

- What populations are associated with the development of otitis media?

Slide 46

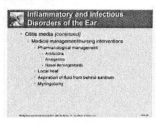

- Otitis media can be chronic or acute. What are the implications associated with chronic otitis media?

- Outline preventive measures to reduce the potential for re-infection.

Slide 47

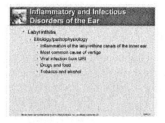

Slide 48

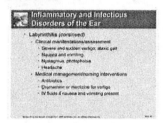

- When caring for the patient experiencing labyrinthitis, what data should the nurse collect and record?

Slide 49

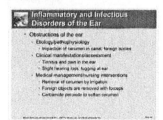

- Obstruction of the ear can be blamed on cerumen in the canal. Given the fact that "wax" is normally present in the ear, how can obstruction result?

- Review habits that should be avoided related to cleaning the ear canal.

Slide 50

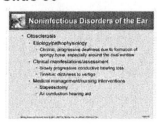

- Otosclerosis is an autosomal dominant inherited disease. Women are affected more frequently than men.

- What tones are most difficult to distinguish for patients with otosclerosis?

- What diagnostic tests will be used to confirm a diagnosis of otosclerosis?

Slide 51

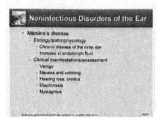

- Ménière's disease is seen more in women ages 30 to 60 years old.
- What data should the nurse collect from the patient suspected of having Ménière's disease?

Slide 52

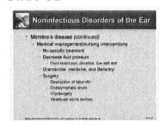

- When Ménière's disease is suspected, what diagnostic tests can be anticipated?
- What will the ordered tests show if a diagnosis of Ménière's disease is confirmed?
- Although there is no specific treatment, there are commonly utilized therapies. What are the goals of the medications and dietary restrictions prescribed?

Slide 53

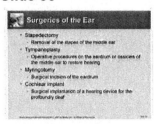

- Surgical intervention might be needed to manage auditory disorders. What common elements will need to be included in the preoperative teaching provided?
- What will be included in the postoperative assessment of the patient?

Slide 54

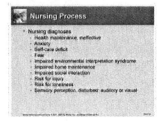

ELSEVIER

Mosby items and derived items © 2011, 2007 by Mosby, Inc., an affiliate of Elsevier Inc.
Some material was previously published.

Adult Health Nursing, 6th ed.
Christensen & Kockrow

TEACHING FOCUS

In this chapter, the student will be introduced to the care of the patient with a neurological disorder. The student will begin by exploring the anatomy and physiology of the neurological system, including the parts and functions of the neuron, the two structural divisions of the nervous system, the location and functions of the parts of the nervous system, and the 12 cranial nerves. The student will explore the physiological changes that occur in the nervous system with aging, the assessment of the nervous system, the prevention of problems of the nervous system, and common laboratory and diagnostic examinations of the nervous system. Finally, the student will have the opportunity to learn the etiology and pathophysiology, clinical manifestations, assessment, diagnostic tests, medical management, nursing interventions, patient teaching, and prognosis for a variety of neurological disorders.

MATERIALS AND RESOURCES

- ☐ Computer/overhead projector (all lessons)
- ☐ White/black board and marker/chalk (all lessons)
- ☐ Unlabeled diagram of a neuron for each student (Lesson 14.1)
- ☐ Ball or other soft object that can be passed around the classroom (Lesson 14.1)
- ☐ Piece of blank, unlined paper for each student (Lesson 14.1)
- ☐ Items such as pencils or fruit that can be used as a small prize (Lesson 14.1)
- ☐ Brief scenarios describing a comatose patient with a head injury, a disoriented older adult, and a patient with a history of migraine headaches (Lesson 14.2)
- ☐ List of neurological tests (Lesson 14.2)
- ☐ Photo of the back that illustrates the spinal cord and the spinal canal; possible sources include the obstetrics department or a childbirth preparation instructor (Lesson 14.2)
- ☐ List of neurological disorders (Lesson 14.3)
- ☐ Assistive devices used by stroke patients (Lesson 14.3)
- ☐ Blank note cards (Lesson 14.3)
- ☐ A full-color image of the brain (Lesson 14.4)

LESSON CHECKLIST

Preparations for this lesson include:
- Lecture
- Prepare a "bingo" game, with bingo cards similar to an ordinary BINGO card, but with squares consisting of short answers about Guillain-Barré, meningitis, encephalitis, and implications of AIDS.
- Obtain the use of the nursing laboratory.

KEY TERMS

agnosia (FAAHN p. 1911, AHN p. 675)

aneurysm (FAAHN p. 1932, AHN p. 696)

aphasia (FAAHN p. 1895, AHN p. 659)

apraxia (FAAHN p. 1925, AHN p. 689)

ataxia (FAAHN p. 1917, AHN p. 681)

aura (FAAHN p. 1912, AHN p. 676)

bradykinesia (FAAHN p. 1919, AHN p. 683)

deep brain stimulation (DBS) (FAAHN p. 1921, AHN p. 685)

diplopia (FAAHN p. 1905, AHN p. 669)

dysarthria (FAAHN p. 1895, AHN p. 659)

dysphagia (FAAHN p. 1908, AHN p. 672)

flaccid (FAAHN p. 1896, AHN p. 660)

Glasgow coma scale (FAAHN p. 1894, AHN p. 658)

global cognitive dysfunction (FAAHN p. 1942, AHN p. 706)

hemianopia (FAAHN p. 1939, AHN p. 703)

hemiplegia (FAAHN p. 1909, AHN p. 673)

hyperreflexia (FAAHN p. 1946, AHN p. 710)

nystagmus (FAAHN p. 1917, AHN p. 681)

paresis (FAAHN p. 1896, AHN p. 660)

postictal period (FAAHN p. 1912, AHN p. 676)

proprioception (FAAHN p. 1897, AHN p. 661)

spastic (FAAHN p. 1896, AHN p. 660)

stroke (FAAHN p. 1930, AHN p. 694)

unilateral neglect (FAAHN p. 1897, AHN p. 661)

ADDITIONAL RESOURCES (AHN)

PPT Ch. 54, 1 through 70 FAAHN (Ch. 14, 1 through 70 AHN)
EILR IC images Ch. 54, 1 through 26 FAAHN (Ch. 14, 1 through 26 AHN)
EILR TB questions Ch. 54, 1 through 41 FAAHN (Ch. 14, 1 through 41 AHN)
EILR Open Book Quiz Ch. 54, 1 through 10 FAAHN (Ch. 14, 1 through 10 AHN)
ESLR Review Questions for the NCLEX® Examination Ch. 54, 54-01 through 54-10 FAAHN (Ch. 14, 14-01 through 14-10 AHN)

Legend

PPT
PowerPoint
Slides

EILR
EVOLVE Instructor
Learning Resources:
Image Collection, Test
Bank, Open Book Quizzes

ESLR
EVOLVE Student
Learning Resources:
Review Questions
for the NCLEX
Examination

SG
Study Guide

NCP CTQ
Nursing Care Plan
Critical Thinking
Question

Class Activities are indicated in **bold italic**.

LESSON 14.1

PRETEST

1. The concept of proprioception refers to which of the following?
   a. Being perceptually unaware of and inattentive to one side of the body
   b. A defect of vision or blindness in half of the visual field
   c. The sensation pertaining to spatial position and muscular activity stimuli originating from within the body
   d. A numbness in the lower extremities associated with reduced environmental temperatures

2. While reviewing a cerebrospinal fluid test result, you note that the lab identified reduced glucose and chloride levels. Based upon your knowledge, you anticipate a diagnosis consistent with:
   a. a bacterial infection.
   b. a viral infection.
   c. a herpes viral infection.
   d. a varicella infection.

3. The _____ cranial nerve is responsible for the sense of smell.
   a. vagus
   b. hypoglossal
   c. acoustic
   d. olfactory

4. After performing the Glasgow coma scale, the patient assessment reveals a score of 13. This score indicates:
   a. a light comatose state.
   b. disorientation.
   c. normal neurological functioning.
   d. a deep comatose state.

5. A physician of a patient who has suffered a mild CVA has recorded in her notes that the patient is experiencing dysarthria. This refers to which of the following occurrences?
   a. Poorly articulated speech
   b. A reduced degree of motor movement abilities
   c. A complete loss of motor movement abilities
   d. Inability to swallow

Adult Health Nursing, 6th ed.
Christensen & Kockrow

6. A patient in a coma, after being in a serious motor vehicle accident, has been diagnosed with a significant neurological impairment. He is lying down, demonstrating decorticate posturing. An assessment of his positioning will reveal:
   a. flaccid upper extremities accompanying tightened lower muscle extremity tone.
   b. flexion of the arms, wrists, and fingers with adduction in the upper extremities.
   c. all four extremities are in rigid extension with hyperpronation of the forearms and plantar extension of the feet.
   d. all four extremities are in rigid flexion with hyperpronation of the forearms and feet.

7. After a seizure, the patient appears groggy and lethargic. These findings are consistent with which stage of the seizure?
   a. The postictal period
   b. The post recovery period
   c. The post aura
   d. The aura phase

8. A patient who has recently been diagnosed with seizures asks why he cannot ever drive again. What is the best response to his question?
   a. "Unfortunately, you are correct."
   b. "Once the seizures are under medical control for a period of time, you might be able to drive."
   c. "It is best you do not drive as the stressors could indeed bring on seizure activity."
   d. "Seizure activity should not hinder your driving ability."

9. An assessment noting diplopia, vertigo, loss of joint sensation, and nystagmus is consistent with which of the following disorders?
   a. Multiple sclerosis
   b. Parkinson's disease
   c. Huntington's disease
   d. Myasthenia gravis

10. When caring for a patient with a diagnosis of trigeminal neuralgia, an area for concern will include:
   a. respiratory insufficiency.
   b. avoidance of skin breakdown.
   c. activation of trigger points.
   d. muscle wasting.

Answers:

1. c	2. d	3. d	4. c	5. a
6. b	7. a	8. b	9. a	10. c

BACKGROUND ASSESSMENT

Question: A patient presents to the physician's office with feelings of stiffness and drawing in her face. A visual inspection of her face reveals a drooping of the mouth and cheek. She states her sense of taste is also significantly reduced. After being seen by the physician, she is diagnosed with Bell's palsy. The patient becomes upset, asking, "Have I had a stroke? What has happened to me?" What information should be provided to the patient?

Answer: The exact cause of Bell's palsy is not known. It is believed to be the result of an inflammatory process of the facial nerve. Other theories support the involvement of the herpes simplex virus. She will need reassurance that she has not had a "stroke." In most cases, the effects of Bell's palsy are not permanent. Most of the treatments are supportive in nature, and the patient can be placed on corticosteroids or antiviral medications. The prognosis is good.

Question: While you are working in the emergency room, a patient arrives after being transported there by his wife in the family car. He states he was hit in the left side of his head with a baseball during a game of "catch" with his son. He says he is probably "OK" but wants to be sure, given the force of the ball's impact. What elements will need to be included in the assessment of his condition? What diagnostic testing will be performed? What medical management interventions do you anticipate?

Adult Health Nursing, 6th ed.

Christensen & Kockrow

Answer: It is a good sign that he is able to move and communicate without obvious impairment. It will be important to determine if he experienced any loss of consciousness. Other important questions determine the occurrence of a headache, nausea, or vomiting. The physical assessment will focus on the presence of bleeding, fluid leakage, level of alertness, and size and reactivity of the pupils. The medical management will be largely determined by the assessment findings. An x-ray, CT, MRI, or PET scan might be performed. The patient could be admitted to the facility for overnight monitoring of his level of consciousness and any later onset clinical manifestations.

CRITICAL THINKING QUESTION

While working the night shift, you are preparing to care for a 78-year-old male patient hospitalized for treatment of a minor skin disorder. The nurse reporting to you states that she has experienced numerous problems providing his care. She indicated he became increasingly confused as the evening wore on and became incontinent. Further, she stated he nearly got burned when a cup of coffee that was clearly in view was knocked over, and he failed to move quickly enough. You have cared for this patient previously and did not have any of the problems experienced by your coworker. Based upon the nurse's report, what do you anticipate to be the problem? What should be the focus of the nursing interventions for your shift?

Guidelines: The patient has no history of this type of behavior. He could be experiencing an increase in disorientation associated with the evening hours of the day. This is a phenomenon that can be seen in older adults. He should have a thorough neurological assessment. His medications should be evaluated for changes or the presence of drugs having side effects associated with disorientation or confusion. The laboratory reports need to be reviewed to evaluate electrolyte imbalances or drug toxicities. The patient's inability to move quickly is a common problem for the older adult. They experience a 1% reduction of neurons annually after age 50. This loss of neurons will manifest as an increase in reaction time. The nursing interventions for the shift should focus on keeping the patient oriented and maintaining a safe environment.

OBJECTIVES	CONTENT	TEACHING RESOURCES
Name the two structural divisions of the nervous system and give the functions of each.	■ Anatomy and physiology of the neurologic system (FAAHN p. 1887, AHN p. 651) □ Structural divisions (FAAHN p. 1887, AHN p. 651)	PPT 2, Ch. 54 FAAHN (Ch. 14 PPT 2 AHN) SG Divisions of the Nervous System, Ch. 54 p. 493 FAAHN (Ch. 14 p. 181 AHN) ▶ Discuss the differences between the divisions of the nervous system. ▶ Discuss the functions of each of the divisions of the nervous system. *Class Activity Divide the class into two groups. One group will be the "central nervous system" and the other, the "peripheral nervous system." Assign each group the task of developing three NCLEX-style questions for its assigned neurological system.* *Note: If the class is large, further subdivide the groups. The questions can be used later for a quiz or exam review.*
List the parts of the neuron and describe the function of each part.	□ Cells of the nervous system (FAAHN p. 1887, AHN p. 651) – Neuron (FAAHN p. 1888, AHN p. 652)	PPT 3, 4, Ch. 54 FAAHN (Ch. 14 PPT 3, 4 AHN) EILR IC Ch. 54 image 1 FAAHN (Ch. 14 image 1 AHN)

Adult Health Nursing, 6th ed.

Christensen & Kockrow

OBJECTIVES	CONTENT	TEACHING RESOURCES
	– Neuromuscular junction (FAAHN p. 1888, AHN p. 652) – Neurotransmitters (FAAHN p. 1888, AHN p. 652) – Neuron coverings (FAAHN p. 1888, AHN p. 652) ☐ Central nervous system (FAAHN p. 1888, AHN p. 652) – Brain (FAAHN p. 1888, AHN p. 652) – Spinal cord (FAAHN p. 1890, AHN p. 654) ☐ Peripheral nervous system (FAAHN p. 1891, AHN p. 655) – Spinal nerves (FAAHN p. 1891, AHN p. 655) – Cranial nerves (FAAHN p. 1891, AHN p. 655) – Autonomic nervous system (FAAHN p. 1891, AHN p. 655)	ESLR Review Questions for the NCLEX Examination Ch. 54 question 1 FAAHN (Ch. 14 question 1 AHN) SG Neuron, Ch. 54 p. 493 FAAHN (Ch. 14 p. 181 AHN) **BOOK RESOURCES** Fig. 54-1 **A,** Diagram of a typical neuron showing dendrites, cell body, and axon. **B,** Myelinated axon, showing a cross-section of concentric layers of the Schwann cell fi lled with myelin (FAAHN p. 1887) (Fig. 14-1 AHN p. 651) ▸ Discuss the two categories of nervous system cells. ▸ Discuss the functions of neurons. *Class Activity* ***Provide each student with an unlabeled diagram of a neuron. Ask each student to label the cell's primary parts.***
Explain the anatomic location and functions of the cerebrum, brainstem, cerebellum, spinal cord, peripheral nerves, and cerebrospinal fluid.	☐ Central nervous system (FAAHN p. 1888, AHN p. 652) – Brain (FAAHN p. 1888, AHN p. 652) – Spinal cord (FAAHN p. 1890, AHN p. 654) ☐ Peripheral nervous system (FAAHN p. 1891, AHN p. 655) – Spinal nerves (FAAHN p. 1891, AHN p. 655) – Cranial nerves (FAAHN p. 1891, AHN p. 655) – Autonomic nervous system (FAAHN p. 1891, AHN p. 655)	PPT 5, 6, Ch. 54 FAAHN (Ch. 14 PPT 5, 6 AHN) EILR IC Ch. 54 images 2, 3 FAAHN (Ch. 14 images 2, 3 AHN) EILR TB Ch. 54 questions 1, 2 FAAHN (Ch. 14 questions 1, 2 AHN) SG Nervous System, Ch. 54 p. 495 FAAHN (Ch. 14 p. 183 AHN) **BOOK RESOURCES** Fig. 54-2 Sagittal section of the brain (note position of midbrain (FAAHN p. 1889) (Fig. 14-2 AHN p. 653) Fig. 54-3 Cerebral cortex (FAAHN p. 1889) (Fig. 14-3 AHN p. 653) Box 54-1 Functions of the Cerebrum (FAAHN p. 1890) (Box 14-1 AHN p. 654) Fig. 54-4 Neural pathway involved in the patellar reflex (FAAHN p. 1891) (Fig. 14-4 AHN p. 655) ▸ Discuss the relationship between the brain and the spinal cord.

OBJECTIVES	CONTENT	TEACHING RESOURCES
		▸ Discuss the divisions and functions of the cerebrum. *Class Activity **Pass a ball around the class. As the ball is passed to a student, ask the student to state a fact about the functions of the cerebrum, brainstem, cerebellum, spinal cord, or spinal nerves. Continue until all students have participated.***
Discuss the parts of the peripheral nervous system and how the system works with the central nervous system .	☐ Peripheral nervous system (FAAHN p. 1891, AHN p. 655) – Spinal nerves (FAAHN p. 1891, AHN p. 655) – Cranial nerves (FAAHN p. 1891, AHN p. 655) – Autonomic nervous system (FAAHN p. 1891, AHN p. 655)	PPT 7, 8, Ch. 54 FAAHN (Ch. 14 PPT 7, 8 AHN) SG Nervous System, Ch. 54 p. 495 FAAHN (Ch. 14 p. 183 AHN) **BOOK RESOURCES** Table 54-1 Cranial Nerves (FAAHN p. 1893) (Table 14-1 AHN p. 657) ▸ Discuss the relationship between the peripheral nervous system and the central nervous system. ▸ Discuss the differences between the peripheral nervous system and the central nervous system. *Class Activity **Provide each student with a piece of blank, unlined paper. Assign each student a component of the peripheral nervous system. Ask half of the students to write the function of the assigned part on the paper. The remaining students will use colored pencils to illustrate the assigned anatomic part. After both groups are finished, ask them to locate their appropriate "match."***
Name the 12 cranial nerves and list the areas they serve.	– Cranial nerves (FAAHN p. 1891, AHN p. 655)	SG Cranial Nerves, Ch. 54 p. 496 FAAHN (Ch. 14 p. 184 AHN) **BOOK RESOURCES** Table 54-1 Cranial Nerves (FAAHN p. 1893) (Table 14-1 AHN p. 657) ▸ Discuss the names of the cranial nerves. ▸ Discuss the role of each of the cranial nerves. *Class Activity **Divide the class into small groups of three to five students. Assign each group to develop a short catchy phrase or saying to remember the name of each of the cranial nerves.*** *Note: **Provide a small prize (fruit or pencils) to the winning team).***

OBJECTIVES	CONTENT	TEACHING RESOURCES
List physiologic changes that occur in the nervous system with aging.	☐ Effects of normal aging on the nervous system (FAAHN p. 1891, AHN p. 655)	PPT 9, Ch. 54 FAAHN (Ch. 14 PPT 9 AHN) EILR TB Ch. 54 question 29 FAAHN (Ch. 14 question 29 AHN) ESLR Review Questions for the NCLEX Examination Ch. 54 question 2 FAAHN (Ch. 14 question 2 AHN) SG Aging, Ch. 54 p. 497 FAAHN (Ch. 14 p. 185 AHN) **BOOK RESOURCES** Review Questions for the NCLEX Examination Ch. 54 question 1 FAAHN (Ch. 14 question 1 AHN) Life Span Considerations, Older Adults: Neurologic Disorder (FAAHN p. 1892) (AHN p.656) ▶ Discuss the implications of aging on the nervous system. ▶ Discuss activities an older adult can perform to improve neurological functioning. *Class Activity Assign each student the task of interviewing an older adult. The adult should be asked what changes he/she has noted in the nervous system with aging.* *Note: The students should be assigned the interview in a prior class. Ask students to review findings in small assigned groups.*
Explain the importance of prevention in problems of the nervous system and give several examples of prevention.	☐ Prevention of neurological problems (FAAHN p. 1892, AHN p. 656)	PPT 10, Ch. 54 FAAHN (Ch. 14 PPT 10 AHN) SG Prevention, Ch. 54 p. 502 FAAHN (Ch. 14 p. 190 AHN) **BOOK RESOURCES** Review Questions for the NCLEX Examination Ch. 54 question 14 FAAHN (Ch. 14 question 3 AHN) Safety Alert! Preventing Neurologic Injuries (FAAHN p. 1893) (AHN p. 657) ▶ Discuss the impact preventative behaviors can have on the health of the nervous system. ▶ Discuss behaviors associated with impaired neurological functioning.

OBJECTIVES	CONTENT	TEACHING RESOURCES
		Class Activity Assign each student a partner. One student will have the role of the nurse and the other will be the patient. Instruct students to role-play patient education for a patient whose lifestyle includes risky behaviors. The pairs can present their skit to other groups in the class.

14.1 Homework/Assignments:

14.1 Instructor's Notes/Student Feedback:

LESSON 14.2

CRITICAL THINKING QUESTION

A 17-year-old male has been hospitalized with neurological changes and an elevated temperature. The physician plans to perform a lumbar puncture. When you approach the parents to sign the consent for the procedure, the mother asks what the test of a tiny amount of fluid can show. The father states his concern because he does not want his son to become paralyzed. It is obvious the patient's family has numerous concerns and the level of anxiety is high. What is a primary goal for the nurse in this situation? What information should they be given?

Guidelines: The family will require emotional support and education. The lumbar puncture is performed to obtain a sample of cerebrospinal fluid to be analyzed. The characteristics of the fluid can aid the physician in assigning a diagnosis. The procedure is brief and involves a needle sheathed by a catheter inserted into the lower back. The sheathed needle is inserted below the bottom of the spinal cord to alleviate the risk of paralysis.

OBJECTIVES	CONTENT	TEACHING RESOURCES
Identify the significant subjective and objective data related to the nervous system that should be obtained from a patient during assessment.	■ Assessment of the neurological system (FAAHN p. 1893, AHN p. 657) ☐ History (FAAHN p. 1893, AHN p. 657) ☐ Mental status (FAAHN p. 1894, AHN p. 658) – Level of consciousness (FAAHN p. 1894, AHN p. 658) – Glasgow coma scale (FAAHN p. 1894, AHN p. 658) – FOUR Score Coma Scale (FAAHN p. 1894, AHN p. 658) ☐ Language and speech (FAAHN p. 1895, AHN p. 659) ☐ Cranial nerves (FAAHN p. 1895, AHN p. 659) ☐ Motor function (FAAHN p. 1896, AHN p. 660) ☐ Sensory and perceptual status (FAAHN p. 1897, AHN p. 661)	PPT 11, Ch. 54 FAAHN (Ch. 14 PPT 11 AHN) EILR IC Ch. 54 image 1 FAAHN (Ch. 14 image 1 AHN) EILR TB Ch. 54 questions 4, 12 FAAHN (Ch. 14 questions 4, 12 AHN) EILR Open Book Quiz Ch. 54 question 1 FAAHN (Ch. 14 question 1 AHN) SG Assessment and Management of Neurological Disorders, Ch. 54 p. 500 FAAHN (Ch. 14 p. 188 AHN) SG Spinal Cord Trauma, Ch. 54 p. 506 FAAHN (Ch. 14 p. 194 AHN) **BOOK RESOURCES** Review Questions for the NCLEX Examination Ch. 54 question 15 FAAHN (Ch. 14 question 15 AHN) Table 54-2 Levels of Consciousness (FAAHN p. 1894) (Table 14-2 AHN p. 658) ▸ Discuss the optimal environment in which a neurological assessment should be performed. ▸ Discuss the components of a mental status examination. ***Class Activity** Demonstrate an assessment of the neurological system on a student volunteer.*

ELSEVIER

Christensen & Kockrow

OBJECTIVES	CONTENT	TEACHING RESOURCES
Differentiate between normal and common abnormal findings of a physical assessment of the nervous system.	■ Assessment of the neurological system (FAAHN p. 1893, AHN p. 657) ☐ History (FAAHN p. 1893, AHN p. 657) ☐ Mental status (FAAHN p. 1894, AHN p. 658) 　– Level of consciousness (FAAHN p. 1894, AHN p. 658) 　– Glasgow coma scale (FAAHN p. 1894, AHN p. 658) 　– FOUR Score Coma Scale (FAAHN p. 1894, AHN p. 658) ☐ Language and speech (FAAHN p. 1895, AHN p. 659) ☐ Cranial nerves (FAAHN p. 1895, AHN p. 659) ☐ Motor function (FAAHN p. 1896, AHN p. 660) ☐ Sensory and perceptual status (FAAHN p. 1897, AHN p. 661)	PPT 11, Ch. 54 FAAHN (Ch. 14 PPT 11 AHN) EILR IC Ch. 54 images 8, 9 FAAHN (Ch. 14 images 8, 9 AHN) EILR TB Ch. 54 questions 13, 37, 39 FAAHN (Ch. 14 questions 13, 37, 39 AHN) ESLR Review Questions for the NCLEX Examination Ch. 54 questions 3, 4 FAAHN (Ch. 14 questions 3, 4 AHN) SG Assessment and Management of Neurological Disorders, Ch. 54 p. 500 FAAHN (Ch. 14 p. 188 AHN) **BOOK RESOURCES** Review Questions for the NCLEX Examination Ch. 54 questions 24 through 26 FAAHN (Ch. 14 questions 24 through 26 AHN) Table 54-4 FOUR Score Coma Scale (FAAHN p. 1896) (Table 14-4 AHN p. 660) ▶ Discuss the differences between the subjective and objective assessment of the neurological system. ▶ Discuss the appropriate terminology to be used when describing a patient's level of consciousness. *Class Activity **Demonstrate assessment of each of the cranial nerves. Utilize a student to do the primary demonstration. After the demonstration, have student pairs perform the same tests.***
Discuss the Glasgow coma scale.	– Glasgow coma scale (FAAHN p. 1894, AHN p. 658)	PPT 11, Ch. 54 FAAHN (Ch. 14 PPT 11 AHN) EILR TB Ch. 54 question 16 FAAHN (Ch. 14 question 16 AHN) SG Glasgow Coma Scale, Ch. 54 p. 500 FAAHN (Ch. 14 p. 188 AHN) **BOOK RESOURCES** Review Questions for the NCLEX Examination Ch. 54 question 7 FAAHN (Ch. 14 question 7 AHN)

Christensen & Kockrow

OBJECTIVES	CONTENT	TEACHING RESOURCES

		Table 54-3 Glasgow Coma Scale: Demonstrating Measurement of Level of Consciousness (FAAHN p. 1895) (Table 14-3 AHN p. 659)
		
		▶ Discuss the components of the Glasgow coma scale.
		
		▶ Discuss the appropriate use of the Glasgow coma scale.
		
		Class Activity Develop a set of brief scenarios:
		   – a comatose patient with a head injury
		   – a disoriented older adult
		   – a patient who has had a history of migraine headaches
		
		Ask students to determine the Glasgow coma scale ranking of each situation.

List common laboratory and diagnostic examinations for evaluation of neurological disorders.	■ Laboratory and diagnostic examinations (FAAHN p. 1897, AHN p. 661)
	
	☐ Blood and urine tests (FAAHN p. 1897, AHN p. 661)
	
	☐ Cerebrospinal fluid (FAAHN p. 1897, AHN p. 661)
	   – Lumbar puncture (FAAHN p. 1897, AHN p. 661)
	
	☐ Other tests (FAAHN p. 1898, AHN p. 662)
	   – Computed tomography scan (FAAHN p. 1898, AHN p. 662)
	
	   – Brain scan (FAAHN p. 1898, AHN p. 662)
	
	   – Magnetic resonance imaging (MRI) scan (FAAHN p. 1898, AHN p. 662)
	
	   – Magnetic resonance angiography (FAAHN p. 1898, AHN p. 662)
	
	   – Positron emission tomography scan (FAAHN p. 1899, AHN p. 663)
		▦ PPT 12 through 14, Ch. 54 FAAHN (Ch. 14 PPT 12 through 14 AHN)
		
		🔗 EILR IC Ch. 54 images 6, 7 FAAHN (Ch. 14 images 6, 7 AHN)
		
		🔗 EILR TB Ch. 54 questions 6, 8, 14, 28, 36 FAAHN (Ch. 14 questions 6, 8, 14, 28, 36 AHN)
		
		🔗 EILR Open Book Quiz Ch. 54 question 2 FAAHN (Ch. 14 question 2 AHN)
		
		🔗 ESLR Review Questions for the NCLEX Examination Ch. 54 question 4 FAAHN (Ch. 14 question 4 AHN)
		
		📖 SG Diagnostic Tests, Ch. 54 p. 498 FAAHN (Ch. 14 p. 186 AHN)
		
		BOOK RESOURCES
		
		Review Questions for the NCLEX Examination Ch. 54 questions 2, 4, 5, 22, 23, 31 FAAHN (Ch. 14 question 2, 4, 5, 22, 23, 31 AHN)
		
		Table 54-3 Glasgow Coma Scale: Demonstrating Measurement of Level of Consciousness (FAAHN p. 1895) (Table 14-3 AHN p. 659)
		
		Fig. 54-6 Position and angle of the needle when lumbar puncture is performed (FAAHN p. 1898) (Fig. 14-6 AHN p. 662)
		
		Fig. 54-7 Tracings of electroencephalogram (FAAHN p. 1899) (Fig. 14-7 AHN p. 663)
		
		▶ Discuss the laboratory blood screenings that

OBJECTIVES	CONTENT	TEACHING RESOURCES
	– Electroencephalogram (FAAHN p. 1899, AHN p. 663) – Myelogram (FAAHN p. 1900, AHN p. 664) – Angiogram (FAAHN p. 1900, AHN p. 664) – Carotid duplex (FAAHN p. 1900, AHN p. 664) – Electromyogram (FAAHN p. 1900, AHN p. 664) – Echoencephalogram (FAAHN p. 1901, AHN p. 665)	can be used to identify a neurological disorder. ▶ Discuss the positioning requirements for the correct performance of the radiological examinations of the neurological system. *Class Activity Assign students to a group of three to five peers. Assign each group a neurological test to investigate. After the groups have completed the exercise, instruct them to present their findings to one other group. Allow 15 minutes for this activity.* *Class Activity Obtain a photo of the back. This photo will need to illustrate the location of the spinal cord and the spinal canal. Demonstrate the correct point of entry for a lumbar puncture. See FAAHN p. 1898 or AHN p. 662.* *Note: This will be helpful in a variety of ways. Many people have the misconception concerning the risk of paralysis associated with a lumbar puncture. This will clear up any concerns held by students as well as allow them the necessary tools to provide informed patient education. A resource for such a tool will include the obstetrics department or childbirth preparation instructor.*
List five signs and symptoms of increased intracranial pressure and why they occur, as well as nursing interventions that decrease intracranial pressure.	■ Common disorders of the neurologic system (FAAHN p. 1901, AHN p. 665) ☐ Headaches (FAAHN p. 1901, AHN p. 665) – Etiology and pathophysiology (FAAHN p. 1901, AHN p. 665) – Clinical manifestations (FAAHN p. 1901, AHN p. 665) – Assessment (FAAHN p. 1901, AHN p. 665) – Diagnostic tests (FAAHN p. 1902, AHN p. 666) – Medical management (FAAHN p. 1902, AHN p. 666) – Nursing interventions and patient teaching (FAAHN p. 1902, AHN p. 666) – Prognosis (FAAHN p. 1903, AHN p. 667)	PPT 14 through 22, Ch. 54 FAAHN (Ch. 14 PPT 14 through 22 AHN) EILR IC Ch. 54 images 8, 9 FAAHN (Ch. 14 images 8, 9 AHN) EILR TB Ch. 54 questions 3, 5, 10, 33, 40 FAAHN (Ch. 14 questions 3, 5, 10, 33, 40 AHN) ESLR Review Questions for the NCLEX Examination Ch. 54 questions 5, 6 FAAHN (Ch. 14 questions 5, 6 AHN) SG Intracranial Pressure (ICP), Ch. 54 p. 503 FAAHN (Ch. 14 p. 191 AHN) **BOOK RESOURCES** Review Questions for the NCLEX Examination Ch. 54 questions 16, 18, 27 FAAHN (Ch. 14 questions 16, 18, 27 AHN) Fig. 54-8 **A,** Unequal pupils, also called anisocoria. **B,** Dilated and fixed pupils, indicative of severe neurologic deficit (FAAHN p. 1905) (Fig. 14-8 AHN p. 669) Fig. 54-9 Decorticate and decerebrate responses (FAAHN p. 1906) (Fig. 14-9 AHN p. 670)

OBJECTIVES	CONTENT	TEACHING RESOURCES
	☐ Neuropathic pain (FAAHN p. 1903, AHN p. 667) – Etiology, pathophysiology, and clinical manifestations (FAAHN p. 1903, AHN p. 667) – Assessment (FAAHN p. 1903, AHN p. 667) – Diagnostic tests (FAAHN p. 1903, AHN p. 667) – Medical management (FAAHN p. 1903, AHN p. 667) – Nursing interventions and patient teaching (FAAHN p. 1904, AHN p. 668) – Prognosis (FAAHN p. 1904, AHN p. 668) ☐ Increased intracranial pressure (FAAHN p. 1904, AHN p. 668) – Etiology, pathophysiology, and clinical manifestations (FAAHN p. 1904, AHN p. 668) – Assessment (FAAHN p. 1905, AHN p. 669) – Diagnostic tests (FAAHN p. 1906, AHN p. 670) – Medical management (FAAHN p. 1907, AHN p. 671) – Nursing interventions and patient teaching (FAAHN p. 1907, AHN p. 671) – Prognosis (FAAHN p. 1908, AHN p. 672)	▸ Discuss the signs and symptoms associated with intracranial pressure. ▸ Discuss potential causes of increased intracranial pressure. ***Class Activity** On the board, have the class develop a nursing care plan for the care of the patient experiencing increased intracranial pressure. The care plan should include nursing diagnoses, interventions, rationales, and goals.*
Discuss various neurological disturbances in motor function and sensory-perceptual function.	☐ Disturbances in muscle tone and motor function (FAAHN p. 1908, AHN p. 672) – Etiology and pathophysiology (FAAHN p. 1908, AHN p. 672) – Clinical manifestations (FAAHN p. 1908, AHN p. 672)	PPT 23, 24, Ch. 54 FAAHN (Ch. 14 PPT 23, 24 AHN) EILR TB Ch. 54 questions 15, 22 FAAHN (Ch. 14 questions 15, 22 AHN) EILR Open Book Quiz Ch. 54 questions 3, 4 FAAHN (Ch. 14 questions 3, 4 AHN) SG Assessment and Management of

Christensen & Kockrow

OBJECTIVES	CONTENT	TEACHING RESOURCES
	– Assessment (FAAHN p. 1908, AHN p. 672) – Diagnostic tests (FAAHN p. 1908, AHN p. 672) – Medical management (FAAHN p. 1908, AHN p. 672) – Nursing interventions (FAAHN p. 1909, AHN p. 673) – Patient teaching (FAAHN p. 1911, AHN p. 675) ☐ Disturbed sensory and perceptual function (FAAHN p. 1911, AHN p. 675) – Etiology and pathophysiology (FAAHN p. 1911, AHN p. 675) – Assessment (FAAHN p. 1911, AHN p. 675) – Medical management (FAAHN p. 1911, AHN p. 675) – Nursing interventions and patient teaching (FAAHN p. 1911, AHN p. 675)	Neurological Disorders, Ch. 54 p. 500 FAAHN (Ch. 14 p. 188 AHN) SG Increased Intracranial Pressure, Ch. 54 p. 503 FAAHN (Ch. 14 p. 191 AHN) SG Seizures, Ch. 54 p. 503 FAAHN (Ch. 14 p. 191 AHN) SG Spinal Cord Trauma, Ch. 54 p. 506 FAAHN (Ch. 14 p. 194 AHN) **BOOK RESOURCES** Health Promotion: The Patient with a Neurologic Disorder (FAAHN p. 1911) (AHN p. 675) ▶ Discuss the medical terminology used to refer to neurological disturbances in motor, sensory, and perceptual functioning. ▶ Discuss the assessment needed to identify neurological disturbances in motor, sensory, and perceptual functioning. *Class Activity Recruit a volunteer. Demonstrate the assessment of neurological disturbances in motor, sensory, and perceptual functioning. Develop a nursing care plan focusing on the interventions needed to meet the needs associated with sensory impairments.*
List four classifications of seizures, their characteristics, clinical signs, aura, and postictal period.	■ Other disorders of the neurologic system (FAAHN p. 1912, AHN p. 676) ☐ Conduction abnormalities (FAAHN p. 1912, AHN p. 676) ☐ Epilepsy or seizures (FAAHN p. 1912, AHN p. 676) – Etiology and pathophysiology (FAAHN p. 1912, AHN p. 676) – Clinical manifestations (FAAHN p. 1912, AHN p. 676) – Assessment (FAAHN p. 1912, AHN p. 676) – Diagnostic test (FAAHN p. 1914, AHN p. 678) – Medical management (FAAHN p. 1914, AHN p. 678)	PPT 25 through 27, Ch. 54 FAAHN (Ch. 14 PPT 25 through 27 AHN) EILR TB Ch. 54 questions 11, 23 FAAHN (Ch. 14 questions 11, 23 AHN) EILR Open Book Quiz Ch. 54 question 5 FAAHN (Ch. 14 question 5 AHN) ESLR Review Questions for the NCLEX Examination Ch. 54 question 7 FAAHN (Ch. 14 question 7 AHN) SG Seizures, Ch. 54 p. 503 FAAHN (Ch. 14 p. 191 AHN) **BOOK RESOURCES** Review Questions for the NCLEX Examination Ch. 54 questions 6, 35 FAAHN (Ch. 14 questions 6, 35 AHN) Table 54-1 Cranial Nerves (FAAHN p. 1893) (Table 14-1 AHN p. 657) Table 54-6 Characteristics of Seizures (FAAHN p. 1913) (Table 14-6 AHN p. 677)

Christensen & Kockrow

OBJECTIVES	CONTENT	TEACHING RESOURCES
	– Nursing interventions and patient teaching (FAAHN p. 1915, AHN p. 679) – Prognosis (FAAHN p. 1916, AHN p. 680)	Patient Teaching: The Patient with Seizures (FAAHN p. 1914) (AHN p. 678) ▸ Discuss the different types of seizures and the manner in which they are classified. ▸ Discuss the stages of the seizure and the nursing care needed in each stage. *Class Activity Divide the students into groups of three to five. Instruct each student to develop three to five NCLEX-style questions relating to seizure disorders. After the questions are completed, use them to play a team game. In the game, assign each student to a team. The instructor will ask the questions to the teams. The team having the most correct answers will win.*

14.2 Homework/Assignments:

14.2 Instructor's Notes/Student Feedback:

LESSON 14.3

CRITICAL THINKING QUESTION

A 49-year-old man contacts the physician's office with complaints of left-side facial numbness and left-side weakness. He reports the entire episode lasted only about 10 minutes. After hearing the complaints, the physician calls the patient in to examine him. A diagnosis of transient ischemic attack (TIA) is made. The physician has requested a full diagnostic workup and orders laboratory testing and a CT scan. The physician indicates there may also be pharmacological or surgical interventions necessary, depending upon the outcome of the diagnostic tests. After the patient is advised of the proposed plan of care, he states, "I don't see why this will be necessary. I am fine now." Based upon your understanding of TIA, is the patient's response appropriate? Because the attack lasted only a few minutes, do all of the tests need to be completed? What should the patient be told?

Guidelines: A TIA occurs in response to a period of cerebral vascular insufficiency. The resulting clinical manifestations have occurred as a result of the reduced blood flow to the brain. Although the attack is indeed limited in duration and there has been a complete return of functioning, a TIA should never be devalued. A TIA is a warning sign and an indication of an underlying problem. TIAs are often precursors of a cerebral vascular attack. The purpose of the diagnostic tests is to determine the location and level of vascular insufficiency. It allows the physician to determine the best course of treatment and preventative therapies. The patient will need education regarding the implications of a TIA, the diagnostic procedures ordered, and potential therapies.

OBJECTIVES	CONTENT	TEACHING RESOURCES
Give examples of six degenerative neurological diseases and explain the etiology and pathophysiology, clinical manifestations, assessment, diagnostic tests, medical management, and nursing interventions for each.	☐ Degenerative diseases (FAAHN p. 1916, AHN p. 680) ☐ Multiple sclerosis (FAAHN p. 1916, AHN p. 680) – Etiology and pathophysiology (FAAHN p. 1916, AHN p. 680) – Clinical manifestations (FAAHN p. 1916, AHN p. 680) – Assessment (FAAHN p. 1917, AHN p. 681) – Diagnostic tests (FAAHN p. 1917, AHN p. 681) – Medical management (FAAHN p. 1917, AHN p. 681) – Nursing interventions (FAAHN p. 1918, AHN p. 682) – Patient teaching (FAAHN p. 1919, AHN p. 683) – Prognosis (FAAHN p. 1919, AHN p. 683) ☐ Parkinson's disease (FAAHN p. 1919, AHN p. 683)	PPT 28 through 42, Ch. 54 FAAHN (Ch. 14 PPT 28 through 42 AHN) EILR IC Ch. 54 images 13 through 16 FAAHN (Ch. 14 images 13 through 16 AHN) EILR TB Ch. 54 questions 20, 21, 30 FAAHN (Ch. 14 questions 20, 21, 30 AHN) EILR Open Book Quiz Ch. 54 questions 6 through 9 FAAHN (Ch. 14 questions 6 through 9 AHN) ESLR Review Questions for the NCLEX Examination Ch. 54 questions 8 through 10 FAAHN (Ch. 14 questions 8 through 10 AHN) SG Diagnostic Tests, Ch. 54 p. 508 FAAHN (Ch. 14 p. 196 AHN) SG Assessment and Management of Neurological Disorders, Ch. 54 p. 500 FAAHN (Ch. 14 p. 188 AHN) **BOOK RESOURCES** Fig. 54-13 Pathogenesis of multiple sclerosis (FAAHN p. 1917) (Fig. 14-13 AHN p. 681)

ELSEVIER

OBJECTIVES	CONTENT	TEACHING RESOURCES
	– Etiology and pathophysiology (FAAHN p. 1919, AHN p. 683) – Clinical manifestations (FAAHN p. 1920, AHN p. 684) – Assessment (FAAHN p. 1921, AHN p. 685) – Diagnostic tests (FAAHN p. 1921, AHN p. 685) – Medical management (FAAHN p. 1921, AHN p. 685) – Nursing interventions (FAAHN p. 1921, AHN p. 685) – Patient teaching (FAAHN p. 1924, AHN p. 688) – Prognosis (FAAHN p. 1924, AHN p. 688) ☐ Alzheimer's disease (FAAHN p. 1924, AHN p. 688) – Etiology and pathophysiology (FAAHN p. 1924, AHN p. 688) – Clinical manifestations (FAAHN p. 1925, AHN p. 689) – Assessment (FAAHN p. 1925, AHN p. 689) – Diagnostic tests (FAAHN p. 1925, AHN p. 689) – Medical management (FAAHN p. 1925, AHN p. 689) – Nursing interventions and patient teaching (FAAHN p. 1925, AHN p. 689) – Prognosis (FAAHN p. 1926, AHN p. 690) ☐ Myasthenia gravis (FAAHN p. 1926, AHN p. 690) – Etiology and pathophysiology (FAAHN p. 1926, AHN p. 690) – Clinical manifestations (FAAHN p. 1928, AHN p. 692) – Assessment (FAAHN p. 1928, AHN p. 692)	Fig. 54-14 Nigrostriatal disorders produce parkinsonism (FAAHN p. 1919) (AHN Fig. 14-14 p. 683) Fig. 54-15 Characteristic appearance of a patient with Parkinson's disease (FAAHN p. 1920) (Fig. 14-15 AHN p. 684) Table 54-8 Medications for Disorders of the Neurologic System (FAAHN p. 1922) (Table 14-8 AHN p. 686) Fig. 54-16 Effects of Alzheimer's disease on the brain (FAAHN p. 1925) (Fig. 14-16 AHN p. 689) Box 54-2 Early Warning Signs of Alzheimer's Disease (FAAHN p. 1926) (Box 14-2 AHN p. 690) Nursing Care Plan 54-1 The Patient with Alzheimer's Disease (FAAHN p. 1927) (NCP 14-1 AHN p. 691) 💡 NCP CTQ 1 through 3 (FAAHN p. 1927) (AHN p. 691) Patient Teaching: Myasthenia Gravis (FAAHN p. 1929) (AHN p. 693) ▸ Discuss assessment of the degenerative neurological disorders. Include both the subjective and objective manifestations. ▸ Discuss the prognosis of each of the disorders. *Class Activity Place each student in a work group. Assign each group a neurological disorder to investigate. Each student group will be required to provide a skit (3 to 5 minutes) demonstrating the challenges faced by those affected with their disorder. At the end of the presentation, the groups will need to present at least three priority nursing diagnoses for their assigned disorder.*

OBJECTIVES	CONTENT	TEACHING RESOURCES
	– Diagnostic tests (FAAHN p. 1928, AHN p. 692) – Medical management (FAAHN p. 1928, AHN p. 692) – Nursing interventions and patient teaching (FAAHN p. 1928, AHN p. 692) – Prognosis (FAAHN p. 1929, AHN p. 693) ☐ Amyotrophic lateral sclerosis (FAAHN p. 1929, AHN p. 693) ☐ Huntington's disease (FAAHN p. 1929, AHN p. 693)	
Discuss the etiology and pathophysiology, clinical manifestations, assessment, diagnostic tests, medical management, and nursing interventions for a stroke patient.	☐ Vascular problems (FAAHN p. 1930, AHN p. 694) ☐ Stroke (FAAHN p. 1930, AHN p. 694) – Etiology and pathophysiology (FAAHN p. 1930, AHN p. 694) – Clinical manifestations (FAAHN p. 1931, AHN p. 695) – Assessment (FAAHN p. 1932, AHN p. 696) – Diagnostic tests (FAAHN p. 1933, AHN p. 697) – Medical management (FAAHN p. 1933, AHN p. 697) – Nursing interventions (FAAHN p. 1935, AHN p. 699) – Patient teaching (FAAHN p. 1936, AHN p. 700) – Prognosis (FAAHN p. 1936, AHN p. 700)	⊠▪ PPT 45 through 47, Ch. 54 FAAHN (Ch. 14 PPT 45 through 47 AHN) ▰ EILR IC Ch. 54 images 17 through 21 FAAHN (Chapter 14 images 17 through 21 AHN) ▰ EILR TB Ch. 54 questions 7, 24 FAAHN (Ch. 14 questions 7, 24 AHN) SG Stroke and Traumatic Brain Injury, Ch. 54 p. 505 FAAHN (Ch. 14 p. 193 AHN) **BOOK RESOURCES** Review Questions for the NCLEX Examination Ch. 54 question 34 FAAHN (Ch. 14 question 34 AHN) Cultural Considerations: Stroke (FAAHN p. 1930) (AHN p. 694) Fig. 54-17 Three types of stroke (FAAHN p. 1931) (Fig. 14-17 AHN p. 695) Fig. 54-18 Manifestations of right-sided and left-sided stroke (FAAHN p. 1933) (Fig. 14-18 AHN p. 697) Fig. 54-19 Spatial and perceptual deficits in stroke (FAAHN p. 1933) (Fig. 14-19 AHN p. 697) Fig. 54-20 Clipping and wrapping of aneurysms (FAAHN p. 1933) (Fig. 14-20 AHN p. 697)

OBJECTIVES	CONTENT	TEACHING RESOURCES
		Fig 54-21 The MERCI Retriever removes blood clots in patients who are experiencing ischemic stroke (FAAHN p. 1934) (Fig. 14-21 AHN p. 698) ▶ Discuss the different types of stroke. Include the populations at highest risk to develop each type. ▶ Discuss the significance of a transient ischemic attack. *Class Activity **Bring to class assistive devices used by stroke patients. Assign students to use the devices for a portion of the class period. To provide the maximum effect, allow students to trade devices. At the end of the class, allow students the opportunity to share their impressions.***
Differentiate between trigeminal neuralgia and Bell's palsy.	☐ Cranial and peripheral nerve disorders (FAAHN p. 1936, AHN p. 700) ☐ Trigeminal neuralgia (FAAHN p. 1936, AHN p. 700) – Etiology and pathophysiology (FAAHN p. 1936, AHN p. 700) – Clinical manifestations (FAAHN p. 1937, AHN p. 701) – Medical management (FAAHN p. 1937, AHN p. 701) – Nursing interventions (FAAHN p. 1937, AHN p. 701) – Prognosis (FAAHN p. 1937, AHN p. 701) ☐ Bell's palsy (peripheral facial paralysis) (FAAHN p. 1937, AHN p. 701) – Etiology and pathophysiology (FAAHN p. 1937, AHN p. 701) – Clinical manifestations (FAAHN p. 1938, AHN p. 702) – Nursing interventions (FAAHN p. 1938, AHN p. 702) – Prognosis (FAAHN p. 1938, AHN p. 702)	PPT 48 through 50, Ch. 54 FAAHN (Ch. 14 PPT 48 through 50 AHN) EILR IC Ch. 54 image 22 FAAHN (Ch. 14 image 22 AHN) EILR TB Ch. 54 question 32 FAAHN (Ch. 14 question 32 AHN) SG Trigeminal Neuralgia and Bell's Palsy, Ch. 54 p. 507 FAAHN (Ch. 14 p. 195 AHN) **BOOK RESOURCES** Review Questions for the NCLEX Examination Ch. 54 questions 10, 32 FAAHN (Ch. 14 question 10, 32 AHN) Fig. 54-22 Pathway of trigeminal nerve and facial areas innervated by each of the three main divisions of this nerve (FAAHN p. 1937) (Fig. 14-22 AHN p.701) Box 54-3 Comfort Measures for Patients with Trigeminal Neuralgia (FAAHN p. 1937) (Box 14-3 AHN p. 701) ▶ Discuss the clinical manifestations of trigeminal neuralgia and Bell's palsy. ▶ Discuss the nursing interventions appropriate for the patient diagnosed with trigeminal neuralgia and Bell's palsy. *Class Activity **Provide each student with a note card. Instruct each student to write a***

OBJECTIVES	CONTENT	TEACHING RESOURCES
	☐ Infection and inflammation (FAAHN p. 1938, AHN p. 702) – Etiology and pathophysiology (FAAHN p. 1938, AHN p. 702) – Assessment (FAAHN p. 1938, AHN p. 702) – Diagnostic tests (FAAHN p. 1938, AHN p. 702) – Nursing interventions and patient teaching (FAAHN p. 1938, AHN p. 702)	*question and answer on the card about trigeminal neuralgia or Bell's palsy. After the students are finished, ask that they trade cards with another student. Allow a few minutes for the cards to be reviewed. After a few minutes, call "time" and instruct the students to exchange cards with another student. Continue this process for at least five "trades."*
Discuss the etiology, pathophysiology, clinical manifestations, assessment, diagnostic tests, medical management, nursing interventions, and patient teaching for GBS, meningitis, encephalitis, and AIDS.	☐ Guillain-Barré syndrome (polyneuritis) (FAAHN p. 1939, AHN p. 703) – Etiology and pathophysiology (FAAHN p. 1939, AHN p. 703) – Clinical manifestations (FAAHN p. 1939, AHN p. 703) – Diagnostic tests (FAAHN p. 1939, AHN p. 703) – Medical management (FAAHN p. 1939, AHN p. 703) – Nursing interventions (FAAHN p. 1940, AHN p. 704) – Prognosis (FAAHN p. 1940, AHN p. 704) ☐ Meningitis (FAAHN p. 1940, AHN p. 704) – Etiology and pathophysiology (FAAHN p. 1940, AHN p. 704) – Clinical manifestations (FAAHN p. 1940, AHN p. 704) – Diagnostic tests (FAAHN p. 1940, AHN p. 704) – Medical management (FAAHN p. 1940, AHN p. 704) – Nursing interventions (FAAHN p. 1940, AHN p. 704) – Prognosis (FAAHN p. 1941, AHN p. 705) ☐ Encephalitis (FAAHN p. 1941, AHN p. 705)	📺 PPT 51 through 60, Ch. 54 FAAHN (Ch. 14 PPT 51 through 60 AHN) 💾 EILR TB Ch. 54 questions 26, 27 FAAHN (Ch. 14 questions 26, 27 AHN) 💾 EILR Open Book Quiz Ch. 54 question 10 FAAHN (Ch. 14 question 10 AHN) 📓 SG Infectious and Inflammatory Disorders of the Neurological System, Ch. 54 p. 507 FAAHN (Ch. 14 p. 195 AHN) **BOOK RESOURCES** Review Questions for the NCLEX Examination Ch. 54 questions 9, 33 FAAHN (Ch. 14 questions 9, 33 AHN) ▶ Discuss the causes, clinical manifestations, and diagnosis of meningitis. ▶ Discuss the nursing interventions associated with a diagnosis of Guillain-Barré syndrome. *Class Activity Develop a "bingo" game. Prepare a card similar to a BINGO card. Each square will have a short (1 to 3 word) answer about Guillain-Barré, meningitis, encephalitis, and implications of AIDS. The student can use Cheerios or squares of paper as game markers. To play the game, ask the students a question. Any student having a correct answer in one of the board squares can cover that spot. Continue to ask questions concerning the desired topics until the first student says, "bingo."*

OBJECTIVES	CONTENT	TEACHING RESOURCES
	☐ West Nile virus (FAAHN p. 1941, AHN p. 705)	
	☐ Brain abscess (FAAHN p. 1942, AHN p. 706)	
	☐ Acquired immunodeficiency syndrome (FAAHN p. 1942, AHN p. 706)	
	– Etiology and pathophysiology (FAAHN p. 1942, AHN p. 706)	
	– Clinical manifestations (FAAHN p. 1942, AHN p. 706)	
	– Diagnostic tests (FAAHN p. 1943, AHN p. 707)	
	– Medical management (FAAHN p. 1943, AHN p. 707)	
	– Nursing interventions (FAAHN p. 1943, AHN p. 707)	
	– Prognosis (FAAHN p. 1943, AHN p. 707)	

14.3 Homework/Assignments:

14.3 Instructor's Notes/Student Feedback:

Christensen & Kockrow

LESSON 14.4

CRITICAL THINKING QUESTION

A 26-year-old female has been admitted to your floor after hitting her head on the windshield during a motor vehicle accident. During the data collection, you notice that she has blood pooling inside of her right ear, the right pupil is smaller than the left, and she is complaining of a headache. When you got the report from the ER nurse, she stated that the patient was being observed for craniocerebral brain injury. The patient is able to communicate with you but said that she passed out during the accident. She states she is very sleepy and asks you to leave so she can go to sleep. What action should you take? What response should you make to the patient? What other signs and symptoms might develop should the patient's condition worsen?

Guidelines: A craniocerebral trauma is the result of trauma to the brain and can cause tension strains and/or shearing forces on the brain tissue. Instruct the patient in firm but gentle directions that she shouldn't get up without help because she could be dizzy or have a tendency to fall. Tell her that you will be in to see her frequently to assess her vital signs and level of consciousness. Other signs and symptoms that might occur are nausea, vomiting, abnormal sensations, loss of consciousness, Battle's sign, and continued changes in the size of the pupils.

OBJECTIVES	CONTENT	TEACHING RESOURCES

Explain the mechanism of injury to the brain that occurs with a stroke and traumatic brain injury.	☐ Vascular problems (FAAHN p. 1930, AHN p. 694)
	
	 ☐ Stroke (FAAHN p. 1930, AHN p. 694)
	
	   – Etiology and pathophysiology (FAAHN p. 1930, AHN p. 694)
	
	 ☐ Trauma (FAAHN p. 1944, AHN p. 708)
	
	 ☐ Head injury (FAAHN p. 1944, AHN p. 708)
	
	   – Etiology and pathophysiology (FAAHN p. 1944, AHN p. 708)
	
	   – Clinical manifestations (FAAHN p. 1944, AHN p. 708)
	
	   – Assessment (FAAHN p. 1945, AHN p. 709)
	
	   – Diagnostic tests (FAAHN p. 1945, AHN p. 709)
	
	   – Medical management (FAAHN p. 1945, AHN p. 709)
	
	   – Nursing interventions (FAAHN p. 1945, AHN p. 709)
	
	   – Patient teaching (FAAHN p. 1946, AHN p. 710)
	
	   – Prognosis (FAAHN p. 1946, AHN p. 710)
	
	 ☐ Spinal cord trauma (FAAHN p. 1946, AHN p. 710)
		PPT 45 through 47, 64 through 66, Ch. 54 FAAHN (Ch. 14 PPT 45 through 47, 64 through 66 AHN)
		
		 EILR IC Ch. 54 image 1 FAAHN (Ch. 14 image 1 AHN)
		
		 SG Stroke and Traumatic Brain Injury, Ch. 54 p. 505 FAAHN (Ch. 14 p. 193 AHN)
		
		 BOOK RESOURCES
		
		 Review Questions for the NCLEX Examination Ch. 54 questions 19, 20, 28 FAAHN (Ch. 14 question 19, 20, 28 AHN)
		
		 Fig. 54-23 **A,** Raccoon eyes and rhinorrhea. **B,** Battle's sign (postauricular ecchymosis) with otorrhea. **C,** Halo or ring sign (FAAHN p. 1245) (Fig. 14-23 AHN p.709)
		
		 Fig. 54-24 Mechanisms of spinal injury (FAAHN p. 1246) (Fig. 14-24 AHN p. 710)
		
		 ▶ Discuss documenting the assessment findings for the patient who has experienced a spinal cord injury.
		
		 ▶ Discuss assessment findings that necessitate contacting the physician.
		
		 Class Activity Obtain a colored image of the brain (FAAHN p. 1889, AHN p. 653). Using a pointer, illustrate to the class the clinical manifestations that will be associated with brain trauma to different locations in the brain.

OBJECTIVES	CONTENT	TEACHING RESOURCES
	– Etiology and pathophysiology (FAAHN p. 1946, AHN p. 710) – Clinical manifestations (FAAHN p. 1946, AHN p. 710) – Assessment (FAAHN p. 1948, AHN p. 712) – Diagnostic tests (FAAHN p. 1948, AHN p. 712) – Medical management (FAAHN p. 1948, AHN p. 712) – Nursing interventions and patient teaching (FAAHN p. 1948, AHN p. 712) – Prognosis (FAAHN p. 1949, AHN p. 713)	
Discuss the etiology and pathophysiology, clinical manifestations, assessment, diagnostic tests, medical management, and nursing interventions for brain tumors, head injury, and spinal trauma.	☐ Brain tumors (FAAHN p. 1943, AHN p. 707) – Etiology and pathophysiology (FAAHN p. 1943, AHN p. 707) – Assessment (FAAHN p. 1943, AHN p. 707) – Diagnostic tests (FAAHN p. 1943, AHN p. 707) – Medical management (FAAHN p. 1943, AHN p. 707) – Nursing interventions (FAAHN p. 1944, AHN p. 708) – Prognosis (FAAHN p. 1944, AHN p. 708) ☐ Trauma (FAAHN p. 1944, AHN p. 708) ☐ Head injury (FAAHN p. 1944, AHN p. 708) – Etiology and pathophysiology (FAAHN p. 1944, AHN p. 708) – Clinical manifestations (FAAHN p. 1944, AHN p. 708) – Assessment (FAAHN p. 1945, AHN p. 709) – Diagnostic tests (FAAHN p. 1945, AHN p. 709) – Medical management (FAAHN p. 1945, AHN p. 709)	▨▦ PPT 61 through 70, Ch. 54 FAAHN (Ch. 14 PPT 61 through 70 AHN) *e* EILR IC Ch. 54 images 23 through 26 FAAHN (Ch. 14 images 23 through 26 AHN) *e* EILR TB Ch. 54 questions 17 through 19, 25, 31, 41 FAAHN (Ch. 14 questions 17 through 19, 25, 31, 41 AHN) SG SG Spinal Cord Trauma, Ch. 54 p. 506 FAAHN (Ch. 14 p. 194 AHN) **BOOK RESOURCES** Review Questions for the NCLEX Examination Ch. 54 questions 11, 13, 14, 17, 21, 29 FAAHN (Ch. 14 questions 11, 13, 14, 17, 21, 29 AHN) Table 54-9 Functional Level of Spinal Cord Injury and Rehabilitation Potential (FAAHN p. 1947) (Table 14-9 AHN p. 711) Fig. 54-25 Pictorial diagram of cause of autonomic hyperreflexia (dysreflexia) and results (FAAHN p. 1948) (Fig. 14-25 AHN p. 712) Box 54-4 Emergency Care for Autonomic Dysreflexia or Hyperreflexia (FAAHN p. 1948) (Box 14-4 AHN p. 712) Fig. 54-26 Patient with Crutchfield tongs inserted into skull to hyperextend (FAAHN p. 1949) (Fig. 14-26 AHN p. 713) ▸ Discuss the psychological implications of a spinal cord or traumatic brain injury.

Christensen & Kockrow

OBJECTIVES	CONTENT	TEACHING RESOURCES
	– Nursing interventions (FAAHN p. 1945, AHN p. 709) – Patient teaching (FAAHN p. 1946, AHN p. 710) – Prognosis (FAAHN p. 1946, AHN p. 710) ☐ Spinal cord trauma (FAAHN p. 1946, AHN p. 710) – Etiology and pathophysiology (FAAHN p. 1946, AHN p. 710) – Clinical manifestations (FAAHN p. 1946, AHN p. 710) – Assessment (FAAHN p. 1948, AHN p. 712) – Diagnostic tests (FAAHN p. 1948, AHN p. 712) – Medical management (FAAHN p. 1948, AHN p. 712) – Nursing interventions and patient teaching (FAAHN p. 1948, AHN p. 712) – Prognosis (FAAHN p. 1949, AHN p. 713)	▶ Discuss the referrals appropriate for the patient who is experiencing a traumatic brain or spinal cord injury. *Class Activity Utilize the nursing lab. Recruiting a student volunteer, demonstrate the positioning for the patient who has had surgical management to treat a craniocerebral or spinal trauma.*
Discuss patient teaching and home care planning for the patient with stroke, multiple sclerosis (MS), Parkinson's disease, and myasthenia gravis.	☐ Multiple sclerosis (FAAHN p. 1916, AHN p. 680) – Patient teaching (FAAHN p. 1919, AHN p. 683) ☐ Parkinson's disease (FAAHN p. 1919, AHN p. 683) – Patient teaching (FAAHN p. 1924, AHN p. 688) ☐ Myasthenia gravis (FAAHN p. 1926, AHN p. 690) – Nursing interventions and patient teaching (FAAHN p. 1928, AHN p. 692) ☐ Stroke (FAAHN p. 1930, AHN p. 694) – Patient teaching (FAAHN p. 1936, AHN p. 700) ☐ Nursing process for the patient with a neurological disorder (FAAHN p. 1949, AHN p. 713)	PPT 28 through 36, 39 through 40 Ch. 54 FAAHN (Ch. 14 PPT 28 through 36, 39 through 40) EILR IC Ch. 54 image 1 FAAHN (Ch. 14 image 1 AHN) EILR TB Ch. 54 question 9 FAAHN (Ch. 14 question 9 AHN) SG Patient Education, Ch. 54 p. 509 FAAHN (Ch. 14 p. 197 AHN) **BOOK RESOURCES** Review Questions for the NCLEX Examination Ch. 54 questions 12, 21, 29 FAAHN (Ch. 14 question 12, 21, 29 AHN) Fig. 54-10 Volar resting splint provides support to wrist, thumb, and fi ngers of patient after cerebrovascular accident (stroke), maintaining them in position of extension (FAAHN p. 1909) (Fig. 14-10 AHN p. 673) Fig. 54-11 Velcro shirtsleeve to facilitate closure (FAAHN p. 1910) (Fig. 14-11 AHN p. 674)

OBJECTIVES	CONTENT	TEACHING RESOURCES
	– Assessment (FAAHN p. 1949, AHN p. 713) – Nursing diagnosis (FAAHN p. 1949, AHN p. 713) – Expected outcomes and planning (FAAHN p. 1950, AHN p. 714) – Implementation (FAAHN p. 1950, AHN p. 714) – Evaluation (FAAHN p. 1950, AHN p. 714)	Fig. 54-12 Long-handled bath sponges (FAAHN p. 1910) (Fig. 14-12 AHN p. 674) ▸ Discuss the assessment of readiness for discharge teaching of the patient and family after a stroke. ▸ Discuss the community resource information that will need to be provided to the patient and family regarding support agencies prior to discharge. *Class Activity Utilize the nursing lab. Solicit a student volunteer and demonstrate the movement, transfer, and safety-related interventions needed when planning the home care of a patient who has been diagnosed with a stroke.*
Performance Evaluation		🔁 EILR TB Ch. 54 questions 1 through 72 FAAHN (Ch. 14 questions 1 through 72 AHN) 🔁 EILR Open Book Quiz Ch. 54 questions 1 through 10 FAAHN (Ch. 14 questions 1 through 10 AHN) 🔁 ESLR Review Questions for the NCLEX Examination Ch. 54 questions 1 through 10 FAAHN (Ch. 14 questions 1 through 10 AHN) 📓 SG Ch. 54 pp. 493-512 FAAHN (Ch. 54 pp. 181-200 AHN) **BOOK RESOURCES** Nursing Care Plan 54-1 The Patient with Alzheimer's Disease (FAAHN p. 1927) (NCP 14-1 AHN p. 691) 💡 NCP CTQ 1 through 3 (FAAHN p. 1927) (AHN p. 691) Review Questions for the NCLEX Examination Ch. 54 questions 1 through 37 FAAHN (Ch. 14 questions 1 through 37 AHN)

14.4 Homework/Assignments:

14.4 Instructor's Notes/Student Feedback:

ELSEVIER

Adult Health Nursing, 6th ed.
Christensen & Kockrow

Slide 1

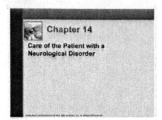

Slide 2

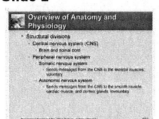

- The nervous system functions as a switchboard for the body. It receives messages from the environment and transfers them to the brain for interpretation and action.

Slide 3

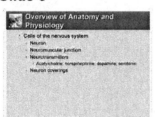

- The basic nerve cell in the body is known as a neuron.

- Neurons act under the "all or none law." Explain this phenomenon.

Slide 4

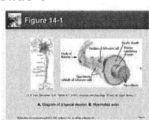

- The neuron is composed of three main structures. These structures are the cell body, the axon, and the dendrites.

- What roles are played by each of the parts?

Slide 5

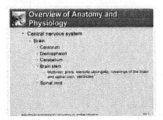

- The central nervous system is one of the divisions of the nervous system. The brain is one of the body's largest organs. What are the functions of each of the structures identified?

- What is the impact on the body if the key areas identified are injured or unable to adequately function?

Mosby items and derived items © 2011, 2007 by Mosby, Inc., an affiliate of Elsevier Inc.
Some material was previously published.
Christensen & Kockrow

Slide 6

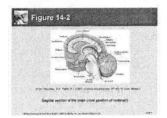

Slide 7

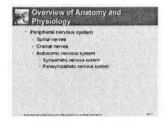

Slide 8

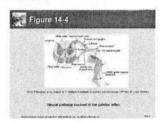

Slide 9

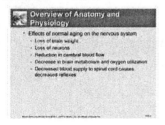

- As the body ages, there is a gradual reduction in the effectiveness of neurological functioning. An estimated 1% loss of neurons occurs after age 50.

- Outline the implications when factoring in this loss for an adult at age 65.

- Ask those who have grandparents to estimate their ages and discuss the implication of a 1% loss in neurons for them.

- What safety implications arise when considering the neurological changes in an older adult?

Slide 10

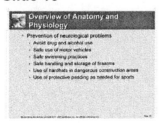

- Some of the disorders in the neurological system are the result of a disease process. Other illnesses occur in response to an injury or are the impact of a chosen lifestyle.

- What populations are associated with unhealthy neurological behaviors?

- What opportunities exist for health teaching in these populations?

Adult Health Nursing, 6th ed.
Mosby items and derived items © 2011, 2007 by Mosby, Inc., an affiliate of Elsevier Inc.
Some material was previously published.
Christensen & Kockrow

Slide 11

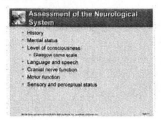

- When collecting neurological data, a comprehensive approach is best. Input from both the patient and family can provide invaluable clues regarding behavior indicative of neurological changes.

- What elements in a patient's health history are beneficial?

- The Glasgow coma scale is performed to assess the patient's level of consciousness. It is important to note that the Glasgow coma scale results are on a potentially changing continuum.

- What factors are assessed in the Glasgow coma scale?

- What techniques can be utilized to review cranial nerve function?

Slide 12

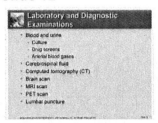

- The patient's direct reports of neurological impairments and changes are combined with diagnostic testing to determine a diagnosis.

- Testing can include serum values or electronic scanning to obtain a physical picture.

- What are the nursing implications for each of the tests listed?

Slide 13

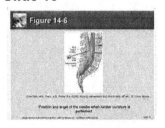

- The lumbar puncture is an invasive exam. It can be done at the patient's bedside.

- A frequently voiced concern relates to the possibility of paralysis if done incorrectly or if the patient moves. Review the reasoning that should be shared with the patient and family as to why paralysis should not be a concern.

Slide 14

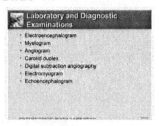

- Diagnostic examinations used for the nervous system often employ scanning techniques to view an area of concern.

- What patient teaching will be needed for each of the listed exams?

Slide 15

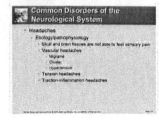

- Headaches are a frequent complaint in both men and women. They can be caused by a variety of events. Headaches are classified according to their underlying cause.

- What population is most at risk of experiencing each of the headache types?

ELSEVIER

Slide 16

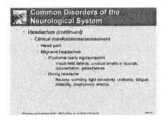

- To diagnose and classify the type of headaches, an accurate accounting of the clinical manifestations is important.

- What data should be collected from the patient regarding the headache?

Slide 17

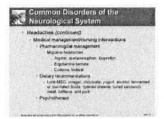

- Treatment options for headaches can be pharmacological or nonpharmacological.

- What nondrug interventions can be employed for managing headaches?

- What is the underlying rationale for each of the interventions?

- Why are caffeine restrictions recommended in headache sufferers and yet caffeine is one of the leading ingredients in migraine relief medications?

Slide 18

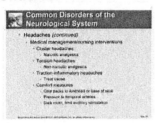

- What is the underlying rationale for each of the interventions?

- Why are narcotic analgesics avoided in patients with tension headaches?

Slide 19

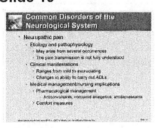

- Neuropathic pain is common. A number of factors may contribute to its development. These factors include postherpetic neuralgia, phantom limb pain, diabetic neuropathies, and trigeminal neuralgia.

- What tests may be implemented to diagnose the disorder?

Slide 20

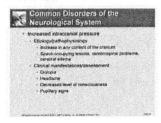

- The structure of the cranium does not allow for expansion as it is housed within the rigid skull. Any increase in the contents will result in an increase in intracranial pressure. What are normal contents of the cranium?

- What are some causes of intracranial pressure?

- Does intracranial pressure occur suddenly with rapid onset or is it slow, taking place over a period of time?

Adult Health Nursing, 6th ed.

Christensen & Kockrow

Slide 21

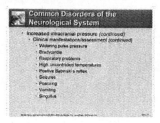

- The onset of symptoms associated with intracranial pressure will vary. They will become increasingly evident as the pressure intensifies.

- Initially the body attempts to compensate for the changes. What actions does the body take into account for the alteration in homeostasis?

- In what order will the signs and symptoms manifest? Why?

- At what point do these clinical manifestations become ominous?

Slide 22

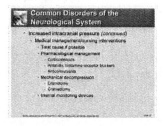

- Once it is identified, there may be limited time to treat intracranial pressure.

- What diagnostic testing can be utilized for increased intracranial pressure?

- Why is prompt treatment such a priority?

- Discuss the use of pharmacological agents in the management of intracranial pressure. What physiological symptoms indicate that the medical interventions have been effective?

- What is the prognosis for increased intracranial pressure?

Slide 23

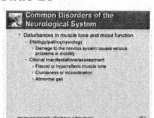

- Patients experiencing neurological system disorders can present with a variety of signs and symptoms. The assessment will be key in making a determination of the exact problem and developing a plan of care.

- Review the assessments that will be performed.

- What types of questions should be asked during the patient interview?

Slide 24

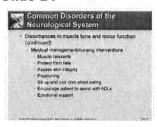

- Safety is a key part of a successful plan of care for the neurologically impaired patient. The risk of injury is great.

- What are priority safety-related goals for the neurologically impaired patient?

Slide 25

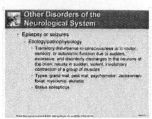

- Seizures affect both men and women of all races and ages.

- Identify some potential causes of seizures.

- Recurrent generalized seizures will result in status epilepticus. Sudden withdrawal from the prescribed anticonvulsant therapies is the #1 cause of its occurrence.

- Status epilepticus is a "9-1-1" event. Emergency intervention is needed to prevent brain damage or death. What events occur during status epilepticus that will result in neurological death?

Adult Health Nursing, 6th ed.

Christensen & Kockrow

Slide 26

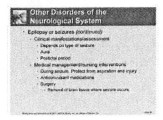

- Seizures have predictable stages. The seizure might begin with an aura (the predictor of the seizure), followed by the ictal phase (seizure), and ending with the postictal period.

- An estimated 50% of people experience auras. An aura is a sensation that indicates impending seizure activity. Auras are individualized and can include psychic, olfactory, visual, auditory, or taste hallucinations.

- What is the value of an aura? What should the patient do after experiencing the aura?

- After the seizure activity ends, a patient might experience a postictal period. The postictal period can be characterized by feelings of fatigue, lethargy, and disorientation.

Slide 27

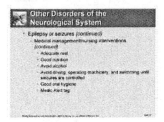

- The diagnosis of a seizure disorder is traumatic to the patient and family. What are the long-range implications of a seizure disorder diagnosis?

- What are the nursing responsibilities when caring for the patient during and after seizure activity?

Slide 28

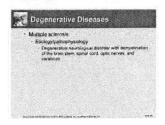

- Multiple sclerosis is a chronic, progressive neurological disease.

- The disease initially begins between the ages of 15 and 50 years.

- Women are affected more than men.

Slide 29

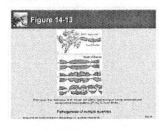

- In multiple sclerosis, the myelin sheath becomes damaged. This loss of myelin integrity results in impaired transmission of nerve impulses.

- What theories do scientists support regarding the cause of multiple sclerosis?

Slide 30

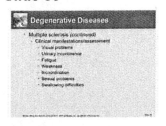

- The clinical manifestations are typically vague and gradually increase in severity and regularity.

- Several body systems are affected as multiple sclerosis progresses.

- The disease is associated with periods of remissions and exacerbations.

- What diagnostic procedures can be implemented when multiple sclerosis is suspected?

Adult Health Nursing, 6th ed.
Christensen & Kockrow

Slide 31

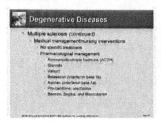

- The prescribed pharmacological treatments will vary among practitioners. Drug therapy will also be affected by the stage and severity of the disease.

- What are goals of nursing interventions when caring for the patient experiencing an exacerbation of multiple sclerosis?

- Outline the prognosis associated with multiple sclerosis.

Slide 32

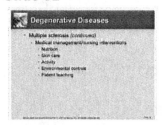

- What are goals of nursing interventions when caring for the patient experiencing an exacerbation of multiple sclerosis?

- Outline the prognosis associated with multiple sclerosis.

Slide 33

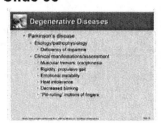

- Parkinson's disease is a chronic neurological disorder. It occurs most frequently in middle-aged and older adults.

- Explain the pathology of the disease.

- There is no known cure.

Slide 34

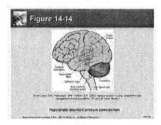

Slide 35

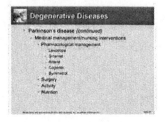

- Treatment goals for Parkinson's disease focus on managing symptoms.

- Long-term drug therapy for the management of the disease can eventually result in an overabundance of side effects. A "drug holiday" might be indicated. Discuss the purpose of the drug holiday.

- Considering the treatment modalities available, what are the implications of a diagnosis of Parkinson's disease for patients and families?

Adult Health Nursing, 6th ed.

Christensen & Kockrow

Slide 36

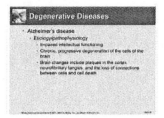

- Alzheimer's disease is a chronic, progressive disease that impacts men and women in equal numbers.

- Review available theories relating to potential causes of Alzheimer's disease.

Slide 37

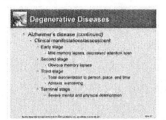

- A series of four stages is used to outline the progression of Alzheimer's disease. The stages chronicle the clinical manifestations being experienced by the patient. As the disease progresses, the characteristics of the stages worsen.

- What are the goals of nursing care for each of the stages?

Slide 38

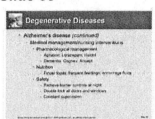

- Presently there is no cure for the disease. Pharmacological therapies focus on controlling symptoms. Nonmedication therapies seek to promote and prolong functioning for the patient.

- What are the psychosocial implications of a diagnosis of Alzheimer's disease?

Slide 39

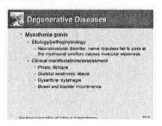

- Myasthenia gravis is a disorder of the nervous system associated with neuromuscular weakness. It is considered an autoimmune disease.

- What is meant by the term "autoimmune"?

- How is an individual affected by an autoimmune disease such as myasthenia gravis?

Slide 40

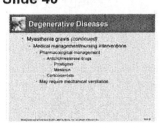

- Myasthenia gravis characteristically has a slow onset, and diagnosis may be difficult or mistaken for other disorders.

- What tests are employed to assess for myasthenia gravis?

Adult Health Nursing, 6th ed.
Christensen & Kockrow

Slide 41

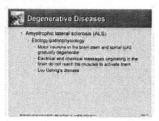

- Amyotrophic lateral sclerosis (ALS) involves the destruction of motor neurons in the brain stem and spinal cord. The loss of motor neurons impairs the body's ability to respond to messages from the brain.

- The disorder is often referred to as Lou Gehrig's disease, named after a professional baseball player who developed the disease in the 1940s.

Slide 42

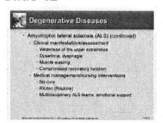

- The progression of ALS is made increasingly difficult because as the body begins to fail, the patient's mind remains intact and fully functioning.

- There is no cure. Therapies seek to manage symptoms and promote functioning.

- What nursing interventions should be incorporated into the care of the patient experiencing ALS?

Slide 43

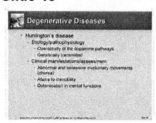

- Huntington's disease is genetically transmitted. It is an autosomal dominant disorder. The children of an affected parent have a 50% chance of inheriting it.

- Given the rate of transmission between parents and children, what genetic counseling should be provided to potential carriers?

Slide 44

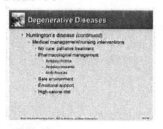

- The disease has no cure. The goals of treatment seek to manage the symptoms and reduce injury.

- What are the primary needs of the patient? How can the nurse meet these needs?

Slide 45

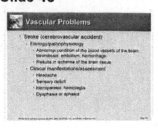

- Stroke is the most prevalent neurological disorder. It ranks as the third leading cause of death in the United States.

- The clinical manifestations of a stroke vary by cause and individual. Some of the more common symptoms can include disturbances in motor activity, intellectual functioning, or communication abilities. What factors can determine the types and degree of impairments that will be experienced?

ELSEVIER

Adult Health Nursing, 6th ed.

Christensen & Kockrow

Slide 46

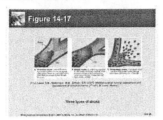

- Strokes are classified by their underlying cause. Strokes can be ischemic, thrombotic, or embolic. How do the types of strokes differ?

Slide 47

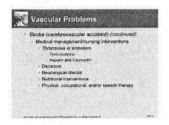

- The greatest chance for a positive prognosis involves early intervention. Currently there are pharmacological interventions, if provided in the early stages, that can improve the patient's chances for recovery. These therapies involve the use of thrombolytics. Explain their uses and parameters for successful intervention.

- What nursing assessments are needed for the patient who has had a stroke?

Slide 48

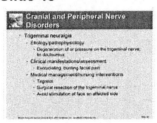

- Trigeminal neuralgia is a disorder of the peripheral nervous system. It is most common in women in middle and late adulthood.

- Patients having trigeminal neuralgia experience severe pain when trigger points along the trigeminal nerve are activated. What activities can cause this pain?

Slide 49

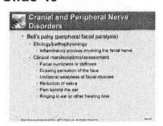

- Bell's palsy occurs as a result of inflammation of the facial nerve (cranial nerve V). No exact cause has been identified.

- What theories concerning a cause of this disease have been identified?

Slide 50

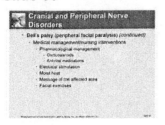

- There is no exact course of therapy to treat Bell's palsy. Medical interventions seek to reduce inflammation and manage symptoms.

- What are the nursing responsibilities in the care of this disorder?

- What is the prognosis for patients diagnosed with Bell's palsy?

ELSEVIER

Adult Health Nursing, 6th ed.

Christensen & Kockrow

Slide 51

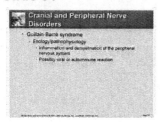

- Guillain-Barré syndrome involves the loss of myelin sheaths in the peripheral nervous system. Myelin acts as insulation for nerves, and the loss of myelin results in alterations of nerve conduction.

- Although no exact cause has been pinpointed, commonality has been noted between at least 50% of people diagnosed. Review this "common ground."

Slide 52

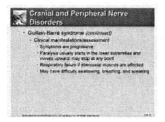

Slide 53

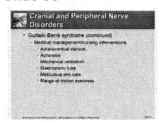

- The vast majority of people diagnosed with Guillain-Barré syndrome will fully recover. What are the goals of treatment during the acute phase of the disease?

Slide 54

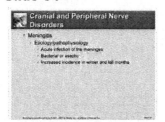

Slide 55

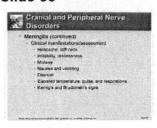

- The clinical manifestations seen in meningitis largely occur as a result of the impact of the inflammatory process on the meninges.

- What diagnostic testing can be used to confirm diagnosis?

Mosby items and derived items © 2011, 2007 by Mosby, Inc., an affiliate of Elsevier Inc.
Some material was previously published.

Adult Health Nursing, 6th ed.
Christensen & Kockrow

Slide 56

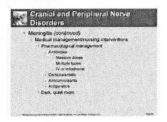

- Treatment of meningitis uses a variety of different classifications of medications.

- What is the desired effect/purpose for the use of each of the potential drug classifications?

- What is the prognosis for the patient diagnosed with meningitis?

Slide 57

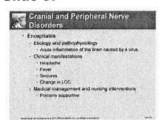

- Encephalitis may be associated with certain seasons and endemic to certain geographic locations. What are potential causes of nonepidemic encephalitis?

- The best prognosis is associated with early diagnosis. What tests may be utilized to confirm a diagnosis?

Slide 58

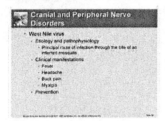

- Certain individuals infected with West Nile virus will become affected with West Nile virus meningitis or encephalitis.

- What is the prognosis for this disease? What population has the most harsh prognosis?

Slide 59

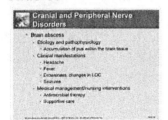

Slide 60

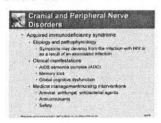

- What opportunistic infections may be associated with this disorder?

- What diagnostic tests may be utilized in the care of the patient suspected of having this condition?

ELSEVIER

Slide 61

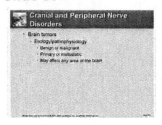

- Brain tumors can originate in the brain tissue or spread there from some other location of the body.

- What terminology would be used to describe those tissues originating in the brain?

- What would tumors that spread to the brain be referred to as?

Slide 62

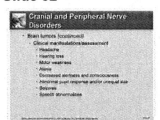

- The clinical manifestations of a brain tumor will vary according to size and location.

Slide 63

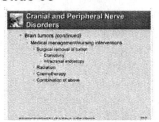

- Management of brain tumors is individualized. The physician and patient chart a path unique to the individual's degree of involvement and personal wishes.

- What nursing care will be needed for the patient after surgical intervention for a brain tumor?

Slide 64

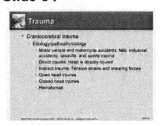

- Trauma to the brain can result in disability or death. It is a major cause of neurological impairment.

- How do acceleration and deceleration injuries differ? Provide examples of each type of injury.

- A hematoma can occur as a result of a brain injury. Compare and contrast an epidural and a subdural hematoma.

Slide 65

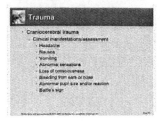

- In addition to the assessment of objective and subjective data, diagnostic tools can be employed to assess a craniocerebral injury. What tests can be anticipated?

Christensen & Kockrow

Slide 66

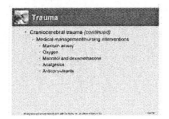

- When a head injury occurs, the priorities employ the ABCs of health care—Airway, Breathing, and Circulation.

- Once the patient has been stabilized, pain management might be needed. Care must be given to medicate the patient while avoiding medications that reduce respirations or mask neurological changes. What are the preferred analgesic medications when caring for the patient who has experienced a head injury? What analgesics should be avoided?

- Anticonvulsants can also be administered. What is the rationale for their use?

Slide 67

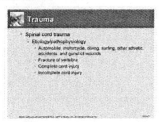

- An estimated 10% of traumatic injuries to the nervous system involve the spinal cord.

- What populations are at greatest risk of spinal cord injury?

- Compare and contrast a complete spinal cord injury with an incomplete spinal cord injury.

Slide 68

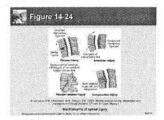

Slide 69

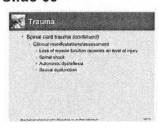

- The level of spinal cord injury will determine the degree of functioning lost. The higher the injury, the greater the loss.

- Outline the types of impairments that would be associated with injuries to the cervical, thoracic, lumbar, and sacral regions.

- Spinal shock is a common early occurrence in most spinal cord injuries. What additional needs might the patient have during this period?

- Autonomic dysreflexia is a serious complication experienced when damage at or above T-6 occurs. Review the signs and symptoms of autonomic dysreflexia. What stimuli can promote this problem?

Slide 70

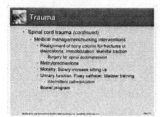

- A spinal cord injury is a traumatic event for the patient and family. What psychosocial supports will be indicated?

- What are the responsibilities of the nurse regarding emotional support?

Slide 71

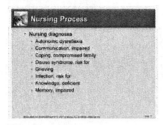

Slide 72

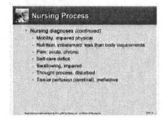

Adult Health Nursing, 6th ed.
Christensen & Kockrow

15 Lesson Plan
Care of the Patient with an Immune Disorder

TEACHING FOCUS

In this chapter, the student will be introduced to the care of the patient with an immune disorder. The student will begin by exploring the physiology of immunity, including the function of natural and acquired immunity, the mechanisms of the immune response, and the differences between humoral and cell-mediated immunity. The student will have the opportunity to learn about the concepts of immunocompetence, immunodeficiency, and autoimmunity, and the factors that affect the development of hypersensitivity. Finally, the student will explore anaphylaxis and its treatment, allergies, steps to prevent transfusion reactions in blood recipients, autoimmune disorders, and immunodeficiency disease.

MATERIALS AND RESOURCES

- ☐ Computer/overhead projector (Lessons 15.1 and 15.2)
- ☐ White/black board and marker/chalk (Lessons 15.1 and 15.2)
- ☐ Blank nursing care plan sheets (Lesson 15.1)
- ☐ Short patient scenarios written on index cards (Lesson 15.1)
- ☐ Copies of tag that accompanies a unit of blood (obtain from a laboratory at a local hospital (Lesson 15.2)
- ☐ Copies of recording sheet used with administration of blood products (obtain from a nursing unit) (Lesson 15.2)

LESSON CHECKLIST

Preparations for this lesson include:
- Lecture
- Contact a speaker's bureau and invite a guest speaker on the topic of living with an autoimmune disorder.

KEY TERMS

adaptive immunity (FAAHN p. 1956, AHN p. 720)

allergen (FAAHN p. 1958, AHN p. 722)

anaphylactic shock (FAAHN p. 1962, AHN p. 726)

antigen (FAAHN p. 1957, AHN p. 721)

attenuated (FAAHN p. 1959, AHN p. 723)

autoimmune (FAAHN p. 1966, AHN p. 730)

autologous (FAAHN p. 1965, AHN p. 729)

cellular immunity (FAAHN p. 1958, AHN p. 722)

humoral immunity (FAAHN p. 1957, AHN p. 721)

hypersensitivity (FAAHN p. 1960, AHN p. 724)

immunity (FAAHN p. 1956, AHN p. 720)

immunization (FAAHN p. 1957, AHN p. 721)

immunocompetence (FAAHN p. 1955, AHN p. 719)

immunodeficiency (FAAHN p. 1966, AHN p. 730)

immunogen (FAAHN p. 1958, AHN p. 722)

immunology (FAAHN p. 1956, AHN p. 720)

immunosuppressive (FAAHN p. 1965, AHN p. 729)

immunotherapy (FAAHN p. 1959, AHN p. 723)

innate immunity (FAAHN p. 1956, AHN p. 720)

lymphokine (FAAHN p. 1957, AHN p. 721)

plasmapheresis (FAAHN p. 1967, AHN p. 731)

proliferation (FAAHN p. 1957, AHN p. 721)

ADDITIONAL RESOURCES (AHN)

PPT Ch. 55, 1 through 39 FAAHN (Ch. 15, 1 through 39 AHN)

EILR IC images Ch. 55, 1 through 3 FAAHN (Ch. 15, 1 through 3 AHN)

EILR TB questions Ch. 55, 1 through 32 FAAHN (Ch. 15, 1 through 32 AHN)

EILR Open Book Quiz Ch. 55, 1 through 10 FAAHN (Ch. 15, 1 through 10 AHN)

ESLR Review Questions for the NCLEX® Examination Ch. 55, 55-01 through 55-10 FAAHN (Ch. 15, 15-01 through 15-10 AHN)

Legend

PPT
PowerPoint
Slides

EILR
EVOLVE Instructor
Learning Resources:
Image Collection, Test
Bank, Open Book Quizzes

ESLR
EVOLVE Student
Learning Resources:
Review Questions
for the NCLEX
Examination

SG
Study Guide

NCP CTQ
Nursing Care Plan
Critical Thinking
Question

Class Activities are indicated in *bold italic*.

LESSON 15.1

PRETEST

1. _____ is the ability of the immune system to mobilize an antibody in response to an antigen.
   a. Cellular immunity
   b. Cell-mediated immunity
   c Immunotherapy
   d. Immunocompetence

2. Which of the following statements concerning innate immunity is correct?
   a. There are no physical barriers with this subcategory of immunity.
   b. Innate immunity involves a nonspecific inflammatory response.
   c. Innate immunity employs T lymphocytes to protect the body.
   d. Innate immunity utilizes humoral immunity.

3. When describing the manner in which B cells work, which of the following is most correct?
   a. B cells are produced in response to antibodies.
   b. B cells reduce in number as they respond to a potential pathogen.
   c. B cells are an active part of the innate immune process.
   d. B cells increase in number as they are called to respond to an antigen.

4. _____ immunity results from the development and continuing presence of antibodies circulating in the plasma.
   a. Humoral
   b. Cell-mediated
   c. Cellular
   d. Histamine-based

5. When caring for a patient with a disorder of the immune system, you are asked what is meant by the term of "antigen." What should be included in your response?
   a. An antigen is able to protect the body from a pathogen.
   b. Antigens allow the body to fight off infection.
   c. The antigens are potential invaders to the body's immune system.
   d. "Antigens" and "antibodies" are interchangeable terms referring to the body's ability to defend itself from disease.

6. Which of the following positions is most appropriate for a patient being treated for an anaphylactic reaction?
   a. Sitting upright
   b. Sitting upright with the legs elevated
   c. Recumbent with legs elevated
   d. Recumbent with the legs lowered

Adult Health Nursing, 6th ed.
Christensen & Kockrow

7. When an autoimmune disorder occurs, which of the following best explains what has taken place?
   a. The immune system's concept of memory has not effectively provided recall about an antigen's exposure.
   b. The humoral immune system has overreacted in response to environmental stimuli.
   c. There has been a decrease in T cell production.
   d. The body has not been able to effectively differentiate its own cells from foreign invaders.

8. A patient who suffered an allergic reaction asks how potential allergens can get into the body and cause the reaction. Which of the following is an accurate statement?
   a. Most allergens enter the body from cuts and other skin openings.
   b. The oral cavity is the portal for most environmental allergens.
   c. The gastrointestinal and respiratory systems are the most common means of entry for allergens.
   d. The most common route of entry for pathogens involves the ingestion of pathogens.

9. Common allergens that could be associated with anaphylaxis include:
   a. milk, chocolate, and peanuts.
   b. walnuts and grapes.
   c. peanuts, shellfish, and wheat.
   d. oats, strawberries, and grapes.

10. At the first sign of anaphylaxis, administration of epinephrine is indicated. What dosage is appropriate?
    a. 0.2 to 0.5 mL epinephrine IM
    b. 0.2 to 0.5 mL epinephrine subcutaneously
    c. 1.5 to 2.0 mL epinephrine IV push
    d. 0.5 to 1.0 mL epinephrine IM

Answers:

1. d	2. b	3. d	4. a	5. c
6. c	7. d	8. d	9. a	10. a

BACKGROUND ASSESSMENT

Question: The body's immune system is organized into levels of defense. When potential pathogens are introduced to the environment, what is involved in the body's first line of defense?
Answer: The initial line of defense involves innate immunity. This type of immunity provides a physical barrier. Organs and tissues involved in this role include the skin and mucous membranes. The skin wards off the invasion of microorganisms from the body's interior. The body's mucous membranes secrete substances that can kill bacteria. Cilia, tears, and natural flora of the intestines and vagina also are active providers of this natural protection.

Question: After experiencing a hypersensitivity reaction to a bee sting, the patient has been seen by the clinic in which you are employed. After being evaluated by the physician, the patient has been given a prescription for a bee sting kit. What are the responsibilities of the nurse in providing care for this patient?
Answer: The kit that has been given to the patient contains epinephrine and tourniquet. The nurse will need to provide education concerning the use of the tourniquet and medication. The tourniquet should be applied if stung. It will prevent spread of the toxins in the bee's venom. The medication is to be injected subcutaneously. The patient will need to have information concerning the appropriate means of providing an injection should the need arise. The patient should also be advised to wear a medical alert bracelet and carry the kit when going outside.

CRITICAL THINKING QUESTION

A 74-year-old patient has come to the physician's office with complaints of flu-like signs and symptoms. After the patient was seen by the physician, you are providing the education concerning follow-up care. The patient states he is tired of being sick all of the time. He reports he has noticed that he has been less able to fight off illness as he has aged. Based upon your knowledge, what factors concerning his age might be related to his concerns?
Guidelines: Studies have shown a reduction in immunity as the body ages. The older adult demonstrates a greater incidence of tumor development and susceptibility to infections. The thymus gland, which has a key role in the immune system, changes with aging. These changes include the reduction in size and activity. Fewer T cells are produced. There is also a reduction in the efficiency of memory cells.

Adult Health Nursing, 6th ed.

Christensen & Kockrow

OBJECTIVES	CONTENT	TEACHING RESOURCES
Differentiate between natural and acquired immunity.	■ Nature of immunity (FAAHN p. 1955, AHN p. 719) ☐ Innate, or natural, immunity (FAAHN p. 1956, AHN p. 720) ☐ Adaptive, or acquired, immunity (FAAHN p. 1956, AHN p. 720)	☒ PPT 2 through 9, Ch. 55 FAAHN (Ch. 15 PPT 2 through 9 AHN) 🖪 EILR IC Ch. 55 images 1, 2 FAAHN (Ch. 15 images 1, 2 AHN) 🖪 EILR TB Ch. 55 question 6 FAAHN (Ch. 15 question 6 AHN) 🖪 EILR Open Book Quiz Ch. 55 questions 1, 2 FAAHN (Ch. 15 questions 1, 2 AHN) 📖 SG Immunity, Ch. 55 p. 513 FAAHN (Ch. 15 p. 201 AHN) **BOOK RESOURCES** Review Questions for the NCLEX Examination Ch. 55 questions 1, 3 FAAHN (Ch. 15 questions 1, 3 AHN) Fig. 55-1 When an infectious agent enters the body, it first encounters elements of the innate immune system (FAAHN p. 1956) (Fig. 15-1 AHN p. 720) Table 55-1 Innate (Natural) and Adaptive (Acquired) Immunity (FAAHN p. 1956) (Table 15-1 AHN p. 720) Fig. 55-2 Organization of the immune system (FAAHN p. 1957) (Fig. 15-2 AHN p. 721) Fig. 55-3 Origin and processing of B and T cells (FAAHN p. 1957) (Fig. 15-3 AHN p. 721) Box 55-1 The Four Rs of the Immune Response (FAAHN p. 1958) (Box 15-1 AHN p. 722) Box 55-2 Review of the Mechanisms of Immune Response (FAAHN p. 1959) (Box 15-2 AHN p. 723) ▶ Discuss the tools used in the process of innate immunity. ▶ Discuss the components of the adaptive immune process. *Class Activity **Divide the students into two teams. One team will be "innate immunity" and the other team will be "adaptive immunity." Instruct each team to develop a series of short questions and answers concerning their assigned immunity. Then, ask each team to quiz its opponents. The team correctly answering the most questions will win.***

OBJECTIVES	CONTENT	TEACHING RESOURCES
Compare and contrast humoral and cell-mediated immunity.	☐ Humoral immunity (FAAHN p. 1957, AHN p. 721) ☐ Cellular immunity (FAAHN p. 1958, AHN p. 722)	PPT 10, 11, Ch. 55 FAAHN (Ch. 15 PPT 10, 11 AHN) EILR IC Ch. 55 image 3 FAAHN (Ch. 15 image 3 AHN) EILR TB Ch. 55 questions 13, 31 FAAHN (Ch. 15 questions 13, 31 AHN) EILR Open Book Quiz Ch. 55 question 1 FAAHN (Ch. 15 question 1 AHN) ESLR Review Questions for the NCLEX Examination Ch. 55 question 2 FAAHN (Ch. 15 question 2 AHN) SG Types of Immunity, Ch. 55 p. 513 FAAHN (Ch. 15 p. 201 AHN) **BOOK RESOURCES** Review Questions for the NCLEX Examination Ch. 55 question 5 FAAHN (Ch. 15 question 5 AHN) Fig. 55-3 Origin and processing of B and T cells (FAAHN p. 1957) (Fig. 15-3 AHN p. 721) Box 55-1 The Four Rs of the Immune Response (FAAHN p. 1958) (Box 15-1 AHN p. 722) Box 55-2 Review of the Mechanisms of Immune Response (FAAHN p. 1959) (Box 15-2 AHN p. 723) ▸ Discuss the process of humoral immunity. ▸ Discuss the process of cellular immunity. *Class Activity Divide the class into four teams. Two teams will confer and then illustrate the concept of humoral immunity on the board. The other two teams will confer and illustrate the concept of cell-mediated immunity on the board. The class members will vote to select the best illustration of each type of immunity.*
Explain the concepts of immuno-competency, immuno-deficiency, and autoimmunity.	■ Nature of immunity (FAAHN p. 1955, AHN p. 719) ■ Complement system (FAAHN p. 1958, AHN p. 722) ■ Genetic control of immunity (FAAHN p. 1958, AHN p. 722)	PPT 3, 12 through 14 Ch. 55 FAAHN (Ch. 15 PPT 3, 12 through 14 AHN) EILR IC Ch. 55 images 1, 2 FAAHN (Ch. 15 images 1, 2 AHN) EILR TB Ch. 55 questions 3, 4, 17, 32 FAAHN (Ch. 15 questions 3, 4, 17, 32 AHN)

OBJECTIVES	CONTENT	TEACHING RESOURCES
	■ Effects of normal aging on the immune system (FAAHN p. 1958, AHN p. 722)	⬛ EILR Open Book Quiz Ch. 55 question 3 FAAHN (Ch. 15 question 3 AHN) ⬛ ESLR Review Questions for the NCLEX Examination Ch. 55 question 3 FAAHN (Ch. 15 question 3 AHN) 📖 SG Immunity Differences, Ch. 55 p. 514 FAAHN (Ch. 15 p. 202 AHN) **BOOK RESOURCES** Life Span Considerations, Older Adult: Immune Disorder (FAAHN p. 1959) (AHN p. 723) ▸ Discuss the theory of immunotherapy. ▸ Discuss the potential continuum of altered immune responses. *Class Activity Distribute blank nursing care plan sheets to the class. Divide students into small groups. Assign the groups the task of creating a care plan addressing the alteration in immunity experienced by older adults.*
Review the mechanisms of immune response.	■ Immune response (FAAHN p. 1959, AHN p. 723)	🖼 PPT 15 through 17, Ch. 55 FAAHN (Ch. 15 PPT 15 through 17 AHN) ⬛ EILR IC Ch. 55 image 1 FAAHN (Ch. 15 image 1 AHN) ⬛ EILR TB Ch. 55 questions 7, 11 through 13, 16 FAAHN (Ch. 15 questions 7, 11 through 13, 16 AHN) ⬛ ESLR Review Questions for the NCLEX Examination Ch. 55 question 1 FAAHN (Ch. 15 question 1 AHN) 📖 SG Organization of the Immune System, Ch. 55 p. 515 FAAHN (Ch. 15 p. 203 AHN) **BOOK RESOURCES** Box 55-1 The Four Rs of the Immune Response (FAAHN p. 1958) (Box 15-1 AHN p. 722) ▸ Discuss the four Rs of the immune response. ▸ Discuss the differences between passive and active immunity. *Class Activity Divide the class into four groups. Using symbols, characters, cartoons (anything but words), each group is to create a picture representation of the "four Rs" related to the immune response.*

Adult Health Nursing, 6th ed.
Christensen & Kockrow

OBJECTIVES	CONTENT	TEACHING RESOURCES
Discuss five factors that influence the development of hypersensitivity.	■ Disorders of the immune system (FAAHN p. 1960, AHN p. 724) ☐ Hypersensitivity disorders (FAAHN p. 1960, AHN p. 724) – Etiology and pathophysiology (FAAHN p. 1960, AHN p. 724) – Assessment (FAAHN p. 1960, AHN p. 724) – Diagnostic tests (FAAHN p. 1961, AHN p. 725) – Medical management (FAAHN p. 1961, AHN p. 725) – Nursing diagnoses (FAAHN p. 1962, AHN p. 726) – Patient teaching (FAAHN p. 1962, AHN p. 726)	PPT 17 through 20 Ch. 55 FAAHN (Ch. 15 PPT 17 through 20 AHN) EILR TB Ch. 55 questions 6, 8, 9, 14, 15, 22, 23 FAAHN (Ch. 15 questions 6, 8, 9, 14, 15, 22, 23 AHN) EILR Open Book Quiz Ch. 55 questions 5, 6, 8, 9 FAAHN (Ch. 15 questions 5, 6, 8, 9 AHN) ESLR Review Questions for the NCLEX Examination Ch. 55 questions 4, 5, 10 FAAHN (Ch. 15 questions 4, 5, 10 AHN) SG Hypersensitivity Development, Ch. 55 p. 515 FAAHN (Ch. 15 p. 203 AHN) **BOOK RESOURCES** Review Questions for the NCLEX Examination Ch. 55 questions 4, 7, 14, 15 FAAHN (Ch. 15 questions 4, 7, 14, 15 AHN) Box 55-3 Factors Influencing Hypersensitivity (FAAHN p. 1961) (Box 15-3 AHN p. 725) Table 55-2 Medications for Immune Disorders (FAAHN p. 1962) (Table 15-2 AHN p. 726) Safety Alert! Treating the Patient with a Hypersensitivity Reaction (FAAHN p. 1962) (AHN p. 726) ▶ Discuss the concept of hypersensitivity disorders. ▶ Discuss the nursing assessment of a hypersensitive reaction. *Class Activity Develop short patient scenarios including specific clinical manifestations of allergic reactions. Write these on index cards. Distribute the cards to 50% of the class. Those students with cards are to be "patients." The remaining students will act as the nurses. Instruct each student to link with a partner and role-play a data collection situation involving an allergic reaction.*

OBJECTIVES	CONTENT	TEACHING RESOURCES
Identify the clinical manifestations of anaphylaxis.	□ Anaphylaxis (FAAHN p. 1963, AHN p. 727) – Etiology and pathophysiology (FAAHN p. 1963, AHN p. 727) – Clinical manifestations (FAAHN p. 1963, AHN p. 727) – Assessment (FAAHN p. 1963, AHN p. 727) – Medical management (FAAHN p. 1963, AHN p. 727) – Nursing interventions and patient teaching (FAAHN p. 1963, AHN p. 727) – Prognosis (FAAHN p. 1964, AHN p. 728)	PPT 21 through 24, Ch. 55 FAAHN (Ch. 15 PPT 21 through 24 AHN) EILR TB Ch. 55 questions 1, 2, 10, 20 FAAHN (Ch. 15 questions 1, 2, 10, 20 AHN) EILR Open Book Quiz Ch. 55 question 7 FAAHN (Ch. 15 question 7 AHN) ESLR Review Questions for the NCLEX Examination Ch. 55 question 6 FAAHN (Ch. 15 question 6 AHN) SG Anaphylaxis, Ch. 55 p. 516 FAAHN (Ch. 15 p. 204 AHN) **BOOK RESOURCES** Review Questions for the NCLEX Examination Ch. 55 questions 9, 18 FAAHN (Ch. 15 questions 9, 18 AHN) Box 55-4 Common Allergens Causing Anaphylaxis (FAAHN p. 1963) (Box 15-4 AHN p. 727) ▶ Discuss the role of the nurse in the care of an anaphylactic reaction. *Class Activity Ask students to list on the board the clinical manifestations of anaphylactic reactions.*
Outline the immediate aggressive treatment of systemic anaphylactic reaction.	□ Anaphylaxis (FAAHN p. 1963, AHN p. 727) – Etiology and pathophysiology (FAAHN p. 1963, AHN p. 727) – Clinical manifestations (FAAHN p. 1963, AHN p. 727) – Assessment (FAAHN p. 1963, AHN p. 727) – Medical management (FAAHN p. 1963, AHN p. 727) – Nursing interventions and patient teaching (FAAHN p. 1963, AHN p. 727) – Prognosis (FAAHN p. 1964, AHN p. 728)	PPT 24, Ch. 55 FAAHN (Ch. 15 PPT 24 AHN) EILR IC Ch. 55 image 1 FAAHN (Ch. 15 image 1 AHN) EILR TB Ch. 55 questions 1, 2, 10, 14, 20 FAAHN (Ch. 15 question 1, 2, 10, 14, 20 AHN) SG Anaphylaxis, Ch. 55 p. 516 FAAHN (Ch. 15 p. 204 AHN) **BOOK RESOURCES** Review Questions for the NCLEX Examination Ch. 55 questions 8, 13 FAAHN (Ch. 15 questions 8, 13 AHN) ▶ Discuss treatment for an anaphylactic reaction. *Class Activity Ask the students to list on the board the nurse's responsibilities in patient education regarding anaphylactic reaction.*

Mosby items and derived items © 2011 by Mosby, Inc., an affiliate of Elsevier Inc.
Some material was previously published.

Christensen & Kockrow

15.1 Homework/Assignments:

15.1 Instructor's Notes/Student Feedback:

Adult Health Nursing, 6th ed.

Christensen & Kockrow

LESSON 15.2

CRITICAL THINKING QUESTION

While caring for a postoperative patient, the physician has ordered a blood transfusion. The patient is to receive 3 units of packed red blood cells. Approximately 15 minutes after the transfusion was initiated, the patient calls out to the nurse's station. He complains of itching all over his body. His temperature was 98.3 when the transfusion initiated, and now it is 99.6. He is flushed, there is a rash on his arms and trunk, and audible wheezes are present. What has happened? What should the nurse do at this time? What will the treatment entail?

Guidelines: The patient is most likely experiencing a moderate blood transfusion reaction. It is the responsibility of the nurse to recognize the event, perform an assessment, contact the physician and the blood bank, and carry out the orders given by the physician. The patient might have the transfusion stopped and saline administered. Medications will be given, including epinephrine or Benadryl. The nurse must document all observations and treatments carried out. The patient will need close observation during the period following the shift.

OBJECTIVES	CONTENT	TEACHING RESOURCES
Discuss the two types of latex allergies and recommendations for preventing allergic reactions to latex in the workplace.	☐ Latex allergies (FAAHN p. 1964, AHN p. 728) – Types of latex allergies (FAAHN p. 1964, AHN p. 728) – Nursing interventions (FAAHN p. 1964, AHN p. 728)	PPT 25 through 27, Ch. 55 FAAHN (Ch. 15 PPT 25 through 27 AHN) EILR TB Ch. 55 question 30 FAAHN (Ch. 15 question 30 AHN) ESLR Review Questions for the NCLEX Examination Ch. 55 question 8 FAAHN (Ch. 15 question 8 AHN) SG Latex Allergies, Ch. 55 p. 517 FAAHN (Ch. 15 p. 205AHN) ▶ Discuss the implications of the increase in latex allergies in health care professionals. ▶ Discuss "warning" signs associated with a latex allergy. *Class Activity Instruct students to individually prepare a list of all of the potential latex allergens in the health care workplace. After the lists are completed, share them aloud.*

Adult Health Nursing, 6th ed.
Christensen & Kockrow

OBJECTIVES	CONTENT	TEACHING RESOURCES
Discuss selection of blood donors, typing and cross-matching, storage, and administration in preventing transfusion reaction.	☐ Transfusion reactions (FAAHN p. 1965, AHN p. 729) ☐ Delayed hypersensitivity (FAAHN p. 1965, AHN p. 729) ☐ Transplant rejection (FAAHN p. 1965, AHN p. 729)	PPT 28 through 35, Ch. 55 FAAHN (Ch. 15 PPT 28 through 35 AHN) EILR TB Ch. 55 questions 24 through 26 FAAHN (Ch. 15 questions 24 through 26 AHN) EILR Open Book Quiz Ch. 55 questions 8, 9 FAAHN (Ch. 15 questions 8, 9 AHN) ESLR Review Questions for the NCLEX Examination Ch. 55 questions 7, 9 FAAHN (Ch. 15 questions 7, 9 AHN) SG Transfusion Reaction, Ch. 55 p. 517 FAAHN (Ch. 15 p. 205 AHN) **BOOK RESOURCES** Review Questions for the NCLEX Examination Ch. 55 questions 2, 10, 12 FAAHN (Ch. 15 questions 2, 10, 12 AHN) ▸ Discuss the causes of a transfusion reaction. ▸ Discuss the role of the nurse in caring for a patient who has experienced a transfusion reaction. *Class Activity Contact a local hospital. Obtain an example of a tag that is on a unit of blood from the laboratory. Obtain a copy of the recording sheet that is used with the administration of blood products from the nursing unit. Make copies of the materials obtained and distribute them to the class. Lead students in the steps required to complete the documentation required for a blood transfusion.*
Explain an immunodeficiency disease.	■ Immunodeficiency disorders (FAAHN p. 1966, AHN p. 730) ☐ Primary immunodeficiency disorders (FAAHN p. 1966, AHN p. 730) ☐ Secondary immunodeficiency disorders (FAAHN p. 1966, AHN p. 730)	PPT 36 through 38, Ch. 55 FAAHN (Ch. 15 PPT 36 through 38 AHN) EILR TB Ch. 55 question 4 FAAHN (Ch. 15 question 4 AHN) EILR Open Book Quiz Ch. 55 questions 4, 17, 18 FAAHN (Ch. 15 questions 4, 17, 18 AHN) SG Immunodeficiency Disease, Ch. 55 p. 518 FAAHN (Ch. 15 p. 206 AHN)

Christensen & Kockrow

OBJECTIVES	CONTENT	TEACHING RESOURCES
		BOOK RESOURCES Review Questions for the NCLEX Examination Ch. 55 question 11 FAAHN (Ch. 15 question 11 AHN) ▶ Discuss and identify diseases that are believed to be immunodeficiency disorders. ▶ Discuss the impairments in immune function that cause an immunodeficiency disease. *Class Activity **Divide the class into five groups. Assign each group the topics of stress, age, malnutrition, radiation, and surgery. Next, instruct each group to use a section of the board to diagram how its assigned topic influences immunodeficiency diseases.***
Discuss the cause of autoimmune disorders.	■ Autoimmune disorders (FAAHN p. 1966, AHN p. 730)	PPT 39, Ch. 55 FAAHN (Ch. 15 PPT 39 AHN) EILR TB Ch. 55 questions 4, 17, 32 FAAHN (Ch. 15 question 4, 17, 32 AHN) SG Autoimmune Disorders, Ch. 55 p. 518 FAAHN (Ch. 15 p. 206 AHN) **BOOK RESOURCES** Review Questions for the NCLEX Examination Ch. 55 question 19 FAAHN (Ch. 15 question 19 AHN) ▶ Discuss what takes place in an autoimmune disorder. ▶ Discuss the diseases that are considered to be autoimmune disorders. *Class Activity **Contact a local speakers' bureau. Invite a guest speaker to the class and ask the speaker to discuss life for someone with an autoimmune disorder.***
Explain plasmapheresis in the treatment of autoimmune diseases.	■ Plasmapheresis (FAAHN p. 1967, AHN p. 731)	EILR Open Book Quiz Ch. 55 question 10 FAAHN (Ch. 15 question 10 AHN) SG Autoimmune Disorders, Ch. 55 p. 518 FAAHN (Ch. 15 p. 206 AHN)

Adult Health Nursing, 6th ed.

Christensen & Kockrow

OBJECTIVES	CONTENT	TEACHING RESOURCES
		BOOK RESOURCES
		Review Questions for the NCLEX Examination Ch. 55 question 16 FAAHN (Ch. 15 question 16 AHN)
		▶ Discuss the candidates that should be considered for plasmapheresis.
		Class Activity Contact a local acute care facility. Ask a member of the transfusion team to come to speak to the class.
Performance Evaluation		🖥 EILR TB Ch. 55 questions 1 through 32 FAAHN (Ch. 15 questions 1 through 32 AHN)
		🖥 EILR Open Book Quiz Ch. 55 questions 1 through 10 FAAHN (Ch. 15 questions 1 through 10 AHN)
		🖥 ESLR Review Questions for the NCLEX Examination Ch. 55 question 1 through 10 FAAHN (Ch. 15 question 1 through 10 AHN)
		📓 SG Ch. 55 pp. 513 through 520 FAAHN (Ch. 15 pp. 201 through 208 AHN)
		BOOK RESOURCES
		Review Questions for the NCLEX Examination Ch. 55 questions 1 through 19 FAAHN (Ch. 15 questions 1 through 19 AHN)

15.2 Homework/Assignments:

15.2 Instructor's Notes/Student Feedback:

Christensen & Kockrow

Slide 1

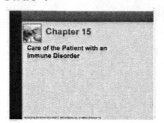

Slide 2

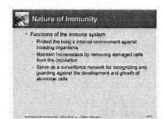

- Immune is a word meaning "free from burden" in Latin. How does the definition correspond to our understanding of the functions of the immune system?

- A healthy functioning immune system is necessary for survival. It is this system that enables the body to protect itself.

- What body parts make up the immune system?

Slide 3

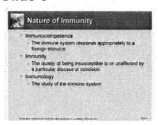

- An appropriately functioning immune system reacts by a process known as immunocompetence.

- What are examples of exposures that will cause immunocompetence?

Slide 4

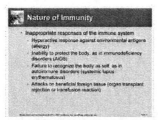

- When the immune system does not work against potential pathogens, homeostasis is affected.

Slide 5

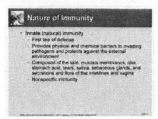

- There are two subclassifications of immunity: innate and adaptive.

- Innate acts as a barrier between the body and the outside world. Its components act as soldiers against potentially invasive microorganisms.

- Does innate immunity always work? What will occur if it does not?

Christensen & Kockrow

Slide 6

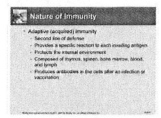

- In the event the body's innate immunity does not effectively handle pathogens, adaptive immunity is the next line of defense.
- This type of immunity has the characteristic of specificity and memory. How do each of these concepts relate to the immune process?

Slide 7

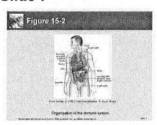

- The body organs identified assist in maintaining the lines of defense. Outline what role each of the listed parts does to aid in this function.

Slide 8

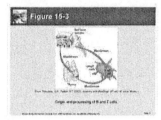

- The process of adaptive immunity utilizes cells in defending the body. A specific type of white blood cell, known as a lymphocyte, is involved. Discuss the differences between T cells and B cells.

Slide 9

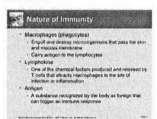

- Adaptive immunity is assisted by helper cells. These cells include macrophages and lymphocytes. How are these cells similar? How do they differ?
- Discuss where these cells are produced. What determines their number?

Slide 10

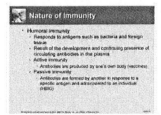

- In humoral immunity, the body produces B cells in response to a challenge by an antigen. The concept of memory is important to the success of humoral immunity.

Adult Health Nursing, 6th ed.
Christensen & Kockrow

Slide 11

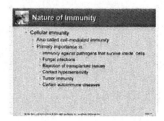

- When potential pathogens are introduced into the body, T cells are activated. This process results in a full cellular response.
- What action is taken by the T cells once activated?
- Is there a specific type of pathogen targeted by the T cells?

Slide 12

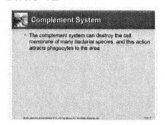

- The complement system is an organized series of enzymatic proteins. These enzymes are "awakened" when the body comes into contact with an antigen.
- What would you liken this process to?
  It is similar to a video game, such as Pac-Man.

Slide 13

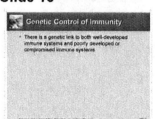

- Theories of immunity support the impact of heredity. What influences can be attributed to immunity? Provide examples of genetics interacting with illness and disease

Slide 14

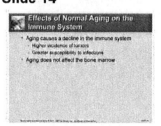

- As the human body ages, there is a natural increase in disease process. What disorders increase with aging?
- What factors associated with growing older can encourage the onset of illness?

Slide 15

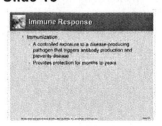

- There are two ways to assist the body to develop immunity. They are immunization and immunotherapy.
- The concept of immunization dates back to the late 1790s.
- Vaccines and toxoids are weakened forms of disease-causing organisms, administered to provide protection from disease.
- Compare and contrast live and dead vaccines.
- For which diseases are vaccines routinely provided?

ELSEVIER

Mosby items and derived items © 2011, 2007 by Mosby, Inc., an affiliate of Elsevier Inc.
Some material was previously published.

Adult Health Nursing, 6th ed.
Christensen & Kockrow

Slide 16

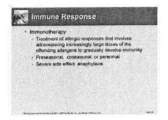

- Immunotherapy is a long-term management option to treat allergies.

- In most cases this therapy is initiated in the physician's office.

- When is home maintenance appropriate? If home maintenance is initiated, what are the responsibilities of the nurse?

- What supplies will be needed in the home if home therapy is ordered?

Slide 17

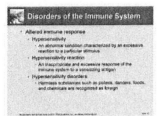

- Immune responses result as the body tries to protect itself.

- What factors can be attributed to a failure in immune response?

Slide 18

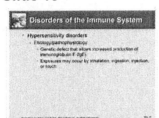

- When hypersensitivity reactions result, what will determine the degree of reaction?

Slide 19

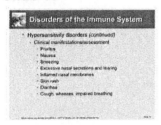

- The types of clinical manifestations seen in a hypersensitivity reaction might vary between individuals.

Slide 20

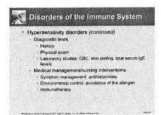

- What information should be collected from the patient concerning the events surrounding a hypersensitivity reaction?

Adult Health Nursing, 6th ed.
Christensen & Kockrow

Slide 21

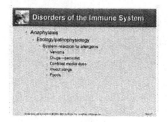

- Anaphylaxis is the most severe type of allergic reaction. It involves the systemic reaction to the allergen.

- Discuss the events that result in the anaphylactic response demonstrated.

Slide 22

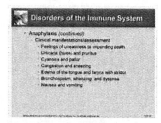

- The onset of symptoms from the time of exposure is rapid.

- Early intervention can often stop the onset of more severe reactions in the patient.

Slide 23

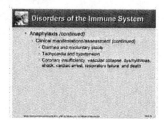

Slide 24

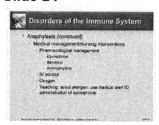

- Upon recognition of anaphylaxis, treatment must begin quickly to reduce complications and potential death.

- What are the actions of the recommended medications?

- How are the medications administered?

- Identify two nursing diagnoses for the patient diagnosed with anaphylaxis.

Slide 25

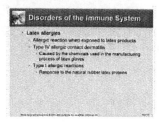

- Latex allergies are growing. What factors can be related to this increase in latex allergies?

ELSEVIER

Mosby items and derived items © 2011, 2007 by Mosby, Inc., an affiliate of Elsevier Inc.
Some material was previously published.

Adult Health Nursing, 6th ed.
Christensen & Kockrow

Slide 26

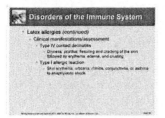

- The identification of people at risk for the development of latex allergies is key in the prevention of allergic reactions.

- What risk factors are associated with the development of a latex allergy?

Slide 27

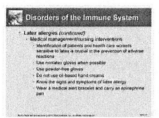

- The development of a latex allergy in a health care worker is serious. What are the responsibilities of the workplace regarding the environment and work supplies?

- Ask if any of the students have latex sensitivities. Further, if there are affirmative responses, ask what the impact has been on their clinical experiences.

Slide 28

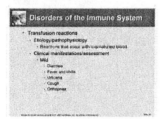

- An allergic reaction due to a blood transfusion is serious.

- What steps can the nurse take to reduce the likelihood of this happening?

Slide 29

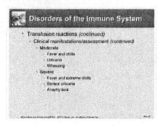

- When a transfusion reaction results, what data must be collected by the nurse?

Slide 30

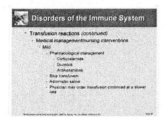

Christensen & Kockrow

Slide 31

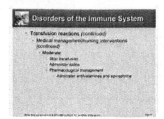

- When a transfusion reaction results, the patient could have an antihistamine and epinephrine administered. How do these medications work? What nursing implications accompany their administration?

Slide 32

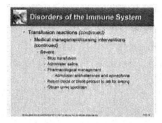

- Care of the patient who has experienced a blood transfusion reaction has several steps. The physician must be notified, the transfusion stopped or slowed, and medications given. What nursing diagnoses are appropriate for this patient?

- What information should be documented in the patient's medical record?

Slide 33

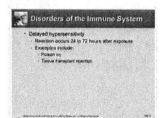

Slide 34

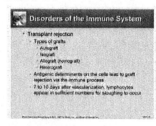

- The introduction of tissue into the body might be done for a variety of reasons.

- What treatment plans utilize tissue transplantation?

- Define each of the tissue types used in transplantation.

Slide 35

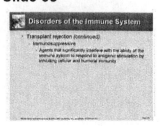

- Pharmacological agents are administered to reduce the risk of tissue rejection.

- What classification of agents can be used?

Adult Health Nursing, 6th ed.

Christensen & Kockrow

Slide 36

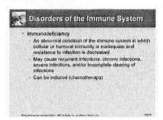

- A healthy, functioning immune system provides the body with protection against pathogens. When the immune system fails to adequately provide protection, illness and disease will result.

- What are examples of immunodeficiency diseases?

Slide 37

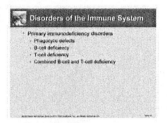

Slide 38

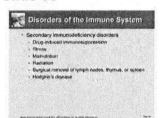

- How do each of the factors listed contribute to immunodeficiency disorders?

Slide 39

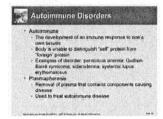

Christensen & Kockrow

TEACHING FOCUS

In this chapter, the student will be introduced to the care of the patient with HIV/AIDS. The student will begin by exploring the agent that causes HIV disease, along with the differences between HIV infection, HIV disease, and AIDS. The student will have the opportunity to learn how HIV is and is not transmitted, the pathophysiology of HIV disease, tests related to HIV disease, and issues related to testing. The student will explore the prevention of HIV infection, patients who are at risk for HIV infection, and the nurse's role in prevention. Finally, the student will explore the nurse's role in caring for the HIV-infected patient, including the multidisciplinary approach, the importance of adherence to treatment, the signs and symptoms of HIV disease, the opportunistic infections associated with AIDS, and the care plan for the patient with AIDS.

MATERIALS AND RESOURCES

- ☐ Computer/overhead projector (Lessons 16.1 and 16.2)
- ☐ White/black board and marker/chalk (Lessons 16.1 and 16.2)
- ☐ Large sheets of unlined paper (Lesson 16.1)
- ☐ Copies of forms used to record HIV testing; obtain from laboratory at a local hospital (Lesson 16.1)
- ☐ Several scenarios describing the concerns of a person living with HIV, written on index cards (Lesson 16.2)
- ☐ Copies of pamphlets used to educate the public about HIV and AIDS; obtain from Department of Health (Lesson 16.2)

LESSON CHECKLIST

Preparations for this lesson include:
- Lecture
- Contact a local HIV treatment center and request a speaker on treatment options available for HIV and AIDS patients and their families.
- Contact a family planning clinic or Department of Health and request a speaker on the role of education in preventing the spread of HIV infection.

KEY TERMS

acquired immunodeficiency syndrome (AIDS) (FAAHN p. 1980, AHN p. 744)

adherence (FAAHN p. 1996, AHN p. 760)

CD_4^+ lymphocyte (FAAHN p. 1978, AHN p. 742)

Centers for Disease Control and Prevention (FAAHN p. 1970, AHN p. 734)

enzyme-linked immunosorbent assay (ELISA) (FAAHN p. 1983, AHN p. 747)

HIV disease (FAAHN p. 1980, AHN p. 744)

HIV infection (FAAHN p. 1980, AHN p. 744)

human immunodeficiency virus (HIV) (FAAHN p. 1970, AHN p. 734)

Kaposi's sarcoma (FAAHN p. 1970, AHN p. 734)

opportunistic (FAAHN p. 1972, AHN p. 736)

phagocytic (FAAHN p. 1980, AHN p. 744)

Pneumocystis jiroveci (formerly *carinii*) pneumonia (FAAHN p. 1970, AHN p. 734)

retrovirus (FAAHN p. 1978, AHN p. 742)

seroconversion (FAAHN p. 1976, AHN p. 740)

seronegative (FAAHN p. 1983, AHN p. 747)

vertical transmission (FAAHN p. 1975, AHN p. 739)

viral load (FAAHN p. 1975, AHN p. 739)

virulent (FAAHN p. 1971, AHN p. 735)

Western blot (FAAHN p. 1983, AHN p. 747)

ADDITIONAL RESOURCES

PPT Ch. 56, 1 through 48 FAAHN (Ch. 16, 1 through 48 AHN)

EILR IC images Ch. 56, 1 through 4 FAAHN (Ch. 16, 1 through 4 AHN)

EILR TB questions Ch. 56, 1 through 30 FAAHN (Ch. 16, 1 through 30 AHN)

EILR Open Book Quiz Ch. 56, 1 through 10 FAAHN (Ch. 16, 1 through 10 AHN)

ESLR Review Questions for the NCLEX® Examination Ch. 56, 56-01 through 56-10 FAAHN (Ch. 16, 16-01 through 16-10 AHN)

Legend

PPT
PowerPoint
Slides

EILR
EVOLVE Instructor
Learning Resources:
Image Collection, Test
Bank, Open Book Quizzes

ESLR
EVOLVE Student
Learning Resources:
Review Questions
for the NCLEX
Examination

SG
Study Guide

NCP CTQ
Nursing Care Plan
Critical Thinking
Question

Class Activities are indicated in **bold italic**.

LESSON 16.1

PRETEST

1. When reviewing the number of total AIDS cases in people age 55 or older, which statement is most accurate?
   a. Fewer than 5% of the reported cases of AIDS are people age 55 or older.
   b. The number of AIDS cases in people older than 55 is greater than the population of age 20 to 35 years.
   c. More than 10% of AIDS cases are reported to be in people age 55 or older.
   d. Between 5% and 10% of AIDS cases have been reported to be in people age 55 or older.

2. Which of the following populations demonstrates the highest rate of HIV seroprevalence?
   a. Hispanics
   b. African Americans
   c. Caucasian Americans
   d. European immigrants

3. The terminology used to describe HIV- and AIDS-related procedures is important. Which of the following terms is most appropriate?
   a. HIV antibody test
   b. AIDS test
   c. AIDS serology examination
   d. AIDS positive

4. What percentage of HIV-positive individuals are considered rapid progressors?
   a. Less than 5%
   b. 5% to 10%
   c. 10% to 15%
   d. More than 15%

5. During seroconversion, which of the following characteristics is correct?
   a. The viral load is low, with a short-term drop in CD4+ cells.
   b. The viral load is low, with a short-term elevation in CD4+ cells.
   c. The viral load is extremely high, with a short-term elevation in CD4+ cells.
   d. The viral load is extremely high, with a short-term drop in CD4+ cells.

6. _____ refers to the development of antibodies from HIV.
   a. Asymptomatic immunodeficiency disease
   b. Seroconversion
   c. Primary HIV infection
   d. Retroconversion

ELSEVIER

Mosby items and derived items © 2011 by Mosby, Inc., an affiliate of Elsevier Inc.
Some material was previously published.

Christensen & Kockrow

7. The initial test used to begin the diagnostic process for HIV infection employs which of the following tests?
   a. Seronegative test
   b. ELISA test
   c. Western blot test
   d. bDNA reaction test

8. When caring for the patient diagnosed with pneumocystis, which of the following medications can be anticipated?
   a. Acyclovir
   b. Amphotericin B + 5-flucytosine
   c. Trimethoprim-sulfamethoxazole
   d. Vancomycin

9. When reviewing the expenses for the care of a person infected with HIV, which of the following is responsible for the largest portion of the health care expenditures?
   a. Medications
   b. Hospitalization
   c. Physician care expenses
   d. Alternative therapies

10. The anticipated lifetime cost of care for the HIV-positive person is:
    a. $ 250,000 to $ 350,000
    b. $ 350,000 to $ 450,000
    c. $ 450,000 to $ 550,000
    d. Exceeds all of these amounts

Answers:

1. d	2. a	3. a	4. c	5. a
6. b	7. b	8. c	9. a	10. d

BACKGROUND ASSESSMENT

Question: You are assigned to care for a hospitalized patient diagnosed with HIV. While you are interacting with the family who resides in the home with the patient, the patient's mother states she has concerns about the safety of the rest of the household. She reports using bleach to sterilize all of the household surfaces. Based on your knowledge, what information should be provided to the family concerning the risk of exposure when sharing the household with a person with HIV?

Answer: The patient's family needs to receive accurate education concerning the transmission of HIV. It is transmitted by infected blood, semen, cervicovaginal secretions, and breast milk. Although the virus has been identified in saliva, urine, tears, and feces, the virus cannot be transmitted by them unless they contain blood. Casual contact is considered safe. Sharing the items in the household does not present a transmission risk.

Question: A patient reports to the physician's office with complaints of a sore throat and evidence of an oral yeast infection. He reports he has experienced repeated infections and skin eruptions over the past several months. After some discussion, he indicates he is concerned about his HIV status. You ask him if he has been tested. He states he has not. When questioned about why he has not yet been tested, the patient states, "I want to. I cannot let anyone know I have been tested because of my position in the community. Besides, if I have HIV, I will die anyway." What information should be provided the patient?

Answer: The testing process is confidential. If the patient is reluctant to be tested by his primary care physician, he should be referred to a community agency. Anonymous testing is also an option. With anonymous testing, people are not required to give identifying information. The test results are tracked and monitored by numbers. The importance is not on where to be tested but simply to be tested. Testing will allow the patient to begin treatment for his condition, if needed. HIV infection is not an automatic indication of immediate death. In many cases, HIV can be successfully managed for a lengthy period of time.

Christensen & Kockrow

CRITICAL THINKING QUESTION

A female patient, age 29, recently diagnosed with HIV, has reported to the community center to receive information concerning available resources. During the intake assessment, the patient indicates she has not yet exhibited any signs and symptoms of the disease. She reports being diagnosed after attempting to donate blood. When asked if she has questions or concerns, she states, "Having AIDS has changed my life. I certainly am not ready to die before my 30th birthday, but I guess I do not have a choice." Based upon your knowledge of the disease process, what misconceptions are held by the patient concerning the illness? What information should be provided to the patient at this time?

Guidelines: Based upon the information provided, the patient most likely has been diagnosed with HIV infection. HIV infection is the terminology used to refer to the disease processes and clinical illness caused by the HIV infection. AIDS is used to describe the final stages of the HIV infection. The period between the diagnosis and death is variable. In some cases, up to 10 years can pass before the onset of symptoms. It is highly probable that this patient will see her 30th birthday. In addition, the patient will need information to demonstrate the enhanced health status that early treatment and intervention make possible.

OBJECTIVES	CONTENT	TEACHING RESOURCES
Describe the agent that causes HIV disease.	■ Nursing and the history of HIV disease (FAAHN p. 1970, AHN p. 734) ☐ Significance of the problem (FAAHN p. 1973, AHN p. 737) – Disease burden (FAAHN p. 1973, AHN p. 737)	⊠■ PPT 2, Ch. 56 FAAHN (Ch. 16 PPT 2 AHN) SG Cause of HIV, Ch. 56 p. 521 FAAHN (Ch. 16 p. 209 AHN) **BOOK RESOURCES** Table 56-1 Diagnostic Criteria for AIDS (FAAHN p. 1972) (Table 16-1 AHN p. 736) Life Span Considerations, Older Adults: HIV Disease (FAAHN p. 1973) (AHN p. 737) Cultural Considerations: HIV Disease (FAAHN p. 1974) (AHN p. 738) ▶ Discuss the history of the identification of HIV. *Class Activity Ask students to write down their personal beliefs concerning the origins of HIV and AIDS. After completion, collect the notes. They can be used to stimulate a discussion.* *Note: It might be helpful to complete this activity before the accompanying lecture.*
Provide the definition of AIDS given in January 1993 by the Centers for Disease Control and Prevention.	■ Nursing and the history of HIV disease (FAAHN p. 1973, AHN p. 737) ☐ Significance of the problem (FAAHN p. 1973, AHN p. 737) – Disease burden (FAAHN p. 1973, AHN p. 737)	⊠■ PPT 3, 4, Ch. 56 FAAHN (Ch. 16 PPT 3, 4 AHN) ⎚ EILR IC Ch. 56 image 1 FAAHN (Ch. 16 image 1 AHN) SG The Cause of HIV, Ch. 56 p. 521 FAAHN (Ch. 16 p. 209 AHN) ▶ Discuss the appropriate terminology for referring to HIV-related patients and disorders.

Adult Health Nursing, 6th ed.

Christensen & Kockrow

OBJECTIVES	CONTENT	TEACHING RESOURCES
		▶ Discuss the role of the CDC in recording the incidence of HIV.
		***Class Activity** Instruct each student to develop two NCLEX-style questions concerning the diagnostic criteria for AIDS. The questions of the entire class will be shared and used as a review.*
Explain the differences among HIV infection, HIV disease, and AIDS.	■ Nursing and the history of HIV disease (FAAHN p. 1973, AHN p. 737) ☐ Significance of the problem (FAAHN p. 1973, AHN p. 737) – Disease burden (FAAHN p. 1973, AHN p. 737)	🔲 EILR TB Ch. 56 questions 4, 5, 13 FAAHN (Ch. 16 questions 4, 5, 13 AHN) 🔲 EILR Open Book Quiz Ch. 56 question 4 FAAHN (Ch. 16 question 4 AHN) 📘 SG The Cause of HIV, Ch. 56 p. 521 FAAHN (Ch. 16 p. 209 AHN) **BOOK RESOURCES** Table 56-3 Proper Terms Related to HIV and AIDS (FAAHN p. 1981) (Table 16-3 AHN p. 745) ▶ Discuss the criteria needed for HIV to be identified as AIDS. ▶ Discuss the history of HIV infection. ***Class Activity** Ask each student to take out a piece of blank paper. Instruct students to list what they believe the differences to be among HIV infection, HIV disease, and AIDS. After completing the task, each student will select a partner. The list will be shared between the pair. To check understanding, allow students to use their books.*
Describe the progression of HIV infection.	■ Nursing and the history of HIV disease (FAAHN p. 1973, AHN p. 737) ☐ Significance of the problem (FAAHN p. 1973, AHN p. 737) – Disease burden (FAAHN p. 1973, AHN p. 737) ☐ Influences on viral load and disease progression (FAAHN p. 1978, AHN p. 742) ☐ Spectrum of HIV infection (FAAHN p. 1980, AHN p. 744) ☐ Acute retroviral syndrome (FAAHN p. 1981, AHN p. 745)	🔲 EILR IC Ch. 56 image 3 FAAHN (Ch. 16 image 3 AHN) 🔲 EILR TB Ch. 56 question 16 FAAHN (Ch. 16 question 16 AHN) 🔲 ESLR Review Questions for the NCLEX Examination Ch. 56 questions 1, 6 through 8 FAAHN (Ch. 16 question 1, 6 through 8 AHN) 📘 SG The Pathology of the HIV Infection, Ch. 56 p. 521 FAAHN (Ch. 16 p. 209 AHN) **BOOK RESOURCES** Fig. 56-2 Spectrum of HIV disease and associated signs and symptoms at various stages of the disease process (FAAHN p. 1980) (Fig. 16-2 AHN p. 744)

Adult Health Nursing, 6th ed.

Christensen & Kockrow

OBJECTIVES	CONTENT	TEACHING RESOURCES
	☐ Early infection (FAAHN p. 1981, AHN p. 745) ☐ Early symptomatic disease (FAAHN p. 1981, AHN p. 745) ☐ AIDS (FAAHN p. 1982, AHN p. 746)	▸ Discuss the concept of seroconversion. ▸ Discuss the timeline between infection by HIV and the onset of symptoms. *Class Activity Provide large sheets of unlined paper to the class. Divide the class into small groups. Instruct each group to illustrate the progression of HIV infection.*

Discuss how HIV is and is not transmitted.	■ Transmission of HIV (FAAHN p. 1974, AHN p. 738)
	
	☐ Sexual transmission (FAAHN p. 1975, AHN p. 739)
	
	☐ Parenteral exposure (FAAHN p. 1976, AHN p. 740)
	
	  – Injecting drug use (FAAHN p. 1976, AHN p. 740)
	
	  – Blood and blood products (FAAHN p. 1976, AHN p. 740)
	
	  – Occupational exposure (FAAHN p. 1976, AHN p. 740)
	
	  – Perinatal (vertical) transmission (FAAHN p. 1977, AHN p. 741)
		▱ EILR TB Ch. 56 question 1 FAAHN (Ch. 16 question 1 AHN)
		
		▱ ESLR Review Questions for the NCLEX Examination Ch. 56 questions 3 through 5 FAAHN (Ch. 16 questions 3 through 5 AHN)
		
		▱ SG Risk for HIV Ch. 56 p. 524 FAAHN (Ch. 16 p. 212 AHN)
		
		BOOK RESOURCES
		Fig. 56-1 Viral load in the blood and the relationship to CD 4+ lymphocyte cell count over the spectrum of HIV disease (FAAHN p. 1975) (Fig. 16-1 AHN p. 739)
		
		Table 56-2 Types of White Blood Cells and their Involvement in HIV Disease (FAAHN p. 1979) (Table 16-2 AHN p. 743)
		
		▸ Discuss the body fluids in which HIV can be found.
		
		▸ Discuss the types of contact associated with the transmission of HIV.
		
		Class Activity Divide the students into small groups. Instruct the groups to discuss and make a list of misconceptions they have heard or personally hold regarding the transmission of HIV.

Describe patients who are at risk for HIV infection.	■ Trends and most affected populations (FAAHN p. 1973, AHN p. 737)	▱ PPT 5, 6, Ch. 56 FAAHN (Ch. 16 PPT 5, 6 AHN) ▱ EILR TB Ch. 56 questions 3, 8, 18, 26, 28 FAAHN (Ch. 16 questions 3, 8, 18, 26, 28 AHN) ▱ EILR Open Book Quiz Ch. 56 question 2 FAAHN (Ch. 16 question 2 AHN) ▱ ESLR Review Questions for the NCLEX Examination Ch. 56 question 2 FAAHN (Ch. 16 question 2 AHN)

Mosby items and derived items © 2011 by Mosby, Inc., an affiliate of Elsevier Inc.
Some material was previously published.

Christensen & Kockrow

OBJECTIVES	CONTENT	TEACHING RESOURCES
		SG Risk for HIV, Ch. 56 p. 524 FAAHN (Ch. 16 p. 212 AHN)
		BOOK RESOURCES
		Cultural Considerations: HIV Disease (FAAHN p. 1974, AHN p. 738)
		Box 56-9 Risk of HIV Transmission Associated with Sexual Practices (FAAHN p. 2008) (Box 16-9 AHN p. 772)
		▶ Discuss behaviors that increase the risk of HIV infection.
		▶ Discuss the information that should be provided to the families of patients living with HIV concerning the risk of infection.
		*Class Activity **Divide the students into pairs. In each pair, one person will act as the patient and the other as the nurse. Instruct each pair to role-play a teaching session geared to provide education to the members of the household of a person living with HIV.***
Discuss the pathophysiology of HIV disease.	■ Pathophysiology (FAAHN p. 1978, AHN p. 742) ☐ Influences on viral load and disease progression (FAAHN p. 1978, AHN p. 742) ☐ Spectrum of HIV infection (FAAHN p. 1980, AHN p. 744) ☐ Acute retroviral syndrome (FAAHN p. 1981, AHN p. 745) ☐ Early infection (FAAHN p. 1981, AHN p. 745) ☐ Early symptomatic disease (FAAHN p. 1981, AHN p. 745) ☐ AIDS (FAAHN p. 1982, AHN p. 746)	PPT 7 through 12, Ch. 56 FAAHN (Ch. 16 PPT 7 through 12 AHN) EILR TB Ch. 56 question 12 FAAHN (Ch. 16 question 12 AHN) EILR Open Book Quiz Ch. 56 question 3 FAAHN (Ch. 16 question 3 AHN) SG The Pathology of the HIV Infection, Ch. 56 p. 521 FAAHN (Ch. 16 p. 209 AHN) ▶ Discuss the replication process of the virus once introduced into the human body. ▶ Discuss the involvement of white blood cells in the pathophysiology of HIV. *Class Activity **Instruct each student to develop two NCLEX-style questions concerning the pathophysiology of HIV. Once completed, collect the questions and mix them up. Redistribute the questions and ask each student to meet with four other students to share the questions. Review.***

Christensen & Kockrow

List signs and symptoms that may be indicative of HIV disease.	■ Spectrum of HIV infection (FAAHN p. 1980, AHN p. 744) □ Acute retroviral syndrome (FAAHN p. 1981, AHN p. 745) □ Early infection (FAAHN p. 1981, AHN p. 745) □ Early symptomatic disease (FAAHN p. 1981, AHN p. 745) □ AIDS (FAAHN p. 1982, AHN p. 746)	PPT 13 through 17, Ch. 56 FAAHN (Ch. 16 PPT 13 through 17 AHN) EILR IC Ch. 56 image 2 FAAHN (Ch. 16 image 2 AHN) EILR TB Ch. 56 question 27 FAAHN (Ch. 16 question 27 AHN) SG The Pathology of the HIV Infection, Ch. 56 p. 521 FAAHN (Ch. 16 p. 209 AHN) **BOOK RESOURCES** Fig. 56-2 Spectrum of HIV disease and associated signs and symptoms at various stages of the disease process (FAAHN p. 1980) (Fig. 16-2 AHN p. 744) Table 56-4 Primary HIV Infection: Signs and Symptoms (FAAHN p. 1981) (Table 16-4 AHN p. 745) Box 56-1 Signs and Symptoms of HIV Infection (FAAHN p. 1982) (Box 16-1 AHN p. 746) ▸ Discuss the incidence of seroconversion syndrome. ▸ Discuss the signs of early infection and their impact on the delay in seeking treatment. *Class Activity Divide the class into three or four teams. Using content covered, ask questions of each team. For each correct answer, award 1 point. After asking 10 to 15 questions, tally the points. The team with the most points wins.* *Note: If the class is large, more teams might be needed. Have the teams raise hands when they have the correct answer, and call on the team who first raised hands. Another option is to ask each team one question at a time.*
Discuss the laboratory and diagnostic tests related to HIV disease.	■ Diagnostic tests (FAAHN p. 1983, AHN p. 747) □ HIV antibody testing (FAAHN p. 1983, AHN p. 747) □ CD_4^+ cell monitoring (FAAHN p. 1983, AHN p. 747) □ Viral load monitoring (FAAHN p. 1983, AHN p. 747)	PPT 18 through 20, Ch. 56 FAAHN (Ch. 16 PPT 18 through 20 AHN) EILR IC Ch. 56 image 1 FAAHN (Ch. 16 image 1 AHN) EILR TB Ch. 56 questions 2, 6, 7, 19 FAAHN (Ch. 16 questions 2, 6, 7, 19 AHN) ESLR Review Questions for the NCLEX Examination Ch. 56 question 9 FAAHN (Ch. 16 question 9 AHN)

ELSEVIER

Adult Health Nursing, 6th ed.

Mosby items and derived items © 2011 by Mosby, Inc., an affiliate of Elsevier Inc.
Some material was previously published.

Christensen & Kockrow

	☐ Resistance testing (FAAHN p. 1985, AHN p. 749) ☐ Other laboratory parameters (FAAHN p. 1985, AHN p. 749)	SG Diagnostic Tests, Ch. 56 p. 523 FAAHN (Ch. 16 p. 211 AHN) **BOOK RESOURCES** Table 56-2 Types of White Blood Cells and their Involvement in HIV Disease (FAAHN p. 1979) (Table 16-2 AHN p. 743) ▸ Discuss the impact of early testing and diagnosis on the successful management and treatment of HIV. ▸ Discuss the testing available to diagnose HIV. ***Class Activity Contact the laboratory at the local hospital. Obtain the forms that are needed to perform HIV testing. Copy and bring the forms to the class. Distribute forms to the class to review and study.***

16.1 Homework/Assignments:

16.1 Instructor's Notes/Student Feedback:

LESSON 16.2

CRITICAL THINKING QUESTION

While working at a hospice, you are caring for a young gay man in the final stages of AIDS. You begin noticing behavioral changes in his sister. She appears tired and, when questioned, she reports abdominal pain, anorexia, and shortness of breath. She also states she has not been sleeping much since finding out that her brother's death is anticipated at any time. Based upon your knowledge, what is being experienced by the patient's sister? What can be done to assist her?

Guidelines: The patient's sister could be experiencing disenfranchised grief. This can result when a loss results that is difficult to publicly acknowledge. HIV and AIDS are still viewed by many members of society as taboo. Allowing the members of the family to ventilate their concerns and feelings will assist them in overcoming this hurdle. Ongoing problems require a referral to a counselor or physician.

OBJECTIVES	CONTENT	TEACHING RESOURCES
Discuss the issues related to HIV antibody testing.	■ Diagnostic tests (FAAHN p. 1983, AHN p. 747) □ HIV antibody testing (FAAHN p. 1983, AHN p. 747)	⚡ EILR Open Book Quiz Ch. 56 questions 5, 9 FAAHN (Ch. 16 questions 5, 9 AHN) 📓 SG Issues with Testing, Ch. 56 p. 525 FAAHN (Ch. 16 p. 213 AHN) **BOOK RESOURCES** Box 56-3 Pretest and Posttest Counseling Associated with HIV-Antibody Testing (FAAHN p. 1984) (Box 16-3 AHN p. 748) ▶ Discuss the recommended frequency for HIV testing. ▶ Discuss common concerns held by the public concerning HIV testing. *Class Activity Divide the students into groups of two or three. Instruct each team to discuss and record what it thinks is the role of the nurse in caring for the person undergoing testing for HIV.*
Describe the multidisciplinary approach in caring for a patient with HIV disease.	■ Therapeutic management (FAAHN p. 1985, AHN p. 749) □ Pharmacological management (FAAHN p. 1985, AHN p. 749) – Opportunistic diseases associated with HIV (FAAHN p. 1985, AHN p. 749) – Antiretroviral therapy (FAAHN p. 1986, AHN p. 750)	⚡ EILR TB Ch. 56 questions 21 through 23 FAAHN (Ch. 16 questions 21 through 23 AHN) ⚡ EILR Open Book Quiz Ch. 56 questions 4, 7 FAAHN (Ch. 16 questions 4, 7 AHN) ⚡ ESLR Review Questions for the NCLEX Examination Ch. 56 question 10 FAAHN (Ch. 16 question 10 AHN) 📓 SG Multidisciplinary Care, Ch. 56 p. 527 FAAHN (Ch. 16 p. 215 AHN)

Mosby items and derived items © 2011 by Mosby, Inc., an affiliate of Elsevier Inc.
Some material was previously published.

OBJECTIVES	CONTENT	TEACHING RESOURCES
	– Alternative and complementary therapies (FAAHN p. 1993, AHN p. 757)	**BOOK RESOURCES** Table 56-7 Pros and Cons of Highly Active Antiretroviral Therapy (HAART) (FAAHN p. 1989) (Table 16-7 AHN p. 753) Table 56-8 Medications for HIV Disease (Antiretrovirals) (FAAHN p. 1989) (Table 16-8 AHN p.753) ▶ Discuss the different disciplines needed to provide comprehensive care to the patient and family living with a HIV diagnosis. ▶ Discuss the health care priorities for a patient diagnosed with HIV. ***Class Activity Instruct students to brainstorm about resources in the local community that are available and needed by the patient and family living with HIV. Allow 3 to 5 minutes for this portion. Next, ask the students to gather in groups of three or four to share ideas. If time permits, allow groups to share findings with the larger class.***
List opportunistic infections associated with advanced HIV disease.	– Opportunistic diseases associated with HIV (FAAHN p. 1985, AHN p. 749)	PPT 22 through 29, Ch. 56 FAAHN (Ch. 16 PPT 22 through 29 AHN) EILR IC Ch. 56 image 4 FAAHN (Ch. 16 image 4 AHN) EILR TB Ch. 56 questions 10, 11 FAAHN (Ch. 16 questions 10, 11 AHN) EILR Open Book Quiz Ch. 56 question 8 FAAHN (Ch. 16 question 8 AHN) SG Opportunistic Infections, Ch. 56 p. 527 FAAHN (Ch. 16 p. 215 AHN) **BOOK RESOURCES** Fig. 56-4 Oral candidiasis (FAAHN p. 1982) (Fig. 16-4 AHN p. 746) Table 56-5 Common Opportunistic Diseases Associated with HIV/AIDS (FAAHN p. 1987) (Table 16-5 AHN p. 751) Table 56-6 Opportunistic Illness Prophylaxis Guidelines (FAAHN p. 1988) (Table 16-6 AHN p. 752) ▶ Discuss the impact of opportunistic infections associated with advanced HIV disease. ▶ Discuss the opportunistic infections by body system associated with advanced HIV disease.

Christensen & Kockrow

OBJECTIVES	CONTENT	TEACHING RESOURCES
		Class Activity Divide students into groups of three to five. Assign each group one opportunistic infection commonly associated with advanced HIV disease. Instruct groups to investigate the signs and symptoms and management of the disease. After this is completed, ask the groups to meet with a group having a different type of infection. Allow each group to share its findings with the class. Only allow 5 minutes for this portion.
Discuss the nurse's role in assisting the HIV-infected patient with coping, grieving, reducing anxiety, and minimizing social isolation.	■ Nursing interventions (FAAHN p. 1993, AHN p. 757) □ Adherence (FAAHN p. 1996, AHN p. 760) □ Palliative care (FAAHN p. 1997, AHN p. 761) □ Psychosocial issues (FAAHN p. 1998, AHN p. 762) □ Assisting with coping (FAAHN p. 1998, AHN p. 762) □ Minimizing social isolation (FAAHN p. 1998, AHN p. 762) – Assisting with grieving (FAAHN p. 1999, AHN p. 763) □ Confidentiality (FAAHN p. 1999, AHN p. 763) □ Duty to treat (FAAHN p. 1999, AHN p. 763) □ Ethical and legal principles (FAAHN p. 1999, AHN p. 763) □ Acute intervention (FAAHN p. 1999, AHN p. 763) – Wasting and lipodystrophy syndromes (FAAHN p. 2001, AHN p. 765) – Neurological complications (FAAHN p. 2003, AHN p. 767) – Management of opportunistic infections (FAAHN p. 2005, AHN p. 769)	⊠ PPT 30 through 39, Ch. 56 FAAHN (Ch. 16 PPT 30 through 39 AHN) ▰ EILR TB Ch. 56 questions 15, 20 FAAHN (Ch. 16 questions 15, 20 AHN) ▰ SG Nurse's Role, Ch. 56 p. 526 FAAHN (Ch. 16 p. 214 AHN) **BOOK RESOURCES** Box 56-5 Nursing Interventions for the Patient with HIV Infection or HIV Disease (FAAHN p. 1986) (Box 16-5 AHN p. 750) Table 56-8 Medications for HIV Disease (Antiretrovirals) (FAAHN p. 1989) (Table 16-8 AHN p. 753) Box 56-4 Nursing Assessment of the Patient with HIV Infection (FAAHN p. 1994) (Box 16-4 AHN p. 758) Box 56-6 Psychological Crisis Intervals in the Course of HIV Disease (FAAHN p. 1998) (Box 16-6 AHN p. 762) Box 56-7 Conducting a Risk Assessment (FAAHN p. 2000) (Box 16-7 AHN p.764) ▸ Discuss concerns of students associated with providing care to HIV-positive patients and their families. ▸ Discuss the rights of the HIV-positive patient to have safe, quality care provided. *Class Activity Develop several scenarios relating to the concerns of a person living with HIV. Write them on small note cards. Divide the students into pairs. Ask one student to be the patient and the other, the nurse. Instruct them to role-play the scenario.*

ELSEVIER

OBJECTIVES	CONTENT	TEACHING RESOURCES
	– Health promotion (FAAHN p. 2005, AHN p. 769)	
Implement a care plan for the patient with AIDS.	■ Nursing interventions (FAAHN p. 1993, AHN p. 757) ☐ Adherence (FAAHN p. 1996, AHN p. 760) ☐ Palliative care (FAAHN p. 1997, AHN p. 761) ☐ Psychosocial issues (FAAHN p. 1998, AHN p. 762) ☐ Assisting with coping (FAAHN p. 1998, AHN p. 762) ☐ Minimizing social isolation (FAAHN p. 1998, AHN p. 762) ☐ Assisting with grieving (FAAHN p. 1999, AHN p. 763) ☐ Confidentiality (FAAHN p. 1999, AHN p. 763) ☐ Duty to treat (FAAHN p. 1999, AHN p. 763) – Ethical and legal principles (FAAHN p. 1999, AHN p. 763) ☐ Acute intervention (FAAHN p. 1999, AHN p. 763) – Wasting and lipodystrophy syndromes (FAAHN p. 2001, AHN p. 765) – Neurological complications (FAAHN p. 2003, AHN p. 767) – Management of opportunistic infections (FAAHN p. 2005, AHN p. 769) – Health promotion (FAAHN p. 2005, AHN p. 769)	PPT 37 through 39, Ch. 56 FAAHN (Ch. 16 PPT 37 through 39 AHN) EILR TB Ch. 56 questions 14, 25, 29, 30 FAAHN (Ch. 16 questions 14, 25, 29, 30 AHN) SG Care Plan, Ch. 56 p. 528 FAAHN (Ch. 16 p. 216 AHN) **BOOK RESOURCES** Table 56-10 Factors Related to Nonadherent Behavior (FAAHN p. 1997) (Table 16-10 AHN p. 761) Nursing Care Plan 56-1 The Patient Who Is HIV Positive (FAAHN p. 2004) (NCP 16-1 AHN p. 768) NCP CTQ 1 through 3 (FAAHN p. 2004) (AHN p. 768) Health Promotion: The Patient Infected with HIV (FAAHN p. 2005) (AHN p. 769) ▶ Discuss the goals of the plan of care for the patient diagnosed with HIV. ▶ Discuss the nursing diagnoses applicable for the patient living with HIV infection. *Class Activity Contact a local HIV treatment center. Ask a speaker to come to class to discuss treatment options available for HIV and AIDS patients and their families in the community.*
Discuss the importance of adherence to HIV treatment.	☐ Adherence (FAAHN p. 1996, AHN p. 760)	**BOOK RESOURCES** Table 56-9 Nursing Activities in HIV Disease (FAAHN p. 1995) (Table 16-9 AHN p. 759) ▶ Discuss factors associated with nonadherent behaviors with the prescribed treatment plan.

ELSEVIER

OBJECTIVES	CONTENT	TEACHING RESOURCES
		▸ Discuss the potential roadblocks for the patient living with HIV in maintaining the prescribed treatment plan. *Class Activity Divide the class into groups of three students. Instruct each group to modify a care plan for the person living with HIV. Each care plan should include three prioritized nursing diagnoses and three nursing interventions.*
Discuss the use of effective prevention messages in counseling patients.	■ Prevention of HIV infection (FAAHN p. 2005, AHN p. 769) ☐ HIV testing and counseling (FAAHN p. 2005, AHN p. 769) ☐ Risk assessment and risk reduction (FAAHN p. 2007, AHN p. 771) ☐ Barriers to prevention (FAAHN p. 2007, AHN p. 771) ☐ Reducing risks related to sexual transmission (FAAHN p. 2007, AHN p. 771) ☐ Reducing risks related to drug abuse (FAAHN p. 2009, AHN p. 773) ☐ Reducing risks related to occupational exposure (FAAHN p. 2009, AHN p. 773) ☐ Other methods to reduce risk (FAAHN p. 2010, AHN p. 774)	PPT 40 through 47, Ch. 56 FAAHN (Ch. 16 PPT 40 through 47 AHN) SG Risk for HIV, Ch. 56 p. 524 FAAHN (Ch. 16 p. 212 AHN) **BOOK RESOURCES** Box 56-8 Prevention Options (FAAHN p. 2006) (Box 16-8 AHN p. 770) Box 56-9 Risk of HIV Transmission Associated with Sexual Practices (FAAHN p. 2008) (Box 16-9 AHN p. 772) ▸ Discuss the availability of testing for HIV in the community. ▸ Discuss the presence of educational programs in the community and their intended audience. *Class Activity Contact the Department of Health. Obtain copies of pamphlets that are used to educate the public concerning HIV and AIDS. Copy and distribute these to the class. Ask the class to review the pamphlets and determine if they are appropriate for their intended audience. After completing the review, ask students to meet in small groups and discuss the messages available to the public.*
Define the nurse's role in the prevention of HIV infection.	■ Prevention of HIV infection (FAAHN p. 2005, AHN p. 769) ☐ HIV testing and counseling (FAAHN p. 2005, AHN p. 769) ☐ Risk assessment and risk reduction (FAAHN p. 2007, AHN p. 771) ☐ Barriers to prevention (FAAHN p. 2007, AHN p. 771)	PPT 40 through 48, Ch. 56 FAAHN (Ch. 16 PPT 40 through 48 AHN) EILR TB Ch. 56 questions 9, 17, 24 FAAHN (Ch. 16 questions 9, 17, 24 AHN) EILR Open Book Quiz Ch. 56 question 10 FAAHN (Ch. 16 question 10 AHN) SG The Cause of HIV, Ch. 56 p. 521 FAAHN (Ch. 16 p. 209 AHN)

Adult Health Nursing, 6th ed.

Christensen & Kockrow

OBJECTIVES	CONTENT	TEACHING RESOURCES
	☐ Reducing risks related to sexual transmission (FAAHN p. 2007, AHN p. 771) ☐ Reducing risks related to drug abuse (FAAHN p. 2009, AHN p. 773) ☐ Reducing risks related to occupational exposure (FAAHN p. 2009, AHN p. 773) ☐ Other methods to reduce risk (FAAHN p. 2010, AHN p. 774) ■ Outlook for the future (FAAHN p. 2010, AHN p. 774)	▸ Discuss populations having the greatest need for education concerning HIV infection. ▸ Discuss the information most needed by the public to prevent HIV infection. **Class Activity** *Invite a nurse to speak to the students concerning their role in education to prevent spread of the HIV infection.* *Note: A source for the speaker could be a local family planning clinic or the Department of Health in the local community.*
Performance Evaluation		🖻 EILR TB Ch. 56 questions 1 through 39 FAAHN (Ch. 16 questions 1 through 39 AHN) 🖻 EILR Open Book Quiz Ch. 56 questions 1 through 10 FAAHN (Ch. 16 questions 1 through 10 AHN) 📖 SG Ch. 56 pp. 521 through 530 FAAHN (Ch. 56 pp. 209 through 218 AHN) **BOOK RESOURCES** Nursing Care Plan 56-1 The Patient Who Is HIV Positive (FAAHN p. 2004) (NCP 16-1 AHN p. 768) 💡 NCP CTQ 1 through 3 (FAAHN p. 2004) (AHN p. 768) Review Questions for the NCLEX Examination Ch. 56 questions 1 through 34 FAAHN (Ch. 56 question 1 through 34 AHN)

16.2 Homework/Assignments:

16.2 Instructor's Notes/Student Feedback:

Slide 1

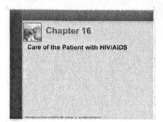

Slide 2

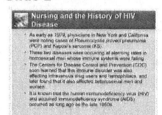

- Although HIV has been known to have been in existence since the 1950s, it was not widely known until the 1980s.

- Ask students when they can first recall having ever heard about HIV.

Slide 3

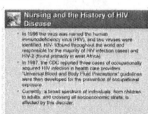

- What influences has the population initially known to be most impacted by HIV had on advances in treatment and research?

- What other elements associated with HIV influenced the perception of the disease?

Slide 4

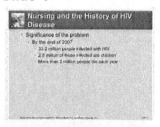

- HIV is a deadly diagnosis. To optimize the prognosis and lengthen the life span, prompt diagnosis and treatment are needed.

- What factors are responsible for many potentially HIV-positive individuals not seeking diagnostic information?

Slide 5

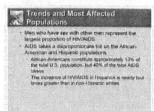

- Disparity is evident between the races regarding the number of new cases.

- The number of cases among African Americans and Hispanics is growing at an alarming rate.

- What factors could explain this phenomenon?

ELSEVIER

Adult Health Nursing, 6th ed.
Christensen & Kockrow

Slide 6

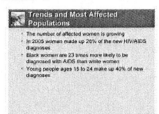

- What factors may be responsible for the disparity of statistics between differing groups of women?

Slide 7

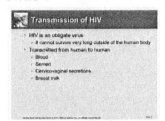

- Research has consistently supported the primary means of disease transmission. It cannot be transmitted via casual contact or by living with an infected person.

- What misconceptions might be held by members of society concerning the transmission of HIV?

Slide 8

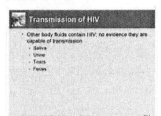

- HIV has also been identified in saliva, urine, tears, and feces. It has not, however, been shown to use those body fluids for transmission to others.

- Reinforce the need for the consistent use of standard precautions.

Slide 9

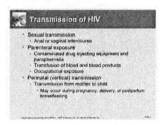

- Occupational exposure is a risk and of concern for all members of the health care team.

- What clinical areas carry the greatest risk?

Slide 10

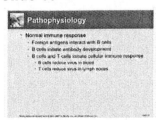

- HIV is a slow retrovirus or lentivirus. A long period of time typically passes between infection and the appearance of signs and symptoms.

- There is an initial body response to restore and maintain health after becoming infected with HIV. The body's own efforts work to manage the infection in both the blood and lymph nodes.

- To what could this body response be compared?

Slide 11

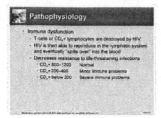

- The CD4 cells are key to the virus' ability to remain active in the body.
- What role do they play?

Slide 12

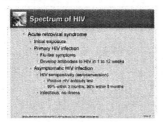

- The term "HIV" has been used to refer to all of the illnesses caused by the virus. Historically, AIDS-related complex and AIDS have been used inappropriately.
- Since beginning this unit, what misconceptions have been identified?
- Direct students to share their own personal misconceptions.

Slide 13

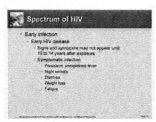

- During the early phase of HIV infection, the individual might not realize he/she has the virus. During this time, there are few clinical manifestations pointing toward HIV.
- How does this lack of knowledge impact the individual's behaviors?
- What identified factors have an influence on the length of time before the patient exhibits symptoms?

Slide 14

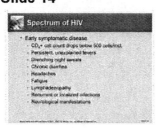

- Although symptoms exist during the early symptomatic period of the disease, there might still be a delay for seeking treatment. The clinical manifestations could be vague or attributed to other factors.
- What populations have a more rapid disease progression?

Slide 15

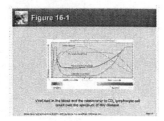

ELSEVIER

Mosby items and derived items © 2011, 2007 by Mosby, Inc., an affiliate of Elsevier Inc.
Some material was previously published.

Adult Health Nursing, 6th ed.
Christensen & Kockrow

Slide 16

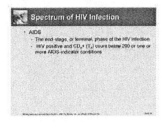

- The CD_4+ count is used as an indicator of the disease's progression. Explain the term CD4+ cell count.

- The Centers for Disease Control and Prevention (CDC) has developed criteria to be used for the classification of the disease process. Review this system.

Slide 17

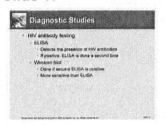

- An early diagnosis of HIV allows for vital treatment to begin. Studies have shown early intervention is closely tied with successful management and increased survival rates.

- ELISA and the Western blot tests are needed to identify a positive HIV status.

- Relay the steps for administration of the ELISA and Western blot test.

Slide 18

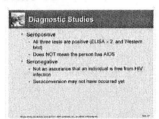

- The terms "seropositive" and "seronegative" are used to illustrate HIV testing outcomes.

- What length of time normally passes between infection and a positive HIV test?

Slide 19

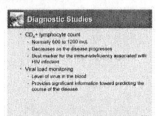

- Once a positive HIV status is established, it is necessary to monitor the CD_4+ count and viral load of the patient's blood.

- What are the nurse's responsibilities concerning the pretest and posttest counseling?

Slide 20

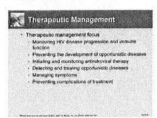

- The words "HIV positive" are considered by many to be a death sentence. To ensure the best possible outcomes for the patient, what are three priorities that should be reflected in patient goals?

ELSEVIER

Adult Health Nursing, 6th ed.

Mosby items and derived items © 2011, 2007 by Mosby, Inc., an affiliate of Elsevier Inc.
Some material was previously published.

Christensen & Kockrow

Slide 21

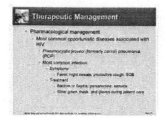

- Management of opportunistic infections is the largest hurdle for patients living with HIV and their health care providers.
- The use of prophylactic medications is employed. What characteristics are needed in the HIV-infected person to begin treatment?
- Discuss goals for the antiretroviral therapies.

Slide 22

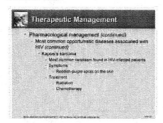

- When medications are prescribed to manage and prevent opportunistic infections, what education should accompany each prescribed course of therapy?

Slide 23

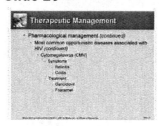

- Compare and contrast the use of "cocktails" and single-drug therapy when managing HIV infection.

Slide 24

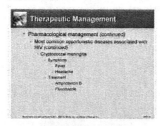

- Previous antiretroviral experience could impact the success of the plan of care. Discuss this impact.

Slide 25

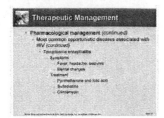

ELSEVIER

Mosby items and derived items © 2011, 2007 by Mosby, Inc., an affiliate of Elsevier Inc.
Some material was previously published.

Adult Health Nursing, 6th ed.
Christensen & Kockrow

Slide 26

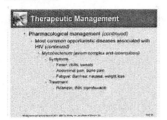

Slide 27

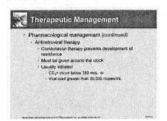

- The use of medications will have numerous implications for both the patient and his family. Identify these issues.

Slide 28

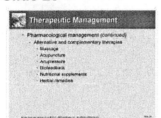

- The use of nonpharmacological therapies in the care of HIV is often employed by patients and recommended by health care providers.

- What information should be provided to the patient concerning the use of alternative therapies by the nurse?

Slide 29

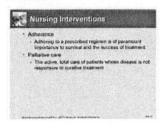

- The treatment regimen to manage HIV infection is complex and often difficult to follow. What factors could reduce the patient's ability/desire to follow the plan of care?

- Disenfranchised grief could be associated with the loss of a family member due to HIV. Explain this concept.

Slide 30

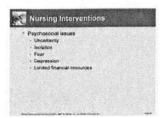

- Any potentially terminal diagnosis is associated with psychosocial issues. Compare the psychosocial concerns of the patient diagnosed with HIV and other terminal illnesses.

ELSEVIER

Adult Health Nursing, 6th ed.

Mosby items and derived items © 2011, 2007 by Mosby, Inc., an affiliate of Elsevier Inc.
Some material was previously published.

Christensen & Kockrow

Slide 31

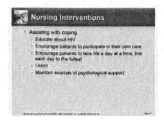

- The diagnosis of HIV is associated with valleys and plateaus.

- Identify events along the path of HIV infection progression that will require increased assistance with coping.

Slide 32

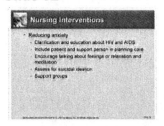

- Open communication is vital to successful case management for the person living with HIV. Who should be included in the treatment plan for the patient?

- Because of the implications of the HIV diagnosis, patients could experience impaired abilities to manage the activities of daily living. Depression is common.

- What clues might exist to alert the nurse of the need for increased intervention or referrals?

Slide 33

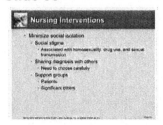

- Unfortunately, some members of society hold misconceptions and are guilty of stereotyping people infected with HIV. Fear of these behaviors can result in the patient avoiding social contacts.

- Discuss the need for support in dealing with the diagnosis of HIV. What resources exist locally to assist patients with an HIV diagnosis?

Slide 34

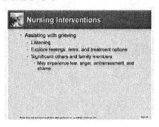

- Being faced with HIV causes individuals to face their own mortality in a potentially accelerated fashion. In addition to the potential for death, there are other losses experienced by the HIV-positive person.

- List some of the emotional losses that might be faced by the HIV-positive person.

Slide 35

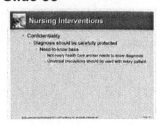

- A source of concern and potential debate by health care providers involves the health care team's right to be apprised of a patient's HIV status.

- Do you feel health care providers have the right to be advised of a patient's positive HIV status? Why or why not?

ELSEVIER

Christensen & Kockrow

Slide 36

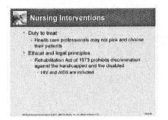

- Patients diagnosed with HIV are entitled to the same quality care as non-HIV-positive patients. Refusal to treat HIV-infected patients is not ethical.

- Ask members of the class what concerns they hold about caring for HIV-positive patients.

Slide 37

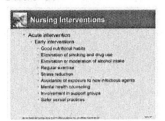

- Beginning treatment interventions early in the progression of HIV will help the patient maintain health status longer.

- Education is needed to inform the patient of health promotion behaviors.

- What topics should be covered? Who should be included in patient education?

Slide 38

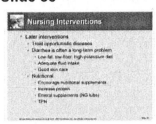

- As the disease progresses, the educational topics will become more complicated. The focus will begin to include the management of opportunistic infections as they result.

- What are two patient-focused goals for the patient relating to education/knowledge during the later stages of the disease?

Slide 39

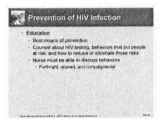

Slide 40

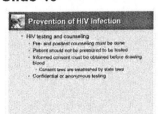

- HIV infection is often asymptomatic in the early stages. Testing is needed to give the patient the knowledge of his/her status to seek treatment to reduce and/or prolong the onset of complications.

- What information is needed by the patient prior to testing?

- What testing sites are available in the community? Is there a fee involved?

Slide 41

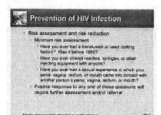

- It is a responsibility of nurses to be aware of risk factors associated with HIV infection. When patients present with behaviors or clinical manifestations associated with an increased incidence of HIV infection, the need for testing must be evaluated.

- Discuss the manner in which the need for further evaluation of potential HIV positive status will need to be introduced.

Slide 42

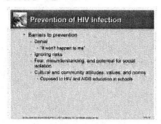

- There are numerous reasons people avoid being tested for HIV infection.

- Failure to be tested increases the risk of transmission and reduces the ability of the body to fight off opportunistic infections related to the delayed initiation of treatment.

- When a person at an increased or high risk for HIV is putting up roadblocks to avoid testing, what can the nurse do?

Slide 43

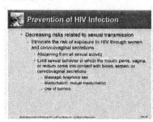

- Eliminating high-risk behaviors can curb the spread of HIV.

- Identify opportunities to provide education to at-risk populations.

Slide 44

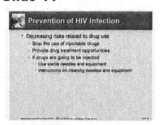

- Users of illegal IV drugs are at an increased risk of HIV. Transmission is possible via contaminated needles.

- Is a needle exchange program available in your community?

Slide 45

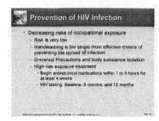

- Health care workers are at an increased risk of exposure to contaminated materials. The use of standard precautions will aid in reducing the incidence of exposure.

- When exposed to potentially contaminated materials or secretions, what steps will the nurse need to take?

Christensen & Kockrow

Slide 46

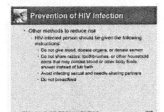

- The person living with HIV infection will need to be responsible to prevent the transmission of his/her infection to others.

- List sources of information available to the patient living with HIV.

Slide 47

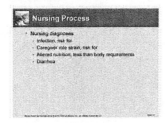

ELSEVIER

Mosby items and derived items © 2011, 2007 by Mosby, Inc., an affiliate of Elsevier Inc.
Some material was previously published.

Adult Health Nursing, 6th ed.
Christensen & Kockrow

TEACHING FOCUS

In this chapter, the student will be introduced to the care of the patient with cancer. The student will begin by exploring risk factors and warning signs of cancer, along with the incidence of cancer in the United States. The student will have the opportunity to learn about the development, prevention, and detection of cancer, along with the terminology used in oncology, the pathophysiology of cancer, and the process of metastasis. The student will explore the diagnostic tests used to identify the presence of cancer, recommended preventive behaviors, tumor classification, tumor lysis syndrome, and guidelines for pain relief. Finally, the student will explore nursing interventions for the patient undergoing various kinds of cancer treatment.

MATERIALS AND RESOURCES

- ☐ Computer/overhead projector (Lessons 17.1 and 17.2)
- ☐ White/black board and marker/chalk (Lessons 17.1 and 17.2)
- ☐ Blank note cards (Lesson 17.1)
- ☐ Pamphlets on screening for cancer from the American Cancer Society (Lesson 17.1)
- ☐ Three scenarios describing patients with cancer (Lesson 17.1)
- ☐ Copies of screening tools used to grade and stage tumors, and copies of forms used to record screening results, from a local oncologist (Lesson 17.2)
- ☐ Large diagram of the human body (Lesson 17.2)
- ☐ Small ball or other soft object that can be passed around the classroom (Lesson 17.2)
- ☐ Pain management scale chart (Lesson 17.2)

LESSON CHECKLIST

Preparations for this lesson include:

- Lecture
- Invite a speaker from the American Cancer Society to discuss screening and diagnostic test recommendations.
- Invite a surgical nurse from a local hospital to discuss steps taken with biopsy samples.

KEY TERMS

alopecia (FAAHN p. 2032, AHN p. 796)
autologous (FAAHN p. 2036, AHN p. 800)
benign (FAAHN p. 2021, AHN p. 785)
biopsy (FAAHN p. 2022, AHN p. 786)
cachexia (FAAHN p. 2037, AHN p. 801)
carcinogen (FAAHN p. 2015, AHN p. 779)
carcinogenesis (FAAHN p. 2015, AHN p. 779)
carcinoma (FAAHN p. 2021, AHN p. 785)
differentiated (FAAHN p. 2021, AHN p. 785)
immunosurveillance (FAAHN p. 2021, AHN p. 785)
leukopenia (FAAHN p. 2028, AHN p. 792)
malignant (FAAHN p. 2021, AHN p. 785)

metastasis (FAAHN p. 2021, AHN p. 785)
neoplasm (FAAHN p. 2021, AHN p. 785)
oncology (FAAHN p. 2014, AHN p. 778)
palliative (FAAHN p. 2025, AHN p. 789)
Papanicolaou's test (smear) (FAAHN p. 2022, AHN p. 786)
sarcoma (FAAHN p. 2021, AHN p. 785)
stomatitis (FAAHN p. 2032, AHN p. 796)
thrombocytopenia (FAAHN p. 2032, AHN p. 796)
tumor lysis lysis syndrome (FAAHN p. 2035, AHN p. 799)

ADDITIONAL RESOURCES (AHN)

PPT Ch. 57, 1 through 25 FAAHN (Ch. 17, 1 through 25 AHN)
EILR IC images Ch. 57, 1 through 3 FAAHN (Ch. 17, 1 through 3 AHN)
EILR TB questions Ch. 57, 1 through 40 FAAHN (Ch. 17, 1 through 40 AHN)
EILR Open Book Quiz Ch. 57, 1 through 10 FAAHN (Ch. 17, 1 through 10 AHN)
ESLR Review Questions for the NCLEX® Examination Ch. 57, 57-01 through 57-10 FAAHN (Ch. 17, 17-01 through 17-10 AHN)

Legend

PPT
PowerPoint
Slides

EILR
EVOLVE Instructor
Learning Resources:
Image Collection, Test
Bank, Open Book Quizzes

ESLR
EVOLVE Student
Learning Resources:
Review Questions
for the NCLEX
Examination

SG
Study Guide

NCP CTQ
Nursing Care Plan
Critical Thinking
Question

Class Activities are indicated in **bold italic**.

LESSON 17.1

PRETEST

1. When counseling a 16-year-old male about the use of smokeless tobacco, he says that because there is no smoke, he does not need to be concerned about lung cancer. What is the best response from the nurse?
   a. "You certainly are correct. Smokeless tobacco is safe for your use."
   b. "Smokeless tobacco is associated with cancer of the liver and pancreas."
   c. "Your risk of mouth, larynx, pharynx, and esophageal cancer will increase with the use of smokeless tobacco."
   d. "It is still not clear what cancer risks are increased by the use of smokeless tobacco."

2. _____ has been identified as a risk factor for the development of breast, prostate, and ovarian cancers.
   a. Obesity
   b. Smoking
   c. Radiation exposure
   d. Chlorine

3. A woman of Japanese descent voices concerns about her risk for breast cancer. What should she be told?
   a. "Breast cancer is common in Japanese women."
   b. "There is little breast cancer found in Japanese women."
   c. "Your risk of developing breast cancer is higher before menopause."
   d. "Breast cancer should not be a concern for you."

4. When preparing to instruct a group of students about making dietary changes to reduce the incidence of breast cancer, which of the following factors is correct?
   a. White cheese should be substituted for yellow cheese whenever possible.
   b. Heavy alcohol intake could increase the risk of breast and uterine cancer.
   c. The daily diet should include four servings of fruits and vegetables.
   d. Cauliflower, carrots, and cantaloupe are the best sources of beta-carotene.

5. When considering the impact of dietary intake on the development of cancer, which of the following statements is correct?
   a. Nearly 70% of cancer-related deaths can be attributed to high-fat and high-fiber diets.
   b. Diets high in fat and low in fiber can be blamed for nearly one third of cancer-related deaths.
   c. Low-protein diets are associated with the development of colon cancers.
   d. High-protein diets are linked to breast cancer.

ELSEVIER

Mosby items and derived items © 2011 by Mosby, Inc., an affiliate of Elsevier Inc.
Some material was previously published.

Adult Health Nursing, 6th ed.
Christensen & Kockrow

6. The teaching care plan for a 23-year-old woman concerning preventative behaviors for the development of cervical cancer should include:
   a. taking oral contraceptive medications to reduce the development of cervical cancer.
   b. reporting signs and symptoms of abdominal swelling, vaginal bleeding, and chronic stomach pain.
   c. avoiding sun exposure between noon and 3 PM.
   d. employing the use of barrier contraceptives with sexual intercourse.

7. Characteristics associated with benign tumors include:
   a. a variable rate of growth.
   b. little resemblance to the parent tissue.
   c. immobility when palpated.
   d. resemblance to parent tissue.

8. The term referring to an uncontrolled or abnormal growth of cells is _____.
   a. metastasis
   b. proliferation
   c. neoplasm
   d. anaplasia

9. A laboratory test has determined that a 59-year-old male undergoing chemotherapy for lung cancer has a platelet count of $100,000/mm^3$, hemoglobin of 15 g/dL, and hematocrit of 44%. Which of the following interventions can be anticipated?
   a. Administration of diphenhydramine
   b. Avoidance of aspirin or aspirin preparations
   c. Administration of Epogen
   d. A transfusion of packed RBCs

10. Tumor lysis syndrome is most likely to occur in which of the following patients?
    a. A 33-year-old female during her first day of chemotherapy for metastatic breast cancer
    b. A 55-year-old man diagnosed with basal cell carcinoma of the lips
    c. A 23-year-old male diagnosed with osteosarcoma and having had his last chemotherapy treatment 10 days ago
    d. A 67-year-old female diagnosed with ovarian cancer and having had a recent hysterectomy

Answers:

1. c	2. a	3. b	4. a	5. b
6. d	7. d	8. c	9. b	10. a

BACKGROUND ASSESSMENT

Question: A 17-year-old female reports to the family planning clinic to have a pelvic examination and consult with the nurse practitioner about the most appropriate method of birth control. During the intake interview, she denies ever having performed a self breast examination. What information should be provided her?

Answer: She is of an age in which she needs to begin monthly self breast examinations. The self-examinations should be performed 2 to 3 days after her menstrual period is over. She should be given information concerning the correct positioning and palpation movements to use in the self examination.

Question: A patient recently heard a discussion about "cancer markers." He asks what they mark and how they work. How would you answer his questions?

Answer: Cancer marker refers to blood studies that evaluate the presence of substances in the body. When these substances are identified, they are often associated with the presence of a malignancy. These tests are not infallible and may be associated with false positives. Two of the most common types are the PSA and the CA-125. The PSA is used to screen for prostate cancer. CA-125 is performed to detect ovarian cancer.

CRITICAL THINKING QUESTION

A 62-year-old man reports to the physician's office for a routine physical examination. He relates his plans to retire from his job in the next few months. He says it is becoming depressing to see so many of his friends and colleagues becoming ill and dying from heart disease and cancer. He states, "It just seems as if cancer gets them as they get older." He then asks if this is just a coincidence or if older people get cancer more frequently. If so, why? What is the correct response to his question?

Guidelines: This gentleman is indeed correct. The incidence of cancer does increase with age. There are more cases of cancer in older adults than in any other age bracket. The reason can be multifaceted. As the body ages, the ability of cells and tissues to regenerate and repair themselves from injuries is reduced. There is a possible reduction in the effectiveness of the immune system and changes in the body's DNA. Unfortunately, some of the warning signals associated with a diagnosis of cancer can mimic signs of aging, and diagnosis might not occur in a timely manner.

OBJECTIVES	CONTENT	TEACHING RESOURCES
Discuss the incidence of cancer as one of the leading causes of death in the United States.	■ Oncology (FAAHN p. 2014, AHN p. 778)	PPT 2, Ch. 57 FAAHN (Ch. 17 PPT 2 AHN) EILR IC Ch. 57 images 1, 2 FAAHN (Ch. 17 images 1, 2 AHN) SG Risk Factors, Ch. 57 p. 531 FAAHN (Ch. 17 p. 219 AHN) **BOOK RESOURCES** Cultural Considerations: Cancer (FAAHN p. 2015) (AHN p. 779) Fig. 57-1 Estimated cancer cases in the United States (2008 estimates) (FAAHN p. 2015) (Fig. 17-1 AHN p. 779) Fig. 57-2 Estimated cancer deaths in the United States (2008 estimates) (FAAHN p. 2016) (Fig. 17-2 AHN p. 780) ▸ Discuss the medical definition of cancer. ▸ Discuss/identify the leading cancers for both men and women. *Class Activity Ask each student to write on a note card what he/she believes is the leading cause of cancer. Review the responses as a group. After that portion of the exercise, ask the students which cancers are more problematic for men and which affect women most often.*
Compare the three most common sites for cancer in men and women.	■ Oncology (FAAHN p. 2014, AHN p. 778)	PPT 2, Ch. 57 FAAHN (Ch. 17 PPT 2 AHN) SG Risk Factors, Ch. 57 p. 531 FAAHN (Ch. 17 p. 219 AHN)

Christensen & Kockrow

OBJECTIVES	CONTENT	TEACHING RESOURCES
		BOOK RESOURCES Cultural Considerations: Cancer (FAAHN p. 2015) (AHN p. 779) Fig. 57-1 Estimated cancer cases in the United States (2008 estimates) (FAAHN p. 2015) (Fig. 17-1 AHN p. 779) Fig. 57-2 Estimated cancer deaths in the United States (2008 estimates) (FAAHN p. 2016) (Fig. 17-2 AHN p. 780)
Discuss development, prevention, and detection of cancer.	■ Development, prevention, and detection of cancer (FAAHN p. 2016, AHN p. 780)	PPT 3 through 5, Ch. 57 FAAHN (Ch. 17 PPT 3 through 5 AHN) EILR TB Ch. 57 question 39 FAAHN (Ch. 17 question 39 AHN) ESLR Review Questions for the NCLEX Examination Ch. 57 question 3 FAAHN (Ch. 17 question 3 AHN) SG Prevention and Detection, Ch. 57 p. 533 FAAHN (Ch. 17 p. 221 AHN) **BOOK RESOURCES** Review Questions for the NCLEX Examination Ch. 43 questions 7, 13, 17 FAAHN (Ch. 3 questions 7, 13, 17 AHN) Health Promotion: Foods to Reduce Cancer Risk (FAAHN p. 2016) (AHN p. 780) Health Promotion: Prevention and Detection of Cancer (FAAHN p. 2020) (AHN p. 784) ▸ Discuss the process of carcinogenesis. ▸ Discuss the impact early detection can have on long-range survival rates. *Class Activity **Give a note card to every student. Ask each of them to list all of the preventive steps they can recall regarding cancer. After a few minutes, review the responses with the class.***
List seven risk factors for the development of cancer.	■ Development, prevention, and detection of cancer (FAAHN p. 2016, AHN p. 780) ■ Hereditary cancers (FAAHN p. 2017, AHN p. 781)	PPT 4 through 7, Ch. 57 FAAHN (Ch. 17 PPT 4 through 7 AHN) EILR TB Ch. 57 questions 32 FAAHN (Ch. 17 questions 32 AHN) EILR Open Book Quiz Ch. 57 questions 1, 31 FAAHN (Ch. 17 questions 1, 31 AHN)

Christensen & Kockrow

OBJECTIVES	CONTENT	TEACHING RESOURCES
	☐ Genetic susceptibility (FAAHN p. 2017, AHN p. 781) ☐ Cancer risk assessment and cancer genetic counseling (FAAHN p. 2017, AHN p. 781)	☑ ESLR Review Questions for the NCLEX Examination Ch. 57 questions 1, 2, 7 FAAHN (Ch. 17 questions 1, 2, 7 AHN) 📖 SG Risk Factors, Ch. 57 p. 531 FAAHN (Ch. 17 p. 219 AHN) ▸ Discuss the risk factors associated with the development of cancer. ▸ Discuss the impact of heredity on the development of cancer. *Class Activity **List the risk factors associated with the development of cancer on the board. Instruct each student to determine his/her own personal risk level.***
Discuss the American Cancer Society's recommendations for preventive behaviors and screening tests for men and women.	■ Cancer prevention and early detection (FAAHN p. 2017, AHN p. 781)	🖼 PPT 8, Ch. 57 FAAHN (Ch. 17 PPT 8 AHN) ☑ EILR TB Ch. 57 questions 12, 24, 33, 40 FAAHN (Ch. 17 questions 12, 24, 33, 40 AHN) ☑ ESLR Review Questions for the NCLEX Examination Ch. 57 questions 5, 6 FAAHN (Ch. 17 questions 5, 6 AHN) 📖 SG Early Cancer Detection, Ch. 57 p. 531 FAAHN (Ch. 17 p. 219 AHN) **BOOK RESOURCES** Review Questions for the NCLEX Examination Ch. 57 question 5 FAAHN (Ch. 17 question 5 AHN) Health Promotion: Foods to Reduce Cancer Risk (FAAHN p. 2016) (AHN p. 780) Table 57-1 (FAAHN p. 2020) (Table 17-1 AHN p. 784) Health Promotion: Prevention and Detection of Cancer (FAAHN p. 2020) (AHN p. 784) ▸ Discuss the role of the nurse when providing education concerning the use of diagnostic tests and screening for cancer. ▸ Discuss the screening tests recommended by the American Cancer Society. *Class Activity **Contact the American Cancer Society and ask to receive pamphlets relating to diagnosis and screening for cancer.***

OBJECTIVES	CONTENT	TEACHING RESOURCES
		Provide these materials to the class for personal use. As the materials are distributed to the class, determine the students' awareness of community-based, cancer-related resources.
State seven warning signs of cancer.	■ Cancer prevention and early detection (FAAHN p. 2017, AHN p. 781)	*E* EILR IC Ch. 57 image 1 FAAHN (Ch. 17 image 1 AHN)
		E EILR TB Ch. 57 questions 11, 28 FAAHN (Ch. 17 questions 11, 28 AHN)
		E EILR Open Book Quiz Ch. 57 question 2 FAAHN (Ch. 17 question 2 AHN)
		SG SG Early Cancer Detection, Ch. 57 p. 531 FAAHN (Ch. 17 p. 219 AHN)
		BOOK RESOURCES
		Box 57-1 Cancer's Seven Warning Signals (FAAHN p. 2017) (Box 17-1 AHN p. 781)
		▶ Discuss the types of cancer that could be implicated by each of the seven warning signs of cancer.
		▶ Discuss the optimal time to teach patients about the seven warning signs of cancer.
		Class Activity Develop a teaching care plan for the seven warning signs of cancer.
Explain common reasons for delay in seeking medical care when a diagnosis of cancer is suspected.	■ Cancer prevention and early detection (FAAHN p. 2017, AHN p. 781)	*E* EILR Open Book Quiz Ch. 57 question 10 FAAHN (Ch. 17 question 10 AHN)
		SG SG Prevention and Detection, Ch. 57 p. 533 FAAHN (Ch. 17 p. 221 AHN)
		▶ Discuss the psychosocial implications of a diagnosis of cancer.
		Class Activity Ask students how they would feel if they personally noted one of the seven warning signs. Ask students why fear is associated with cancer. Impress upon the students the impact of anxiety when deciding to seek health care.
Define the terminology used to describe cellular changes, characteristics of malignant cells, and types of malignancies.	■ Pathophysiology of cancer (FAAHN p. 2021, AHN p. 785) □ Cell mechanisms and growth (FAAHN p. 2021, AHN p. 785) □ Description, grading, and staging of tumors (FAAHN p. 2021, AHN p. 785)	▦ PPT 8, 9, Ch. 57 FAAHN (Ch. 17 PPT 8, 9 AHN)
		E EILR TB Ch. 57 questions 27, 29, 41 FAAHN (Ch. 17 questions 27, 29, 41 AHN)
		E ESLR Review Questions for the NCLEX Examination Ch. 57 question 4 FAAHN (Ch. 17 question 4 AHN)

Adult Health Nursing, 6th ed.

Christensen & Kockrow

OBJECTIVES	CONTENT	TEACHING RESOURCES
	– Extent of disease classification (FAAHN p. 2022, AHN p. 786)	SG Malignant Cells, Ch. 57 p. 534 FAAHN (Ch. 17 p. 222 AHN) **BOOK RESOURCES** Review Questions for the NCLEX Examination Ch. 57 questions 25, 27 FAAHN (Ch. 17 questions 25, 27 AHN) ▸ Discuss the concept of differentiation. ▸ Discuss the naming of cancer types. ***Class Activity Develop three case scenarios describing cancers. Present these cancer descriptions to the class. Allow the student to determine the names, classification, and staging for each scenario. Include how metastasis influences the staging and classification process.***
Describe the pathophysiology of cancer, including the characteristics of malignant cells and the nature of metastasis.	■ Pathophysiology of cancer (FAAHN p. 2021, AHN p. 785) ☐ Cell mechanisms and growth (FAAHN p. 2021, AHN p. 785)	PPT 10 through 12, Ch. 57 FAAHN (Ch. 17 PPT 10 through 12 AHN) EILR TB Ch. 57 questions 5, 23 FAAHN (Ch. 17 questions 5, 23 AHN) EILR Open Book Quiz Ch. 57 question 3 FAAHN (Ch. 17 question 3 AHN) SG Malignant Cells, Ch. 57 p. 534 FAAHN (Ch. 17 p. 222 AHN) **BOOK RESOURCES** Review Questions for the NCLEX Examination Ch. 43 questions 2, 16, 24, 31 FAAHN (Ch. 3 questions 2, 16, 24, 31 AHN) Table 57-2 (FAAHN p. 2021) (Table 17-2 AHN p. 785) ▸ Discuss the characteristics of benign tumors. ▸ Discuss the characteristics of malignant tumors. ***Class Activity Ask for student volunteers. Ask each volunteer to go the board and illustrate the manner in which they visualize how cancer is spread.***

17.1 Homework/Assignments:

17.1 Instructor's Notes/Student Feedback:

LESSON 17.2

CRITICAL THINKING QUESTION

A 34-year-old patient undergoing chemotherapy for breast cancer has begun to notice hair loss. Tearfully, she brings her concerns to your attention. She has numerous concerns. She asks if all of her hair will be falling out and when it will return. During the interaction, she also asks if there are any preventive steps she can take to avoid the hair loss. How should you best respond to her concerns? Guidelines: Honesty must be tempered with compassion and empathy. Areas that should be covered include the cause of the hair loss, anticipated regrowth potential and implications, and methods to protect the scalp and existing hair. Alopecia can occur as a side effect of chemotherapy. Unfortunately, it is not preventable. Hair loss, in response to the drug therapy, is not permanent. When new growth does occur, hair could be a different color or texture.

OBJECTIVES	CONTENT	TEACHING RESOURCES
Describe the process of metastasis.	☐ Cell mechanisms and growth (FAAHN p. 2021, AHN p. 785)	▣ PPT 10, Ch. 57 FAAHN (Ch. 17 PPT 10 AHN) SG Malignant Cells, Ch. 57 p. 534 FAAHN (Ch. 17 p. 222 AHN) ▸ Discuss the growth progression associated with malignant cells. ▸ Discuss the impact of malignancy and the subsequent metastasis on the body's organs and system. *Class Activity Post a large diagram of the human body. Using a pointer, outline the manner in which cancer is spread throughout the body.*
Define the systems of tumor classification: grading and staging.	☐ Description, grading, and staging of tumors (FAAHN p. 2021, AHN p. 785) – Extent of disease classification (FAAHN p. 2022, AHN p. 786)	▣ PPT 11, 12, Ch. 57 FAAHN (Ch. 17 PPT 11, 12 AHN) EILR TB Ch. 57 questions 9, 34 through 38 FAAHN (Ch. 17 questions 9, 34 through 38 AHN) SG Tumor Staging, Ch. 57 p. 535 FAAHN (Ch. 17 p. 223 AHN) **BOOK RESOURCES** Review Questions for the NCLEX Examination Ch. 57 questions 32, 34 FAAHN (Ch. 17 questions 32, 34 AHN) Box 57-2 (FAAHN p. 2021) (Box 17-2 AHN p. 785) ▸ Discuss the use of the tumor, nodes, metastasis classification (TNM) system.

Adult Health Nursing, 6ᵗʰ ed.
Christensen & Kockrow

OBJECTIVES	CONTENT	TEACHING RESOURCES
		Class Activity **Contact a local pathology office. Ask for copies of the screening tools used to grade and stage tumors. Contact a local oncologist. Ask for a copy of the types of forms utilized to record screening results. Bring these tools to class. They can be passed around the class and questions answered.**
List common diagnostic tests used to identify the presence of cancer.	■ Diagnosis of cancer (FAAHN p. 2022, AHN p. 786) ☐ Biopsy (FAAHN p. 2022, AHN p. 786) ☐ Endoscopy (FAAHN p. 2023, AHN p. 787) ☐ Diagnostic imaging (FAAHN p. 2023, AHN p. 787) – Computed tomography (FAAHN p. 2023, AHN p. 787) – Radioisotope studies (FAAHN p. 2023, AHN p. 787) – Ultrasound testing (FAAHN p. 2023, AHN p. 787) – Magnetic resonance Imaging (MRI) (FAAHN p. 2024, AHN p. 788) – Positron emission tomography (FAAHN p. 2024, AHN p. 788) ☐ Laboratory tests (FAAHN p. 2024, AHN p. 788) – Measurement of alkaline phosphatase blood levels (FAAHN p. 2024, AHN p. 788) – Serum calcitonin level (FAAHN p. 2024, AHN p. 788) – Carcinoembryonic antigen serum level (FAAHN p. 2024, AHN p. 788) – Blood markers (FAAHN p. 2024, AHN p. 788) – Stool examination for blood (FAAHN p. 2025, AHN p. 789)	⊠▬ PPT 13 through 15, Ch. 57 FAAHN (Ch. 17 PPT 13 through 15 AHN) *e* EILR IC Ch. 57 image 3 FAAHN (Ch. 17 image 3 AHN) *e* EILR TB Ch. 57 questions 2, 3, 7, 30 FAAHN (Ch. 17 questions 2, 3, 7, 30 AHN) *e* EILR Open Book Quiz Ch. 57 questions 4, 5 FAAHN (Ch. 17 questions 4, 5 AHN) SG Diagnostic Tests, Ch. 57 p. 537 FAAHN (Ch. 17 p. 225 AHN) **BOOK RESOURCES** Review Questions for the NCLEX Examination Ch. 57 questions 4, 12, 28, 29 FAAHN (Ch. 17 questions 4, 12, 28, 29 AHN) ▸ Discuss the recommendations for cancer screening tests. ▸ Discuss the education needed for patients planning to undergo a screening for cancer. ▸ Discuss the incidence of false positives that can accompany the use of cancer markers. *Class Activity* **Invite a speaker from the American Cancer Society to meet with the class to discuss preventive health screening and diagnostic test recommendations.**

Christensen & Kockrow

OBJECTIVES	CONTENT	TEACHING RESOURCES
Explain why biopsy is essential in confirming a diagnosis of cancer.	☐ Biopsy (FAAHN p. 2022, AHN p. 786)	⊠ PPT 13, 14, Ch. 57 FAAHN (Ch. 17 PPT 13, 14 AHN) SG Diagnostic Tests, Ch. 57 p. 537 FAAHN (Ch. 17 p. 225 AHN) **BOOK RESOURCES** Fig. 57-3 Types of biopsy (FAAHN p. 2023) (Fig. 17-3 AHN p. 787) ▶ Discuss the implications for each of the types of biopsy. ▶ Discuss nursing care for the patient who has had a biopsy. *Class Activity Invite a surgical nurse from a local hospital to speak to the class about the steps taken with the biopsy sample after the physician has obtained it.*
Describe nursing interventions for the individual undergoing surgery, radiation therapy, chemotherapy, bone marrow, or peripheral stem cell transplantation.	■ Cancer therapies (FAAHN p. 2025, AHN p. 789) ☐ Surgery (FAAHN p. 2025, AHN p. 789) – Nursing interventions (FAAHN p. 2026, AHN p. 790) ☐ Radiation therapy (FAAHN p. 2026, AHN p. 790) – External radiation therapy (FAAHN p. 2026, AHN p. 790) – Internal radiation therapy (FAAHN p. 2027, AHN p. 791) ☐ Chemotherapy (FAAHN p. 2027, AHN p. 791) – Hematopoietic system (FAAHN p. 2027, AHN p. 791) – Integumentary system (FAAHN p. 2032, AHN p. 796) – Gastrointestinal system (FAAHN p. 2032, AHN p. 796)	⊠ PPT 16 through 19, Ch. 57 FAAHN (Ch. 17 PPT 16 through 19 AHN) ⚡ EILR TB Ch. 57 questions 1, 6, 8, 10, 13 through 16, 18 through 22, 26 FAAHN (Ch. 17 questions 1, 6, 8, 10, 13 through 16, 18 through 22, 26 AHN) ⚡ EILR Open Book Quiz Ch. 57 questions 6 through 8 FAAHN (Ch. 17 questions 6 through 8 AHN) ⚡ ESLR Review Questions for the NCLEX Examination Ch. 57 questions 7 through 10 FAAHN (Ch. 17 questions 7 through 10 AHN) SG Nursing Interventions, Ch. 57 p. 540 FAAHN (Ch. 17 p. 228 AHN) **BOOK RESOURCES** Review Questions for the NCLEX Examination Ch. 57 questions 1, 3, 8 through 11, 15, 18 through 23, 30 FAAHN (Ch. 17 questions 1, 3, 8 through 11, 15, 18 through 23, 30 AHN) Communication: Nurse-Patient Therapeutic Dialogue Prior to Modified Radical Mastectomy (FAAHN p. 2026) (AHN p. 790) Box 57-3 (FAAHN p. 2028) (Box 17-3 AHN p. 792)

ELSEVIER

Mosby items and derived items © 2011 by Mosby, Inc., an affiliate of Elsevier Inc.
Some material was previously published.

Adult Health Nursing, 6th ed.

Christensen & Kockrow

OBJECTIVES	CONTENT	TEACHING RESOURCES
	– Tumor lysis syndrome (FAAHN p. 2035, AHN p. 799) ☐ Biotherapy (FAAHN p. 2036, AHN p. 800) ☐ Bone marrow transplantation (FAAHN p. 2036, AHN p. 800) ☐ Peripheral stem cell transplantation (FAAHN p. 2037, AHN p. 801)	Table 57-4 Medications for Symptom Control of Cancer Treatment (FAAHN p. 2033) (Table 17-4 AHN p. 797) ▸ Discuss the differences between radiation therapy and chemotherapy. ▸ Discuss the side effects and needed nursing care associated with radiation therapy and chemotherapy. *Class Activity Assign groups of five students each a topic that includes surgical management of cancer, radiation therapy for cancer, chemotherapy, bone marrow transplants, and stem cell transplants. After doing research, each group will provide a 5-minute presentation to the class about its topic. The presentation should relate to the nursing care and nursing implications of each of the treatment options.*
Describe the major categories of chemotherapeutic agents.	☐ Chemotherapy (FAAHN p. 2027, AHN p. 791) – Hematopoietic system (FAAHN p. 2027, AHN p. 791) – Integumentary system (FAAHN p. 2032, AHN p. 796) – Gastrointestinal system (FAAHN p. 2032, AHN p. 796) – Tumor lysis syndrome (FAAHN p. 2035, AHN p. 799)	▰ EILR TB Ch. 57 question 4 FAAHN (Ch. 17 question 4 AHN) ▨ SG Chemotherapeutic Agents, Ch. 57 p. 535 FAAHN (Ch. 17 p. 223 AHN) **BOOK RESOURCES** Table 57-3 Medications for Chemotherapy (FAAHN p. 2029) (Table 17-3 AHN p. 793) Safety Alert! Neutropenic Precautions (FAAHN p. 2031, AHN p. 795) Table 57-4 Medications for Symptom Control of Cancer Treatment (FAAHN p. 2033) (Table 17-4 AHN p. 797) ▸ Discuss the six different categories of chemotherapeutic agents. ▸ Discuss the common side effects associated with each of the categories of chemotherapeutic agents. *Class Activity Pass a small ball around the classroom. As the ball is passed to a student, ask a question concerning chemotherapy. After the student responds, the ball is passed until all students have responded to another classmate.*

Explain the etiology/ pathophysiology, medical management, and nursing interventions for tumor lysis syndrome.	– Tumor lysis syndrome (FAAHN p. 2035, AHN p. 799)	EILR TB Ch. 57 question 25 FAAHN (Ch. 17 question 25 AHN) EILR Open Book Quiz Ch. 57 question 9 FAAHN (Ch. 17 question 9 AHN) SG Tumor Lysis Syndrome, Ch. 57 p. 541 FAAHN (Ch. 17 p. 229 AHN) ▸ Discuss the types of cancers at highest risk for the development of tumor lysis syndrome. ▸ Discuss the clinical manifestations associated with tumor lysis syndrome. *Class Activity Divide the class into groups of three or four students. Ask each group to develop two or three questions concerning tumor lysis syndrome. Assign differing aspects of the syndrome to work on. Areas include the etiology/ pathophysiology, clinical manifestations, medical management, and nursing interventions. Use the completed questions as a review for the entire class.*
Discuss six general guidelines for the use of pain relief measures for the patient with advanced cancer.	■ Advanced cancer (FAAHN p. 2037, AHN p. 801) ☐ Pain management (FAAHN p. 2037, AHN p. 801) ☐ Nutritional therapy (FAAHN p. 2038, AHN p. 802) – Malnutrition (FAAHN p. 2038, AHN p. 802) – Anorexia (FAAHN p. 2038, AHN p. 802) – Altered taste sensation (FAAHN p. 2038, AHN p. 802) ☐ Communication and psychological support (FAAHN p. 2038, AHN p. 802) ☐ Terminal prognosis (FAAHN p. 2039, AHN p. 803)	PPT 21 through 25, Ch. 57 FAAHN (Ch. 17 PPT 21 through 25 AHN) EILR TB Ch. 57 questions 17, 31 FAAHN (Ch. 17 questions 17, 31 AHN) ESLR Review Questions for the NCLEX Examination Ch. 57 questions 6, 14, 33 FAAHN (Ch. 17 question 6, 14, 33 AHN) SG Pain, Ch. 57 p. 539 FAAHN (Ch. 17 p. 227 AHN) **BOOK RESOURCES** Evidence-Based Practice: The Burden of Illness for Cancer Survivors (FAAHN p. 2040, AHN p. 804) ▸ Discuss the pain management options for the patient diagnosed with cancer. ▸ Discuss the clinical implications associated with the pharmacological interventions used to control pain in the cancer patient.

Adult Health Nursing, 6ᵗʰ ed.

Christensen & Kockrow

		*Class Activity **Obtain a pain management scale chart from a local facility. Distribute copies of the scale to students. Then, using these scenarios, ask each student to document the pain on a sheet of paper incorporating the use of a pain scale tool.***
		  – ***a 28-year-old man who's had a bone marrow transplant***
		  – ***a 58-year-old man with lung cancer (stage III)***
		  – ***a 40-year-old woman with breast cancer (stage IV)***
		
		After finishing the task, ask several volunteers to stand and read their entries.

Performance Evaluation		📀 EILR TB Ch. 57 questions 1 through 40 FAAHN (Ch. 17 questions 1 through 40 AHN) 📀 EILR Open Book Quiz Ch. 57 questions 1 through 10 FAAHN (Ch. 17 questions 1 through 10 AHN) 📀 ESLR Review Questions for the NCLEX Examination Ch. 57 questions 1 through 10 FAAHN (Ch. 17 questions 1 through 10 AHN) 📖 SG Ch. 57 pp. 531-544 FAAHN (Ch. 17 pp. 219-232 AHN) **BOOK RESOURCES** Review Questions for the NCLEX Examination Ch. 57 questions 1 through 34 FAAHN (Ch. 17 questions 1 through 34 AHN)

17.2 Homework/Assignments:

17.2 Instructor's Notes/Student Feedback:

ELSEVIER

Christensen & Kockrow

Slide 1

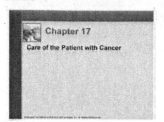

Slide 2

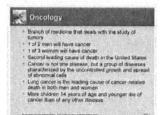

- The word cancer often results in feelings of fear and helplessness. Cancer is a serious, life-threatening, and potentially life-ending disease.

- Statistically speaking, every American will experience or know someone who is faced with a cancer diagnosis.

- Review the racial/cultural influences that exist regarding the incidence of cancer.

Slide 3

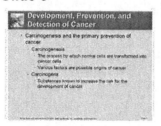

- As studies continue to increase the knowledge about cancer and its causes, there is an increase in attention to eliminate or reduce one's contact with risk-causing elements.

Slide 4

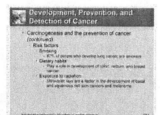

- Risk factors are consistent between varying types of cancer. For example, smoking is associated with an increased risk of not only lung cancer, but also cancer of the kidney, mouth, pharynx, larynx, esophagus, pancreas, uterus, and cervix.

- Why would nutritional habits impact the rate of cancer development?

- What are some potential misconceptions about the risk factors associated with a cancer diagnosis?

Slide 5

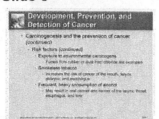

- The environment may also harbor potential carcinogens. Rubber fumes, chlorine, and dust from cotton, coal, nickel, and asbestos can increase the risk of cancer.

- What types of cancer can increase due to environmental exposure to these chemicals?

- What populations are exposed to these potential dangers most frequently?

ELSEVIER

Slide 6

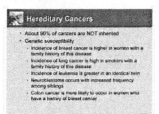

- Cancer is also related to the question of "nature versus nurture." An estimated 10% of cancers are inherited. Why do some families experience an increase in cancer development?

Slide 7

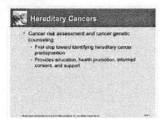

Slide 8

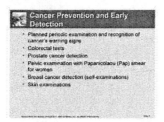

- The American Cancer Society has recommendations for the implementation of screening practices for both men and women.

- How do the screening recommendations differ between the sexes?

- In addition to having diagnostic testing done, what behavior changes can an individual initiate to reduce the incidence of cancer?

Slide 9

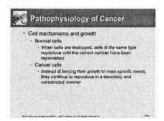

Slide 10

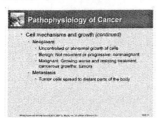

- When cancer occurs, there is an increase of abnormal cellular growth. What characteristics of these malignant cells result in problems for the body? *Cancerous cells compete with the body's normal cells for space and nutrition. As the cancerous cells continue to accumulate, they can impede the body's passages and interfere with normal organ functions.*

ELSEVIER

Adult Health Nursing, 6th ed.

Christensen & Kockrow

Slide 11

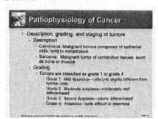

- Malignant tumors are named according to the type of originating tissue and location in the body.

- Grading is used to classify the degree of differentiation noted in the cancerous tissue. Explain the concept of differentiation.

Slide 12

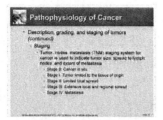

Slide 13

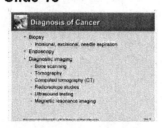

- When the presence of cancer is suspected, diagnostic testing is performed to locate the disease. Biopsies are performed to obtain a sample of tissue from the body.

- Visualization studies can also be utilized to view the area of suspicion.

Slide 14

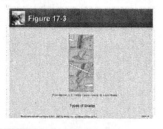

- There are four types of biopsies.

- Discuss each of the four biopsy types. How do the nursing care interventions differ for each of the types?

Slide 15

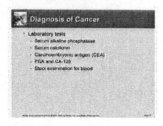

- When cancer occurs, there could be changes in the body's normal blood chemistry. The use of "cancer markers" can be employed as a screening tool.

- What impact does the presence of cancer have on the readings of serum alkaline phosphatase, serum calcitonin, carcinoembryonic antigen, PSA, and CA-125?

- What factors can cause false positives?

ELSEVIER

Mosby items and derived items © 2011, 2007 by Mosby, Inc., an affiliate of Elsevier Inc.
Some material was previously published.

Adult Health Nursing, 6th ed.
Christensen & Kockrow

Slide 16

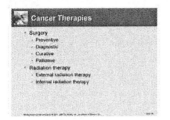

- Surgery can have many goals. Outline the desired outcomes for each of the surgical rationales.

- Radiation is used to reduce the size of a tumor. How do internal and external radiation differ?

Slide 17

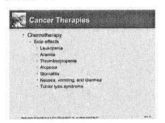

- The use of drug therapy to reduce or slow cancerous cell growth is known as chemotherapy.

- How do chemotherapeutic agents work?

- There are numerous side effects associated with the use of chemotherapy. What body systems are most affected by chemotherapy? Why?

- What are the nursing responsibilities for the care of the patient experiencing side effects associated with chemotherapy?

Slide 18

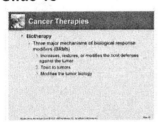

- Biotherapy is defined as treatment with agents derived from biologic sources or affecting biologic responses. It was previously known as immunotherapy.

Slide 19

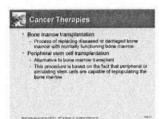

- Bone marrow transplantation is used to treat a variety of diseases. When successful, bone marrow transplantation can increase the individual's rate of survival. What are sources of bone marrow for a transplant?

- Where are stem cells obtained?

- What ethical implications are associated with bone marrow or stem cell transplants?

Slide 20

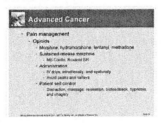

- The pain associated with a diagnosis of cancer can be severe and unrelenting. It is usually an indicator of advanced disease states.

- What responsibilities does the nurse have relating to pain management in the oncologic patient?

- Identify some of the more common issues faced by nurses when attempting to manage the cancer patient's pain.

Slide 21

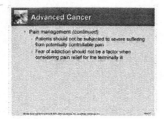

Slide 22

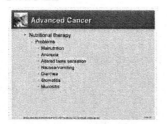

- The cancer patient is at an increased risk for the development of nutritional problems. What factors associated with cancer increase this risk?

- Outline the assessment and interventions indicated for each of the nutritional complications.

Slide 23

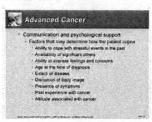

- Lead an open discussion about the implications of a diagnosis of cancer.

Slide 24

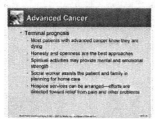

- What attributes will positively or negatively affect a patient's response to cancer.

Slide 25

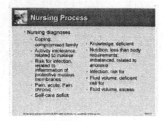